A MANUAL OF LABORATORY DIAGNOSTIC TESTS

Third Edition

A MANUAL OF LABORATORY DIAGNOSTIC TESTS

Third Edition

Frances Talaska Fischbach, R.N., B.S.N., M.S.N.
Associate Clinical Professor in Health Restoration
University of Wisconsin-Milwaukee
School of Nursing
Milwaukee, Wisconsin

Inservice Educator
Clement Zablocki Veterans Administration
Medical Center
Milwaukee, Wisconsin

Former Associate Professor
University of Wisconsin-Milwaukee
Milwaukee, Wisconsin

J. B. Lippincott Company   Philadelphia
London   Mexico City   New York
St. Louis   São Paulo   Sydney

Sponsoring Editor: Diana Intenzo
Coordinating Editorial Assistant: Mary Murphy
Manuscript Editor: Lorraine Smith
Indexer: Ann Cassar
Design Coordinator: Anita Curry/Anne O'Donnell
Cover Design: Kevin Curry
Production Manager: Kathleen P. Dunn
Production Coordinator: Ken Neimeister
Compositor: Bi-Comp, Incorporated
Printer/Binder: R. R. Donnelley & Sons Company

Third Edition

5 6

Library of Congress Cataloging in Publication Data

Fischbach, Frances Talaska.
    A manual of laboratory diagnostic tests.

    Includes bibliographies and index.
    1. Diagnosis, Laboratory—Handbooks, manuals, etc.
2. Diagnosis—Handbooks, manuals, etc.   I. Title.
[DNLM: 1. Diagnosis, Laboratory.   QY 25 F528m]
RB38.2.F57 1988   616.07'5   87-16848
ISBN 0-397-54686-6

Any procedure or practice described in this book should be
applied by the health-care practitioner under appropriate
supervision in accordance with professional standards of care
used with regard to the unique circumstances that apply in each
practice situation. Care has been taken to confirm the accuracy of
information presented and to describe generally accepted
practices. However, the author, editors, and publisher cannot
accept any responsibility for errors or omissions or for
consequences from application of the information in this book and
make no warranty, express or implied, with respect to the contents
of the book.

Every effort has been made to ensure that drug selections and
dosages are in accordance with current recommendations and
practice. Because of ongoing research, changes in government
regulations, and the constant flow of information on drug therapy,
reactions, and interactions, the reader is cautioned to check the
package insert for each drug for indications, dosages, warnings,
and precautions, particularly if the drug is new or infrequently
used.

To my former classmates at St. Mary's Hospital
School of Nursing, Rochester, Minnesota

PREFACE

This third edition of *A Manual of Laboratory Diagnostic Tests* is intended to be a comprehensive and up-to-date diagnostic reference manual for health-care practitioners and a teaching/learning tool for students in a variety of health-care areas: nursing, medicine, dentistry, medical assistants, medical technology, radiologic technology, physical therapy, and others. The preparation of this third edition is based on critical comments and suggestions from those who have read and used previous editions: practitioners, educators, and students, as well as on extensive library, laboratory, and hospital research.

The decision to include new tests takes into consideration trends and issues in diagnostic health care and practice. For example, there is a definite tendency to substitute newer for older technologies. There has been a marked reduction over the past decade in the use of contrast radiology, with the exception of computed tomography (CT scan) and cardiac catheterizations. The number of cardiac catheterizations, especially for persons with myocardial infarction, has been on the rise, as has the use of Holter monitors. In what may be a possible substitution of one technology for another in regard to contrast x-ray filming, there is a significant growth rate in the use of diagnostic ultrasound.

An important issue is the cost of health care. It is interesting to note that in studies done to determine whether or not changes in clinical practice had contributed to rising hospital costs, it was found that there was little change in total use of services from the 1970s to the 1980s. Findings showed that use of laboratory services remained the same and that, contrary to "conventional wisdom," laboratory tests did not contribute to rising costs. Moreover new imagery techniques were commonly substituted for older, more invasive procedures.

This edition also reflects a definite trend to report laboratory test data in Système International (SI) units. This is a common practice in much of the world where such units are used on a daily basis in patient care and in research studies and publications. However, the underlying reason for advocating change to SI units is that biological components react on a molar basis *in vivo*.

Normal values in this edition are reported in both conventional units and, whenever available, in units of the SI system. Alerts are given for panic (crisis or critical) laboratory values that have life and death significance to the patient and need to be reported to the attending physician immediately.

Many major changes have been made in this edition, beginning with a new introductory chapter on care-giver responsibilities. This new chapter is divided into pre- and post-test responsibilities. Emphasis is on knowledge, safety, infection control, ethical and legal implications, individualized pre- and post-test assessment and care planning, coordination of tests and activities of daily living, guidelines for disclosure of findings of serious disease, follow-up based on test results, after-care to detect and prevent complications, and documentation of diagnostic processes.

The framework for the third edition highlights knowledge and communication as the keys to prevention of diagnostic test errors as well as explanation of benefits and risks. Special considerations are made for those persons with special needs: for example, those with diabetes or ostomies, the elderly, and those receiving chemotherapy.

The information in all chapters starting with "Blood Studies" was carefully updated using material that has been gathered from many sources. Respected experts were interviewed and consulted. As in other editions, all new methods that involved patients were personally observed by the author and/or research assistants. All chapters were revised, reorganized, and/or retitled to reflect current practice. Many parts were completely rewritten. For example, "Amniotic Fluid Studies" was retitled "Prenatal Diagnosis and Tests of Fetal Well-Being" so that hormone and stress testing, fetoscopy, and chorionic villus sampling could be included.

More than 125 new tests were added. Included is a section in "Chemistry Studies" on therapeutic drug monitoring to manage individual drug therapy and to detect drug toxicity. A section in "Urine Studies" focuses on drug investigation and witnessed urine sampling to detect drug usage.

Significant alterations were made in the appendices. The section on drugs that affect tests was removed because, with so many drugs interfering with test outcomes, this is one area of medicine that is constantly changing. The reader is alerted to the fact that drugs *do* affect testing methods or outcome and is urged to consult a current reference concerning medications and their possible influence on optimum test results. Some specific drug information does remain in the "Interfering Factors" paragraphs. For example, in the section discussing blood in urine, the "Interfering Factors" lists "drugs that are toxic to the kidney;" "drugs that cause actual bleeding," and so on.

The new Appendix One for the third edition is a table of vitamins, giving reference range, critical range, and significance of values. The new Appendix Two is a table of minerals, also giving reference and critical ranges, types of specimen, and clinical significance of increased or decreased values.

This edition retains a concise, consistent format, with the resulting easy retrievability of up-to-date information on commonly ordered diagnostics.

I wanted to write a text that would be comprehensive in scope, one that would emphasize care-giver responsibilities for pre- and post-test phases. This revision is based on current trends in diagnostics and on principles that reflect ethical behavior, such as the value of human life and the sanctity of the individual. I hope the reader concludes that I have achieved my purpose.

Frances Talaska Fischbach, R.N., B.S.N., M.S.N.

ACKNOWLEDGMENTS

I want to give special thanks and recognition to my research assistants—Jack Fischbach, Julie Erickson, Ann Shafranski Fischbach, and Gloria Shutte Boge; to Frances Talaska for information management; to Kathie Gordon and Margaret Fischbach for typing of the manuscript; to Jeanne Hough Ewens for help in condensing and selecting materials for publication, and to Corrine Strandell for assistance in compiling the tables in the appendices.

I would also like to acknowledge the following persons for providing information, help, and encouragement in manuscript preparation: S. Arnold, M.D.: Mary Jane Bates; Peggy Beyer; Victor Buendia; Julie Burgireno; Karen Burns; James Cates, M.D.; Kedar Chintapalli, M.D.; Carol Colasocco; James Cooper; Sally Creagan; Rod Doering; Marshall B. Dunning; Jacquelyn Eggbrecht; Maria M. de Elejalde; Rafael de Elejalde, M.D.; Dorothy Carlson Fischbach; Teresa Giersch Fischbach; Sister Mary Lou Fischbach; Mary Garroth; Hugh Garthwaite; Dolaine Genthe; Nina Genthe; William Genthe; Eugene Gottfried, M.D.; Keith Hadley, M.D.; Mary Fischbach Johnson; Donna Soik Karweick; Edwin Ketola; Carol Knott; Emmy Lou Koehler; Joanne Krumberger; John R. Milbrath, M.D.; Cheryl Miller; Don Nelson; Barbara Niemczyski; Allan Perris; Timothy Philipp; Linda Pohl; Randle Pollard, M.D.; James Roberts; Mary Pat Schmidt; John T. Schmitz, M.D.; Irene Schreck; Eric Schreiber, M.D.; Jean Schultz; Kathy Seely; Gerald Sedmak; Ed Seisse, M.D.; Adolph Stofl, M.D.; John Wertsch, M.D., and Linda Wolf.

Gratefully remembered are those dear persons who helped with the first and second editions, especially Timothy Philipp, Charles Kerr, Theresa Philipp, Mary Fischbach Johnson, and Margaret Fischbach.

Appreciation is also due the staff of the laboratory, radiology, and special diagnostic departments of various hospitals in Milwaukee: Veterans, Milwaukee County Medical, St. Mary's, Froedtert, Columbia, and St. Joseph's, and San Francisco General Hospital in San Francisco. I also appreciate the use of their manuals for reference.

I sincerely value the expert editorial support of Diana Intenzo, Mary Murphy, and Lorraine Smith during the preparation of the manuscript.

CONTENTS

A MANUAL OF LABORATORY DIAGNOSTIC TESTS

Third Edition

CARE-GIVERS' RESPONSIBILITIES

1

Introduction

Because the delivery of health care involves so many types of personnel, the care-giver must have a working knowledge of other professional endeavors, including the role of diagnostic evaluation. Diagnostics is just one large area of activity the care-giver must understand in this era of high technology. Laboratory and diagnostic tests are tools. By and of themselves, they are almost useless, but in conjunction with a pertinent history and physical examination, they may confirm a diagnosis or provide valuable information about a patient's status and response to therapy.

Preparing patients for diagnostic or therapeutic procedures and providing follow-up care have long been accepted parts of professional practice. Professionals today need to be expert in developing meaningful care plans and in helping patients adjust their daily activities to meet the requirements of the tests. Responsibility can be divided into the pre- and post-test phase of diagnostic care.

Pretest Phase
1. Basic knowledge. Know abbreviations, purpose, and procedures of tests.
   (a) It is especially important to know admission test results. The plan of care is developed or changed on the basis of test results.
   (b) The primary care-giver also needs to be alert to critical laboratory test values that have immediate life and death significance to the patient and to report these findings to the attending physician immediately. Know your institution's policy about prompt reporting and appropriate filing of results.
   (c) It is also important to know how to gather diagnostic information from the charts. Keep in mind that you must always look at the most recent laboratory data first to determine the current status, then work backward in the chart to note trends in the data.
2. History and assessment
   Obtain a relevant history and individualized assessment. The history should identify contraindications to testing, allergies to contrast substances used, such as iodine, and persons who are undergoing a procedure for the first time. Assessment should include the patient's need for information and methods of coping; identify patients who are afraid and unable to cope with confined spaces, since some procedures involve this consideration. It is necessary to document this data and to note any questions the patient may ask.

3. Correct procedures
   (a) Order tests correctly. Requests should be submitted on appropriate forms. Information should be complete, accurate, and legible.
   (b) When appropriate, ensure that all specimens are correctly obtained, handled, labeled, and delivered to the appropriate department. For example, generally it is not acceptable to draw blood from an extremity in which an intravenous line (IV) is infusing. Use infection control procedures for patients in isolation.
4. Proper coordination of activities
   Coordinate patient activities and testing to avoid conflicts with meal times, medications, lengthy treatments, and other diagnostic tests.
   (a) Be ever aware of patients who are not allowed to receive anything orally (NPO) and know when to give medications prior to specific tests. Schedule tests that involve contrast substances so that they do not invalidate the succeeding tests.
   (b) Take action to minimize stress and anxiety, fear, nausea, and vomiting.
5. Minimizing interference
   (a) Care-giver actions that affect or interfere with accurate test results include

   Incorrect specimen collection and handling
   Wrong preservative or lack of necessary preservative
   Delayed delivery of a collected specimen to the laboratory
   Old specimens that may contain destroyed cells and may increase or decrease test results
   Incorrect or incomplete patient preparation
   Hemolysis of blood samples; this is a preventable problem
   Incomplete collection, especially of timed urine collection
   Incorrect labeling of specimens

   (b) Patient factors that affect or interfere with accurate test results include

   Diet preparation
   Current drug history
   Illness
   Plasma volume
   Position or activity at time specimen was obtained
   Postprandial status (time since patient ate last)
   Time of day
   Pregnancy
   Age and sex
   Lack of patient knowledge
   Stress

6. Avoiding errors
   Knowledge and communication are keys to prevention of error in diagnostic testing.
   (a) The primary care-giver should be aware of how the test is carried out and have a basic understanding of how the results are measured. Patients and their families (when appropriate) should be knowledgeable about tests to be performed and preparation necessary for correct test results. Any dietary restrictions or collection of multiple or timed specimens should be communicated to patients and staff.
   (b) The other side of the coin is that too often personnel in the diagnostic departments do not coordinate their activities for the good of the patient. Technologists complain that specimens are not marked correctly or that specimens are lost or otherwise ineptly handled by the nursing or medical staff. Patients are not always correctly or completely prepared for the examination or the testing personnel are not informed of changes in orders.
7. Proper preparation
   Prepare the patient properly.
   (a) Be aware of clinical considerations of special patients such as ostomy patients, diabetics, and the elderly. How well the patient is prepared may well affect the outcome of the tests. For example, patients need to be aware of when they can eat and drink and how much they are permitted to eat before certain tests.
   (b) Realize that fear is experienced on the part of the patients who are undergoing diagnostic procedures. Help the patient to use imagery and relaxation techniques to reduce anxiety during the examination.
   (c) When giving patients information, be sure that the person can read any written materials you give him and can hear what you have to say (hearing aid turned on or adjusted as needed).
8. Patient education
   Educate patient and family about tests.
   (a) Patients need both sensory and objective information about the purpose and procedure of tests. They need this information so they can create an image in their minds of what is going to occur. Well thought-out descriptions enable patients to form a realistic schema of what will be experienced.
   (b) Sensory information helps to interpret a situation that is completely different from anything experienced in the past. Subjective features would be physical sensations; objective features would be characteristics of a diagnostic situation such as length of procedure. The cause of sensations should be discussed so that the person is less apt to misinterpret and falsely conclude that something has gone wrong.

9. Protocols

Develop protocols for testing that encompass pretest and comprehensive follow-up care. Guidelines for giving patients preparatory information should be developed and followed.

(a) Prepare patients only for those aspects of the procedure that are noticed by the majority of patients. Care-givers can work together to develop a pattern of responses, using a list to evaluate patients when testing is completed to determine what aspects most persons noticed and what words were used to describe sensations that were experienced.

10. Patient independence

Plan care so that the patient maintains as much control of the diagnostic phase as possible. Patients should be included in decisions, beginning with diagnostic procedures. The uncertain and stressful diagnostic period of care can be reduced by helping patients to participate in as much of this phase as is possible. Because anxiety is usually so high during the diagnostic period, the person may not hear the instructions and explanations you give about the test procedure. The patient's understanding of instruction must be validated. Inform the patient of the diagnostic plan, of the day-to-day time frame for conducting the tests, and of how the person can comply to ensure reliability and successful completion of the tests.

11. Test results

It is vital to know the meaning of normal or reference values. It can be misleading to give normal ranges in published materials because definitely there will be some variation from laboratory to laboratory. Theoretically, "normal" could refer to health, to the ideal or average value, or to the types of distribution, such as Gaussian. Keep in mind that the reported reference range for a test varies with the method used for testing as well as with the population tested. Each laboratory must provide its own normal range for the particular testing method it uses and for the special population in which the set of values is described.

12. SI values

Values will be given in conventional units and in units of the Système International d'Unités (SI), when available. The SI system is currently in use by most of the world. Clinical laboratories will need to tabulate their own "panic values" expressed in SI units, with "panic values" indicating values reflecting life or death situations. The biggest difference in laboratory reports affected by SI is that the concentration is written as amount per volume (moles or millimoles per liter) rather than as a mass per volume (grams or milligrams per deciliter or 100 milliliters). Sometimes there will be a change in numbers; sometimes they will stay the same. Chloride stays the same (95–105 MEq./liter, conventional, and 95–105 mmol./liter, SI). See Tables 1-1 and 1-2.

Table 1-1
Seven Fundamental Units of SI

Physical Quantity/Property	Base Unit	SI Symbol
1. Length	Meter	m
2. Mass	Kilogram	kg
3. Time	Second	s
4. Amount of substance	Mole	mol
5. Thermodynamic temperature	Kelvin	K
6. Electric current	Ampere	A
7. Luminous intensity	Candela	cd

13. Margins of error
    The care-giver needs to know that, if a patient has a battery of chemistry tests such as sequential multiple analyzers (SMAC) or multiple sequential screening panel (MSSP), the possibility is great that some tests will be abnormal due purely to chance. This is because a significant margin of error arises from the arbitrary setting of limits. We know that if a laboratory test is considered normal up to the 95th percentile, then 5 times out of 100, a test will show an abnormality even though a patient is not ill. If the person has two tests performed, the probability that both will be within the normal range is 0.95 × 0.95 or 90.25%. This means that 9.75 times out of 100 a test will show an abnormality even though the person has no underlying disorder. With three tests, the probability that all three will have results within the normal range is 0.95 × 0.95 × 0.95 or 85.7%. The point is that if the patient has a group of tests performed on one blood sample, the possibility is great that some of the tests will be abnormal, due purely to chance.
14. Legal implications
    (a) Always be aware of the legal implications of diagnostic testing, such as patient's right for information, instances when a legal

Table 1-2
Seven Representative Derived Units of SI

Derived Unit	Name & Symbol	SI Symbol
1. Area	Square meter	m^2
2. Volume	Cubic meter	m^3
3. Force	Newton (N)	$kg\ m\ s^{-2}$
4. Pressure	Pascal (Pa)	$kg\ m^{-1}\ s^{-2}\ (N/M^2)$
5. Work, energy	Joule (J)	$kg\ M^2\ s^{-2}\ (N/M)$
6. Density	Kilogram per cubic meter	kg/m^3
7. Frequency	Hertz (Hz)	s^{-1}

consent form must be signed, explanation to patient and/or significant other of risks inherent in such tests as angiography and amniocentesis, as well as documentation, which is vital.

(b) A team approach to diagnostics is essential for responsible patient care. It is the attending physician's role to inform the patient about test results, as well as alternatives and medical and surgical actions for follow-up. It is the purview of all other caregivers to provide information and clarification, and to give support to patient and family, especially with abnormal test results.

15. Ethical considerations

Be aware of ethical considerations such as confidentiality of information, reporting of infectious diseases, and the dehumanizing effects of some diagnostic procedures. Patients and family need to know both benefits and risks of testing, and to recognize the right to accept or refuse diagnostic tests. Care-givers also need to be warned of risks in obtaining and handling specimens.

Post-Test Care

1. Abnormal test results

It is important to recognize abnormal test results, their meaning, and the possible effects on the patient; for example, know when test results indicate serious disease, shortened life span, or the need for amputation of a limb. Help the patient and family understand what a positive or negative test result means.

2. False results

Know what is meant by false-positive and false-negative results. Drugs are a big factor that can result in negative or positive results, depending on the testing methods, or that can actually cause a positive or negative result. In the Venereal Disease Research Laboratories (VDRL) test for syphilis, a number of persons will have positive tests, even though they do not have syphilis. This is an example of false-positive tests. On the other hand, false-negatives also occur. The electrocardiogram (ECG) is not a sensitive test for coronary disease *prior* to myocardial infarction. In other words, coronary disease is not detected by this particular test. This is why a person can have a normal ECG one day and a myocardial infarction the next. There can be extreme psychological and social consequences of being identified as having a serious disease such as Acquired Immune Deficiency Syndrome (AIDS) or syphilis because of false-positive test results.

3. Follow-up care

Follow up consistently on test results. Follow-up care should include discharge instructions based on test results and infection control measures, such as site care after cardiac catheterization. Be sure the patient understands medical and surgical management and is allowed time for ventilation and discussion. Also, clarify the meaning of test results. A patient who has just been diagnosed as having anemia or diabetes has vastly different problems from the patient with a cerebral aneurysm or bone cancer. This includes a variety of patient problems that need to be dealt with in a highly individualized manner and that also need to be consistently recorded.

4. Safety measures
Aftercare to detect and prevent complications should assure patient safety and well-being. Post-test assessment should include evaluating the patient's appearance in relation to abnormal test results and determining if the patient is accepting or not accepting the significance of the test results, as in the patient who is identified as having a chronic disease. For example, patients with chemical and electrolyte imbalances that are associated with decreased mental alertness and sensorial disturbances need to be protected from possible injury. Also, patients who have had barium need to know the importance of completely evacuating the contrast medium. In the elderly, often the first sign of fecal impaction may be fainting, so close observation is necessary for all older persons following radiographic studies using barium such as upper and lower gastrointestinal (GI) series. Infection control measures should be followed when portals of infection have been established, as after cardiac catheterization, and whenever infectious diseases have been confirmed.

5. Documentation
Document the diagnostic process. This documentation, which has legal, budgetary, insurance, and diagnostic related grouping (DRG) implications, should include a recorded history and physical assessment for indications and contraindications to testing as well as the patient's or family's need for information. The record should indicate that the patient was informed about the purpose and effect of the test and was offered an explanation (when appropriate) of the value, risks, expected results, and alternative methods available. The length of time the patient was involved in the testing procedure should always be recorded, as well as how the procedure was tolerated, when and how specimens were collected, and if any difficulties occurred in obtaining samples. A brief review of post-test assessment and follow-up care and recommendations for patient well-being and safety should also be included in the documentation. It is most important to record and report adverse effects of contrast media. Determine whether contrast media was used in the test and chart that you assessed for presence or absence of reaction signs.

6. Disclosure guidelines
   Develop accepted guidelines for informing a patient of a diagnosis of serious disease (how much to reveal and how to reveal the diagnosis).
   Guidelines:
   (a) The physician is the person who has the responsibility for informing the patient. The nurse or medical assistant is the person who has the responsibility for arranging the conference with patient, doctor, family, and nurse, and for enlisting the help of the family. It is necessary that the diagnosis (such as cancer) should not be kept a secret from the patient so that the person will not be stigmatized or isolated.
   (b) It is far better to reveal the diagnosis and explain the illness to the individual, discussing what has been found, and the approach to treatment.
   (c) Disclosure prevents a conspiracy of silence from developing. Persons should not be deceived.
   (d) The most effective method of revealing the diagnosis is to tell the patient and family together. Resist protective relatives' occasional insistence that the patient cannot take the truth.
7. Patient response to outcome
   (a) Be able to use wisely crisis intervention skills in the event that the findings indicate a very serious disease such as leukemia or advanced heart disease. The impact on a person finding out that he has AIDS has been graphically described as "an amputation of the future" for the person involved. Many persons whose diagnostic tests confirm cancer experience sheer terror and have reported that their whole lives passed before them during the immediate confirmation stage.
   (b) Recognize initial patient responses to learning of the diagnosis of diseases that threaten lifestyle and self-image. In a typical pattern, the immediate response lasts several days, and then is followed by a secondary response that may last several weeks.

Immediate Response	*Secondary Response*
Acute emotional turmoil, shock, disbelief about diagnosis.	Insomnia, anorexia, difficulty in concentration, depression, difficulty in performing work-related responsibilities
Feelings of anxiety will usually last several days as the person assimilates the information.	Depressed feelings may last several weeks as the person begins to incorporate the information and to participate realistically in a treatment plan.

8. Comfort measures
   Give comfort if outcome reveals a chronic or life-threatening disease. Help patient work through anxiety and depression. Point out to patient that concerns and fears related to the diagnosis are to be expected. Positive interventions the care-giver can focus on include helping patient and family cope with necessary alterations in lifestyle and self-concept when unexpected life events occur. Emphasize that risk factors associated with many disorders can be reduced, such as overweight, unrelieved stress and worry, lack of exercise, poor sleep habits, poor nutrition, and high alcohol intake.

BLOOD STUDIES

2

Introduction

Composition

The average person has about 5 liters of blood (5 to 6 qt.) that may be separated into 3 liters of plasma and 2 liters of cells. The plasma is a liquid derived from the intestines and organs of the body, and the cells compose the solids formed mainly by the bone marrow. The normal adult's blood volume is estimated at one-thirteenth of his total body weight.

The blood can be thought of as a tissue serving many functions. Without plasma, cells cannot circulate, and without cells, the vascular fluid alone cannot maintain life.

The cells are classified as white cells (leukocytes), red cells (erythrocytes), and platelets (thrombocytes); white cells are further divided into granulocytes, agranulocytes, and their related subclassifications:

A. Erythrocytes (red blood cells)
B. Leukocytes (white blood cells)
   1. Granulocytes (granular leukocytes)
      (a) Neutrophils
      (b) Eosinophils
      (c) Basophils
   2. Agranulocytes (agranular leukocytes)
      (a) Lymphocytes
      (b) Monocytes
C. Thrombocytes or platelets

The cells vary in size, with the white cells being the largest, the red cells next, and the platelets the smallest. Red cells greatly predominate; for every 500 red cells there are approximately 30 platelets and only one white cell.

Blood Disorders

Disorders of the red blood cells (RBCs) are grouped into *anemias* (severe reductions in circulating red blood cells due to blood loss, production and destruction disorders), and *polycythemias* (abnormal increases in circulating red cells).

Disorders of the leukocytes are termed either as *leukocytosis* (an increased number of cells) or *leukopenia* (a decreased number of cells). Since there are numerous types of white blood cells (WBCs), variations in the counts of the different types of cells may reflect a wide range of disorders, including infection, leukemia, agranulocytosis, or granulocytopenia. Decreased counts of platelets or thrombocytes result in thrombocytopenia, which can become manifest in hemorrhage.

The production of red cells, platelets, and white cells is referred to as *hematopoiesis* and occurs mainly in bone marrow. Under normal conditions, only mature cells enter the bloodstream from the bone marrow. In pathologic states, a variety of immature cells can be found in the circulating blood.

Therefore, examination of the blood and bone marrow constitutes the major means of determining certain types of blood disorders. The procedures involved in obtaining the specimens are skin puncture of finger, toe, or heel, venipuncture, and bone marrow aspiration.

COLLECTION PROCEDURES
Skin Puncture

Capillary blood is preferred for a peripheral blood smear.

1. Capillary blood is obtained from
   (a) The tip of a finger or earlobe in adults
   (b) The great toe or heel in infants
   (c) The tip of the finger in infants over 1 year old
2. Puncture site is washed with disinfectant (70% alcohol), dried with sterile gauze, and skin in punctured no deeper than 2 mm. with a sterile disposable lancet. If povidone-iodine [Betadine] is used, it must be allowed to dry thoroughly to be effective.
3. First drop of blood is wiped away with sterile gauze and subsequent drops are collected in a microtube and slides.

Clinical Alert

1. Avoid squeezing the extremity to obtain blood, because doing this will alter the composition of the blood.

Venipuncture

Venipuncture is a procedure necessary for most tests that require anti-coagulation and large quantities of blood. It is the puncturing of a vein with a needle attached to a syringe.

1. Venous blood is usually obtained from the antecubital vein, although veins in other sites may be chosen. There is no variation in blood values if specimens are obtained from different veins.
2. A tourniquet is placed and tightened on the upper arm to cause venous congestion and prevent venous return.

Note: A blood pressure cuff that is inflated to a level between systolic and diastolic pressure can be used as a tourniquet.

3. The patient is asked to make a fist and to open and close his hand several times.
4. The puncture site is cleansed with 70% alcohol and dried with sterile gauze. If povidone-iodine (Betadine) is used, it must be allowed to dry thoroughly.
5. The vein is cleanly punctured with either a sterile needle and syringe or a Vacutainer system.

   Note: The size of needle and syringe is determined by the amount of blood needed as well as the size and integrity of the vein to be used. Furthermore, many hospitals use the Vacutainer system because it is cheaper. The Vacutainer system consists of a vacuum tube (Vacutainer tube), a holder, and a multisample collecting needle.

6. After the vein is entered, blood will fill the vacuum tubes of the Vacutainer system. However, if a needle and syringe are used, gentle suction with the syringe is needed to obtain the specimen. Excessive suction can collapse the vein.
7. Remove needle and apply sterile gauze with pressure to stop bleeding. Cover puncture site with an adhesive bandage.
8. The anticoagulant needed is dependent on the test to be performed. In general, most hematology tests use ethylene diamine tetraacetic acid (EDTA) anticoagulant. The tests are done on well-mixed whole blood. Even slightly clotted blood invalidates the test.

Clinical Alert

1. If oozing from the puncture site is difficult to stop, elevate area and apply a pressure dressing. Stay with the patient until bleeding stops.
2. Never draw blood for any laboratory test from the same extremity that is being used for IV medications, IV fluids, or blood.
3. In patients with leukemia or agranulocytosis and in others with lowered resistance, the finger-stick and earlobe puncture are more likely to cause infection than venipuncture. If a capillary sample is necessary in these patients, the cleansing agent should remain in contact with the skin for at least 7 to 10 minutes. Alcohol is not bacteriocidal; povidone-iodine (Betadine) is the cleansing agent of choice on leukemic patients.

If a Betadine swab is used, the skin is scrubbed, allowed to dry (this can take up to 2 minutes), and then wiped off with alcohol and dried with sterile gauze.

4. If difficulty is encountered in obtaining blood
   (a) Warm the extremity (this must be done for all blood gases).
   (b) Allow the extremity to remain in a hanging position for some time.

5. Hematomas can be prevented by
   (a) Using good technique
   (b) Releasing the tourniquet before the needle is removed
   (c) Applying sufficient pressure over the puncture site after completion of the procedure

Prolonged use of a tourniquet causes stasis of blood, produces hemoconcentration, and causes other changes that make the blood unsuitable for blood gases, blood count, blood *p*H, and some clotting.

Bone Marrow Aspiration

Normal Appearance
Rust red color, thick fluidlike consistency with visible amounts of fatty material, and pale gray white marrow fragments.

Explanation of Test
Bone marrow is that organ located within cancellous bone and in cavities of long bones. A smear is made from a bone marrow aspiration or biopsy to see if the bone marrow is performing its function of manufacturing normal red and white cells and platelets. The developmental stages of the most immature cells, relative to those ready to be released into the circulating blood can be seen (Table 2-1).

Indications for Test
A bone marrow smear is of particular help in diagnosing (a) aplastic anemia, (b) pernicious anemia, (c) leukemia, (d) purpura, and (e) agranulocytosis. It is even more helpful in determining hematopoiesis. However, a bone marrow smear does not always provide specific or even relevant information and is not diagnostically sufficient in and of itself. The presence or the suspicion of a blood disorder is not always an indication of the need to study the bone marrow. The decision to employ this procedure is made for each patient on the basis of the history, physical examination, and examination of his peripheral blood.

Table 2-1
Bone Marrow Normal Range

Formed Cell Elements	Normal (Mean %)	Range (%)
Undifferentiated cells	0.0	0.0–1.0
Reticulum cells	0.4	0.0–1.3
Myeloblasts	2.0	0.3–5.0
Promyelocytes	5.0	1.0–8.0
Myelocytes		
Neutrophilic	12.0	5.0–19.0
Eosinophilic	1.5	0.5–3.0
Basophilic	0.3	0.0–0.5
Metamyelocytes		
Neutrophilic	25.6	17.5–33.7
Eosinophilic	0.4	0.0–1.1
Basophilic	0.0	0.0–0.2
Segmented granulocytes		
Neutrophilic	20.0	11.6–30.0
Eosinophilic	2.0	0.5–4.0
Basophilic	0.2	0.0–3.7
Monocytes	2.0	1.6–4.3
Lymphocytes	10.0	3.0–20.7
Megakaryocytes	0.4	0.0–3.0
Plasma cells	0.9	0.1–1.7
Erythroid series		
Pronormoblasts	0.5	0.2–4.2
Basophilic normoblasts	1.6	0.25–4.8
Polychromatic normoblasts	10.4	3.5–20.5
Orthochromatic normoblasts	6.4	3.0–25
Promegaloblasts	0	0
Basophilic megaloblasts	0	0
Polychromatic megaloblasts	0	0
Orthochromatic megaloblasts	0	0
Myeloid : erythroid ratio (M : E) ratio of WBC to nucleated RBC	3.0–4.1	6.1–2.1

(Platt WR: Color Atlas and Textbook of Hematology. Philadelphia, JB Lippincott, 1969)

Procedure

1. Patient is positioned on his back or side according to site selected. The posterior iliac crest is the preferred site in all patients over the age of 12 to 18 months. Other sites include the anterior iliac crest, sternum, spinous vertebral processes T10 through L4, ribs, and tibia in children.

   The sternum usually is not used in children because the cavity is too shallow, danger of mediastinal and cardiac perforation is too great, and observation of procedure is associated with apprehension and lack of cooperation.

2. The area is shaved, if necessary, cleansed, and draped as for any minor surgical procedure.

3. A local anesthetic of procaine or lidocaine is injected. The infiltration of the medication is accompanied by pain from needle insertion and a burning sensation.
4. A short, rigid, sharp-pointed needle with stylet is introduced through the periosteum into the marrow cavity. The stylet is removed from the needle and 0.2 to 0.5 ml. of marrow fluid is aspirated.

   When the bone marrow is entered, a feeling of pressure is experienced. Moderate discomfort, which only lasts a few seconds, *may* be felt when aspiration is done, especially if the iliac crest is the chosen site. There is no way to prevent or lessen this discomfort.
5. After the needle is removed, pressure is applied to the site until any bleeding ceases and a small sterile dressing is applied to the puncture site. Slides are usually smeared at the bedside.
6. Total procedure time is approximately 20 to 30 minutes.
7. Label specimen container with patient's name, date, and room number, and take it immediately to the laboratory.

Clinical Implications
1. A specific and diagnostic bone marrow picture is associated with many diseases. The report indicates the presence, absence, and ratio of cells that are characteristic of the suspected disease. However, bone marrow interpretation is a complicated task and requires considerable training and experience. Only a highly trained hematologist can be expected to evaluate a marrow specimen accurately.
2. Bone marrow examination may reveal
   (a) Leukemia
   (b) Deficiency states including vitamin B_{12}, folic acid, iron, and pyridoxine
   (c) Toxic states producing marrow depression or destruction
   (d) Neoplastic diseases in which the marrow is invaded by tumor cells
   (e) Agranulocytosis (a decrease in the production of certain types of white cells). This occurs when the bone marrow activity is severely depressed, usually due to radiation therapy and drugs used in cancer therapy, and means that the patient can be in danger of death due to overwhelming infection.
   (f) Platelet disorders

Patient Preparation
1. A legal permit must be signed.
2. Instruct the patient about the procedure, purpose, benefits, and risks of the test.
3. Reassure the patient that many persons are extremely fearful about this test, especially if they have had it done previously.

4. Advise the patient that analgesics or sedatives may be ordered.
5. If the iliac crest is the site used, prepare the patient for pain by having him hold a pillow and bite into it if pain is experienced.

Patient Aftercare
1. Observe for bleeding at the puncture site, signs of shock, and continued pain, which may indicate fracture.
2. Recommend bed rest for 30 minutes; then normal activities may be resumed.
3. Administer analgesics or sedatives if necessary. Slight soreness over the puncture site area for 3 to 4 days after procedure is normal and is no cause for alarm.

Clinical Alert
1. Bone marrow aspiration is usually contraindicated in patients with hemophilia and other bleeding dyscrasias. However, the importance of further information that could be obtained by this method should be weighed against the risks.
2. Complications include bleeding and sternal fractures. Osteomyelitis and death due to injury to heart or great vessels are rare but do occur.
3. Pressure over the puncture site will control excessive bleeding that sometimes occurs in patients with thrombocytopenia and other bleeding disorders.

Hemogram

A hemogram includes platelet count, white blood count (WBC), red blood count (RBC), hematocrit (HCT), and indices. Complete blood count (CBC) is a hemogram plus differential count.

Complete Blood Count (CBC)

Explanation of Test
The CBC is a basic screening test in all patients and is one of the most frequently ordered laboratory procedures. The significant findings in the CBC give valuable information about the patient's diagnosis, prognosis, response to treatment, and recovery. The CBC consists of

White blood count (WBC)
Differential white cell count (Diff)

Red blood count (RBC)
Hematocrit (Hct)
Hemoglobin (Hgb)
Red blood cell indices
  Mean corpuscular volume (MCV)
  Mean corpuscular hemoglobin (MCH)
  Mean corpuscular hemoglobin concentration (MCHC)
Stained red cell examination (film or peripheral blood smear)
Platelet count (often included in CBC)

These tests will be described in detail in following pages.

White Blood Cell Count (WBC) (Leukocyte Count)

Normal Values
5–10^3/μl.   or 5–10^9/liter

Leukocyte Function
The main function of leukocytes is to fight infection, defend the body by phagocytosis against invasion by foreign organisms, and to produce, or at least transport and distribute, antibodies in the immune response. Behaving as separate yet related systems, the various types of leukocytes serve different functions. These functions will be discussed in detail in subsequent test descriptions.

Types of Leukocytes
Leukocytes, or white blood cells, are divided into two main groups: granulocytes and agranulocytes. These are further classified as follows:

Granulocytes		Agranulocytes	
Band neutrophils	0%–5%	Lymphocytes	20%–40%
Neutrophils	60%–70%	Monocytes	2%–6%
Eosinophils	1%–4%		
Basophils	0.5%–1%		

The granulocytes receive their name from the granules that are present in the cytoplasm of neutrophils, basophils, and eosinophils. However, each of these cells also contains a multilobed nucleus, which accounts for their also being called *polymorphonuclear leukocytes*. In laboratory terminology, they are often called "polys" (PMNs)

   The agranulocytes, which consist of the lymphocytes and monocytes, do not contain granules and have nonlobular nuclei. They are not necessarily spherical; thus, the term *mononuclear leukocytes* is applied to these cells.

Leukocyte Formation

Since granulocytes and monocytes are formed in the red bone marrow, all of these cells can be considered myelogenous. The lymphocytes are formed in the lymphatic tissue, which includes the spleen, thymus, and tonsils. After formation they are transported in the blood to the different regions, organs, or tissues of the body where they are needed. Vitamins, folic acid, and amino acids are used by the body in the formation of the leukocytes.

The endocrine system is an important regulator of the number of leukocytes in the blood. Hormones affect production of the leukocytes in the blood-forming organs, their storage and release from the tissue, and their disintegration. A local inflammatory process exerts a definite chemical effect on the mobilization of the leukocytes.

The life span of leukocytes varies from 13 to 20 days, after which the cells are destroyed in the lymphatic system; many are excreted from the body in fecal matter.

Granulocyte Development

Granulocytes develop through the following progression:

1. Myeloblasts (immature cells normally found in bone marrow); increased numbers found in granulocytic leukemia
2. Promyelocytes (immature cells normally can be found in blood in granulocytic [myelocytic] leukemia)
3. Myelocytes (found in the bone marrow)
4. Metamyelocytes (cells found in granulocytic [myelocytic] leukemia or severe infection)
5. "Bands" (neutrophils in early stages of maturity; increased numbers found in blood when leukocyte count is elevated [stabs])
6. "Polys" (mature cells sometimes referred to as "segs" [segmented neutrophils])

Staining Properties

Neutrophils, basophils, and eosinophils are distinguished from one another by the staining properties of the granules in their cytoplasm.

Neutral staining reaction: Neutrophils
Acid stain reaction: Eosinophils
Basic stain reaction: Basophils

Agranulocyte Development

Agranulocytes develop through the following progression:

Lymphocytes
1. Lymphoblast (immature cell found in lymphocytic leukemia)
2. Prolymphocyte (immature cell found in lymphocytic leukemia)
3. Lymphocyte (mature cell)

Monocytes
1. Monoblasts
2. Promonocytes (immature cells seen in monocytic leukemia)
3. Monocyte (mature cell)

Explanation of Test

Measurement of the total number of circulating leukocytes is an important procedure in the diagnosis and prognosis of the disease process, because specific patterns of leukocyte response can be expected in different types of diseases. It is known that certain diseases are accompanied by a specific type of white blood cell increase or decrease that is proportional to the severity of the signs and symptoms of the disease.

Since leukocytes are affected by so many diseases, the leukocyte count serves as a useful guide to the severity of the disease process. The differential count (count of the numbers of different types of leukocytes; see page 25) will identify certain persons with increased susceptibility to infection. A leukocyte-function test may be done to determine the white blood cells' ability to phagocytize and destroy bacteria.

Leukocytes and differential counts by themselves are of little value as aids to diagnosis unless the results are related to the clinical condition of the patient; only then is a correct and useful interpretation possible. Serial examinations have diagnostic and prognostic value. Disorders of the WBC are often associated with changes in the red blood cells and platelet counts. The stained red cell examination is done with the differential count. The same blood slide is examined to detect variations in structure, size, shape, color, and content of the red blood cells.

Procedure

1. A venous anticoagulated EDTA blood sample of 7 ml. or a finger-stick sample is obtained.
2. The time when specimen was obtained is recorded (*e.g.*, 7:00 A.M.).
3. Blood is processed either manually or in an automated piece of equipment such as the Coulter counter. Results obtained by such methods are reported.

Clinical Implications

A. *Leukocytosis* (white blood cell count above 10,000/μl.)
  1. Leukocytosis is usually due to an increase of only *one* type of white cell and is given the name of the type of cell that shows the main increase.
     (a) Neutrophilic leukocytosis or neutrophilia
     (b) Lymphocytic leukocytosis or lymphocytosis
     (c) Eosinophilic leukocytosis or eosinophilia
     (d) Monocytic leukocytosis or monocytosis
     (e) Basophilic leukocytosis or basophilia

2. An increase in circulating leukocytes is rarely due to a proportional increase in leukocytes of all types. When it occurs it is usually due to hemoconcentration.
3. In certain diseases (such as measles, pertussis, and sepsis), the increase of leukocytes is so great that the blood picture suggests leukemia. *Leukocytosis of a temporary nature is distinguished from leukemia, in which the leukocytosis is permanent and progressive.* The absence of anemia helps to distinguish severe infections from leukemia. The bone marrow is diagnostic.
4. Leukocytosis occurs in acute infections in which the degree of increase of white cells depends on
   (a) The severity of the infection
   (b) The patient's resistance
   (c) The patient's age
   (d) Marrow efficiency and reserve
5. Other causes of leukocytosis include
   (a) Hemorrhage
   (b) Trauma or tissue injury as occurs in surgery
   (c) Malignant disease, especially of the GI tract, liver, bone, and metastasis
   (d) Toxins, uremia, coma, eclampsia
   (e) Drugs, especially ether, chloroform, quinine, adrenalin
   (f) Serum sickness
   (g) Circulatory disease
   (h) Tissue necrosis
   (i) Leukemia (in acute leukemia there is an increase in the total WBC with a decrease in normal-appearing cells)
6. Occasionally leukocytosis is found when there is no evidence of clinical disease. Such findings suggest the presence of
   (a) Occult disease or
   (b) Physiologic leukocytosis due to excitement and other causes, but unrelated to disease
7. Steroid therapy modifies the leukocyte response.
   (a) When ACTH is given to a healthy person, leukocytosis occurs.
   (b) When ACTH is given to a patient with severe infection, the infection can spread rapidly without producing the expected leukocytosis; thus, what would normally be an important sign in obscured.
B. *Leukopenia* (a decrease of white blood cells below 4000)
   Occurs during and following
   1. Viral infections
   2. Hypersplenism
   3. Bone-marrow depression due to
      (a) Drugs

    (1) Antimetabolites
    (2) Barbiturates
    (3) Benzine
    (4) Antibiotics
    (5) Antihistamines
    (6) Anticonvulsives
    (7) Antithyroid drugs
    (8) Arsenicals
    (9) Cancer chemotherapy (causes a decrease in leukocytes; leukocyte count is used as a link to disease)
  (b) Heavy metals
  (c) Radiation
  (d) Agranulocytosis
  (e) Acute leukemia
  (f) Pernicious and aplastic anemia
  (g) Multiple myeloma
  (h) Alcoholism
  (i) Diabetes

Note: Alcoholism and diabetes tend to decrease mobilization of leukocytes; this may contribute to increased susceptibility to pneumonia and other infections.

Clinical Alert

1. WBC below 500 (<500 WBC) represents a panic value
2. Agranulocytosis (marked neutropenia and leukopenia) is extremely dangerous and is often fatal because the body is unprotected against invading agents. Without treatment, death usually occurs three to six days after agranulocytosis appears. Patients who exhibit this disorder must be protected from infection by means of reverse isolation techniques with strictest emphasis on hand-washing technique.

Clinical Considerations
In prolonged severe granulocytopenia

1. Give no fresh fruits or vegetables because the kitchen, especially in a hospital, may be a source of food contamination. When leukocytes are low, a person can get pseudomonas or fungal infection from fresh fruits and vegetables.
2. Use minimal bacteria diet or commercially sterile diet. All food must be served from a single serving or a new package.
3. Consider leukemia diet. See dietary department for restrictions such as cooked food only and careful food preparation.

Interfering Factors
1. Hourly rhythm: There is an early-morning low level and late-afternoon high peak.
2. Age: In newborns and infants the count is high (10,000–20,000) and gradually decreases in children until the adult values are reached at about age 21.
3. Food, exercise, emotions: Eating, moderate physical activity, emotional upheaval, and pain will cause a slight increase in values.
4. Phase of reproductive cycle: Menstruation, last month of pregnancy, and obstetrical labor will cause an increase in values.
5. Stress: Fever, convulsions, anesthesia, paroxysmal tachycardia following severe electric shock, and prolonged cold baths will cause an increase in values.
6. Chronic leukemia: Count may be falsely low in chronic lymphatic leukemia due to increased fragility of the cells. Many smudge cells and cell fragments seen.
7. Drugs: There are many drugs that can cause increased or decreased numbers of leukocytes.

Differential White Blood Cell Count (DIFF)
(Differential Leukocyte Count)

Normal Values

	Relative Values	Absolute Values (No./µl.)
Neutrophils	60%–70% (56% average)	3000–7000
Eosinophils	1%–4% (2.7% average)	50–400
Basophils	0.5%–1% (0.3% average)	25–100
Lymphocytes	20%–40% (34% average)	1000–4000
Monocytes	2%–6%	100–600

Explanation of Test
The total leukocyte count of the circulating white blood cells is differentiated according to the five types of leukocyte cells, each of which performs a specific function.

Cell	These Cells Function to Combat
Neutrophils	Bacterial infections, inflammatory disorders, stress, certain drugs
Eosinophils	Allergic disorders and parasitic infestations
Basophils	Blood dyscrasias and myeloproliferative diseases
Lymphocytes	Viral infections (measles, rubella, chicken pox, infectious mononucleosis)
Monocytes	Severe infections, as the infection is controlled

The differential count is expressed as a percentage of the total number of white cells. The distribution of the number and type of cells and the degree of increase or decrease are diagnostically significant.

The differential count expressed in percent is the *relative* number of each type of leukocyte in the blood. The absolute number of each type of leukocyte is obtained mathematically by multiplying the percentile value of one type of leukocyte by the total leukocyte count.

Formula

$$\begin{array}{ccc} \text{Absolute value} & \text{Relative value} & \text{Total WBC count} \\ \text{WBC/mm.}^3 \quad = & (\%) \quad \times & \text{(cells/mm.}^3) \end{array}$$

The differential count alone has a limited value; it must always be interpreted in relation to the total leukocyte count. The reason for this interpretation can be explained in the following way: If the percentage of one type of cell is increased, it can be inferred that cells of that type are relatively more numerous than normal, but it is not known if this reflects an absolute decrease in cells of another type or an actual absolute increase in the number of cells that are relatively increased. On the other hand, if the relative percentile values of the differential are known and if the total leukocyte count is known, it is possible to calculate absolute values that are not subject to misinterpretation.

Segmented Neutrophils (Polymorphonuclear Neutrophils, PMNs, "Segs," or "Polys")

Normal Values
50%–60% of total white cell count
3000–7000/mm.^{3}
0–3% of the total count of stabs or band cells

Background
The neutrophils are the most numerous and most important type of white cells in the body's reaction to inflammation. They constitute a primary defense against microbial invasion through the process of phagocytosis. These cells can also cause some damage to body tissue by their release of enzymes and endogenous pyrogens.

In their immature stage of development they are referred to as "stab" or "band" cells. The term "band" stems from the appearance of the nucleus that has not assumed the lobed shape of the mature cell.

Clinical Implications
A. *Neutrophilia,* or neutrophilic leukocytosis, is an increased percentage of circulating neutrophils.
   1. Conditions causing neutrophilia
      (a) Bacterial and parasitic infections

    (b) Metabolic disturbances such as diabetic and uremic coma, gout, and eclampsia

    (c) Blood disorders such as hemorrhage, granulocytic leukemia, and myeloproliferative disorders

2. Instances when the presence of early and immature neutrophils is the only indication that infection is present

    (a) In elderly persons or in instances when the infection is overwhelming, there can be an increase in immature neutrophils with little or no leukocytosis (degenerative shift to the left)

    (b) On the other hand, absence of severe infection indicates a poor prognosis

    (c) In pernicious anemia and chronic morphine addiction, only adult or mature hypersegmented neutrophils are associated with increased neutrophils

3. An increase in mature cells (known as a "shift to the right," as in liver disease and megaloblastic anemia due to vitamin B_{12} or folic-acid deficiency) can occur

    (a) In hemolysis

    (b) With drugs such as digitalis, mercury, ACTH, sulfonamides, arsenicals, potassium chlorate, benzene, venoms

    (c) With tissue breakdown as in burns, myocardial infarction, tumors, gangrene, or pus formation; hemolytic transfusion reactions, after surgery, after cancer of liver, GI tract, and bone marrow

    (d) With allergies

B. *Comparison between neutrophilia and total WBC*

1. Increase in percentage of neutrophils represents severity of infection. Total WBC indicates the patient's power of resistance.

2. If leukocyte count and percentage of neutrophils increase proportionately, there is a moderate infection with good resisting power by the patient.

3. If the neutrophil count is increased to a notably greater extent than the total count, no matter how low the count, there is either a lost resistance or severe infection.

4. In general, the degree of neutrophilia is proportionate to the amount of tissue involved in the inflammation. The neutrophilia-promoting substances are probably derived from necrotic cells.

5. The more the body is able to localize the infection, the more localized is the process and the more pronounced is the neutrophilia.

C. *Shift to the left*

1. Any stimulus that causes an increase in neutrophils also causes early and immature neutrophils to be released into the blood. An increase in these cells is known as a "shift to the left" and is an indication of a regenerative response.

2. Conditions causing an increase in percentage of stabs or band cells
   (a) Infectious states
   (b) Chemotherapeutic drugs
   (c) Disorders of cell production such as leukemia characterized by rapid proliferation of leukocytes
   (d) Toxemias
   (e) Hemorrhage
   (f) Chronic neutropenia in children
D. *Neutropenia* (a decreased percentage of neutrophils)
   1. Neutropenia is due either to decreased cell production or increased cell disappearance (sequestration).
   2. Conditions causing neutropenia
      (a) Acute viral infections such as influenza, infectious hepatitis, measles, mumps, poliomyelitis
      (b) Blood diseases such as aplastic and pernicious anemia, agranulocytosis, and acute lymphoblastic leukemia
      (c) Toxic agents
      (d) Hormonal diseases such as Addison's disease, thyrotoxicosis, and acromegaly.
      (e) Neutropenia, instead of an expected neutrophilia, may occur in massive infections, especially in debilitated patients.
E. *Morphologic alterations of neutrophils*
   1. Toxic granulation—dark blue granules in cytoplasm indicative of severe infection or other toxic conditions
   2. Döhle bodies—light blue inclusions in cytoplasm found in severe infections
   3. May–Hegglin anomaly—large blue inclusion bodies found along with giant platelets
   4. Pelger–Huët anomaly—hereditary, autosomal dominant condition involves failure of normal segmentation of neutrophils—all neutrophils are "band"- or "dumbbell"-shaped
   5. Chédiak–Higashi syndrome—autosomal recessive disorder, characterized by large granules in neutrophils

Clinical Alert

A neutropenia of less than 500 increases dramatically a patient's susceptibility to bacterial infections. If this occurs, institute necessary measures to protect the patient.

Interfering Factors
   1. Age
      (a) Children respond to infection with a greater degree of neutrophilic leukocytosis than adults.

    (b) Some elderly patients respond weakly or not at all, even when the infection is severe.
2. Resistance
    (a) People of any age who are weak and debilitated may fail to respond with a significant neutrophilia.
    (b) When an infection becomes overwhelming, the patient's resistance is exhausted and as death approaches, the number of neutrophils decreases greatly.
3. Steroids
    Tissue resistance is weakened when ACTH is given to a person suffering from a severe infection, so that the expected neutrophilia does not occur.
4. Myelosuppressive chemotherapy
5. Marrow efficiency and reserve

Eosinophils

Normal Values
1%–4% of total leukocyte count (relative value) or
50–250/mm.^{3} (absolute value) or
50–250 10^6/liter

Background
Although not too much is known about its function, the eosinophil is capable of phagocytosis. Eosinophils become active in the later stages of inflammation and ingest antigen–antibody complexes. These cells are also active in allergic reactions and parasitic infections. The number of eosinophils in the blood is increased in these conditions.

Explanation of Test
1. Used to diagnose allergic infections, severity of infestations with worms and other large parasites, and the response to treatment.
2. Also the basis for the Thorn test, which is used to evaluate the adrenal response to ACTH (see pg. 31).

Procedure
1. Note the time the blood sample is obtained (*e.g.*, 3:00 P.M.).
2. If the count is done separately, a blood sample of 7 ml. is obtained.
3. A manual white blood count is performed, 100 cells counted, and the percentage of eosinophils is reported.

Clinical Implications
A. *Eosinophilia*—an increase of circulating eosinophils greater than 5% or more than 500
    1. Causes
        (a) As response to hyperimmune, allergic, and degenerative reactions

(b) There is a relative and absolute increase in eosinophils in association with the antigen–antibody reactions seen in the following conditions:
  (1) Allergies
  (2) Parasitic disease such as trichinosis and tape worm
  (3) Addison's disease
  (4) Lung and bone cancer
  (5) Chronic skin infections such as psoriasis, pemphigus, and scabies
  (6) Myelogenous leukemia
  (7) Hodgkin's disease
  (8) Polycythemia
  (9) Subacute infections
  (10) Familial eosinophilia (rare)
  (11) Polyarteritis nodosa
  (12) Many tumors
B. *Eosinopenia*—a decrease in the amount of circulating eosinophils
  1. Usually due to an increased adrenal steroid production that accompanies most conditions of bodily stress.
  2. Associated with
    (a) Infectious mononucleosis
    (b) Hypersplenism
    (c) Congestive heart failure
    (d) Cushing's syndrome
    (e) Aplastic and pernicious anemia
    (f) Use of certain drugs—ACTH, epinephrine, and thyroxin
    (g) Infections with neutrophilia
  3. Eosinophils disappear early in pyogenic infections when there is a leukocytosis with a marked shift to the left (increase in immature white cells).
C. *Eosinophilic myelocytes*
  In the differential count, all the eosinophils are placed in one group, except the eosinophilic myelocytes, which are counted separately because they have a greater significance, being found only in leukemia or leukemoid blood pictures.

Interfering Factors
1. Hourly rhythm
  (a) The normal eosinophil count is lowest in the morning, then rises from noon until after midnight.
  (b) For this reason, serial eosinophil counts should be repeated at the same time in the afternoon each day.
2. Stress
  Stressful situations, such as in burns, postoperative states, lupus erythematosus, electroshock, eclampsia, and labor will cause a decreased count.

3. Steroid therapy
   (a) Eosinophilia can be masked by steroid use; infections can be fatal.
   (b) It is not clear why eosinophils disappear promptly from the blood following injection of ACTH.

Thorn ACTH Test

Background
In 4 hours, administration of ACTH produces a decrease of 50% or more in the eosinophil count in persons with a normally functioning adrenal cortex.

Explanation of Test
Useful in diagnosing Addison's disease as a test of adrenal cortex reserve before surgical procedures, and as a test to distinguish functional hypopituitarism from organic disease of the adrenal cortex.

Procedure
1. No food after 8 P.M.; water only allowed
2. A venous blood sample is drawn in the morning and an eosinophil count is done.
3. ACTH (25 mg.) is injected intramuscularly to stimulate the adrenal cortex. (Note the time of administration, *e.g.*, 8 A.M.)
4. Four hours later a second venous sample is obtained and eosinophil count is again recorded.

Clinical Implications
If adrenal cortex insufficiency is present, as in Addison's disease, the second eosinophil count will be decreased less than 20%.

Basophils

Normal Values
0.5%–1.0% of the total leukocyte count or
25–100/mm.^{3}

Background
Basophils comprise a small percentage of the total leukocyte count—about 0.5%. Their function is not clearly understood, although they are considered to be phagocytic and to contain heparin, histamines, and serotonin. Tissue basophils are also called *mast cells;* like basophils they store and produce heparin, histamine, and serotonin. Normally,

they are not found in peripheral blood and are rarely seen in healthy bone marrow.

Explanation of Test

Basophil counts are used to study allergic reactions. There is a positive correlation between high basophil counts and high concentrations of blood histamines.

Clinical Implications

A. *Increased count* (basophilia)
  1. Associated most commonly with granulocytic and basophilic leukemia and myeloid metaphasia
  2. Associated less commonly with
     (a) Chronic inflammation
     (b) Polycythemia vera
     (c) Chronic hemolytic anemia
     (d) Following splenectomy
     (e) The healing phase of inflammation
     (f) Following radiation
B. *Decreased count*
  Associated with
  1. Acute allergic reactions
  2. Hyperthyroidism
  3. Stress reactions such as myocardial infarction and bleeding peptic ulcer
  4. Hypersensitivity reactions such as urticaria and anaphylactic shock
  5. Following prolonged steroid therapy
C. *Numbers of tissue mast cells*
  Associated with
  1. Rheumatoid arthritis
  2. Urticaria
  3. Anaphylactic shock
  4. Hypoadrenalism
  5. Lymphoma
  6. Macroglobulinemia
  7. Mast cell leukemia
  8. Lymphoma invading bone marrow
  9. Urticaria pigmentosa

Monocytes (Monomorphonuclear Monocytes)

Normal Values

2%–6% of total leukocyte count relative value or
100–600/mm.^{3}

Background

These agranulocytes, the monomorphonuclear monocytes, are the body's second line of defense against infection and are the largest cells of normal blood. A histiocyte is a *fixed tissue macrophage*. Histiocytes, which are large macrophagic phagocytes, are classified as monocytes in a differential leukocyte count. Histiocytes and monocytes are thought to be capable of reversible transformation from one to the other.

These phagocytic cells of varying size and mobility remove injured and dead cells, microorganisms, and insoluble particles from the circulatory blood. Monocytes escaping from the upper and lower respiratory tracts and the gastrointestinal and genitourinary organs perform a scavenger function, clearing the body of debris. These phagocytic cells are able to produce the antiviral agent called *interferon*.

Monocytes are known to circulate in certain conditions in which their macrophagic properties act specifically—tuberculosis, leprosy, lipid storage disease, and subacute bacterial endocarditis (infectious leukocytosis).

Procedure

A blood sample of 7 ml. is obtained.

Clinical Implications

A. *Monocytosis*—an increase in the number of monocytes
1. Present during recovery stage from acute infections—a favorable sign
   (a) Present in tuberculosis—unfavorable
2. Viral infections
   (a) Infectious mononucleosis
   (b) Chickenpox, mumps
3. Subacute bacterial endocarditis
4. Parasitic infections
   (a) Malaria
   (b) Amebic dysentery
5. Rickettsial infections
6. Collagen diseases
7. Hematologic disorders
   (a) Monocytic leukemia
   (b) Granulocytic leukemia
   (c) Lymphoma—Hodgkin's disease
   (d) Multiple myeloma
8. Phagocytic monocytes (macrophages) may be found in small numbers in the blood in many conditions:
   (a) Severe infections
   (b) Lupus erythematosus

(c) Hemolytic anemias
(d) Agranulocytosis
(e) Thrombocytopenic purpura
B. *Decreased monocyte count* (not usually indentified with specific diseases)
   1. Prednisone treatment
   2. Hairy cell leukemia

Lymphocytes (Monomorphonuclear Lymphocytes)

Normal Values
20%–40% of total leukocyte count (relative value) or 1000–4000/mm.^{3}

Explanation of Test
These agranulocytes are small, motile cells that migrate to areas of inflammation in both the early and late stages of the inflammation process. They may possibly convert to tissue macrophages and plasma cells. These cells are the source of serum immunoglobulins and of cellular immune response and play an important role in immunologic reactions. It is believed that lymphocytes are responsible for the storage of immunologic memory. This means that a second contact with an antigen elicits an accelerated and increased response. The cells are found in the blood in infectious leukocytosis at the recovery stage of disease.

Procedure
Lymphocytes are counted as part of the differential count

Clinical Implications
A. *Lymphocytosis* (an increase in the amount of circulating lymphocytes)
   1. Above 9000/mm.^{3} in infants and young children
      Above 7000/mm^3 in older children
      Above 4000/mm^3 in adults
   2. *Conditions causing or associated with lymphocytosis*
      (a) Infectious lymphocytosis
         (1) Occurs mainly in children
         (2) 95% are small, mature lymphocytes
      (b) Infectious mononucleosis
         (1) Caused by Epstein–Barr virus
         (2) Most common in adolescents and young adults
         (3) Characterized by atypical lymphocytes–Downey cells–large, deeply indented, with deep blue (basophilic) cytoplasm
         (4) Differential diagnosis—positive heterophil test

    (c) Cytomegalovirus infection
    (d) Most viral upper respiratory infections, atypical pneumonia
    (e) Other viral diseases—mumps, rubella, rubeola
    (f) Infectious hepatitis
    (g) Some bacterial infections such as tuberculosis, brucellosis and syphilis, pertussis
    (h) Lymphatic leukemia and lymphocytic lymphosarcoma
    (i) Toxiplasmosis
    (j) Radiation
    (k) Lead intoxication
    (l) Stress

B. *Lymphopenia* (a decrease in the amount of circulating lymphocytes) Occurs
    (a) In Hodgkin's disease
    (b) In lupus erythematosus
    (c) After administration of ACTH and cortisone
    (d) After burns or trauma
    (e) In chronic uremia
    (f) In Cushing's syndrome
    (g) In early acute radiation syndrome

Clinical Alert

A decreased lymphocyte count of less than 500 means that a patient is dangerously susceptible to infection, especially viral infections. *Institute measures to protect patient from infection.*

Morphologic Forms of Lymphocytes

A. *Virocytes* (also called *stress lymphocytes* or *atypical lymphocytes*)
    1. Small atypical cells that appear in viral diseases such as viral hepatitis, viral pneumonia, and viral upper respiratory tract infections
    2. May also be found in numerous nonviral conditions
        (a) Fungoid and protoxoid infections
        (b) Autoimmune states
        (c) Allergic reactions
        (d) After transfusions and tissue grafts
    3. When seen in stress response, are called *stress lymphocytes*
    4. May be found in apparently healthy children

Note: Any amount of atypical lymphocytes is reported.

B. Downey-type cells—Large atypical infectious mononucleosis
C. *Transformed lymphocytes*
    1. Examples
        (a) Lymphocytoid cells that may be seen in macroglobulinemia

(b) Türk's cells and Rieder's cells that are seen in acute lymphatic leukemia

(c) Vacuolated lymphocytes that are seen in lipidosis

2. Culturing of lymphocytes in laboratory

(a) Stimulates small lymphocytes to transform into large atypical cells that produce immunoglobulins

(b) Transformation response is impaired in culturing of lymphocytes from patients with

(1) Hodgkin's disease

(2) Lymphatic leukemia

(3) Lymphocytosis

(4) Agammaglobulinemia

(c) Transformation response increased in sarcoidosis

3. Other uses of transformation test are to determine histiocompatibility of recipient and donor for tissue grafts.

(a) Lymphocytes from donor not related to recipient stimulate the production of up to 3% of transformed lymphocytes in recipient.

(b) Lymphocytes from siblings react less strongly.

(c) No reaction occurs on cultures from fraternal twins.

Red Blood Cell Count (RBC)
(Erythrocyte Count)

Normal Values

Values vary according to individual laboratory standards.

Men: 4.2–5.4 $10^6/\mu l$ (average 4.8) or 4.2–5.4 10^{12}/liter
Women: 3.6–5.0 $10^6/\mu l$ (average 4.3) or 3.6–5.0 10^{12}/liter

Background
Erythrocyte Function
The main function of the red blood cell or erythrocyte is to carry oxygen from the lungs to the body tissue and to transfer carbon dioxide from the tissues to the lungs. This process is achieved by means of the *hemoglobin* in the red cells that combines easily with oxygen and carbon dioxide. The combination of hemoglobin and oxygen gives arterial blood a bright red appearance. Since venous blood has a low oxygen content it appears dark red.

To enable the maximum amount of hemoglobin to be utilized, the red cell is shaped like a biconcave disk, which affords more surface area for the hemoglobin to combine with oxygen. The cell is also able to change its shape when necessary to allow for passage through the smaller capillaries.

Erythrocyte Formation

Red blood cells are formed in the red bone marrow (erythropoiesis). Normally the mature erythrocyte, without nucleus, is the major cell released into the circulation. Frequently, when the hematopoietic (bloodforming) system is faced with a heavy demand for red blood cell replacement (due to hemorrhage or disease), immature blood cells are released into the blood system.

The mature erythrocyte, once released into the circulation, has a life span of about 120 days. When worn out, it is removed from the circulation by phagocytes in the spleen, liver, and red bone marrow (reticuloendothelial system).

Millions of red blood cells are destroyed daily, while millions are formed to replace them. To maintain health, the number of erythrocytes and the amount of hemoglobin they contain must remain fairly constant.

If the number of red cells in the blood is reduced, the bone marrow can increase its rate of production. The trigger of this increased production is the decrease of oxygen in the body system, which stimulates the production of erythropoietin, a hormone that in turn stimulates the production of red blood cells.

Explanation of Test

The RBC determines the total number of red blood cells or erythrocytes found in a cubic millimeter of blood. It is an important measurement in the determination of anemia or polycythemia.

Procedure

Automated electronic devices are generally used to determine the number of red blood cells.

Clinical Implications

A. *Decreased values*
1. Anemias
   Due to
   (a) Decreased red blood cell production
   (b) Increased red blood cell destruction (hemolytic)
   (c) Blood loss
   (d) Dietary insufficiency of iron and certain vitamins, especially B_6, B_{12}, and folic acid, which are essential in the production of erythrocytes
2. Diseases of bone marrow function
   (a) Hodgkin's disease
   (b) Multiple myeloma
   (c) Leukemia
3. Pernicious anemia
4. Lupus erythematosus

5. Addison's disease
6. Rheumatic fever
7. Subacute endocarditis

B. *Increased values*
1. Polycythemia vera
2. Secondary polycythemia
   (seen in erythropoietin-secreting tumors, in renal disorders such as hypernephroma and renal cysts, and in cancer of the liver)
3. Severe diarrhea
4. Dehydration
5. Acute poisoning
6. Pulmonary fibrosis
7. During and immediately following hemorrhage

Interfering Factors

Physiological Variation

1. Posture: When blood sample is obtained from a healthy person in a recumbent position, the count is lower than normal. (If the patient is anemic, the count will be even lower.)
2. Exercise: Extreme exercise and excitement produce higher counts than those obtained under basal conditions. Counts obtained under these conditions are of doubtful clinical value.
3. Dehydration: Hemoconcentration in dehydrated adults due to severe burns, untreated intestinal obstruction, and severe, persistent vomiting may obscure significant anemia.
4. Age: The normal RBC of a newborn is higher than that of an adult with a rapid drop to the lowest point in life at 2 to 4 months. The normal adult level is reached at age 14 and is maintained until old age, where there is a gradual drop.
5. Altitude: The higher the altitude, the greater the increase in RBC. Decreased oxygen content of the air stimulates the RBC to rise (erythrocytosis).
6. Pregnancy: There is a normal decrease in RBC when the body fluid increases in pregnancy with the normal number of erythrocytes becoming more diluted.
7. There are many drugs that may cause *reduced* RBCs.
8. Among the drugs that may cause *increased* RBCs are gentamicin and methyldopa.

Reticulocyte Count

Normal Values

Men: 0.5%–1.5% of total erythrocytes or 0.005-0.015
Women: 0.5%–2.5% or 0.005–0.025

Children: 0.5%–4% of total erythrocytes or 0.005–0.040
Infants: 2%–5% of total erythrocytes or 0.020–0.050
Reticulocyte index = 1.0
Absolute reticulocyte count = % reticulocytes × erythrocyte count
25–85 × 10^3 cells/μl or 25–85 × 10^9 cells/liter

Background

A *reticulocyte* is a young, immature, nonnucleated cell of the erythro-cyte series formed in the bone marrow. As an immature red cell it contains reticular material (from the dissolving nucleus) that will stain a gray blue when tested in the laboratory. Reticulum is present in newly released blood cells and lasts about 4 days before the cell reaches its full mature state. Normally a small number of these cells is found in the circulating blood (about 0.5% to 1.5% of the total red blood count, see the normal value). The number of reticulocytes per 1000 erythro-cytes yields the reticulocyte count.

In order for the reticulocyte count to be meaningful, it must be viewed in relation to the total number of erythrocytes.

Explanation of Text

A reticulocyte count is used

1. To differentiate anemias due to bone marrow failure from those due to hemorrhage or hemolysis (red cell destruction)
2. To check the effectiveness of treatment in pernicious anemia and the recovery of bone marrow function in aplastic anemia
3. To determine the effects of radioactive substances on exposed workers

Procedure

A small blood sample is mixed with a supravital stain such as brilliant cresyl blue. After the stain is allowed to react with the blood (the reticulum can be stained only while the cells are viable), a blood smear is prepared with this mixture and scanned under a microscope.

Clinical Implications

A. *Increased levels*

An increased count (reticulocytosis) means that hyperactive eryth-rocyte production is occurring as the bone marrow replaces cells lost or prematurely destroyed. Identifying reticulocytosis may lead to the recognition of an otherwise occult disease such as hidden chronic hemorrhage or unrecognized hemolysis (sickle cell anemia and thalassemia). Increased levels are observed in the following conditions:

1. Hemolytic anemias
2. Sickle cell disease
3. Metastatic carcinoma
4. Leukemia

5. Three to four days following hemorrhage
6. Hereditary spherocytosis
7. After splenectomy
8. Following treatment of anemias (therapeutic diagnostic test)
   (a) Increase may be used as an index of the effectiveness of treatment.
   (b) After adequate doses of iron in iron-deficiency anemia, the rise in reticulocytes may exceed 20%.
   (c) There is a proportional increase when pernicious anemia is treated by transfusion or vitamin B_{12} therapy.

B. *Decreased levels*
A decreased reticulocyte count means that bone marrow is not producing enough erythrocytes.
Found in
1. Iron-deficiency anemia
2. Aplastic anemia (a persistent deficiency of reticulocytes suggests a poor prognosis)
3. Untreated pernicious anemia
4. Chronic infection
5. Radiation therapy

Interfering Factors
The reticulocyte count is normally increased in pregnancy and infants.

Hematocrit (HCT); Packed Cell Volume (PCV)

Normal values
Men: 40%–54% packed red cell volume (varies widely) or 0.40–0.54 volume fraction
Women: 37%–47% or 0.37–0.47
Newborn (both genders): 50%–62% or 0.50–0.62
Microhematocrit (done on small amount of blood, usually drawn from finger prick)
Men: 45%–47% packed red cell volume or 0.45–0.47 volume fraction
Women: 42%–44% or 0.42–0.44
Infants: 44%–62% or 0.44–0.62

Explanation of Test
The purpose of this test is to determine the space occupied by packed red blood cells. The results are expressed as the percentage of red cells in a volume of whole blood. The word *hematocrit* means "to separate blood," which underscores the mechanism of the test, since the plasma and blood cells are separated by centrifugation.

Procedure
The tube used in this test is a capillary hematocrit tube, which is two-thirds filled with venous blood to which an anticoagulant has been added. The tube is then centrifuged to separate the cellular elements from the plasma. The height of the packed cells in the tube indicates the hematocrit. The measure is recorded in terms of the volume of cells found in 100 ml. of blood and is expressed as a percentage of the total amount of blood centrifuged.

Clinical Implications
1. *Increased values* found in
    (a) Erythrocytosis
    (b) Polycythemia
    (c) Severe dehydration
    (d) Shock, when the hemoconcentration rises considerably
2. *Decreased values* found in
    (a) Anemia—An hematocrit of 30 or less means the patient is moderately to severely anemic.
    (b) Leukemia
    (c) Hyperthyroidism
    (d) Cirrhosis
    (e) Acute, massive blood loss
    (f) Hemolytic reaction—This condition may be found in
        (1) Transfusion of incompatible blood
        (2) Reaction to chemicals or drugs
        (3) Reaction to infectious agents
        (4) Reaction to physical agents *e.g.*, severe burn or prosthetic heart valves
3. The hematocrit may or may not be reliable immediately after even a moderate loss of blood and immediately after transfusions. For example, even though Hgb and Hct are accepted ways of monitoring how a patient is coming along after treatment, they can be considered unreliable if the patient is continuing to lose blood; however, Hct is a good indicator of how much blood has been lost up to the time the blood sample is obtained.
4. Hematocrit may be normal following acute hemorrhage. During the recovery phase, the Hct and RBC will drop remarkably.
5. Usually, the hematocrit parallels the RBC when the cells are of a normal size. As the number of normal-sized erythrocytes increases, so does the hematocrit.
    (a) However, for the patient with microcytic or macrocytic anemia, this relationship does not hold true.
    (b) If a patient has an iron-deficiency anemia with small red cells, the hematocrit decreases because the microcytic cells pack to a smaller volume. The RBC, however, may be normal.

Interfering Factors

People living in high altitudes will have high values, the same as in Hgb.

1. Normally, the value slightly decreases in the physiologic hydremia of pregnancy.
2. The normal values for the hematocrit vary with the age and sex of the individual. The normal value for infants is higher because the newborn has many macrocytic red cells. Hcts in females are usually slightly lower than in males.
3. There is also a tendency toward lower values in men and women after age 50, corresponding to lower values for erythrocyte counts in this age group.

Hemoglobin (Hgb)

Normal Values

Women: 12–16 g./dl. or 1.86–2.48 nmol./liter
Men: 13.5–17.5 g./dl. or 2.09–2.71 nmol./liter
Newborn (both genders): 14–20 g./dl.
Varies widely according to the standard used.

Background

Hemoglobin, the main component of erythrocytes, serves as the vehicle for the transportation of O_2 and CO_2. It is composed of (1) amino acids that form a single protein called *globin*, and (2) a compound called *heme*, which contains iron atoms and the red pigment porphyrin.

The iron pigment is that portion of the hemoglobin that combines readily with oxygen and gives blood its characteristic red color.

Each gram of hemoglobin can carry 1.34 ml. of oxygen. The oxygen-combining capacity of the blood is directly proportional to the hemoglobin concentration rather than to the RBC, since some red cells contain more hemoglobin than others. This is why hemoglobin determinations are more important in the evaluation of anemia than the RBC.

While oxygen transport is the main function of hemoglobin, it also serves as one of the primary buffer substances in the extracellular fluid and helps maintain acid-base balance by the process called *chloride shift*. Chloride moves or shifts in and out of the red blood cells according to the level of oxygen in the blood plasma. For each chloride ion that enters the red blood cell, a bicarbonate ion is released. Thus, a hemoglobin measurement is important in determining acid–base balance.

Explanation of Test

The hemoglobin determination test is used to
1. Screen for disease associated with anemia
2. Determine the severity of anemia
3. Follow the response to treatment for anemia

Procedure

A venous blood EDTA* sample of 2 ml. is obtained. Automated electronic devices are generally used to determine the Hgb; however, a manual colorimetric procedure is also widely used.

Clinical Implications

A. *As an indication of anemia*
   1. It is difficult to say explicitly what hemoglobin level represents the presence of anemia per se, because of the variable adaptability and efficiency of the body in response to blood hemoglobin concentrations.
   2. An arbitrary level of 12 g. is acceptable.
      (a) This level must be evaluated along with the erythrocyte count.
      (b) If the erythrocytes are normal in size (normocytic) and contain normal amounts of hemoglobin (normochromic), the erythrocyte count and the hemoglobin concentrations give compatible information.
   3. The total amount of circulating hemoglobin is of greater physiologic importance than the number of erythrocytes because the symptoms of anemia are caused by an insufficient amount of circulating hemoglobin.
B. *Decreased levels of hemoglobin* found in
   1. Anemia states (especially iron-deficiency anemia)
   2. Hyperthyroidism
   3. Cirrhosis of the liver
   4. Severe hemorrhage
   5. Hemolytic reactions due to
      (a) Transfusions of incompatible blood
      (b) Reactions to chemicals and drugs
      (c) Reactions to infectious agents
      (d) Reactions to physical agents (severe burns and artificial heart valves)
      (e) Various systemic diseases
         (1) Hodgkin's disease
         (2) Leukemia
         (3) Lymphoma

* Ethylene diamine tetraacetic acid—anticoagulant

(4) Systemic lupus erythematosus
(5) Carcinomatosis
(6) Sarcoidosis
(7) Renal cortical necrosis
C. *Increased levels of hemoglobin* found in
  1. Hemoconcentration of the blood (any condition such as poly-cythemia and severe burns in which the number of circulating erythrocytes rises above normal)
  2. Chronic obstructive pulmonary disease
  3. Congestive heart failure
D. *Variance in levels of hemoglobin*
  1. After transfusions, hemorrhages, burns. (Hgb and Hct are both high during and immediately after hemorrhage.)
  2. Hgb and Hct give valuable information in an emergency situation if interpreted not in an isolated fashion but in conjunction with other pertinent laboratory data. There are very few tests in laboratory medicine that can be regarded as diagnostic all on their own.

Interfering Factors

1. People living at high altitudes will have increased values, as in hematocrit values.
2. Excessive fluid intake will cause a decreased value.
3. Normally, the value is higher in infants before active erythropoiesis begins.
4. Hemoglobin levels are normally decreased in pregnancy.
5. Drugs that may cause *increased* levels of hemoglobin include gentamicin and methyldopa.
6. There are many drugs that may cause *decreased* levels of hemoglobin.

Clinical Alert

Panic value is <5.0 g./dl.; leads to heart failure and death.

Red Blood Cell Indices

Background

The red blood cell indices are used to define the size and hemoglobin content of the red blood cell. They consist of the mean corpuscular volume (MCV), mean corpuscular hemoglobin (MCH), and mean corpuscular hemoglobin concentration (MCHC). In most laboratories,

Table 2-2
Morphologic Classification of Anemias

Type of Anemia	Blood Constants	
	MCV (μm.³ or fl.)	MCHC (g.Hb/dl.RBC/ or mmol./liter)
Microcytic hypochromic	60–87	20–30
Macrocytic normochromic	103–160	32–36
Normocytic normochromic	87–103	32–36
Microcytic normochromic	60–87	32–36

(Bauer, JD et al: Bray's Clinical Laboratory Methods, 8th ed. St. Louis, CV Mosby, 1974)

these percentages will be recorded in all hemoglobins and hematocrits (H and H). These tests are determined on the same blood sample used for hemoglobin, hematocrit, and RBC count.

Explanation of Test
The red blood cell indices are used as an aid in differentiating anemias. When these are used together with an examination of the red cells on the stained smear, a clear picture of red cell morphology may be ascertained.

On the basis of the red blood cell indices, the erythrocytes can be characterized as normal in every respect, or as abnormal in volume or hemoglobin content. In deficient states, the anemias can be classified by cell size as macrocytic, normocytic, simple microcytic, or by cell size and color as microcytic hypochromic (Table 2-2).

Mean Corpuscular Volume (MCV)

Normal Values
87–103 fl./red cell or μm.³/red cell
(Higher values in infants and newborns)

Explanation of Test
This description of individual cell size is the best index for classifying anemias and is based on the visual or electronic counting of erythrocytes. It is an index that expresses the volume occupied by a single red cell and is a measure in cubic microns of the mean volume. The MCV indicates whether the red blood cell appears normocytic, microcytic, or macrocytic. If the MCV is less than 87 mm.³, the red cells are microcytic. If the MCV is greater than 103 mm.³, the red cells are macrocytic. If the MCV is within the normal range the red blood cells are normocytic.

Procedure
The volume of the red blood cells is calculated from the red blood cell count, which measures the number of cells per mm.^{3} of blood, and from the hematocrit, which measures the proportion of the blood occupied by the red blood cells and is expressed as volume rather than percent.

Clinical Implications
A. *Decreased values* found in
   1. Iron-deficiency anemia
   2. Thalassemia
   3. Anemia of chronic blood loss
   4. Chlorasis
B. *Increased values* found in
   1. Liver diseases
   2. Alcoholism
   3. Sprue
   4. Antimetabolite therapy
   5. Deficiency of folate or vitamin B_{12}
   6. Pernicious anemia (early)

C. *Unreliable values*
   1. It is possible to have a wide variation of cells (macrocytes and microcytes) in the blood smear and still have a normal MCV. This happens because the MCV is a calculated value rather than a direct measurement.
   2. In sickle cell anemia and other anemias characterized by abnormal erythrocyte shape, the MCV is of doubtful value because the hematocrit is not reliable in these diseases.

Mean Corpuscular Hemoglobin Concentration (MCHC)

Normal Values
31–37 g.Hb/dl RBC or 41.81–57.4 mmol. Hb/liter RBC

Explanation of Test
This test is a measure of the average concentration of hemoglobin in the red blood cells. For a given MCHC, the smaller the cell, the higher the concentration. The percentage represents grams of hemoglobin per 100 ml. of whole blood.
   This test is most valuable in evaluating therapy for anemia because the two most accurate hematological determinations (hemoglobin and hematocrit, not RBC) are used in the calculation of this test.

Procedure
The MCHC is a calculated value. It is an expression of the average concentration of hemoglobin in the red blood cells and as such, it gives the ratio of the weight of hemoglobin to the volume of the red blood cell.

$$\text{Formulas:} \quad \frac{\text{Hb (g./dl.)} \times 100}{\text{Hct (\%)}} \quad \text{or } \% \text{ Hb/cell} \div 100$$

Clinical Implications
A. *Decreased values*
1. A decreased MCHC signifies that a unit volume of packed RBCs contains less hemoglobin than normal, or that hemoglobin has been replaced by erythrocytic stomal material as in
   (a) Iron deficiency
   (b) Macrocytic anemias, chronic blood loss anemia
   (c) Pyridoxine-responsive anemia
   (d) Thalassemia
2. Hypochromic anemia is characterized by an MCHC of 30 or less.
B. *Increased values*
1. An increased MCHC usually indicates spherocytosis.
2. MCHC is not increased in pernicious anemia.
C. *Full saturation*
Occurs at about 30% (greater values are rarely observed)

Mean Corpuscular Hemoglobin (MCH)

Normal Values
26–34 picograms (pg.)/cell or 0.40–0.53 fmol./cell
(Normally higher in newborns and infants)

Explanation of Test
The MCH is a measure of the average weight of hemoglobin in the red blood cell. This index is of value in diagnosing severely anemic patients, but it is not as useful as MCHC because it uses the red cell count in its calculations, and the red cell count is not always accurate.

The MCH is expressed as picograms of hemoglobin per red blood cell.

Procedure
The MCH is a calculated value. It is an expression of the average weight of hemoglobin in the red blood cell.

Clinical Implications

1. An increase of the MCH is associated with macrocytic anemia.
2. A decrease of the MCH is associated with microcytic anemia.

Stained Red Cell Examination (Film)
(Stained Erythrocyte Examination)

Normal Values
Size: Normocytic (normal size—7–8 microns)
Color: Normochromic (normal)

Shape: Normocyte (biconcave disk)
Structure: Normocytes or erythrocytes (anucleated cells)

Explanation of Test

The stained film examination is the best means of studying the blood to determine variations and abnormalities in erythrocyte size, shape, structure, hemoglobin content, and staining properties. It is useful in diagnosing blood disorders such as anemia, thalassemia, and leukemia. This examination also serves as a guide to therapy and as an indicator of harmful effects of chemotherapy and radiation.

Procedure

A blood sample EDTA of 7 ml. is collected. A stained blood smear is studied under a microscope to determine size, shape, and other characteristics of the RBC.

Clinical Implications

A. *Variations in staining, color, and red cell inclusion*
   Normally, the erythrocytes have a tendency to absorb acid stains. The depth of staining is a rough guide to the amount of hemoglobin in the erythrocyte.
   1. *Normochromic cells* are those erythrocytes that are normal in hemoglobin content and color (stains pinkish orange, with a pale central area).
   2. *Hypochromic cells*
      (a) When the amount of hemoglobin is diminished, the central area that is normally pale becomes larger and paler and stains a lighter color.
      (b) Hypochromic cells usually appear in most of the anemias and are an indication that the bone marrow is regenerating to meet the demand for circulating red blood cells in the blood. MCHC is decreased.
   3. *Basophilic stippling* (the inclusion variation that occurs most frequently)
      (a) Term refers to the fine blue granules enclosed in the cell; they usually represent reticulocytes.
      (b) Basophilic stippling will appear in the stained-film examination of every patient who has symptoms of lead poisoning.
      (c) Except in lead poisoning, basophilic stippling indicates a serious blood disorder, usually related to excessive regeneration of erythrocytes or some impairment of hemoglobin synthesis. It is present in severe pernicious anemia, leukemia, and, less commonly, in other forms of anemia.
   4. *Polychromatophilia* (polychromesia)
      (a) Cells that do not take an acid stain, and instead stain with a basic stain to shades of blue; they usually represent reticulocytes.

(b) Cells that stain in this manner are most numerous in acute blood-loss anemia and hemolytic anemias due to increased erythropoietic activity.
5. *Parasitized RBCs* (malarial stippling)
    (a) Term applied to the fine granular appearance of erythrocytes that harbor the parasites of tertiary malaria.
    (b) The very fine granules, Schüffner's dots, stain purplish red.
6. *Nucleated red blood cells* (normal red blood cells do not have a nucleus)
    (a) The variations in structure that are counted and reported as nucleated red blood cells (NRBC) per 100 WBC.
    (b) *Metarubrictye* is another term for a nucleated erythrocyte.
    (c) The presence of NRBCs is an indication of a severe anemia and indicates that the body is making an excessive demand on the bloodforming organs to regenerate erythrocytes (increased erythropoietic activity).
7. *Other inclusion variations*
    (a) Howell–Jolly bodies (nuclear remnants, which appear after removal of the spleen)
    (b) Cabot rings (indicate severe anemia)
B. *Variations in shape*
  1. *Normocytes* are cells that are normal in size and shape (biconcave disc).
  2. *Poikilocytosis* is the presence of erythrocytes showing abnormal variations and irregularities in shape.
     (a) The cause of abnormally shaped RBCs is defective cell formation, usually due to an irreversible alteration of the cell membrane. It is nonspecific, but it is usually associated with severe anemia and with active erythroid regeneration or extreme dullary hematopoiesis. The hemoglobin content also varies greatly.
     (b) Erythrocytes that vary from the normal shape are present in most types of anemia, including severe anemia, and are numerous and most bizarre. Irregularities in shape are especially conspicuous in leukemia and pernicious anemia.
     (c) The abnormally shaped cells most commonly seen are
        (1) *Target cells*
           (a.) Erythrocytes that are thinner than normal with a small amount of hemoglobin in the center (*leptocytes*).
           (b.) Numerous in chronic anemias, liver disease, hemoglobin C disease, and thalassemia, also called *hereditary leptocytosis*.
        (2) *Spherocytes*
           (a.) Erythrocytes that are a little smaller than normal and are round rather than biconcave in shape.

  (b.) Their presence is associated with
    (1.) Hereditary spherocytosis
    (2.) Congenital hemolytic anemia
 (3) *Sickle cells*
  (a.) Erythrocytes that assume a crescent or sickle shape due to the presence of the abnormal hemoglobin (Hgb S)
  (b.) They occur in the hemolytic anemias.
 (4) *Schistocytes*
  (a.) Fragmented erythrocytes with extremely bizarre shapes (triangular or spiral)
  (b.) They occur in the hemolytic anemias.
  (c.) Found in disseminated intravascular coagulation (DIC) syndrome due to fibrin deposits
  (d.) Associated with artificial heart valves

C. *Variations in size*
Normal values: 7–8 microns
Anisocytosis
1. Terms used to identify abnormal variations in size of erythrocytes
2. Due to abnormal cell development caused by
 (a) Congenital structural defects
 (b) Lack of folic acid
 (c) Lack of vitamin B_{12} and iron
3. *Microcytes*
 (a) Abnormally small erythrocytes (6 microns)
 (b) Microcytosis is associated with
  (1) Iron-deficiency anemia (3) Thalassemia major
  (2) Spherocytic anemia   (4) Chronic blood loss
4. *Macrocytes*
 (a) Are abnormally large erythrocytes (9 microns)
 (b) Macrocytosis is associated with pernicious anemia and folic acid deficiency anemia. In pernicious anemia, anisocytosis is extremely pronounced with megalocytes present.
 (c) Cells of larger than normal size are normally seen in newborns.
 (d) Liver disease

Clinical Alert

Marked abnormalities in size and shape of red blood cells without a known cause are an indication for more complete blood studies.

Red Cell Size Distribution Width (RDW)

Normal Values
8.5–11.5 microns

Explanation of Test
This measurement, determined by an automated method, is helpful in the investigation of some hematologic disorder and in monitoring response to therapy. The RDW is essentially an indication of the degree of anisocytosis. The size of red cells shows a normal distribution curve.

Procedure
The RDW is determined and calculated by the analyzer using the MCV and red blood cell count.

Clinical Implications
Changes in coefficients of variation (CV) occur in

(a) Pernicious anemia (CV = 12.9%)
(b) Posthemorrhagic anemia (CV = 9.9%)

Fetal Red Cells (Fetal–Maternal Bleed)

Normal Values
Negative

Explanation of Test
A fetal red cell test is done to detect fetal cells in the maternal circulation. The detection of fetal erythrocytes is important in diagnosing anemia of the newborn when it is suspected that a severe loss has occurred from the fetus, but also when there is a serious risk of the mother becoming immunized against the fetal red cell groups, as when an Rh-negative or Du-negative woman delivers or miscarries. In these instances, the mother's blood should be collected immediately after delivery and examined for fetal cells.

Procedure
A venous blood EDTA sample of 5 ml. is obtained from the mother. The amount of fetal blood that has escaped into the maternal circulation can be roughly calculated using this formula: ml. fetal blood = HgF cells × 50.

Clinical Implications
1. If the fetal blood loss into the circulation exceeds 35 ml., more than one vial of RhoGAM is required. One vial of RhoGAM will neutralize about 30 to 35 ml. of Rh-positive blood.

2. The efficiency of RhoGAM can also be judged by the disappearance of hemoglobin F-containing cells following its administration. If the fetal cells have not disappeared 12 to 24 hours after administration of the first dose, more RhoGAM is required.

OTHER ERYTHROCYTE TESTS

Erythrocyte Fragility (Osmotic Fragility and Autohemolysis)

Osmotic Fragility

Normal Values
Fragility
Hemolysis begins at 0.45%–0.39% saline solution.
Hemolysis ends at 0.33%–0.30% saline solution.

Background
A dramatic increase in the rate of RBC destruction can result in anemia. It is important to know if the increased destruction is due to unusual fragility of the erythrocytes that makes them susceptible to easy damage.

Explanation of Test
Osmotic fragility is determined by exposing red cells to a hypotonic sodium chloride solution, which causes water to enter the cell more rapidly than it leaves. As a result, the cell swells and at some point ruptures, causing the hemoglobin to disperse (hemolysis).

In the fragility test the red cells are exposed to a hypotonic solution of varying strength, ranging from 0.7% to 0.3%. In each solution the cells will swell to some extent. The point at which hemolysis begins is noted along with the point at which it is completed. If the cells burst in relatively high salt concentrations, they are identified as having increased fragility. Those that burst in lower salt concentrations have decreased fragility.

Clinical Implications
A. *Increased fragility* (>0.5%) occurs in
   1. Hereditary spherocytosis
   2. Hemolytic jaundice
   3. Autoimmune anemia (ABO and Rh incompatibility)
   4. Chemical poisons
   5. Burns

B. *Decreased fragility* (<0.3%) occurs in

1. Obstructive jaundice
2. Thalassemia
3. Sickle cell anemia
4. Iron-deficiency anemia

5. Polycythemia vera
6. Liver disease
7. Splenectomy (following)

Decreased fragility indicates that red cells are excessively flat.

Autohemolysis

Normal Values
0.4–4.5
0–0.7 glucose added
0–15 ATP added

Background
Autohemolysis is determined by measuring the amount of spontaneous hemolysis that will occur in blood over a 24- to 48-hour period under special laboratory conditions. Normal blood undergoes very little spontaneous hemolysis in the laboratory.

Explanation of Test
In the test, adenosine triphosphate (ATP) and glucose are added to blood that is incubated for 24 to 48 hours. The results are helpful in differentiating between hereditary spherocytosis and congenital nonspherocytic hemolytic anemia.

1. In hereditary spherocytosis there is a marked diminishing of hemolysis.
2. In congenital nonspherocytic hemolytic anemias, the hemolysis diminishes to a much lesser degree.

Heinz Bodies; Heinz–Ehrlich Body Stain
(Beutler's Method)

Normal Values
Negative in healthy individuals

Explanation of Test
These tests are ordered to detect the presence of Heinz–Ehrlich bodies in the red blood cells. Heinz bodies are granules that contain precipitated denatured hemoglobin. Their presence is usually associated with hemolytic anemias and indicates some injury to the erythrocyte due to

some type of oxidative activity that interferes with the normal functioning of hemoglobin, such as occurs in patients with glucose-6-phosphate dehydrogenase deficiency (G6PD).

G6PD is an enzyme that accounts for a small portion of glucose metabolized by erythrocytes. When red cells are exposed to an oxidative substance, greater amounts of glucose must be metabolized. A deficiency of G6PD will hamper the red cells' ability to metabolize the necessary additional glucose and will result in hemolysis of the erythrocyte and formation of Heinz bodies.

Clinical Implications
1. G6PD deficiency is indicated if more than 40% of the cells have five or more Heinz bodies. Affected individuals are often of Dutch, German, or French ancestry.
2. Heinz bodies are also found in splenectomized patients who had unstable hemoglobin syndromes or thalassemia prior to surgery.
3. Heinz bodies are associated with acute hemolytic crisis and may be associated with methemoglobinemia.
4. Drugs related to hemolytic anemias
   (a) In hemolytic anemias caused by drug poisoning, 50% to 75% of the erythrocytes may contain Heinz bodies.
   (b) Drugs that have an oxidating activity interfere with the normal functioning of hemoglobin in some individuals.
   (c) Drugs that cause this effect include
      (1) Those used in treatment of malaria
      (2) Sulfonamides
      (3) Antipyretics and analgesics
      (4) Nitrofurans such as Furadantin and Furacin
      (5) Phenolhydrazine
      (6) Tolbutamide
      (7) Large doses of vitamin K

RED CELL ENZYME TESTS

Glutathione Reductase (GR)

Normal Levels
9–13 U./g. of hemoglobin

Explanation of Test
This is one of the red cell enzyme screening tests done to detect the cause of congenital nonspherocytic anemia. A few instances of mild hemolytic anemia have been reported in patients with genetic deficiency in erythrocyte levels of GR. Some have been instances of chronic hemolysis and others have been drug induced (*e.g.*, with primaquine).

Procedure

A venous blood sample of at least 3 ml. is obtained. EDTA is added.

Clinical Implications

A *deficiency* of glutathione reductase is associated with

(a) Congenital nonspherocytic hemolytic anemia exhibiting either X-chromosome-linked or autosomal-recessive modes of inheritance
(b) Panocytopenia
(c) Thrombocytopenia
(d) Hypoplastic anemia
(e) Oligophrenia
(f) Gaucher's disease
(g) Alpha-thalassemia

Glucose-6-Phosphate Dehydrogenase (G6PD)

Normal Values

Quantitative: 8.6–18.6 U./g. hemoglobin
Screen: G6PD activity within normal limits; G6PD activity deficient

Explanation of Test

This is one of the tests used to diagnose hereditary enzyme-deficient hemolytic anemia. Hemolytic disease has been associated with deficiencies of nearly 20 erythrocytic enzymes. The most commonly encountered is a deficiency of glucose-6-phosphate dehydrogenase (G6PD). There are more than 50 variants of this sex-linked (X chromosome) condition.

Procedure

A venous blood sample of at least 5 ml. is obtained. EDTA is added. A precise assay of G6PD activity of hemolysate involves measuring the rate at which NADP is reduced in the presence of glucose-6-phosphate.

Clinical Implications

1. A *decreased level* is associated with G6PD deficiency, which is a sex-linked disorder. Affected males inherit the abnormal gene from their mothers who are almost always asymptomatic carriers. In some cases of this disorder there is lifelong hemolysis, but more commonly the condition is asymptomatic and results only in susceptibility to acute hemolytic episodes that may be triggered by drugs such as primaquine, sulfonamides, and antipyretics, by ingestion of fava beans, or by viral or bacterial infection.
2. The major types of G6PD deficiency are
   (a) Type A, found in blacks
   (b) Mediterranean type, found in both Caucasians and Orientals such as Greeks, Sardinians, and Sephardic Jews

(c) Rare, congenital nonspherocytic anemia
(d) Nonimmunologic hemolytic disease of the newborn
3. G6PD levels are *increased* in

(a) Pernicious anemia
(b) Werlhof's disease
(c) Hepatic coma
(d) Hyperthyroidism

(e) Myocardial infarction
(f) Chronic blood loss
(g) Other megaloblastic anemias

Pyruvate Kinase (PK)

Normal Values
2.0–8.8 U./g. hemoglobin

Explanation of Test
This is one of the red cell enzyme tests done to determine the cause of hemolytic anemia. Persons with hemolytic anemia due to pyruvate kinase deficiency have no distinguishing clinical features. PK deficiency is the most frequent and important form of hemolytic anemia due to deficiency of glycolytic enzymes in the erythrocyte.

Procedure
A venous blood sample of at least 2 ml. is obtained, to which EDTA is added. The enzyme activity can be assayed by measuring the ability of hemolysate to form pyruvate from ADP and phosphoenolpyruvate.

Clinical Implications
Pyruvate deficiency may be associated with

1. Congenital inherited nonspherocytic hemolytic anemia with icterus and splenomegaly. These persons will be homozygously affected. The parents of affected patients will be heterozygotes.
2. Acquired type is due to
   (a) Drug ingestion
   (b) Metabolic liver disease

2,3-Diphosphoglycerate (2,3-DPG)

Normal Values
Men: 4.2–5.4 μmol./ml. of packed cells
        9.2–17.4 μmol./ml. of hemoglobin
Women: 4.5–6.1 μmol./ml. of packed cells
        8.4–18.8 μmol./g. of hemoglobin

Explanation of Test

This measurement is used in the investigation of anemia. An increase in 2,3-DPG decreases oxygen binding capacity of hemoglobin so that increased amounts of oxygen are released and become available to tissues at lower oxygen tensions. The oxygen affinity of red cells is inversely proportional to 2,3-DPG concentration.

Procedure

A venous blood sample of at least 3 ml. is obtained.

Clinical Implications

1. *Increased levels* are associated with
   (a) Hypoxia, as in cardiac disease, anemia, and lung disease
   (b) Thyrotoxicosis
   (c) Pyruvate kinase deficiency
   (d) Uremia
2. *Decreased values* are associated with acidosis.

Interfering Factors

1. Increase in value occurs in high altitudes.
2. Decrease in value occurs in stored blood-bank blood.

Erythrocyte Sedimentation Rate (ESR)

Normal Values

Method	Values		
Westergren	Men	0–15 mm./hr.	
	Women	0–20 mm./hr.	
	Children	0–10 mm./hr.	
Cutler	Men	0–8 mm./hr.	
	Women	0–10 mm./hr.	
	Children	4–13 mm./hr.	
Wintrobe	Men	0–9 mm./hr.	
	Women	0–15 mm./hr.	
	Children	0–13 mm./hr.	
Smith	Adults	0–10 mm./hr.	

Explanation of Test

Erythrocyte sedimentation rate (ESR) is the rate at which erythrocytes settle out of unclotted blood in one hour. This test is based on the fact that inflammatory and necrotic processes cause an alteration in blood proteins, resulting in an aggregation of red cells, which make them heavier and more likely to fall rapidly when placed in a special vertical test tube. The faster the sedimentation rate or settling of cells, the higher the ESR. (As indicated in the listing above, the range of normal values will differ depending on the method or type of tube used.)

Sedimentation is due to the surface changes of the erythrocytes that cause them to clump or aggregate together in a column-like manner (rouleau formation). These changes are related to alterations in the plasma, particularly in the physical state of the plasma proteins.

This test is useful in diagnosing occult disease, in differential diagnosis, and in following individual cases. It is most often used as a gauge for determining the progress of an inflammatory disease, rheumatic fever, rheumatoid arthritis, respiratory infections, and acute myocardial infarction. It is a nonspecific test (not considered diagnostic for any particular disorder).

In many diseases the ESR rate is normal; in a variety of disease states the rate is rapid, and in some cases it is proportional to the severity of the disease. An abnormal rate indicates a pathologic state rather than a functional disturbance.

Procedure

An anticoagulated venous sample of 7 ml. is suctioned into a graduated capillary tube and allowed to settle for 1 hour. The amount of settling is the patient's ESR.

Clinical Implications

A. *Increased values found in*
   1. All of the collagen diseases
   2. Infections
   3. Inflammatory diseases
   4. Carcinoma
   5. Acute heavy metallic poisoning
   6. Cell or tissue destruction
   7. Toxemia
   8. Syphilis
   9. Nephritis
   10. Pneumonia
   11. Severe anemia
   12. Rheumatoid arthritis
B. *Decreased values* found in
   1. Polycythemia vera
   2. Sickle cell anemia
   3. Congestive heart failure
   4. Hypofibrinogenemia due to any cause
C. *Varied values* found in
   1. Acute disease—The change in rate may lag behind the temperature elevation and leukocytosis for 6 to 24 hours, reaching a peak after several days.

2. Convalescence—The increased rate tends to persist longer than the temperature or the leukocytosis.
3. Unruptured acute appendicitis—Even when suppurative or gangrenous, the rate is normal, but if abscess or peritonitis develops, the rate increases rapidly.
4. Musculoskeletal conditions
    (a) In rheumatic, gonorrheal, and acute gouty arthritis, the rate is significantly increased.
    (b) In osteoarthritis the rate is slightly increased.
    (c) In neuritis, myositis, and lumbago, the rate is within normal range.
5. Cardiovascular conditions
    (a) In myocardial infarction the ESR is increased.
    (b) In angina pectoris the rate is not increased.
6. Malignant diseases
    (a) In multiple myeloma, lymphoma, and metastatic cancer, the rate is very high
    (b) However, there is little correlation between the degree of elevation of the ESR and the prognosis in any one case.

Interfering Factors
1. The blood sample should not be allowed to stand more than 2 hours before the test is started because the rate will increase.
2. In refrigerated blood the sedimentation rate is greatly increased. Refrigerated blood should be allowed to return to room temperature before the test is performed.
3. Factors leading to increased rate
    (a) The presence of fibrinogen, globulins, and cholesterol
    (b) Pregnancy after 12 weeks until about the fourth week postpartum
    (c) Young children
    (d) Menstruation
    (e) Certain drugs
4. Factors leading to reduced rates
    (a) High blood sugar
    (b) High albumin level
    (c) High phospholipids
    (d) Decreased fibrinogen level in the blood in newborns
    (e) Certain drugs

TESTS FOR HEMOGLOBIN DISORDERS

Normal Values
Hemoglobin A: >95% or 0.95
Hemoglobin A_2: 2.5%–4.0% or 0.025–0.040

Hemoglobin F: <2% or 0.020
No abnormal variants

Hemoglobin Electrophoresis
Normal and abnormal hemoglobins can be detected by electrophoresis, which matches hemolyzed red cell material against standard bands for the various hemoglobins known.

There are many different types of hemoglobin that result from variations in the amino acid structure of the globin portion of the hemoglobin. The most common form of normal hemoglobin found in the adult is hemoglobin A_1. Two other normal hemoglobins found only in trace amounts in the adult are A_2 and F (fetal hemoglobin).

Of the various types of abnormal hemoglobin (hemoglobinopathies), the best known are hemoglobin S, which is responsible for sickle cell anemia, and hemoglobin C, which may result in a mild hemolytic anemia. The most common abnormality is a significant increase in hemoglobin A_2, diagnostic of α-thalassemia minor. The α-thalassemia trait is in and of itself a harmless condition. A large number of variants (more than 350) of hemoglobin have been recognized. They are identified by capital letters such as HbA or G-Philadelphia.

Interfering Factors
The results may be questionable if a blood transfusion has been given in the preceding 4 months.

Fetal Hemoglobin (Hemoglobin F) (Hb F)
(Alkali-Resistant Hemoglobin)

Normal Values
Adults: 0%–2% or 0–0.020
Newborns: 60%–90% or 0.60–0.90
Before age 2: 0%–4% or 0–0.040

Explanation of Test
Fetal hemoglobin, also called hemoglobin F, is a normal hemoglobin that is manufactured in the red blood cells of the fetus and infant and composes 50% to 90% of the hemoglobin in the newborn. The remaining portion of the hemoglobin in the newborn is made up of hemoglobin A_1 and A_2, the adult types.

In laboratory testing, hemoglobin F is the only hemoglobin known to be alkali-resistant. Adult hemoglobin does not resist alkali denaturation when analyzed in the laboratory.

Under normal conditions, the manufacture of fetal hemoglobin is replaced by the manufacture of adult hemoglobin during the first year of life. But if hemoglobin F persists and comprises more than 5% of the hemoglobin after 6 months of age, an abnormality should be expected, especially thalassemia. Therefore, determination of hemoglobin F is useful in the diagnosis of thalassemia, an inherited abnormality in the manufacture of hemoglobin, characterized by microcytic, hypochromic anemia.

Procedure
A venous blood EDTA sample of 7 ml. is used in determining a patient's hemoglobin type(s). Since the different hemoglobins differ in molecular configuration, they are separated by applying a sample on a cellulose acetate support medium and passing current through this system for a given time. Because of their different molecular configurations, different hemoglobins migrate at different rates.

Clinical Implications
Increased values found in

1. Thalassemia
2. Hereditary familial fetal hemoglobinemia
3. Spherocytic anemia
4. Sickle cell anemia
5. Hemoglobin H disease
6. Anemia, as a compensatory mechanism
7. Leakage of fetal blood into the maternal blood stream
8. Aplastic anemia
9. Acute leukemia
10. Myeloproliferative disorders

In *thalassemia minor*, continued production of fetal hemoglobin may occur on a minor scale with values of 5% to 10%. In *thalassemia major*, the values may reach 40% to 90%. This continued production of hemoglobin F leads to a severe anemia. In thalassemia minor, the patient usually lives; in thalassemia major, death usually occurs.

Interfering Factors
If analysis of specimen is delayed for more than 2 to 3 hours, the specimen may falsely appear to have higher quantities of hemoglobin F.

Hemoglobin S (Sickle Cell Test) (Sickledex)

Normal Values
Adult: 0

Background
Sickle cell anemia is caused by an abnormal form of hemoglobin, known as *hemoglobin S*. In this condition, hemoglobin becomes more

viscous and tends to precipitate or bond in such a way as to cause the red cells to sickle in shape. The abnormally shaped cells are unable to pass freely through the capillary system, resulting in increased viscosity of the blood and sluggish circulation. This can cause a backup of cells in the capillary system, resulting in a stoppage of blood supply to certain organs.

Sickle cell disorder is genetically transmitted by a recessive gene. When two such genes are present, sickle cell anemia results.

Explanation of Test
This blood measurement is routinely done as a screening test for sickle cell disorder (anemia/trait) or to confirm these disorders. The purpose of the test is to detect the presence of hemoglobin S, an inherited, recessive gene. An examination is made of the erythrocytes for the sickle-shaped forms characteristic of sickle cell anemia or trait. This is done in the laboratory by removing oxygen from the erythrocyte. In erythrocytes with normal hemoglobin the shape is retained, but erythrocytes containing hemoglobin S will assume a sickle shape. However, the distinction between sickle cell trait and sickle cell disease is done by electrophoresis, which identifies a hemoglobin pattern.

Clinical Implications
Positive test
1. Means that great numbers of erythrocytes have assumed the typical sickle-cell (crescent) shape.
2. Positive tests are 99% accurate.
A. *Sickle cell trait*
1. As an example, definite confirmation of sickle cell trait in a given person by hemoglobin electrophoresis reveals the following A/S heterozygous pattern:
   Hgb S 20%–40%
   Hgb A$_1$ 60%–80%
   Hgb F small amount
2. This means that the patient has inherited a normal Hgb A gene from one parent and an Hgb S gene from the other.
3. This patient does not have any clinical manifestations of the disease, but some of the children of this patient may inherit the disease if the person's mate has the same recessive gene pattern.
4. The diagnosis of sickle cell trait does not affect longevity and is not accompanied by signs and symptoms of sickle cell anemia.
B. *Sickle cell anemia*
1. Definite confirmation of sickle cell anemia by hemoglobin electrophoresis reveals the following S/S homozygous pattern:
   Hgb S 80%–100%
   Hgb F makes up the rest
   Hgb A 0%

2. This means that an abnormal S gene has been inherited from both parents.
3. Such a patient has all the clinical manifestations of the disease.

Interfering Factors
1. False negatives occur in
   (a) Infants before 3 months
   (b) Polycythemia
   (c) Protein abnormalities
2. False positives occur up to 4 months after transfusions with RBCs having sickle cell trait.

Clinical Alert
1. A positive Sickledex test must be confirmed by electrophoresis
2. A positive diagnosis of this disorder has genetic implications.
3. A person with sickle cell disease should avoid situations in which hypoxia may occur such as
   (a) Traveling to high-altitude regions
   (b) Traveling in an unpressurized aircraft
   (c) Performing very strenuous exercise
4. Because of general anesthetics and the state of shock-creating hypoxia, surgical or maternity patients with sickle cell disease need very close observation.

Methemoglobin (Hgb M); Sulfhemoglobin; Carboxyhemoglobin

Background
While abnormalities in the globin portion of the hemoglobin are responsible for hemoglobinopathies such as sickle cell anemia, the ability of the heme portion of hemoglobin to combine with elements other than oxygen can lead to such complexes as methemoglobin, sulfhemoglobin, and carboxyhemoglobin.

Methemoglobin

Normal Values
2% of total hemoglobin or 0.020
0.06–0.24 g./dl. or 9.3–37.2 μmol/liter

Explanation of Test

This test is used to diagnose hereditary or acquired methemoglobinemia (Hgb M), with the suspected patient having symptoms of anoxia or cyanosis without evidence of cardiovascular or pulmonary disease.

Methemoglobin is formed when the iron in the heme portion of deoxygenated hemoglobin is oxidized to a ferric form rather than a ferrous form. In the ferric form, oxygen and iron cannot combine. The formation of methemoglobin is a normal process and is kept within bounds by the reduction of methemoglobin to hemoglobin. Methemoglobin causes a shift to the left of the oxyhemoglobin dissociation curve.

When a high concentration of methemoglobin is produced in the erythrocytes, it reduces the capacity of the red blood cells to combine with oxygen. Thus, anoxia and cyanosis result. When these symptoms appear without evidence of cardiovascular or pulmonary disease, the erythrocytes are examined in an effort to diagnose methemoglobinemia that may be either hereditary or acquired.

Clinical Implications

A. *Hereditary methemoglobinemia*
   1. The Hgb M content may be as high as 40% of the total hemoglobin structure.
   2. Associated with polycythemia (but not with hemolytic anemia)
   3. Possible family history
   4. Treatment includes intravenous methylene blue and oral ascorbic acid.
B. *Acquired methemoglobinemia*
   1. Associated with
      (a) Black water fever
      (b) Paroxysmal hemoglobinuria
      (c) Clostridia infection
      (d) Ingestion of colored wax crayons or chalk
      (e) Exposure to excessive radiation
   2. Most common cause is toxic effect of drugs or chemicals

(a) Aniline dyes and derivatives	(e) Phenacetin
(b) Sulfonamides	(f) Chlorates
(c) Nitrates and nitrites	(g) Benzocaine
(d) Acetanilid	(h) Lidocaine

   3. Exposure to these agents is not always obvious.
      (a) May result from eating Polish sausage and spinach, which are rich in nitrite and nitrate
      (b) Nitrate may also be absorbed from silver nitrate used to treat extensive burns.

(c) Excessive intake of Bromo-Seltzer is a common cause of methemoglobinemia. (The patient appears cyanotic, but otherwise feels well.)

Clinical Alert

Because fetal hemoglobin is more easily converted to methemoglobin than adult hemoglobin, infants are more susceptible than adults to methemoglobinemia, caused by drinking well water containing nitrites. Bismuth preparations for diarrhea may also be reduced to nitrites by bowel action.

Sulfhemoglobin

Normal Values
Very small amount

Background
Sulfhemoglobin is an abnormal hemoglobin pigment produced by the combination of inorganic sulfides with hemoglobin.

Clinical Implications
1. Once sulfhemoglobin is formed, it remains stable and is irreversible, disappearing with the red blood cells after completion of the 120-day life span of the erythrocyte.
2. Sulfhemoglobin is observed in patients who take oxidant drugs such as phenacetin (excessive intake of Bromo-Seltzer).

Carboxyhemoglobin; Carbon Monoxide

Normal Values
0%–2.3% of total hemoglobin or 0–0.023
In heavy smokers: 4%–5% or 0.04–0.05

Background
Carboxyhemoglobin is formed when hemoglobin is exposed to carbon monoxide. The affinity of hemoglobin for carbon monoxide is 218 times greater than for oxygen. Carbon monoxide poisoning causes anoxia because the carboxyhemoglobin formed does not permit hemoglobin to combine with oxygen, and that which does bind is not readily released to the tissues.

Clinical Implications
1. Since carboxyhemoglobin is not capable of transporting oxygen, hypoxia results. A toxic level is greater than 20%.
2. Death may result from anoxia and irreversible tissue changes.

3. Carboxyhemoglobin produces a cherry red or violet color of the blood and skin.
4. The most common cause of carbon monoxide toxicity is automobile exhaust fumes, although smoking is a minor cause.
5. Sixty percent saturation with carbon monoxide is usually fatal.

Clinical Alert

1. With values of 10%–20%, the person may be asymptomatic.
2. 20%–30%—headache, nausea, vomiting, loss of judgment
3. 30%–40%—tachycardia, hyperpnea, hypotension, confusion
4. 50%–60%—loss of consciousness
5. 60%—convulsion, respiratory arrest, death

Myoglobin (Mb)

Normal Values
Blood: 30–90 ng./ml. or nmol./liter

Background
Myoglobin is the oxygen-binding protein of striated muscle. It resembles hemoglobin, but it is unable to release oxygen except at extremely low tension. Injury to skeletal muscle will result in release of myoglobin.

Explanation of Test
Blood tests that measure myoglobin are used as an index of damage in myocardial infarction and to detect muscle injury or prediction of disease exacerbation in polymyositis.

Procedure
A venous blood sample of at least 5 ml. is obtained.

Clinical Implications
A. *Increased blood values* are associated with
   1. Myocardial infarction   3. Polymyositis
   2. Other muscle injury

Haptoglobin (Hp)

Normal Values
83–267 mg./dl. or 0.83–2.67 g./liter

Background
Haptoglobin, a transport glycoprotein synthesized solely in the liver, is structurally similar to hemoglobin. It is the first line of defense for the preservation of iron (located in the heme portion of hemoglobin) in the human body.

Explanation of Test
Measurement of haptoglobin is used primarily as a confirmatory test for the presence of increased intravascular hemolysis. Haptoglobin will increase in any condition that causes tissue damage or repair such as infections and cancer. In this way, it correlates very well with the findings of erythrocyte sedimentation rate. On the other hand, a decrease in haptoglobin in most persons with normal liver function is most likely due to an increased consumption. This means that any disease state that can cause an increased in intravascular hemolysis will most likely cause a decrease in haptoglobin. The concentration of haptoglobin is inversely related to the degree of hemolysis as well as the length of time of the hemolytic episode.

Procedure
A venous blood sample of at least 2 ml. is obtained, centrifuged, and the serum assayed for haptoglobin by a radial immunodiffusion methodology. A single determination is of limited value.

Clinical Implications
1. *Levels are decreased in acquired disorders* such as
   - (a) Transfusion reactions
   - (b) Erythroblastosis fetalis
   - (c) Systemic lupus erythematosus
   - (d) Autoimmune hemolytic anemia
   - (e) Prosthetic heart valves
   - (f) Malarial infestation
   - (g) PNH
   - (h) Hepatocellular disease
   - (i) Thrombotic thrombocytopenic purpura
   - (j) Drug-induced hemolytic anemia (methyldopa)
   - (k) Uremia
   - (l) Hypertension
2. *Levels are also decreased in some inherited disorders* such as
   - (a) Sickle cell disease
   - (b) G6PD deficiency
   - (c) Hereditary spherocytosis
   - (d) Thalassemia and related disorders
   - (e) Hp O-O found in adult blacks
3. *Levels are increased* in
   - (a) Infection (acute and chronic)
   - (b) Neoplasia
   - (c) Biliary obstruction
   - (d) Nephritis
   - (e) Granulomatous disease
   - (f) Adrenal steroid therapy
   - (g) Ulcerative colitis
   - (h) Peptic ulcer
   - (i) Arterial disease
   - (j) Acute rheumatic disease
   - (k) Myocardial infarction (after)

Hemoglobin Bart's

Normal Values
None in children and adults; 0–trace in newborns

Explanation of Test
This test is done to determine the percent of Bart's abnormal hemoglobin in cord blood and to identify α-thalassemia hemoglobinopathies. Bart's is an unstable hemoglobin with high oxygen affinity.

Procedure
A sample of cord blood is obtained, and a hemoglobin electrophoresis is performed.

Clinical Implications
Increased levels are associated with stillborn infants with homozygous α-thalassemia.

Paroxysmal Nocturnal Hemoglobinuria (PNH)
(Screening Acid Serum Test, Presumptive Acid Serum Test, Ham Test–Acidified Serum Lysis Test)

Normal Values
Negative

Background
PNH is a rather uncommon disease characterized by the intermittent appearance of hemoglobin in the urine that is more marked during and after sleep. The actual cause of the disease is unknown. It is known that the red cells appear to be sensitive to the increase of carbon dioxide that occurs during sleep, which lowers the pH of the plasma. The plasma is darker in the morning than during the rest of the day because of hemolysis.

Explanation of Tests
These tests are carried out to make a definitive diagnosis of paroxysmal nocturnal hemoglobinuria (PNH). The basis of these tests is that the cells peculiar to PNH have membrane defects, making them extra sensitive to complement in the plasma. Under certain conditions in the laboratory, osmotic lysis of the cells is demonstrated by activating the serum complement by slightly acidifying the serum (Ham's test) or by means of an osmotic solution of sucrose. Cells from patients with PNH will undergo marked hemolysis after 15 minutes in the laboratory test.

Procedure
1. A venous blood sample of 20 ml. is obtained.
2. The patient's red cells are mixed with normal serum and also with

the patient's own serum, acidified, incubated at 37°C, and examined for hemolysis. Normally, there should be no lysis of the red cells in this test.

Clinical Implications
1. These tests are almost never positive in any other disease than PNH and are seldom negative in patients with PNH.
2. The tests are performed on patients who have hemoglobinuria, bone marrow aplasia (hypoplasia), or undiagnosed hemolytic anemias.

Interfering Factors
False-positive results may be obtained when blood contains large numbers of spherocytes.

TESTS OF OTHER BLOOD COMPONENTS
Vitamin B$_{12}$ (VB$_{12}$)

Normal Values
VB$_{12}$: 160–1300 pg./ml. or 118–959 pmol./liter
VB$_{12}$ (unsaturated binding capacity): 1000–2000 pg./ml.

Background
Vitamin B$_{12}$, also known as the antipernicious anemia factor, is necessary for the production of red blood cells. In man it is obtained only from ingesting animal protein and requires an intrinsic factor for absorption. Both vitamin B$_{12}$ and folic acid are dependent on a normally functioning intestinal mucosa for their absorption and are important in the normal adult for the production of red blood cells. Levels of vitamin B$_{12}$ and folate are usually tested in conjunction with one another because the diagnosis of macrocytic anemia requires measurement of both B$_{12}$ and folate.

Transcobalamin is the B$_{12}$ carrier in the blood. Usually, it is only about one-fourth saturated with the vitamin. The importance of transcobalamin II was confirmed in two siblings who rapidly developed severe megaloblastic anemia in association with a congenital absence of this protein.

Explanation of the Test
This determination is helpful in the differential diagnosis of anemia and conditions marked by high turnover of myeloid cells, as in the leukemias. When binding capacity is measured, it is the unsaturated fraction that is determined. The measurement of unsaturated vitamin B$_{12}$ binding capacity (UBBC) is valuable in distinguishing between untreated polycythemia vera and other conditions in which there is an elevated hematocrit.

Procedure
1. A fasting venous blood sample of at least 5 ml. is obtained.
2. The specimen must be obtained before an injection of vitamin B_{12} is administered.

Clinical Implications
1. *Decreased levels* of less than 100 pg./ml. of vitamin B_{12} are associated with
   (a) Pernicious anemia
   (b) Malabsorption syndromes
   (c) Fish tapeworm infestation
   (d) Primary hypothyroidism
   (e) Loss of gastric mucosa as in gastrectomy and stomach cancer
2. Decreased unsaturated binding capacity is associated with hepatic cirrhosis and hepatitis.
3. *Increased levels* of greater than 1100 pg./ml. of vitamin B_{12} are associated with
   (a) Chronic granulocytic leukemia
   (b) Myelomonocytic leukemia
   (c) Other myeloproliferative diseases such as polycythemia vera
   (d) Liver disease
   (e) Some cases of cancer, especially with liver metastasis
4. Unsaturated binding capacity is also increased in polycythemia vera.

Interfering Factors
Increased values are associated with pregnancy and oral contraceptives.

Patient Preparation
1. Explain purpose and procedure of test.
2. Advise that overnight fasting from food is necessary. Water is permitted.

Clinical Alert

This test is contraindicated in persons who have recently received therapeutic or diagnostic doses of radionuclides.

Folic Acid (Folate)

Normal Values
3.0–2.5 ng./ml. or nmol./liter

Folic acid is needed for the normal function of red and white blood cells and is required for the production of cellular genes. Folic acid is a more potent growth promoter than vitamin B_{12}, although both are dependent on the normal functioning of intestinal mucosa for their absorption. Although fulfilling a different requirement, folic acid, like B_{12}, is required for DNA production. Folic acid is formed by bacteria in the intestines, is stored in the liver, and is present in foods such as eggs, milk, leafy vegetables, yeast, liver, fruits, and other elements of a well-balanced diet.

Explanation of Test

This test is indicated in the differential diagnosis of a hemolytic disorder and in the investigation of folic acid deficiency in altered use. When folic acid absorption is blocked, the liver and body stores of folic acid are depleted, and blood cell production and maturation are affected. If folic acid is deficient, large red cells are produced with shortened life span and impaired oxygen-carrying capacity. Deficiency of folic acid also causes white abnormalities related to altered DNA or RNA synthesis. It takes several weeks for folate deficiency to develop. The folic acid level must remain at a decreased level for 20 weeks or more before anemia develops. The test is usually done in conjunction with vitamin B_{12} levels.

Procedure

A fasting venous sample of 10 ml. is obtained. The specimen must be obtained before any injections of vitamin B_{12} are given.

Clinical Implications

1. The *major* causes of *increased* folic acid are
   (a) Inadequate intake
   (b) Malabsorption of folic acid
   (c) Excessive utilization of folic acid by the body
   (d) Drugs that are folic antagonists (interfere with nucleic acid synthesis) such as
       (1) Anticonvulsants
       (2) Aminopterin and methotrexate used in leukemia treatment
       (3) Antimalarials
       (4) Alcohol
2. *Decreased* folic acid levels are associated with
   (a) Megaloblastic anemia
   (b) Hemolytic anemia
   (c) Liver disease associated with
       (1) Alcoholism
       (2) Malabsorption syndrome
   (d) Sprue
   (e) Celiac disease

(f) Idiopathic steatorrhea
(g) Malignancies
(h) Malnutrition
(i) Drugs mentioned above
(j) Elderly persons with inadequate diets
(k) Hyperthyroidism
(l) Vitamin C deficiency
(m)Febrile states
(n) Chronic dialyses
3. Anemias due to folic acid deficiency include
(a) Megaloblastic anemia of pregnancy because of fetal requirements for folate
(b) Nutritional megaloblastic anemia by occurring in
(1) Infancy
(2) Early childhood
(3) Infections
(4) Old age
(It occurs more commonly when infections or diarrhea increase folate requirements)
(c) Macrocytic hemolytic anemia
(d) Macrocytic anemia due to liver disease associated with alcoholism

Clinical Alert

Elderly persons or those having inadequate diets in this country
are known to develop folate-deficient megaloblastic anemia.

Patient Preparation
Instruct patient about fasting from food for 8 hours before testing.
Water is permitted.

Ferritin

Normal values
Men: 15–300 mg./ml. or μg/liter
Women: 12–150 mg./ml. or μg/liter

Explanation of Test
This measurement is a good indicator of available iron stores; ferritin
is the primary iron storage compound in the body. It is useful in differentiating iron deficiency anemia from the secondary anemias of

chronic disease, such as infection or malignancy when ferritin is usually normal or elevated.

Procedure

A venous blood sample of 6 ml. is obtained.

Clinical Implications

1. Increases are associated with:
   (a) Iron overload as in hemochromatosis, hemosiderosis, and certain liver diseases.
   (b) All anemias except those secondary to blood loss or iron loss associated with hemosiderinuria.
   (c) Other disorders
       (1) Acute myeloblastic and lymphoblastic leukemia
       (2) Inflammatory diseases
       (3) Alcoholic and inflammatory liver disease
       (4) Hodgkin's disease
       (5) Breast cancer
2. Decreases are associated with iron deficiency.

Interfering Factors

1. An iron depletion state with a decreased ferritin is common during menstruation, female reproduction, and in children.
2. Idiopathic hemochromatosis and transfusion may be associated with high serum ferritin levels.

Histiocyte Smear

Normal Values

None, not normally found in circulating blood

Explanation of Test

A blood smear is examined to identify and count the number of histiocytes present. Histiocytes or reticulum cells are not blood cells but tissue cells derived from reticuloendothelial tissue. Histiocytes are not normally found in the blood but are known to circulate in the blood in certain conditions in which their macrophagic properties act specifically, as in tuberculosis, leprosy, subacute endocarditis, and lipid storage diseases. Histiocytes may be classified as monocytes in a differential leukocyte count.

Procedure

1. Usually, four blood smears are taken from a puncture site.
2. The earlobe is rubbed for 1 to 2 minutes, wiped with alcohol, and pricked with a needle.
3. Obtaining a venous blood sample is the other procedure method.

Clinical Implications
Histiocytes are found in

(a) Subacute bacterial endo-
     carditis
(b) Typhoid fever
(c) Hemolytic anemia
(d) Hodgkin's disease
(e) Reticulum cell sarcoma
(f) Severe diarrhea in children

(g) Tuberculosis
(h) Leprosy
(i) Fat storage disease
(j) Lymphoma
(k) Some parasitic diseases
(l) Histiocytic leukemia

Sudan Black B Stain (SBB) for Phospholipids

Normal Values
Lymphocytes will not stain with this method. Granulocytic cells will
stain with this method. Normal blood is used as a control.

Explanation of Test
This technique is used in the diagnosis of leukemia. The Sudan B Stain
is useful in differentiating acute granulocytic leukemia from acute lymphocytic leukemia. Lymphocytes and lymphoblasts (immature lymphocytes) do not stain with SBB and are said to be sudanophobic. Cells
of the granulocytic and monocytic series contain granules that take the
stain and are said to be sudanophilic.

Sudan Black B also stains a wide variety of lipids including neutral
fats, phospholipids, and steroids.

Procedure
A bone marrow aspirate must be taken and a slide prepared from bone
marrow. Aspirate is stained with Sudan Black stain and scanned under
a microscope.

Clinical Implications
1. Positive staining of primitive cells indicates myelogenous origin of
   cells.
2. The test is SBB positive in acute granulocytic leukemia.
3. The test is SBB negative in acute lymphocytic leukemia.

Periodic Acid–Schiff Stain (PAS)

Normal Values
Granulocytes stain PAS positive
Agranulocytes stain PAS negative

Explanation of Test
This staining technique is used to identify reactions to amyloid, a glycoprotein, and to classify immature cells of the blood and bone marrow.

The PAS reaction for glycogen is one of the histological methods that are helpful in the diagnosis of amyloid diseases such as acute lymphocytic leukemia and erythroleukemia. Amyloidosis is a disease process of unknown cause, characterized by waxy deposits in the liver, kidney, spleen, heart, skin, and alimentary tract. This staining technique is also useful in differentiating erythemic myelosis from sideroblastic anemia.

Methods used other than PAS are metachromatic methyl and crystal violet, thioflavine T, and Congo red.

Procedure
A bone marrow aspirate must be taken and a slide prepared, stained with PAS stain, and scanned under the microscope.

Clinical Implications
1. The test is *positive* in
   (a) Acute lymphocytic leukemia
   (b) Erythroleukemia
   (c) Severe iron-deficiency anemia
   (d) Thalassemia
   (e) Amyloidosis
   (f) Strongly positive lymphocytes in the circulatory blood suggest malignant lymphomas
2. Blast cells that stain Schiff positive are
   (a) Erythroblasts of erythroleukemia
   (b) Thalassemia sideroblastic anemia
   (c) Mucin
   (d) Hyaline
   (e) Basement membranes
   (f) Fungus
   (g) Amyloid
   (h) Glycogen
   (i) Gaucher's cells
   (j) Megakaryocytes

Interfering Factors
Results of test reflect the adeptness and skill of the laboratory technician.

Leukocyte Alkaline Phosphatase Stain (LAP); Alkaline Phosphatase Stain

Normal Values
30–130 units of precipitated dye/neutrophil (each laboratory establishes its own range)

Explanation of Test

This test is usually ordered to differentiate granulocytic leukemia from leukemoid or myeloid reactions. The enzyme, alkaline phosphatase, is present in leukocytes; enzyme activity is represented by granulation in the cytoplasm of neutrophilic granulocytes. High concentrations of this enzyme will be found in normal white blood cells and low to negative concentrations in leukemic leukocytes.

Procedure

A venous blood sample or peripheral finger stick is obtained and a blood smear is prepared. The blood smear is fixed in cold formalin–methanol, then the smears are placed in an incubating solution. At this point, the alkaline phosphatase present in the white cells liberates naphthol, which couples with fast blue RR to form an insoluble brown black compound. The smear is then counterstained. The degree of reactivity is determined by scoring each neutrophil according to the amount of precipitated dye present.

Interfering Factors

Value is normally increased in pregnancy.

Clinical Implications

1. In chronic granulocytic anemia, the range is from 0 to 13, meaning that none or little alkaline phosphatase activity is demonstrable.
2. *Values below normal* may be found in
   (a) Acute and chronic granulocytic leukemia
   (b) Paroxysmal nocturnal hemoglobinuria
   (c) Aplastic anemia
   (d) Infectious mononucleosis
   (e) Hereditary hypophosphatasia
   (f) Many infections
   (g) Idiopathic thrombocytopenia purpura
   (h) Sarcoidosis (occasional)
   (i) Granulocytopenia (occasional)
3. *Values above normal* may be found in
   (a) Neutrophilic leukemoid reactions. (A leukemoid reaction is a blood picture that looks like leukemia but is not.)
   (b) Polycythemia vera
   (c) Thrombocytopenia infection
   (d) Myelofibrosis

Buffy Coat Smear and Acid Phosphatase Tartrate Inhibitor

Normal Values
Atypical mononuclear cells
Megakaryocytes
Metamyelocytes and myelocytes
Normal white cell components

The buffy coat of the blood of healthy people contains these cells.

Explanation of Test
This diagnostic smear of the leukocytes is most commonly done on leukemic and cancer patients with metastatic relapse to the bone marrow. The purpose is to search for either cells or tumor cells. This is not a test *per se*. A buffy coat smear is indicated when the number of white cells is very low and is done to concentrate the white cells. The detection of tartrate-resistant acid phosphatase in the lymphoid cells of leukemic reticuloendotheliosis can be helpful in its differentiation from chronic lymphocytic leukemia, lymphosarcoma cell leukemia, and lymphomas.

Procedure
A venous blood sample of 5 ml. is obtained, and a finger stick may also be done.

Clinical Implications
1. Abnormal cells such as tumor cells and LE cells are an indication of
   (a) Leukemia
   (b) Cancer metastatic to the bone
   (c) Lupus erythematosus (The LE prep is one example of the use of buffy coat smears.)
2. Hairy cell leukemia or leukemic reticuloendotheliosis (Tartrate-resistant acid phosphatase cells are indicative of this.)

Erythropoietic Porphyrins; Erythrocyte Total

Normal Value
30 mg./dl. red cells

Background
The porphyrins of red blood cells are, in most cases, protoporphyrin and uroporphyrin.

Explanation of Test
This determination is useful in identifying metabolic disorders of the red blood cells and in detecting and differentiating the porphyrins

along with tests that measure increased porphyrin excretion in urine and feces. Porphyrin disorders, which may be either genetically determined or acquired, result from metabolic defects in heme biosynthesis. Porphyrin disorders are separated into erythropoietic and hepatic types according to the site of the biochemical and pathologic lesion.

Procedure
A venous blood sample is obtained. Washed red blood cells from this specimen are examined.

Clinical Implications
Increased erythrocyte protoporphyrin is associated with
1. Protoporphyria
2. Intoxication porphyria that can be caused by heavy metals, halogenated solvents, and many drugs

Serum Viscosity

Normal Values
1.10–1.22 centipoise

Background
As a flowing liquid, blood is considered a suspension of particles (erythrocytes, leukocytes, and platelets) in plasma. Viscosity is affected by the hematocrit, size of red blood cells, and protein composition of plasma. In macroglobulinemia, increased serum viscosity is produced by IgM molecules, which have a high molecular weight and an unusual shape that increases their intrinsic viscosity. Viscosity is further increased by the tendency of IgM molecules to aggregate.

Explanation of Test
This test is important in the diagnosis of serum hyperviscosity syndromes associated with myeloma or macroglobulinemia. Delayed diagnosis can result in a fatal outcome of a treatable disorder. Because only a few of the many manifestations may be present, this syndrome should be considered in any unexplained coma, bizarre neurological disorder, hemorrhagic sign, or retinal vein segmentation along with any other classic manifestation of hyperviscosity such as hemorrhage. Also, preoperative measurements of viscosity and volume can be used to avoid complications of surgery in all persons with identified monoclonal gammopathies.

Procedure
A venous blood sample of 10 ml. is obtained.

Clinical Implications

1. Increased serum viscosity is associated with
   (a) Hyperviscosity syndrome
   (b) Waldenström's macroglobulinemia
   (c) Multiple myeloma (usually IgA)
2. The relationship between relative viscosity of blood and hematocrit is nearly linear for hematocrit values above 40%. Above 40% the relative viscosity becomes progressively greater.
3. The relative viscosity of blood is also affected by the size of the red blood cell. At a given level of red blood cell count, microcytosis decreases and macrocytosis increases the viscosity.

Clinical Alert

Hyperviscosity syndromes are often benefited by plasmapheresis.

TESTS OF COAGULATION AND HEMOSTASIS

Introduction

A wide variety of laboratory tests are available to determine the nature and extent of coagulation disorders. These tests are generally related to the physiologic response of the body to bleeding disorders and to injury of blood vessels. Blood flows through a vascular system that is lined by endothelium. When vascular damage occurs, there is immediate reflex vasoconstriction. In large vessels, this vasoconstriction may be the main mechanism of hemostasis. In smaller vessels, vasoconstriction serves to narrow the vessel and to reduce the area that must be occluded by the hemostatic plug. The tissue injury leads to exposure of the subendothelial tissues, and it is to these tissues that the platelet adheres.

Mechanism of Hemostasis

Several mechanisms arrest bleeding: (1) the skin, subcutaneous tissue, and muscle comprise the body's first line of defense and may be considered the extravascular resistance to bleeding; (2) blood vessel walls contract to reduce the quantity of blood flowing through them and this response is the vascular resistance to bleeding; (3) platelets adhere to each other and to the damaged endothelium and initiate clotting factors, and (4) the clotting factors of the blood react by a cascading mechanism to generate thrombin and to deposit fibrin. Platelet response plus the clotting factor reactions comprise the intravascular resistance to bleeding (Table 2-3).

(*Text continues on page 82.*)

Table 2-3
The Complex Chain of Reactions Occurring in Coagulation

In the circulating blood there appears to be a balance between the factors acting to stimulate the formation of thrombin and the forces acting to delay its formation. This balance maintains blood in its fluid state. When the blood vessels are injured or when blood is removed from a vessel, the balance is upset and coagulation occurs. A number of coagulation factors have been identified that are involved in four progressive stages of clotting. The Roman numerals assigned to the coagulation factors identify their order of discovery rather than their involvement in the stages of clot formation.

Stage	Components of Stages	Clotting Factors*
		INTERNATIONAL NOMENCLATURE
Stage I (3–5 min)		Factor I = Fibrinogen
Phase I—Platelet Activity Platelets serve as a source of thromboplastin.	90% of all coagulation disorders are due to defects in Phase I. Platelet counts <1,000,000/mm.^{3} indicate moderate interference with Phase I activity.	Factor II = Prothrombin (vitamin K functions in the production of prothrombin) Factor III = Tissue thromboplastin Factor IV = Calcium ions
Phase II—Thromboplastin (Factor III, an enzyme thought to be liberated by damaged cells, is formed by six different factors plus calcium.)	Calcium Factor V Factor VIII Factor IX ⎬ are involved in this formation of tissue thromboplastin (intrinsic prothrombin Factor X activation) Factor XI Factor XII	Factor V = Platelet phospholipids & calcium ions Factor VI = This factor is no longer considered to be a distinct part of coagulation Factor VII = A coenzyme (stable factor)

Stage II (8–15 sec)
Prothrombin, Factor II, is converted to thrombin in the presence of *calcium*.

Factor II
Factor X
Factor VII
Factor V
} are involved in this conversion of fibrinogen to fibrin

Factor VIII = Antihemophilic globulin
Factor IX = Christmas factor (hemophilia)
Factor X = Stuart–Prower factor. Factor X must be activated to convert prothrombin to thrombin
Factor XI = Plasma thromboplastin antecedent (PTA)
Factor XII = Hageman factor
Factor XIII = Fibrin stabilizing factor (FSF)

Stage III (1 sec)
Thrombin interacts with fibrinogen (Factor I) to form the framework of the clot.

At the end of Stage III, Factor XIII functions in the stabilization of the clot.

Stage IV
Fibrinolytic system (antagonistic system to the clotting mechanism; check and balance system is activated)

Removal of fibrin clot through fibrinolysis. Plasminogen is converted to plasmin, which breaks clot into fibrin split products.

* Note: The 13 clotting factors of the blood are proteins. They are present in the blood plasma in an inactive form.

The entire system of coagulation and fibrinolysis (removal of fibrin clot) is kept in balance by a number of natural inhibitors. Thrombin acts as an activator of platelet aggregation but also attacks Factor V and Factor VIII, eventually limiting the coagulation process. A number of antithrombins have been identified—the most important one is probably fibrin itself, which adsorbs thrombin and removes it from the circulation. Antiplasminogen activators and antiplasmins help to control the fibrinolytic activity.

Laboratory diagnostic tests are usually effective in determining the cause of a hemorrhagic disorder. However, judged by the result of laboratory tests, patients can still appear normal and yet have a history of bleeding.

Bleeding does not necessarily indicate a hemorrhagic disorder due to defective hemostasis, nor does the absence of current bleeding rule out an existing hemorrhagic disorder. It is important to remember that the most common cause of hemorrhaging of any sort is thrombocytopenia, the deficiency of platelets. Liver disease, uremia, thrombocytopenia, and DIC disease, as well as the administration of Coumadin (warfarin sodium) and heparin, account for most of the hemorrhagic disorders seen in routine medical practice. Hemophilia is seen infrequently.

Disorders of Hemostasis

A. *Congenital vascular abnormalities*
   Defects of the blood vessel itself are poorly defined and difficult to test. Hereditary telangiectasia is the most commonly recognized. Laboratory studies are all normal so diagnosis must be made chemically.
B. *Acquired vascular abnormalities*
   1. Schönlein–Henoch purpura in allergic response to infection or drugs
   2. Vitamin C deficiency related to inadequate cementing substance between the muscular endothelial cells
   3. Senile purpura due to loss of elastic tissue
   4. Purpura associated with steroid therapy and easy bruising in females
   5. Vascular damage due to rickettsial diseases, septicemia, or amyloidosis
C. *Quantitative platelet abnormalities*
   1. Thrombocytopenia (decreased platelet count)
      (a) Decreased production
      (b) Increased use or destruction of platelets
      (c) Hypersplenism

2. Thrombocytosis (elevated platelet level—normal reactive response)
   (a) Hemorrhage
   (b) Iron-deficiency anemia
   (c) Inflammation
   (d) Splenectomy

Clinical Alert

Increased platelets can cause a tendency toward thrombosis.

---

3. Thrombocythemia (platelet counts greater than one million/mm^3)
   (a) Granulocytic leukemia
   (b) Polycythemia vera
   (c) Myeloid metaplasia

Clinical Alert

When platelets are so greatly increased, they do not function properly and can cause hemorrhage episodes.

D. *Qualitative platelet abnormalities*
   1. Glanzmann's thrombasthenia, a hereditary autosomal-recessive disorder that can produce severe bleeding, especially with trauma and surgical procedures.
   2. Platelet factor 3 differences associated with aggregation, adhesion, or release defects
      (a) Storage-pool disease
      (b) Bernard–Soulier syndrome
      (c) May–Hegglin anomaly
      (d) Wiskott–Aldrich syndrome
   3. Conditions and drugs such as
      (a) Dialysis
      (b) Aspirin and other anti-inflammatory agents, dypyridamole, and prostaglandin E
E. *Congenital coagulation abnormalities*
   1. Hemophilia A and B (deficiencies of Factors VIII and IX)
   2. Rare autosomal recessive traits such as Hemophilia C
   3. Autosomal dominant traits such as von Willebrand's disease
F. *Acquired coagulation abnormalities*
   1. Circulatory anticoagulant activity
      (a) Hemophilia

    (b) Rheumatoid arthritis
    (c) Immediate postpartum period
    (d) Systemic lupus erythematosus
    (e) Multiple myeloma
2. Vitamin D deficiency
    (a) Oral anticoagulants
    (b) Biliary obstruction and malabsorption syndrome
    (c) Intestinal sterilization by antibiotics and in newborns
3. Disseminated intravascular coagulation in which there is continuous generation of thrombin that consumes the other clotting factors and thus causes bleeding
4. Primary fibrinolysis is the isolated activation of the fibrinolytic mechanism without prior coagulation.
    (a) Streptokinase therapy
    (b) Rarely in electroshock, severe liver disease, and cancer of prostate
5. Liver disease, where the extent of coagulation abnormalities depends on the severity of the disease

Disseminated Intravascular Coagulation (DIC)

Disseminated intravascular coagulation (DIC) is a syndrome characterized by uncontrolled formation and deposition of fibrin thrombi. It is an acquired hemorrhagic disease in which there is continuous generation of thrombin that causes depletion "consumption" of the coagulation factors and thus causes bleeding. Fibrinolysis is activated in DIC, which further compounds the hemostatic defect caused by the consumption of clotting factors.

    Multiple coagulation test abnormalties found in DIC that cause uncontrolled bleeding include

Prothrombin time (PT) prolonged	Platelet count decreased
PTT or APTT prolonged	Fibrinolysin test increased
Bleeding time prolonged	Fibrin split products positive
Fibrinogen decreased	

Factor analysis abnormalities found in DIC include

Factor II, V, VIII, X decreased
Fibrinopeptide increased

    DIC is not a primary disease but, rather, a secondary condition caused by another factor. In order to treat DIC, the underlying disease must be uncovered.

The causative factors of DIC include

Septicemia
Malignancies and cancer
Obstetric emergencies (*e.g.*, abruptio placentae)
Cirrhosis of liver
Sickle cell disease
Trauma and crushing injuries
Malaria
Incompatible transfusion
Cold hemoglobinurea and paroxysmal nocturnal hemoglobinuria
Abnormal protein or collagen diseases

In acute DIC, the treatment to stop the uncontrolled bleeding is the use of heparin. Seemingly paradoxically, the heparin blocks thrombin formation, thus blocking consumption of the other clotting factors and causing bleeding to stop. The underlying condition must then be treated to arrest the DIC.

Laboratory Investigation

Generally, a set routine of coagulation studies is followed. Enough blood is collected at one time to provide the specimens needed for the various tests.

1. Usually, at least 20 ml. of blood is obtained using the two-syringe technique.
   (a) In the first syringe 5 ml. of blood is obtained, and this specimen is discarded.
   (b) In the second syringe 15 to 20 ml. of blood is obtained, and this specimen is examined.
2. Coagulation studies, also called *coagulation profiles, coag panels*, or *coagulograms,* are indicated
   (a) In screening of preoperative patients
   (b) With coagulation disorder symptoms such as
       (1) Easy or spontaneous bruising
       (2) Prolonged bleeding
       (3) Heavy or unexplained nosebleeds
       (4) Excessive menstrual flow
       (5) Family history of abnormal heavy bleeding
       (6) GI bleeding

The following sequence of tests is recommended in the investigation of a hemorrhagic disorder (see Table 2-4).

1. Tests for vascular function and platelet function
   (a) Bleeding time
   (b) Capillary fragility test or Rumpel–Leede test

(*Text continues on page 88.*)

Table 2-4
Laboratory Tests to Measure Hemostasis

Name of Test	Vascular Function	Platelet Function	Stage 1	Stage 2	Stage 3	Stage 4
Tourniquet test	x	x				
Bleeding time	x	x				
Platelet count		x				
Platelet adhesiveness		x				
Platelet aggregation		x				
Aspirin tolerance		x				
Platelet factor 3 assay		x				
Clot retraction		x				
Prothrombin consumption		x	x			
Lee–White clotting time		x	x			
Siliconized clotting time		x	x			
Activated clotting time			x			
Recalcification time		x	x			
Activated recalcification time		x	x			
Partial thromboplastin time			x			
Activated partial thromboplastin			x			
Thromboplastin generation test			x			
Hicks–Pitney test			x			

Prothrombin time—Quick			x
Thrombotest*			x
Stypven time*			x
Circulating anticoagulant factor I.D. substitution		x	x
Factor assay		x	x
Thrombin time	x	x	
Reptilase time	x	x	
Fibrinogen assay	x	x	
Factor XIII assay	x	x	
Whole blood clot lysis	x		
Dilute blood clot lysis	x		
Euglobulin lysis time	x		
Fibrin plate lysis	x		
Serial thrombin time	x	x	
Plasminogen assay	x		
Protamine sulfate	x	x	
Ethanol gelatin	x	x	
TRCH II†	x		
Staph clumping	x		
Latex agglutination for FSP	x		

* Monitors oral and coagulant therapy
† Tanned red cell hemagglutination inhibition immunoassay
These tests measure all facets of hemostasis: vascular function, platelets, and clotting factors.
(Based on table in Kennedy J: Laboratory Investigation of Hemostasis. Dade Monograph. Miami, American Hospital Supply, 1973)

2. Tests of platelet function
    (a) Platelet count   (c) Platelet aggregation studies
    (b) Bleeding time   (d) Clot retraction
3. Tests for overall clotting ability
    (a) Activated partial thromboplastin time
    (b) Fibrinogen determination
4. Tests of stage I
    (a) Activated partial thromboplastin time
    (b) Prothrombin consumption
    (c) Platelet function time tests
5. Tests of stage II
    (a) Prothrombin time
6. Tests of stage III
    (a) Fibrinogen level
    (b) Thrombin time
7. Tests of stage IV
    (a) Euglobulin lysis   (c) Partial thromboplastin time
    (b) Clot lysis test   (d) Fibrin split products
8. Tests for circulating anticoagulants

Four primary screening tests are performed in the initial laboratory
investigation of suspected coagulation disorders

1. Platelet count, size, and shape
2. Bleeding time provides information about the ability of platelets to
    perform their normal function and the ability of the capillaries to
    constrict their walls.
3. Partial thromboplastin time determines the overall ability of the
    blood to clot (PTT).
4. Prothrombin time measures the activity of second stage clotting
    factors (PT).

Other commonly ordered tests include

1. Clot retraction
2. Fibrinogen level
3. Factor assays (definitive coagulation studies of a specific factor)
    such as Factor VIII hemophilia
4. Fibrinolysis. When specific factor has been determined to be low or
    absent, a factor assay is done in some laboratories. This will give
    the specific percentage of the factor present. When the problem has
    been suspected of being in the fibrinolytic system, specific tests
    provide the most reliable and precise means of establishing an ac-
    curate diagnosis. These tests will be performed only in certain labo-
    ratories. They are

(a) Euglobulin clot lysis—identifies increased plasminogen activator activity (Plasmin is *not* usually present in the blood plasma.)
(b) Factor XIII–fibrin stabilizing factor
(c) Fibrin split products such as protamine sulfate test

Clinical Alert

1. All patients who are known to have hemorrhagic or bleeding tendencies, or who are being examined through coagulation studies, should be observed closely, and a careful drug history and family history of bleeding should be obtained.
2. If multiple vials are being drawn, samples for coagulation studies should be drawn last.

Assessment of Patient

1. Examine skin for bruising on extremities and other parts of the body that patient cannot easily see.
2. Record the appearance of petechiae that may occur after a blood pressure reading or application of tourniquet for venipuncture. These may be the first indication of a bleeding tendency.
3. Note bleeding from the nose or gums.
4. Estimate quantity of blood appearing in vomitus or expectoration, urine, stools, and increased menstrual flow.
5. Record bleeding from injection sites.
6. Intracranial bleeding may develop. Watch for symptoms associated with cerebrovascular disease and increased intracranial pressure.
7. Determine whether the patient has a history of taking coumarin drugs and aspirin in any form.
8. Procedure alert: When a blood sample is obtained for prothrombin time, PTT, and TT, sodium citrate is the anticoagulant of choice.

Coagulant Factors (Factor Assay)

Normal Values
Factor VII: 65%–135% of normal or 65–135 Aμ
Factor VIII: 55%–145% of normal or 55–145 Aμ
Factor IX: 60%–140% of normal or 60–140 Aμ
Factor X: 45%–155% of normal or 45–155 Aμ
Factor XI: 65%–135% of normal or 65–135 Aμ
Factor XII: 50%–150% of normal or 50–150 Aμ
Ristocetin–Willebrand Factor: 45%–140% of normal or 45–140 Aμ

Factor XIII Inhibitor: Negative
Factor VIII-Related Antigen: 45–185% of normal or 45–185 Aμ

Explanation of Test
This test of specific factors of coagulation is done in the investigation of inherited and required bleeding disorders. For example, tests of Factor VIII–related antigen are used in the differential diagnosis of classic hemophilia and von Willebrand's disease in cases where there is no family history of bleeding and when bleeding times may be borderline or abnormal. A test for ristocetin cofactor is done to help diagnose von Willebrand's disease by determining the degree or rate of platelet aggregation that is taking place.

Procedure
A venous blood sample of 5 ml. is obtained. Sodium citrate is anticoagulant added. Blood is drawn from a normal nonrelated person at the same time to serve as a control.

Clinical Implications
A. *Inherited deficiencies*
  1. All of the specific factors—VII, VIII, IX, X, XI, and XII—may be deficient on a familial basis, for example
    (a) Factor VII is decreased in hypoproconvertinemia (autosomal recessive).
    (b) Factor VIII is decreased in classic hemophilia A and von Willebrand's disease (inherited autosomally).
    (c) Factor IX is decreased in Christmas disease or hemophilia B (sex-linked recessive).
    (d) Factor XI is decreased in hemophilia C, occurring predominantly in Jews, and is autosomal dominant.
B. *Acquired disorders*
  2. Factor VII is also decreased in acquired disorders such as
    (a) Liver disease
    (b) Treatment with coumarin drugs
    (c) Hemorrhagic disease of the newborn
    (d) Kwashiorkor
  3. Factor VIII increases are associated with
    (a) Late normal pregnancy
    (b) Thromboembolic conditions
    (c) Coronary artery disease
    (d) Postoperative period
    (e) Rebound activity after sudden cessation of coumarin
    (f) Hyperthyroidism
    (g) Myeloma
    (h) Macroglobulinemia

(i) Hypoglycemia
(j) Cushing's syndrome

4. Factor IX levels are decreased in
   (a) Uncompensated cirrhosis (40% of cases)
   (b) Nephrotic syndrome
   (c) Development of circulating anticoagulants against Factor IX
   (d) Normal newborn
   (e) Dicumarol and related anticoagulant drugs cause a decrease after 48 to 72 hours of treatment

5. Factor XI decreased levels are associated with
   (a) Liver disease
   (b) Intestinal malabsorption of vitamin K
   (c) Occasional development of circulatory anticoagulants against Factor IX
   (d) Congenital heart disease
   (e) Paroxysmal nocturnal hemoglobin

6. Factor XII level is decreased in the nephrotic syndrome.

7. Factor VIII inhibitors (anticoagulants capable of specifically neutralizing a coagulation factor and thereby disrupting hemostasis) are associated with
   (a) Hemophilia A
   (b) Immunologic reactions

8. Factor VIII–related antigen is low in von Willebrand's disease and normal in hemophilia.

9. Ristocetin cofactor is decreased in von Willebrand's disease and Bernard–Soulier disease, an intrinsic platelet defect.

10. Factor X is increased during normal pregnancy.

11. Factor XI is decreased in newborns and with use of anticoagulant therapy.

12. Factor XII is decreased in newborns and in normal pregnancy and increased after exercise.

13. Factor XIII levels are decreased (in)
    (a) Postoperative patients
    (b) Liver disease
    (c) Persistent increased fibrinogen levels
    (d) Myeloma
    (e) Lead poisoning
    (f) Pernicious anemia
    (g) Agammaglobulinemia

Clinical Alert

For meaningful results, avoid Coumadin for two weeks and heparin therapy for two days before testing.

Bleeding Time (Duke and Ivy Methods)

Normal Values
3–10 minutes in most laboratories
  Duke method < 8 minutes (usually 1–3 minutes)—earlobe
  Ivy method 2–9.5 minutes—forearm

Explanation of Test
Bleeding time measures the primary phase of hemostasis: the interaction of the platelet with the blood vessel wall and the formation of the hemostatic plug. This is one of the four primary screening tests for coagulation disorders. A small stab wound is made in either the earlobe or forearm; the bleeding time is recorded, and a measurement is made of the rate at which a platelet clot is formed. The duration of bleeding from a punctured capillary depends upon the quantity and quality of platelets and the ability of the blood vessel wall to constrict.

The bleeding time test is of significant value in detecting vascular abnormalities and of moderate value in detecting platelet abnormalities or deficiencies. Its principal use today is in the diagnosis of von Willebrand's disease, an inherited defective molecule of Factor VIII, and a type of pseudohemophilia. It has been established that aspirin may cause bleeding in some normal persons, but the bleeding time has not proved to be consistently valuable in identifying such persons. While the bleeding time is classically recognized as prolonged in thrombocytopenia, the test is an indirect method of identifying the condition. A stained red cell examination and platelet count are more effective than bleeding time in confirming the diagnosis of thrombocytopenia.

Procedure
Two procedures are followed, the Duke method and the Ivy method.

Duke Method
In the modified Duke method, the area used for puncture is just above the rounded, fatty portion of the earlobe, which is highly vascular.

1. The ear is quickly pierced with a hemolet ("ear sticker") to make a wound 1–2 mm. deep.
2. A stopwatch is started. Pressure should not be exerted on the ear to initiate bleeding.
3. The blood should be allowed to fall freely on 4″ × 4″ gauze sponges or filter paper.
4. The blood is blotted every 30 seconds until all bleeding has stopped. The wound itself is not disturbed.

Ivy Method
In the Ivy method, the area three finger-widths below the antecubital space is cleansed with alcohol and allowed to dry.

1. A blood pressure cuff is placed on the arm above the elbow and inflated to 40 mm. of mercury.
2. A cleansed area of the forearm without superficial veins is selected. The skin is stretched laterally and tautly between the thumb and forefinger.
3. The skin is punctured with a sterile disposable device to a uniform depth of 5 mm. and width of 1 mm.
4. A stopwatch is started. The edge of a 4" × 4" filter paper is used to blot the blood through capillary action by gently touching the drop every 30 seconds. The wound itself is not disturbed. The blood pressure gauge is removed when bleeding stops spontaneously and a sterile dressing is applied.

The results of both procedures are reported in this way: The end point is reached when blood is no longer blotted from the ear or forearm puncture.

Clinical Implications

1. Bleeding time is prolonged when the level of platelets is decreased or when the platelets are qualitatively abnormal, as in
   (a) Thrombocytopenia
   (b) Platelet dysfunction syndromes
   (c) Decrease or abnormality in plasma factors such as von Willebrand's factor and fibrinogen
   (d) Abnormalities in walls of the small blood vessels
   (e) Vascular defects
   (f) Severe liver disease
   (g) Leukemia
   (h) Aplastic anemia
   (i) DIC disease
2. Bleeding time can be either normal or prolonged in von Willebrand's disease. It will definitely be prolonged if aspirin is administered prior to testing.
3. A single prolonged bleeding time does not prove the existence of hemorrhagic disease because a larger vessel may have been punctured. The puncture should be done twice (on the opposite ear or opposite arm) and the average of the bleeding times taken.
4. Bleeding time is normal in patients with coagulation disorders other than platelet dysfunction or vascular disease

Interfering Factors

1. The normal range may vary when the puncture is not of standard depth and width.
2. Touching the incision during the test will break off any fibrin particles and prolong the bleeding time.
3. Heavy alcohol consumption (as in alcoholics) may cause bleeding time to be increased.

4. Prolonged bleeding time will result from the ingestion of 10 g. of aspirin (acetylsalicylic acid) up to 5 days before the test.
5. Other drugs that may cause the bleeding time to be increased include
   (a) Dextran
   (b) Streptokinase–streptodornase (used as fibrinolytic agent)
   (c) Mithramycin
   (d) Pantothenyl alcohol

Patient Preparation
1. Explain the purpose and procedure of the test to patient.
2. Warn patient to take no aspirin or drugs that contain aspirin for at least 5 days before the test.
3. Advise outpatients not to drink alcoholic beverages before coming for test.

Clinical Alert

If the puncture site is still bleeding beyond 15 minutes, the test should be discontinued by applying pressure to area. Report to physician.

Tourniquet Test (Rumpel-Leede Positive Pressure Test; Capillary Fragility Test; Negative Pressure Test)

Normal Values
Occasional petechiae or none
   Positive pressure test—Occasional (5–10) petechiae
   Negative pressure test—1–2 petechiae or none

Explanation of Test
This test is done to demonstrate a defect of capillary fragility that is due to an abnormality in the capillary walls or thrombocytopenia. Positive or negative pressure is applied to various areas of the body by a blood pressure cuff or a suction cup. The degree of increased capillary fragility is reflected in the number of petechiae (nonraised, round red spots) appearing in a given area of observation.

   The forearm, wrists, hands, and fingers are examined for petechiae. The distribution of petechiae is usually irregular and no effort is made to count the number in a given area. The test is graded 1+ to 4+, depending on whether there are few or many spots.

Procedure
1. In the positive pressure tourniquet test, a blood pressure cuff is applied to the upper arm and inflated to 70 to 90 mm. of mercury or

to midway between the patient's systolic and diastolic pressure. The inflated cuff is removed after 5 minutes. The arm, wrist, and hand are then inspected for petechiae.

2. In the negative pressure test, a lubricated suction cup 2 cm. in diameter is applied to the skin of the upper arm. Pressure is applied to the skin for 1 minute. The suction cup is released and 5 minutes later the skin is inspected for petechiae. (This is not commonly done, but a description is included here because it is referred to in the literature about bleeding disorders.)

Clinical Implications

1. Increased petechiae formation occurs most commonly in thrombocytopenia and less commonly in (a) thrombasthenia, (b) vascular purpura, (c) senile purpura, and (d) scurvy.
2. The number and size of petechiae are roughly proportional to the bleeding tendency and possibly to the degree of thrombocytopenia. However, the test can be positive because of capillary fragility in the presence of a normal platelet count.
3. Results will be normal in coagulation disorders and vascular disorders.
4. Positive 1+ is a few petechiae over anterior forearm.
   2+ is many petechiae over anterior forearm.
   3+ is multiple petechiae over the whole arm and top of hand.
   4+ is confluent petechiae in all areas of arm and top of hand.

Interfering Factors

1. Menstruation: Capillary fragility is normally increased before menstruation.
2. Infectious disease: Capillary fragility is increased in measles and influenza.
3. Age: Women over 40 with decreasing estrogen levels may have a positive test that is not indicative of a coagulation disorder.
4. Readministration: Repetition of the test on same arm within 1 week of the first test may lead to error.
5. Variation: Results may vary because of differences in texture, thickness, and temperature of the skin.

Patient Preparation

Explain purpose and procedure of the test.

Clinical Alert

Do not repeat this test on the same arm for at least 1 week because the results will be unreliable. Use the opposite arm for a repeat test.

Thrombin Time; Thrombin Clotting Time

Normal Values
Fifteen seconds or control ±5 sec. However, there are so many modifications of this test that "normals" vary widely. Check your laboratory values.

Explanation of Test
Stage III defects of fibrinogen abnormalities can be detected by this method. It is a valuable test for detecting hypofibrinogenemia and may also be used for control of heparin therapy. The test measures the time needed for plasma to clot in the laboratory when thrombin is added. Normally, a clot is formed instantly; if not, a fibrinogen deficiency is present (Figure 2-1).

Procedure
If the test is used to monitor heparin therapy, blood is drawn 1 hour before administration of anticoagulant. A 7 ml. venous blood sample is obtained and an anticoagulant, sodium citrate, is added to the syringe.

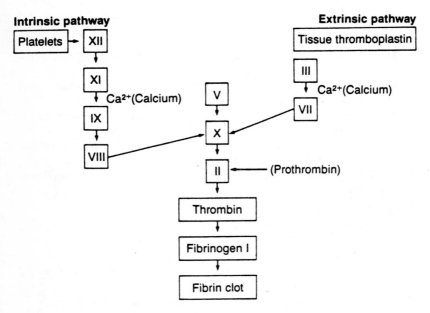

Figure 2-1
Mechanism of fibrin clot formation.

Clinical Implications

1. No clot will form if afibrinogenemia is present.
2. A small visible clot will form in hypofibrinogenemia, but the thrombin clotting time is prolonged.
3. A thrombin curie can be set up to determine the exact amount of fibrinogen present.
   - (a) Normal values—200–400 mg./dl. or 2.0–4.0 g./liter
   - (b) Elevated values occur in pregnancy and inflammation
   - (c) Low values found in DIC and liver disease
4. The thrombin time is also prolonged.
   - (a) Anticoagulant therapy when heparin is present in the blood
   - (b) In the dysproteinemias such as multiple myeloma

Partial Thromboplastin Time (PTT); Activated Partial Thromboplastin Time (APTT)

Normal Values

PTT: 30–45 seconds
APTT: 16–25 seconds

The basis of this test is fibrin clot formation. Normal ranges vary with phospholipid used.

Explanation of Test

The PTT, which is a one stage clotting test, is an important and sensitive screening test for coagulation disorders and is of most value in detecting deficiencies of Stage II clotting mechanism. Specifically, it is used to detect deficiencies of the components of the intrinsic thromboplastin system. This method will detect not only those abnormalities that are identified by the whole blood clotting time, and some that might be missed by the whole blood clotting time, but will also reveal abnormalities characterized by defects in the second stage of the coagulation mechanism. The PTT is sometimes preferred over the coagulation time test for monitoring heparin therapy.

Note: PTT and APTT test for the same functions. Deficiency of Factor VII is not measured in this test system. The APTT is a modified PTT that is used frequently to monitor heparin therapy because it is a more sensitive test than PTT.

The APTT is also used to detect circulating anticoagulants. Both classic hemophilia A and hemophilia B can be complicated by the presence of circulating anticoagulants. These circulating anticoagulants are antibodies, most of which are induced in hemophiliacs by the transfusion of plasma from normal persons. The prolonged PTT of hemophiliacs can be corrected by transfusions, but if the anticoagulants (inhibitors of clotting) develop, the PTT again becomes prolonged.

Procedure

1. A venous sample of 7 ml. is obtained, using sodium citrate added as an anticoagulant in the syringe. A blue top Vacutainer is used.
2. Do not draw from a heparin lock or heparinized catheter.

   Note: The PTT and APTT are essentially the same test. What applies to one applies to the other. The A = activated. The APTT is slightly more sensitive.

Clinical Implications

A. *APTT*
   1. The APTT is prolonged in all coagulation defects of Stage I.
   2. The APTT is usually prolonged in von Willebrand's disease and is accompanied by a consistently diminished Factor VIII level.
   3. The APTT and prothrombin time will detect approximately 95% of coagulation abnormalities. When APTT is performed in conjunction with a prothrombin time (PT), a further clarification of coagulation defects is possible. For example, a normal PT and an abnormal PTT mean that the defect lies within the first stage of the clotting mechanism.
B. *Causes of prolonged APTT* are
   1. Hemophilia
   2. Vitamin K deficiency
   3. Liver disease
   4. Presence of circulating anticoagulants
   5. DIC disease (chronic or acute)
C. *Shortened APTT occurs*
   1. Extensive cancer, except when the liver is involved
   2. Immediately after acute hemorrhage
   3. Very early stages of DIC
D. *Circulating anticoagulants*
   Usually occurs as an inhibitor of a specific factor (*e.g.*, Factor VIII). Most commonly seen in the development of anti–Factor VIII or anti–Factor IX in 5%–10% of hemophiliacs. Anticoagulants that develop in the treated hemophiliac are detected by prolonged APTT. Circulating anticoagulants also can be detected in some cases.
   1. Following repeated plasma transfusions
   2. Drug reactions
   3. Tuberculosis
   4. Chronic glomerulonephritis
   5. Systemic lupus erythematosus
   6. Rheumatoid arthritis

Clinical Alert

APTT > 100 sec. signifies spontaneous bleeding.

E. Heparin Therapy: Protocols and APTT Tests
   1. Heparin combines in the blood with an alpha-globulin (heparin cofactor) for a potent antithrombin.
   2. The intravenous injection of heparin will provide an immediate anticoagulant effect, so it is used when rapid effects are desired.
   3. Because heparin does not remain in the blood very long, the APTT time is measured before each injection.
   4. The APTT is ordinarily maintained at two to two and one half times the normal limit.
   5. To evaluate the effect of heparin, the blood is tested
      (a) Before therapy is started for baseline
      (b) One hour before next dose is administered
      (c) Dependent upon the status of patient (*i.e.*, if there are signs of bleeding); during heparin therapy
   6. Protamine sulfate is the antidote for heparin overdose and hemorrhage.

Prothrombin Time (Pro Time; PT)

Normal Values
10–14 seconds or 100% (each laboratory will set its own normals); will vary with type of thromboplastin used.

Explanation of Test
Prothrombin is a protein produced by the liver and is used in the clotting of blood. Production of prothrombin depends on an adequate intake and absorption of vitamin K. During the clotting process, prothrombin is converted to thrombin. The prothrombin content of the blood will be reduced in patients with liver disease.

Prothrombin time is one of the four most important screening tests used in diagnostic coagulation studies. It directly measures a defect in Stage II of the clotting mechanism. The clotting ability of five plasma coagulation factors (prothrombin, fibrinogen, Factor V, Factor VII, and Factor X) is measured; this ability is referred to as the "prothrombin time." This test is commonly ordered in conjunction with the management of Coumadin anticoagulant therapy.

Procedure
1. 7 ml. venous blood is drawn.
2. A calcium-binding anticoagulant (sodium citrate) is added to the sample or drawn in a blue top Vacutainer.

Oral Anticoagulant Therapy

Oral anticoagulant drugs such as Coumadin and dicumarol (4-hydroxy-coumarin) are commonly used to treat blood clots. However, heparin is used first in treatment because it is rapid acting and also because it partially lyses the clot.

1. These drugs act in the liver to delay coagulation by interfering with the action of vitamin K–dependent factors (II, VII, IX, and X). Coumadin is an indirect anticoagulant; heparin is a direct anticoagulant.
2. Drug therapy delays coagulation and causes the pro time to increase due to *decreased* Factors II, VII, IX, and X.
3. The usual procedure is to run a prothrombin time test every day; after the pro time is determined, the dosage of the anticoagulant is adjusted and administered.
4. Coumadin requires 16 to 48 hours to cause a measurable change in the pro time.

Drug Therapy and Pro Time Protocols

1. Cardiac patients are usually maintained at a pro time of two to two and one half times normal.
2. In the treatment of blood clots, the pro time is maintained within the above range. If the pro time drops below this range, the treatment may be ineffective and old clots may expand or new clots may form. If the pro time rises above 30 seconds, hemorrhage may occur.

Clinical Implications

1. Conditions accompanied by an increased pro time include
   (a) Prothrombin deficiency
   (b) Vitamin K deficiency
   (c) Hemorrhagic disease of the newborn
   (d) Liver disease (*e.g.*, alcoholic hepatitis)
   (e) Anticoagulant therapy
   (f) Biliary obstruction
   (g) Salicylate intoxication
   (h) Hypervitaminosis A
   (i) DIC disease

Interfering Factors

1. Diet: Excessive amounts of green, leafy vegetables will increase the body's absorption of vitamin K.
2. Alcohol: Pro time is increased due to liver disease.
3. Diarrhea and vomiting: These conditions will increase pro time.
4. Quality of venipuncture: It is important that a clean and careful venipuncture is done, otherwise the pro time can be shortened.
5. There are many drugs known to cause increases or decreases in pro time.

Patient Preparation

1. Explain the purpose and frequency of the test. Patients on long-term anticoagulant therapy must understand the need for regular monitoring through frequent blood testing. *Do not refer to anticoagulants as "blood thiners."* One explanation might be: "Your blood will be tested periodically to determine the pro time, which is an indication of how quickly the blood clots." The dose of the anticoagulant will be increased, decreased, maintained, or discontinued on the basis of this test.
2. Caution the patient to avoid self-medication. Explain that many drugs, including medicines available without a prescription, can either increase or decrease the effect of the anticoagulants and alter the results of the test.
3. Instruct the patient never to start or stop taking any drug without the doctor's permission, for this will affect the pro time.

Clinical Alert

1. If pro time is excessively prolonged (>40 seconds), vitamin K is administered intramuscularly. Ordinarily, intramuscular injections are contraindicated during anticoagulant therapy because large painful hematomas may form at the injection site. As values get into danger zones (>30) assess carefully for bleeding, including (a) craniotomy checks, (b) lung auscultation, especially of the upper lobes, (c) occult blood in the urine, using Hemastix (a cellulose strip, saturated with a peroxide and orthotolidine).
2. Patients who are being monitored by pro time for long-term anticoagulant therapy should not take any drugs unless absolutely necessary.
3. When unexpected changes in anticoagulant doses are required to maintain a stable pro time, or when there is a consistent change in pro time, a drug interaction should be suspected.
4. Blood for pro time should be drawn for a baseline and prior to administration of anticoagulants.
5. Protamine sulfate is the antidote for heparin.

Platelet Count

Normal Values

150,000–350,000/mm.^{3} or 150–350 10^9/liter

Phase platelets—the normal value, also as above, can be slightly higher than, or the same as, the standard method. This is the preferred method.

Background
Platelets (or thrombocytes) are the smallest of the formed elements in the blood. These cells are nonnucleated, round or oval, flattened, disk-shaped structures. Platelet activity is necessary for blood clotting.

Function of Platelets
1. Coagulation/clotting of blood
2. Vascular integrity and vasoconstriction
3. Adhesion and aggregation activity in the formation of a platelet plug that occludes (plugs) breaks in small vessels.
4. Ability to take up, store, transport, and release vasoactive amines, platelet factor 3, and thromboxane A_2.

Platelet Formation
Platelet (thrombocyte) development takes place primarily in the bone marrow and possibly in the lungs. Thrombocytes are fragments of megakaryocytes, the largest of all bone marrow cells. The life span of a platelet is approximately 7.5 days. Normally, two-thirds of all the body platelets are in the circulating blood and one-third are in the spleen.

Explanation of Test
This test is indicated when the platelet count is below normal on a peripheral blood smear. This measurement is helpful in evaluating bleeding disorders that occur in liver disease, thrombocytopenia, uremia, and with anticoagulant therapy. This test is also used in following the course of diseases and disorders associated with bone marrow failure as in leukemia, aplastic anemia, and the use of toxic drugs.
   Other tests to study platelet function include:

1. Clot retraction—a rough measurement of platelet function
2. Bleeding time—measures activity of platelets, adhesiveness, and platelet factor 3 content or release
3. Prothrombin consumption test—detects a significant decrease of platelet factor 3
4. Special platelet function tests such as platelet aggregation

   The platelet count is the most important platelet test because thrombocytopenia is the most common bleeding disease.

Procedure
A venous blood sample of 7 ml. is obtained and an anticoagulant (EDTA) is added to the syringe.

Clinical Implications
1. *Abnormally increased numbers* of platelets (thrombocythemia/ thrombocytosis) occur in

(a) Cancer
(b) Chronic myelogenous and granulocytic leukemia
(c) Polycythemia vera
(d) Splenectomy
(e) Trauma
(f) Asphyxiation
(g) Rheumatoid arthritis
(h) Iron-deficiency and posthemorrhagic anemia
(i) Acute infections
(j) Heart disease
(k) Cirrhosis
(l) Chronic pancreatitis
(m)Tuberculosis

In 50% of those patients who exhibit an unexpected increase in platelets, a malignancy will be found. This malignancy is usually disseminated, advanced, or inoperable.

2. *Abnormally decreased numbers* of platelets (thrombocytopenia) occur (in)
(a) Idiopathic thrombocytopenic purpura
(b) Pernicious, aplastic, and hemolytic anemias
(c) After massive blood transfusion
(d) Pneumonia
(e) Allergic conditions
(f) Exposure to DDT and other chemicals
(g) During cancer chemotherapy
(h) Infection
(i) Lesions involving the bone marrow
(j) Toxic effects of many drugs.

Note: The dose of any drug does not have to be high to have a toxic effect. The development of toxic thrombocytopenia depends on the ability of the body to metabolize and secrete the toxic substance.

(k) DIC
(l) Bernard–Soulier syndrome

Clinical Alert

Panic values—A *decrease in platelets* of <20,000 mm.^{3} is associated with a tendency to

(a) Spontaneous bleeding
(b) Prolonged bleeding time
(c) Petechiae
(d) Ecchymosis

Note: The precise number of platelets necessary for hemostasis is not firmly established. Generally, platelet counts of greater than 50,000 mm.^{3} are not associated with spontaneous bleeding. Those occasional patients with platelet counts in the 50,000 to 100,000 range will bleed excessively during surgical procedures.

Interfering Factors
1. Normally decreases first day of an infant's life
2. Normally increases at high altitudes
3. Normally increases after strenuous exercise and excitement
4. Normally increases in winter
5. Normally decreases before menstruation

> **Note:** These physiologic variations in the number of platelets in the blood indicate the balance between their production and their utilization loss or destruction.

Clinical Alert

Observe patients with serious platelet deficits for signs and symptoms of GI bleeding, hemolysis, hematuria, petechiae, vaginal bleeding, epistasis, and bleeding from gums. When hemorrhage is apparent, use emergency measures to control bleeding and notify attending physician.

Mean Platelet Volume

Normal Values
8–10 fL.
25. μm. in diameter

Explanation of Test
This test provides information about platelet size by an automated method. A stained blood film is also a method of testing that reveals that platelets are of different sizes. This test is done in the investigation of various hematologic disorders such as thrombocytopenic purpura, leukemia, and study of alcoholics under treatment.

Note: Adhesive platelets will be larger than nonadhesive platelets.

Procedure
The mean platelet volume is determined and calculated by an analyzer.

Clinical Implications
1. *Increases* in proportion of platelets exceeding 2.5 μm. in diameter occur in
   (a) Idiopathic thrombocytopenia purpura (autoimmune) in apparent remission
   (b) Systemic lupus erythematosus
   (c) DIC
   (d) Megaloblastic anemia due to vitamin B_{12} deficiency
   (e) Rheumatic heart disease with valve impairment
   (f) Diabetes with retinopathy
   (g) Prosthetic heart valve plus rheumatic heart disease
   (h) Microglobulinemia
2. *Decreases* occur in
      Wiskott–Aldrich syndrome

Clot Retraction

Normal Values
After 1 hour the blood clot appreciably shrinks or retracts from the sides of the test tube and becomes more firm. The clot maintains its molded shape when it is removed from the container in which it has formed. Clot retraction is nearly complete in 4 hours and definitely completed in 24 hours. If clot retraction is normal and complete, approximately half the total volume is clot and the other half is serum.

Explanation of Test
This test is a rough measurement and is used to confirm a platelet problem such as thrombocytopenia.

In this test, blood is allowed to clot in a test tube without an anticoagulant. This test is based on the fact that whole blood that clots normally will retract or recede from the sides of its container, resulting in the separation of transparent serum and the contracted blood clot. Since platelets play a major part in the mechanism of clot retraction, this reaction is impaired when platelets are decreased or function abnormally. This reaction is also influenced by the fibrinogen content of the plasma, the ratio of the plasma volume to red cell mass, and the activity of a retraction-promoting principle in the serum. Results are determined at 1 hour and at 24 hours.

Procedure
1. About 5 ml. of venous blood is collected in a tube without anticoagulant.
2. Clot begins separating from tube walls in 30 minutes to 1 hour; clot usually separates completely in 12 to 24 hours.
3. For 72 hours the retracted clot does not change appreciably.

Clinical Implications
There is a distinct parallel between the quality of the clot and the number of platelets. A defective clot is soft and soggy, is readily torn, and, after removal from its container, flattens out as a shapeless mass from which serum continues to ooze.

1. *Poor or decreased clot retraction* occurs in
   (a) Thrombocytopenia
   (b) Von Willebrand's disease when platelets are deficient in quality
   (c) Disorders due to increase in red cell mass
2. *Clot retraction appears to be increased* in severe anemia and hypofibrinogenemia as a result of small clot formation occurring from an increase in plasma volume.

Interfering Factors
1. If the hematocrit is high because of polycythemia or hemocontraction, clot retraction will be decreased.
2. In increased fibrinolysis the clot will lyse in 10 to 30 minutes, and it will appear that no retraction has taken place.

Prothrombin Consumption Test (PCT); Serum Prothrombin Time

Normal Values
15 seconds or more, measured 1 hour after coagulation
>80% consumed in 1 hour

Explanation of Test
In this test, a measurement is made of the prothrombin remaining in the serum after the coagulation of whole blood. After a clot has formed, 25% or less of prothrombin should remain in the serum. A patient with a defect in Stage I will not convert as much prothrombin to thrombin in coagulation; thus, a great deal of prothrombin may be left in the serum.

The PCT is used to diagnose a defect in the intrinsic clotting mechanism. This measurement, also called serum prothrombin time, is one of the most accurate tests used to detect Stage I deficiencies. The outstanding advantage of PCT is its sensitivity to a clinically significant decrease of platelet factor 3. It is not often used because of the length of time the test takes.

Procedure
A venous blood sample of 7 ml. is obtained. No anticoagulant is added to the syringe.

Clinical Implications
1. Decreased values below 15 seconds indicate a deficiency of Factors VIII and IX and platelets or the presence of a circulatory anticoagulant.
2. A shortened PCT indicates a deficiency of platelets and factors that are necessary for production of intrinsic thromboplastin and may indicate the presence of anticoagulants or inhibitors.
3. Shortened PCT is probably due to a deficiency of any one of the factors required in Stages I and II of coagulation (a pro time is done in conjunction with PCT) to rule out Stage II deficiencies.
4. Because normal platelet function is necessary for the generation of plasma thromboplastin, there is no point in doing a PCT when thrombocytopenia is present.
5. A shortened PCT may be associated with the following:
   (a) Circulating anticoagulants (d) Thrombocytopenia
   (b) Hemophilias   (e) Thrombocytopathies
   (c) Hypoprothrombinemia   (f) DIC disease

Interfering Factors
Hemolysis of red cells due to excessive suction in drawing the blood, or in rough handling of the blood, can give results over 35 seconds.

Plasminogen/Plasmin

Normal Values
6.1 plus or minus 2.3 CTA units (CTA = Committee on Thrombolytic Agents)

Explanation of Test
These measurements of fibrinolysis are done to determine the level of plasminogen, the inactive precursor of plasmin, and of the active enzyme plasmin, which has the ability to dissolve formed fibrin clots. The test is useful during streptokinase therapy in arterial thrombosis.

The concentration of plasminogen is expressed in CTA plasma units.

Procedure
A venous blood sample of 5 ml. is obtained. Sodium citrate is added.

Clinical Implications
1. Plasminogen levels fall variably in preeclampsia and eclampsia.
2. Plasmin can activate complement. There is an interrelationship between coagulation, kinin generation, fibrinolysis, and complement activation.

Aspirin Tolerance

Normal Values
Mean values after aspirin ingestion: 9½ minutes with a range of 4 minutes to 21 minutes. Drops are frequently larger after aspirin.

Explanation of Test
This test is an aid in the diagnosis of von Willebrand's disease and other platelet function abnormalities.

Procedure
The bleeding time test is done by any standardized method, immediately before and 2 hours after an adult has ingested 10 to 15 grams of aspirin. Platelet adhesiveness tests can be run at the same time as the bleeding times.

Interfering Factors
A marked response is also seen in persons who are simply hypersensitive to aspirin.

Clinical Implications
Values are *increased* in disorders such as von Willebrand's disease and hemophilia.

Clinical Alert
1. The aspirin tolerance test should not be done if initial bleeding time is significantly prolonged (>10 minutes).
2. The test is also contraindicated in severe hemophilia when extremely prolonged bleeding times after aspirin may occur and when there may be considerable difficulty in stopping the bleeding.

Fibrinolysis/Euglobulin Lysis Time

Normal Values
Euglobulin lysis—no lysis of plasma clot at 37° for 3 hours. Clot observed for 24 hours.

Explanation of Test
This is one of the tests employed to evaluate a fibrinolytic crisis. No one single test has been universally accepted for the complete diagnosis and management of fibrinolytic states.

Fibrinolysis, which occurs without any sign of intravascular coagulation, is extremely rare. Usually seen is secondary fibrinolysis, which follows and occurs simultaneously with intravascular coagulation. This secondary type of fibrinolysis is thought to be a protective mechanism that the body possesses to protect itself against generalized clotting.

Procedure
A venous blood sample of 5 ml. is obtained. Sodium citrate is added.

Clinical Alert

A lysis time of less than 1 hour signifies that abnormal fibrinolysis is occurring.

Clinical Implications
1. *Increased fibrinolysis* occurs (with)
   (a) 48 hours after surgery (The fibrinolytic activity continues to increase for the next 6 days.)
   (b) Incompatible blood transfusions
   (c) Cancer of prostate or pancreas
   (d) Cirrhosis (some cases)
   (e) During lung surgery
   (f) Obstetric complications such as antepartum hemorrhage, amniotic embolism, septic abortion, death of fetus, and hydatidiform mole
   (g) Thrombocytopenic purpura
   (h) Extracorporeal circulation
   (i) Leukemia
2. *Decreased fibrinolysis* occurs in
   (a) Diabetes
   (b) First 48 hours after surgery
   (c) Premature infants

Interfering Factors
1. Increased fibrinolysis occurs with
   (a) Exercise
   (b) Increasing age
   (c) Hyperventilation
   (d) Steroids and ACTH
2. Decreased fibrinolysis occurs (in)
   (a) Arterial blood, when compared with venous blood. This difference is greater in arteriosclerosis (especially in young persons)
   (b) Postmenopausal females
   (c) Normal newborns

(d) On the day following severe unaccustomed exercise by persons out of shape
(e) Obesity
3. Fibrin degradation products interfere with fibrinolysis.
(a) False negatives can occur if fibrinolysis is far advanced.
(b) False positives can be caused by very low fibrinogen levels.

Fibrin Split Products (FSP);
Fibrin Degradation Products (FDP)

Normal Values
Negative 4 μg./ml.

Explanation of Test
This test is done to determine the degree of consumptive coagulopathy in disorders such as positive tests for DIC, thromboembolic disorders, and renal diseases. When fibrin is split by plasmin, positive tests for fibrin degradation or split products, identified by letters S, Y, D, and E, are produced. These products have an anticoagulant action and inhibit clotting when there is an excess in the circulation.

Procedure
A venous blood sample of at least 4.5 ml. is obtained.

Clinical Implications
Increased values are associated (with)

1. Any condition associated with disseminated intravascular coagulation syndrome (DIC)
2. Venous thrombosis
3. Hypoxia
4. Following thoracic and cardiac surgery and renal transplantation
5. Portacaval shunt
6. Incompatible blood transfusion
7. Acute leukemia
8. Infections
9. Burns
10. Some snake bites
11. Heat stroke
12. Pulmonary embolism
13. Prolonged coma due to hypnotic drugs

Interfering Factors
Since all of the laboratory methods are sensitive to fibrinogen as well as FDP, it is essential that no unclotted fibrinogen be left in the serum

preparation. Special care must also be taken with blood containing a therapeutic heparin. False-positive reactions could result if any fibrinogen is present.

Platelet Adhesion

Normal Values
50,000 to 18,000/mm.^{3} (depends on method used)
25% to 60% retention (also depends on methodology)
25% to 58% adherence

Explanation of Test
This measurement is done to detect abnormalities in platelet adhesion. The test is indicated in persons who have had no exposure to aspirin for 2 to 3 weeks and who have a prolonged bleeding time. This test is based on the fact that *in vivo* adhesion to collagen is an important part of platelets' function in hemostasis.

Procedure
Two procedures can be done:

1. Platelet *in vivo*
   (a) A wound is made as in the Ivy bleeding time method, and platelet counts are taken at intervals on the blood issuing from the wound.
   (b) The venous platelet count is compared to those from the wound, and the difference is expressed as percent platelet adhesiveness.
2. Platelet adhesiveness *in vitro*
   (a) A venous blood sample of 5 ml. is obtained. Sodium citrate is added. The specimen is kept at room temperature.
   (b) The platelet count is determined and compared to the venous platelet count and is expressed as percent adhesiveness or percent retention.

Clinical Implications
1. *Adhesiveness is increased* in
   (a) Surgery, trauma, and burns (increases after 48 hours to reach peak values about the tenth day)
   (b) Acute infection
   (c) Cancer (some cases)
   (d) Diabetes
   (e) Atherosclerosis
   (f) Hyperlipidemia
   (g) Homocystinuria
   (h) Multiple sclerosis

2. *Adhesiveness is decreased* in
   (a) Glanzmann's thrombasthenia
   (b) Von Willebrand's disease
   (c) Congential heart disease
   (d) Glycogen storage disease
   (e) Bernard–Soulier giant platelet disease
   (f) Myeloproliferative disorders
   (g) Uremia
   (h) Drug-induced platelet dysfunction

Interfering Factors
Increased adhesiveness occurs with

1. Exertion
2. Increasing age
3. Seasonal variations, greater in springtime
4. Diurnal variations, greater in afternoon
5. Use of some oral contraceptives

Decreased adhesiveness occurs with use of aspirin.

Platelet Aggregation

Normal Values
Visible platelet aggregates form in less than 5 minutes.

Explanation of Test
This procedure is carried out to detect abnormalities in platelet aggregation. Platelets have surface-binding sites for adenosine diphosphate (ADP), a natural biologically active platelet aggregating substance. ADP is added to a platelet mixture and the rate of aggregation and the percentage of aggregation are measured.

Clinical Alert

If the aggregation is abnormal, platelet function is impaired.

Procedure
A venous blood sample of 5 ml. is obtained. Sodium citrate is the anticoagulant. The blood must be kept at room temperature—never refrigerate.

Clinical Implications
Aggregation is reduced in

(a) Infectious mononucleosis
(b) Idiopathic thrombocytopenic purpura

(c) Acute leukemia
(d) Von Willebrand's disease
(e) Hereditary giant platelet syndrome of Bernard–Soulier
(f) Aspirin use
(g) Glanzmann's thrombasthenia

Heparin Neutralization

Normal Values
Interpretative report of the micrograms of circulating heparin.

Explanation of Test
This test is done to measure the amount of circulating heparin and to determine if heparin is responsible for the prolongation of the thrombin time.

Procedure
A venous blood sample of 5 ml. is obtained. In the laboratory, varying concentrations of heparin are added to normal control plasma until its thrombin time equals the thrombin time of the patient's plasma. Protamine sulfate, which neutralizes heparin, is then added to both plasmas to observe the effect of its neutralization capacity.

Clinical Implications
1. If the patient's prolonged thrombin time is shortened by the addition of protamine sulfate, it can be assumed that the prolongation is due to heparin.
2. Prolonged thrombin time due to fibrinogen split products or fibrin polymerization inhibitors will not be corrected by protamine sulfate.

Fibrinopeptide-A (FPA)

Normal Values
0.6–1.9 mg./ml.

Explanation of Test
This measurement is the most sensitive assay done to determine thrombin action. FPA reflects the amount of active intravascular blood clotting as in subclinical disseminated intravascular coagulation (DIC), which is common in patients with leukemia of various types and may be associated with tumor progression. Serial measurements of fibrinopeptide-A are used by some researchers to identify a relapse of acute leukemia.

Procedure
A venous blood sample of 9 ml. is obtained. Discard sample if not obtained by a clean venipuncture.

Interfering Factors
1. A traumatic venous puncture results in falsely elevated levels.
2. The biological half-life is 5 minutes, which imposes limitations on the interpretation of a negative FPA test.

Clinical Implications
1. Levels are increased in
   (a) DIC
   (b) Leukemic patients at time of initial diagnosis or during relapse after remission
   (c) Early treatment phase of leukemia
2. Levels are decreased when clinical remission of leukemia is achieved with chemotherapy.

Clinical Alert

1. DIC occurs commonly in association with death of tumor cells in acute promyelocytic leukemia. For this reason, heparin is used prophylactically and in association with the initiation of chemotherapy for promyelocytic leukemia. In contrast, DIC rarely occurs during the treatment of acute myelomonocytic leukemia and acute lymphocyte leukemia.

Fibrinogen

Normal Values
Thrombin time, semiquantitative: 200–400 mg./dl. or 2.0–4.0 g./liter

Explanation of Test
This test is done to investigate abnormal PT, APTT, and TT as well as to screen for disseminated intravascular coagulation (DIC) and fibrin–fibrinogenolysis.

Procedure
A venous blood sample is obtained.

Clinical Implications
1. Increased values occur in
   (a) Hepatitis   (c) Cancer
   (b) Multiple myeloma   (d) Uremia

(e) Pregnancy
(f) Menstruation
(g) Postsurgery
(h) Compensated DIC

(i) Inflammation such as rheumatic fever, pneumonia, tuberculosis, and septicemia
(j) Nephrosis
(k) Burns

2. Decreased values occur in
(a) Liver disease
(b) DIC
(c) Hereditary afibrinogenemia
(d) Dysfibrinogenemia

BIBLIOGRAPHY

Bauer JD: Clinical Laboratory Methods, 9th ed. St. Louis, CV Mosby, 1982
Beck W: Hematology, 4th ed. Cambridge, MA, MIT Press, 1981
Bonie EJW, Kwaan HC: Thrombosis. Philadelphia, WB Saunders, 1982
Brown BA: Hematology: Principles and Procedures, 4th ed. Philadelphia, Lea &
Febiger, 1984
Dade Monograph, Miami:
Kennedy J: Fibrinogen, Fibrin, and Fibrinolysis, 1974
Collins L: Fibrinogen and Fibrinolysis, 1970
Collins L: Coagulation Factors, 1971
Kennedy J: Laboratory Investigation of Hemostasis, 1973
Hutchinson D: Platelet Function, Disorders, and Testing, 1979
Gurewich V: Disseminated Intravascular Coagulation, 1979
Davidsohn I, Henry JB: Todd–Sanford–Davidsohn Clinical Diagnosis and Man-
agement by Laboratory Methods, 7th ed. Philadelphia, WB Saunders, 1984
Halsted CH, Halsted JA (eds.): The Laboratory in Clinical Medicine, 2nd ed.
Philadelphia, WB Saunders, 1981
Isselbacher KJ, et al (eds.): Harrison's Principles of Internal Medicine, 11th ed.
New York, McGraw–Hill, 1987
Kapff CT, Jandl JH: Blood: Atlas and Source Book of Hematology. Boston,
Little, Brown & Co., 1981
Miale JB: Laboratory Medicine: Hematology, 6th ed. St. Louis, CV Mosby, 1982
Platt WR: Color Atlas and Textbook of Hematology, 2nd ed. Philadelphia, JB
Lippincott, 1979
Sonnenwirth AC, Jarrett L (eds.): Gradwohl's Clinical Laboratory Methods and
Diagnosis, 8th ed. St. Louis, CV Mosby, 1980
Sren NC: Hematology: An Atlas and Diagnostic Guide. Philadelphia, WB Saun-
ders, 1983
Wallerstein RO: Differentiating common anemias. Consultant 20(8):65–66, 1980
Wintrobe MM: Clinical Hematology, 8th ed. Philadelphia, Lea & Febiger, 1981
Zucker F et al: Atlas of Blood Cells, Vols. 1 and 2. Philadelphia, Lea & Febiger,
1981

URINE STUDIES

Introduction

Overview of Urine Formation

Urine, a very complex fluid, is composed of 95% water and 5% solids. It is the end product of the metabolism carried out by billions of cells, resulting in an average urinary output of 1 to 1½ liters (approximately 1.5 qt.) per day, which is dependent on fluid intake. A wide variety of waste products formed in the metabolic processes of the body are carried away in the urine.

The formation of urine takes place in the kidneys, the two small fist-sized organs located outside the peritoneal cavity on each side of the spine at about the level of the last thoracic and upper two lumbar vertebrae. The kidneys, along with the skin and respiratory system, are the chief excretory organs of the body. Each kidney is a highly discriminating organ that maintains the internal environment by selectively excreting or retaining various substances according to specific body needs. The importance of urine formation and excretion as a regulating function is profoundly emphasized in situations in which kidney function is suddenly lost. Under these circumstances, death occurs within a few days.

The main functional unit of the kidney is the nephron. There are about one million nephrons per kidney, each composed of two main parts: a glomerulus, which is essentially a filtering system, and a tubule through which the filtered liquid passes. Each glomerulus consists of a capillary network surrounded by a membrane called *Bowman's capsule*, which continues on to form the beginning of the renal tubule. The afferent arteriole carries blood from the renal artery into the glomerulus, where it divides to form a capillary network. These capillaries reunite to form the efferent arteriole through which blood leaves the glomerulus. The blood vessels then follow the course of the tubule, forming a surrounding capillary network.

There is a tremendous flow of blood through the kidneys. It is believed that 25% of the blood from the left heart passes through the kidneys. One liter of urine can be thought of as the end result of more than 1000 liters of blood passing through the kidneys. The blood enters the glomerulus of each nephron by passing through the afferent arteriole into the glomerular capillaries.

Urine formation begins in the glomerular capillaries, with dissolved substances passing into the proximal tubule as a result of the force of blood pressure in the large afferent arteriole and the pressure in Bowman's capsule. As the filtrate passes along the tubule, more solutes are added by excretion from the capillary blood and secretions from the tubular epithelial cells. Solutes and water pass back into the blood by tubular reabsorption. Urine concentration and dilution take place in the renal medulla. The kidney has the remarkable ability to produce dilute or concentrated urine according to the needs of the individual and to regulate sodium excretion. Blood chemistry, blood pressure, fluid balance, nutrient intake, and state of health are key elements in metabolism. They are also key elements in establishing the character of urine.

Urine contains thousands of dissolved substances, although the three principal constituents are water, urea, and sodium chloride. More solids are excreted from the body in the urine than by any other method. Its composition depends greatly on the quality and the quantity of the excreted waste material. Some constituents of the blood, such as glucose, have a renal threshold; that is, a certain elevated level must be reached in the blood before this constituent will be excreted in the urine. Almost all substances found in the urine are also found in the blood, although in different concentrations. Urea, for example, is present in the blood, but at a much lower concentration than in the excreted urine.

URINE TESTING

Urinalysis is an essential procedure for hospital admissions and physical examinations. It is one of the most useful indicators of health and disease, and it is especially helpful in the detection of renal or metabolic disorders. It is an aid in diagnosing and following the course of treatment in diseases of the kidney and urinary system and in detecting disorders in other parts of the body such as metabolic or endocrinic abnormalities in which the kidneys function normally.

Laboratory Testing
In the laboratory, urinalysis is carried out by technologists who always visually examine specimens and then test them. Dipsticks are used for a number of tests. The Clinitek Reflectance Photometer is an example of a semiautomated instrument for use in routine urinalysis and other tests.

Dipsticks
While laboratory facilities allow for a wide range of urine tests, modern tablets, tapes, and dipstick tests are available for urinalysis. These devices are useful because they do not require a laboratory and can be read directly by patients as well as by clinicians, physicians, and technologists.

Similar in appearance to blotter paper, dipsticks are actually miniature laboratories. These chemically impregnated reagent (reactive) strips allow for quick determination of the following properties of urine: pH, protein, glucose, ketones, bilirubin, hemoglobin (blood), nitrite, leukocyte esterase and urobilinogen. The tip of the dipstick is impregnated with chemicals that react with specific substances in the urine to produce colored end products. In some tests, the depth of color produced is related to the concentration of the substance in the urine. Color standards are provided against which the color can be compared. The reaction rates of the impregnated chemicals are standard for each dipstick, and color changes must be matched at the correct time after each stick is dipped into the urine specimen. These matching methods are included in the instructions that accompany each type of dipstick. When more than one reaction is arranged on a single stick (*e.g.,* pH, protein, glucose), the chemical reagents for each test are separated by a water-permeable barrier made of plastic.

In addition to dipsticks there are other reagent strips, chemical tablets, and treated slides for special determinations such as bacteria, PKU, mucopolysaccharide, salicylate, and cystinuria.

Procedure
1. Use fresh urine.
2. Dip a reagent strip in well-mixed urine, remove, and compare each reagent area with the corresponding color chart on the bottle label at the number of seconds specified on the bottle (*e.g.,* 30 seconds). Hold the strip close to the color blocks and match carefully.
3. Read directions from the manufacturer.

Interfering Factors
1. If dipsticks are kept too long in the urine or urine stream, the chemicals impregnated in the cellulose may be overly dissolved, resulting in an inaccurate reading.
2. If the chemicals in each impregnated pad become mixed, the readings will be inaccurate.

Clinical Alert
1. Precise timing is essential or the color change is meaningless. For example, glucose and ketone test areas are so sensitive that over-timing by only 1 to 3 seconds will demonstrate falsely high amounts of the substance.
2. The frequent review of the instruction sheet accompanying the bottles of dipsticks must be done by all who test urine. This is because manufacturers change procedures and interfering substances are updated frequently.
3. When not in use, the container for the tablets, tapes, or dipsticks should be tightly closed to keep the reagents dry. If the dipsticks, tapes, or tables absorb moisture from the air before

they are used, they will not give correct results. The desiccant should remain in the container.
4. Certain drugs give false-positive reactions.

TYPES OF URINE SPECIMENS

During the course of 24 hours, the composition of urine continuously changes. For this reason, various types of urine specimens are collected for urinalysis.
Single, random specimen
Timed, short-term specimen
Timed, long-term specimen (12- or 24-hr.)

Single, Random Specimen

Most testing is done on a random specimen of urine freshly voided by the patient. Since the composition of urine changes over the course of the day, the time of day when the specimen is collected may influence the findings. The first voided morning specimen is particularly valuable, for it is usually concentrated and more likely to reveal abnormalities and formed substances. Since the chemical testing involved in urinalysis measures the concentration of substances, the results will vary whether or not the urine is dilute. Significant cellular abnormalities will be missed in dilute urine that is collected during the day. Morning specimens are more concentrated and are also relatively free of dietary influences and of changes due to physical activity since they are collected after a period of fasting.

Procedure

1. The patient is instructed to void directly into a clean, dry container or into a clean, dry bedpan and then transfer the specimen directly into an appropriate container. Women should always have a clean, voided specimen if a microscopic examination is ordered.
2. Specimens from infants and young children can be collected in a disposable collection apparatus consisting of a plastic bag with an adhesive backing around the opening that can be fastened to the child so that voiding is done directly into the bag.
3. All specimens should be covered and sent immediately to the laboratory.
4. If a urine specimen is likely to be contaminated with vaginal dis-

charge or menstrual blood, then a clean specimen must be obtained using the same procedure for bacteriologic examination (see section on collection of specimens for culture in Chapter 7, Microbiological Studies).

Interfering Factors

1. Glycosuria appears more often after meals.
2. Proteinuria may occur following strenuous activity or upon assuming an upright position.
3. Hemoglobin may appear in the urine following exertion.
4. In urinary infections the number of bacteria in the urine varies during the day.
5. Feces, vaginal secretion, and menstrual fluid can contaminate the specimen.
6. If the specimen is kept unrefrigerated for more than 1 hour before analysis, changes in the constitution of the urine may occur.
   (a) Bacteria in the urine "split" the urea, converting it to ammonia and producing an alkaline urine.
   (b) Casts decompose in urine after several hours.
   (c) Red blood cells are lysed by hypotonic urine.
   (d) Very low or very high pH may affect cellular components.

Clinical Alert

1. If the specimen is kept for more than 1 hour before analysis, it should be refrigerated to avoid changes in the urine.
2. If the specimen is contaminated by feces or vaginal discharge, a clean voided specimen must be obtained.

Timed, Long-Term Specimen (24-hr.)

Explanation of Test

Some diseases or conditions require that a 24-hour urine specimen be collected in order to evaluate truly and accurately the kidney function. Substances excreted by the kidney are not excreted at the same rate or in the same amounts during various periods of the day and night. Therefore, a random urine specimen would not give an accurate picture of the processes taking place. For measurement of total urine protein, creatinine, electrolytes, and so forth, more accurate information is obtained from urine collected over a 24-hour period. This involves collecting the specimen in a suitable receptacle and either adding a preservative to it or keeping it refrigerated.

Procedure
1. At the beginning of the collection of a 24-hour timed urine specimen (or any timed specimen), the patient is asked to void, the specimen is *discarded*, and the time noted.
2. The time the test begins is placed on the label along with the time the collection should end.
3. All urine passed over the next 24 hours is collected in a large container (usually made of polyethylene), labeled with the patient's name, and marked for the particular test ordered. It is not necessary to measure urine unless explicitly stated for individual tests.
4. To conclude the collection, the patient must void 24 hours after the first voiding. Urine from this last voiding must be added to the specimen in the container.

   Note: Since the patient may not always be able to void on command, a last specimen should be obtained as close as possible to the stated end of time for the final test and the exact time marked on the bottle.
5. Storage
   (a) In the hospital, nonrefrigerated tests may be kept in a soiled utility room or in the patient's bathroom.
   (b) If refrigeration is necessary, the urine specimen must be refrigerated immediately after the patient has voided or it should be placed in an iced container.

Clinical Implications
1. Responsibility for the collection of urine specimens should be assigned to a specific person.
2. All persons instructing a patient about 24-hour urine collections should make certain that the patient understands that he must void and empty his bladder at the time the 24-hour collection is to start and that this specimen is to be discarded.
3. Do not predate and pretime the laboratory slips, for it is rare for patients to urinate on the hour.
4. It cannot be stressed enough that the marking of exact time is crucial and that it is not important whether this is 15 or 30 minutes more or less than 24 hours, provided the information is accurate.
5. The patient should be reminded to try to urinate near the end of the collection period.
6. Whenever a preservative has to be used (such as the hydrochloric acid preservative used for 24-hour urine collection of vanillylmandelic acid), the patient should be warned to take precautions against spilling any liquid from the container.
7. Patients who are using bedpans should be instructed to void before having a bowel movement. Otherwise they may forget and urinate into the pan while having a bowel movement, thus spoiling the urine collection.

Interfering Factors
1. Failure of the patient or attending personnel to comprehend the procedure is the most common source of error.
2. Toilet paper in the collection container may decrease the actual amount of urine saved or possibly contaminate the specimen in some way.
3. Feces in the collection container also may contaminate the specimen. For this reason, patients who are using bedpans should be instructed to void before having a bowel movement.

Patient Preparation
Most 24-hour urine specimens are started in the morning.

1. Empty the bladder completely on awakening in the morning and discard this urine specimen. Record the time the discarded specimen was voided (7:08 A.M.), and begin the test (7:08 A.M.)
2. Save all urine passed during the rest of the day and night. Also save the first specimen of urine passed the next morning.
3. The bedpan, urinal, or the collection bottle itself can be used for each voiding.
4. It is most important that *all* urine be saved and placed in the container. Ideally, the container should be stored in the refrigerator.
5. Test results are calculated on the basis of a 24-hour output, and unless all urine is saved, results will not be accurate. (This is particularly important, for this test is expensive, complicated, and necessary for the evaluation and treatment of the patient's condition.)
6. The urine voided the next morning (as close to 7:00 A.M. as possible) is added to the collection container, and the 24-hour test is terminated. Write down the time of this last voiding.

ROUTINE URINALYSIS (UA) AND RELATED TESTS

Normal Values

General Characteristics and Measurements	Chemical Determinations	Microscopic Examination of Sediment
Color: yellow–amber— indicates a high specific gravity and small output of urine.	Glucose: negative	Casts negative: occasional hyaline casts
	Ketones: negative	
	Blood: negative	Red blood cells negative or rare
	Protein: negative	
Turbidity: clear to slightly hazy	Bilirubin: negative	Crystals negative
Specific gravity: 1.015–1.025 with a normal fluid intake	Urobilinogen: 0.1–1	White blood cells negative or rare
pH: 4.6–4.8—average person has a pH of about 6 (acid)	Nitrate for bacteria: negative	
	Leukocyte esterase: negative	

Explanation of Test

Urinalysis is the means of determining the various properties of urine: color, odor, turbidity, specific gravity, pH, glucose, ketones, blood, protein, bilirubin, urobilinogen, nitrate, and leukocyte esterase, as well as any abnormal constituents revealed by microscopic examination of the sediment. A 10 ml. urine specimen is usually sufficient for conducting these tests.

Specific Gravity (S.G.)

Normal Values

1.003–1.035 (usually between 1.010 and 1.025) S.G.
1.025–1.030 + (concentrated urine) S.G.
1.001–1.010 (dilute urine) S.G.

Explanation of Test

Specific gravity is a means by which the kidneys' ability to concentrate urine is measured. The test is conducted by comparing the weight of urine against the weight of distilled water, which has a specific gravity of 1.000. Since urine is a solution of minerals, salts, and compounds dissolved in water, the specific gravity is obviously greater than 1.000. The relative difference between the specific gravity and the specific gravity of urine reflects the degree of concentration of the urine specimen; specific gravity correlates roughly with osmolality.

The range of urine specific gravity depends on the state of hydration and varies with urine volume and the load of solids to be excreted. When fluid intake is restricted or increased, under standardized conditions, specific gravity measures the concentrating and diluting abilities of the kidney. Loss of these capacities is an indication of renal dysfunction.

Procedure

1. Refractometer
   (a) Specific gravity is most frequently determined with a refractometer or total solids meter (TS). The refractive index (RI) is the ratio of light velocity to the specific gravity of the urinometer.
2. Specific gravity can be tested using a multiple dipstick that has a separate reagent area for specific gravity.
3. Specimen collection
   (a) For regular urinalysis testing, a random specimen is used. One to two milliliters is needed for testing with a refractometer.
   (b) When evaluation of specific gravity is ordered separately from the urinalysis, the patient should fast for 12 hours before the specimen is collected.

Clinical Implications

A. *Normal*
   Specific gravity varies inversely with urine excretion (decrease in volume; increase in specific gravity).
   Examples of conditions in which this relationship is affected
   1. Diabetes: increased volume; increased specific gravity
   2. Hypertension: normal volume; decreased specific gravity
   3. Early chronic renal disease: increased volume; decreased specific gravity
B. *Low specific gravity* (1.001–1.0010)
   1. Diabetes insipidus
      (a) Low specific gravity and large urine volume.
      (b) Due to absence of antidiuretic hormone (ADH). ADH triggers kidney absorption of water; without it kidneys produce excessive amounts of urine (sometimes 15–20 liters a day).
   2. Glomerulonephritis and pyelonephritis (but not in acute disease). Specific gravity can be low in glomerulonephritis when disease occurs.
      (a) Decreased volume, low specific gravity
      (b) Tubular damage affects kidneys' ability to concentrate urine.
   3. Severe renal damage
      Fixed low specific gravity (1.010) that varies little from specimen to specimen.
C. *Increased specific gravity*
   1. Diabetes mellitus or nephrosis
      Abnormally large amounts of glucose and protein increase the specific gravity up to 1.050.
   2. Occurs in instances of excessive water loss (dehydration, fever, vomiting, diarrhea)

Interfering Factors

1. Specific gravity is highest in the morning specimen.
2. Specific gravity is elevated whenever there is an excessive loss of water.
3. Radiopaque contrast media used in radiographs of urinary tract and dextrin may cause false positives.
4. Temperature of urine specimens affects specific gravity when specific gravity is measured in urine removed from the refrigerator. Specific gravity will be falsely higher.
5. Highly buffered alkaline urine may also cause a low reading.
6. Elevated readings may occur in the presence of moderate (100–750) mg./dl. of protein.

Concentration

Normal Values
Methods of concentration testing

Fishberg test: specific gravity of 1:024 or higher on one specimen and up to 300 ml. of urine

Mosenthal's test: 1.020 and at least a seven-point difference between the lowest and highest specific gravity

Volhard's test: 1.025 or higher with osmolality showing rise above 800 on at least one specimen in the afternoon.

Explanation of Test
This test is carried out in patients with suspected renal disease and measures the kidneys' ability to concentrate urine after liquids have been withheld from the diet for a number of hours. The goal of the test is to see if the kidneys can produce urine with a specific gravity greater than 1.020.

In health, specific gravity normally ranges from 1.003 to 1.035 or higher. When fluids are restricted in accordance with this test, the urine produced is more concentrated and has a specific gravity higher than 1.020 to 1.025. Kidney dysfunction can result in *isothenuria* (urine specific gravity remains consistently at 1.010) or *hyposthenuria* (urine specific gravity is less than 1.008). Whenever a more precise measurement is indicated, osmolality of urine can be determined. Osmolality is a measure of the number of particles in a given weight.

Procedure
A. *Pretest preparation*
   1. All diuretics should be stopped 48 to 72 hours prior to the test and during the test.
   2. An adequate protein diet and normal hydration should be followed for 3 days before the test.
   3. No medications should be given.
B. *Test procedure*
   1. The test begins at 6:00 P.M. after which time no fluids are permitted until the test is completed ("dry" foods are permitted).
   2. At 10:00 P.M., the patient voids, *discards* the specimen, and may retire.
   3. The next morning, urine specimens are collected at 6:00 A.M., 7:00 A.M., and 8:00 A.M. Keep specimens separate. (Normally, kidneys concentrate urine at twice the rate during the night as during waking hours.) If patient voids during the night, save this urine and send it to the laboratory in a separate labeled container.

4. The volume of each urine specimen and total volume of all three specimens are measured and recorded.
5. The specific gravity or osmolality (see pgs. 125 and 129) of each specimen is measured.

Clinical Implications

1. A specific gravity of less than 1.020 on all specimens indicates renal disease. With severe involvement the specific gravity is persistently 1.010 or less.
   (a) Total loss of urinary concentrating ability with fixed specific gravity near 1.010 or osmolality between 300 and 400 mOsm/kg. is not seen until very late in the course of renal disease.
   (b) Abnormal concentration levels generally reflect progressive inability of the kidneys to increase the osmotic pressure of urine above that of the glomerular filtrate in chronic renal failure.
2. A normal finding does not necessarily rule out active kidney disease.
3. A specific gravity of 1.020 occurs in
   (a) Potassium deficiency
   (b) Hypercalcemia due to sarcoidosis
   (c) Bone disease (multiple myeloma; vitamin D intoxication or sensitivity)
   (d) Hyperparathyroidism
   (e) Renal parenchymal disease, such as pyelonephritis, which damages the tubules
   (f) Acute renal disease
4. The urine may be abnormally concentrated for a day or so after injection of dyes used in intravenous pyelograms (IVP).
5. Edema, sweats, diarrhea, and fever interfere with the water tests.
6. Concentration tests are meaningless in patients taking diuretics.
7. Patients who have been markedly overhydrated for several days prior to testing may have impaired concentration if dehydration is then imposed.

Interfering Factors

The test is unreliable when the patient is pregnant, is on low salt or protein diets, or suffers from severe water or electrolyte imbalance, chronic liver disease, edema from renal disease, or heart failure. In these conditions the tubules may be unable to concentrate urine.

Patient Preparation

1. Explain the purpose and procedure of the test to the patient.
2. Instruct the patient to completely empty the bladder at each voiding.

Clinical Alert
1. The fluid deprivation required in this test may be contraindicated in some patients with heart disease or early renal failure.
2. Accidental or deliberate fluid intake during the night will interfere with the results. Reschedule the test if this occurs.

Osmolality

Normal Values
After 12-hr. fluid restriction: 850 osmol./kg.

Background
Osmolality, a more exact measurement of urine concentration than specific gravity, depends on the number of particles of solute in a unit of solution, whereas specific gravity depends on both the quantity and precise nature of the particles in the unit. Protein, sugar, and IV contrasts elevate urine specific gravity disproportionately more than the elevate osmolality.

Explanation of Test
Whenever a more precise measurement than specific gravity is indicated in the evaluation of the concentration and diluting ability of the kidney, this test is done. The measurement of urine osmolality during water restriction is an accurate test of decreased kidney function. It is also used in the differential diagnosis of diabetes insipidus (compulsive water drinking).

Procedure
1. A high protein diet is prescribed for 3 days.
2. On the evening before the test, a dry supper is eaten and no liquids drunk until the test is over.
3. At approximately 6:00 A.M., the patient empties the bladder and returns to bed. This urine is not saved.
4. The test urine specimen is collected at 8:00 A.M., the sample is labeled and sent to the laboratory, and the proceedings are entered on the patient's record. The test is then completed.

Clinical Implications
1. *Increased* in
   (a) Postsurgery
   (b) Hepatic cirrhosis
   (c) Congestive heart failure
   (d) Addison's disease
   (e) IV sodium
   (f) High protein diets
   (g) Inappropriate ADH secretion

2. *Decreased* in
   (a) Aldosteronism   (d) Hypercalcemia
   (b) Diabetes insipidus   (e) Compulsive water drinking
   (c) Hypokalemia   (f) IV 5% dextrose and water

Patient Preparation
1. Explain the purpose and procedure of the test to the patient.
2. No liquids are to be taken with the evening meal before the test. No food or liquids should be taken after the evening meal until the test is completed.

Patient Aftercare
Provide the patient with foods and fluids as soon as the 8:00 A.M. urine sample is obtained.

Color

Normal Values
Yellow is the normal color of urine. The specific gravity ranges from 1.011 to 1.019 and the urine output is 1 to 1½ liters per day.
Straw colored urine is normal and indicates a low specific gravity, usually under 1.010. (The exception is a patient with a 4 + sugar; urine is very light and looks like water, but the specific gravity is high.)
Amber colored urine is normal and indicates a high specific gravity and a small output of urine. Specific gravity is above 1.020 and output is less than 1 liter per day.

Explanation of Test
Urine specimens may vary in color from pale yellow to dark amber. The intensity of the normal amber color may be related directly to the concentration or specific gravity of the urine. The color of normal urine is primarily due to urochrome (pigments that are present in the diet or formed from the metabolism of bile). Due to the presence of abnormal pigments, the color of urine changes in many disease states.

Procedure
Observe color of urine specimen.

Clinical Implications
1. A nearly *colorless* urine may be due to
   (a) Large fluid intake
   (b) Reduction in perspiration
   (c) Chronic interstitial nephritis
   (d) Untreated diabetes mellitus
   (e) Diabetes insipidus
   (f) Alcohol ingestion

     (g) Diuretic therapy

     (h) Nervousness

2. An *orange-colored* urine may be due to

     (a) Concentrated urine

     (b) Restricted fluid intake

     (c) Excess sweating

     (d) Fever

     (e) Small quantities of bile pigment

3. A *brownish yellow or greenish yellow* color may indicate bilirubin in the urine.

     (a) However, not all dark urines contain bilirubin.

     (b) Stale urine containing bilirubin may be green due to an oxidation of the bilirubin to biliverdin.

     (c) Bilirubin crystals in the sediment may cause the urine to have an opalescent appearance.

     (d) *Yellow foam* may be due to biliverdin bile pigment.

     (e) *Green foam* may be due to biliverdin bile pigment.

4. A *red or reddish dark brown* color may indicate hemoglobinuria and may be due to blood, porphyrins, hemoglobin, myoglobin.

5. A *port wine* color may be due to porphyrins or a mixture of methemoglobin and oxyhemoglobin.

6. *Dark brown* urine may be due to prophyrias, melanin.

     (a) May indicate a melanotic tumor

     (b) Is sometimes associated with Addison's disease

7. *Brown black* urine may be due to a great deal of hemoglobin, lysol poisoning, or melanin.

8. *Black* urine results from alkaptonuria, a disease of tyrosine metabolism, which causes the urine to turn black on standing.

9. *Smoky* color may be due to red blood cells.

Interfering Factors

1. The color of normal urine darkens on standing. This is due to the oxidation of urobilinogen to urobilin. Decomposition starts in 30 minutes. Many people erroneously call it bilirubin. A trained eye can detect slight increases in urobilinogen.

2. Some foods cause the urine to change color.

     (a) Beets will turn the urine *red*.

     (b) Rhubarb can cause the color to be *brown*.

3. Many drugs cause the urine to change color.

     (a) Cascara and senna laxatives in acid urine will turn the urine *reddish brown;* in alkaline urine they will turn the urine *red*.

     (b) *Orange* may be due to phenazopyridine (Pyridium), amidopyrine.

     (c) *Orange to orange red* may be due to Pyridium, ethoxazene.

     (d) *Orange to purple red* may be due to chlorzoxazone.

(e) *Orange yellow* in alkaline urine may be due to salicylazosulfa-pyridine, anisindione, or phenindione.
(f) *Rust yellow to brownish* may be due to sulfonamides, nitrofuran-toins.
(g) *Pink to red or red brown* may be due to Dilantin (diphenylhydan-toin), Doxidan (dioctyl calcium sulfosuccinate), Ex-Lax (phenolphthalein) and phenothiazine (thiodiphenylamine).
(h) *Magenta* may be due to Ex-Lax.
(i) *Red* may be due to amidopyrine, Pyridium, Neotropin, Pronto-sil, aniline dyes, PSP and BSP dyes in alkaline urine, phenol-phthalein and Pyridium in acid urine, or Desferal (deferox-amine).
(j) *Purple red* may be due to Ex-Lax in alkaline urine.
(k) *Dark brown* may be due to phenolic drugs, phenylhydrazine.
(l) *Brown black* may be due to Jecotofer, cascara.
(m) *Bright yellow* may be due to riboflavin or Pyridium in alkaline urine.
(n) *Blue or green* may be due to methylene blue and amitriptyline.
(o) Urine that *darkens* on standing may be due to antiparkinsonian agents such as levodopa or Sinemet.
(p) *Dark colored* urine may be due to iron salts.
(q) *Pink to brown* may be due to phenothiazine tranquilizer.
(r) *Pale blue* may be due to Dyrenium (triamterene).

Clinical Alert

If the urine is a red color, do not assume drug causation. Check the urine for hemoglobin.

Odor

The characteristic odor of normal, freshly voided urine is due to the presence of volatile acids.

Normal Values
Fresh urine from most healthy persons has an aromatic odor.

Clinical Implications
1. The sweet smell of acetone can be recognized in diabetic ketosis.
2. Heavily infected urine has a particularly unpleasant odor.
3. An inherited disorder of amino acid metabolism is characterized by the passage of urine in infants that smells like maple syrup. This condition is maple sugar urine disease.

Interfering Factors
1. Some foods, such as asparagus, produce characteristic odors.
2. After urine stands for a long time, ammonia with its characteristic pungent odor is formed by bacterial activity and the decomposition of urea in the specimen.

pH

Normal Values
Average range: 4.6–8
Average pH is about 6 (acid)
(The pH of normal urine can vary widely.)

Background
The symbol "pH" expresses the exact strength of the urine as a dilute acid or a base solution and measures the free hydrogen ion (H^+) concentration in the urine. (The lower the pH, the greater the acidity.) pH, therefore, is an indication of the renal tubules' ability to maintain normal hydrogen ion concentration in the plasma and extracellular fluid. The kidneys maintain normal acid–base balance primarily through the reabsorption of sodium and the tubular secretion of hydrogen and ammonium in exchange. Secretion of an acid or alkaline urine by the kidneys is one of the most important mechanisms of the body for maintaining a constant body pH.

Urine becomes increasingly acidic as the amount of sodium and excess acid retained by the body increases. Alkaline urine, usually containing bicarbonate–carbonic acid buffer, is normally excreted when there is an excess of base or alkali in the body.

Ingestion of different foods and sodium bicarbonate also affects the urinary pH. The usual diet, rich in animal protein, produces an acid urine (pH less than 7).

Control of pH
Control of urinary pH is important in the management of several diseases including bacteriuria and renal calculi and in drug therapy in which streptomycin or Mandelamine (methenamine mandelate) is administered.

A. *Renal calculi*
   Renal stone formation is partially dependent on the pH of urine. Patients being treated for renal calculi are frequently given diets or medication to change the pH of the urine so kidney stones will not form.
   1. Calcium phosphate, calcium carbonate, and magnesium phosphate stones develop in alkaline urine. In such instances the urine must be kept acid.

2. Uric acid, cystine and calcium oxalate stones precipitate in acid urines. In the treatment of these urinary calculi, the urine should be kept alkaline.

B. *Drug treatment*
   1. Streptomycin, neomycin, and kanamycin are effective in genitourinary tract infections provided the urine is *alkaline*.
   2. During sulfa therapy, an *alkaline* urine should help prevent formation of sulfonamide crystals.
   3. Urine should also be kept persistently *alkaline* in control of salicylate intoxication (excretion is enhanced) and during blood transfusions.

C. *Clinical conditions*
   The urine should be kept *acid* in the treatment of urinary tract infections and persistent bacteriuria and in the management of those urinary calculi that develop in alkaline urine.

D. *Diet*
   1. A diet that emphasizes citrus fruits and most vegetables, particularly legumes, will help keep the urine alkaline.
   2. A diet high in meat and cranberry juice will keep the urine acid.

Explanation of Test

Urine pH is an important screening test for diagnosing renal disease, respiratory disease, and certain metabolic disorders. It is also used to monitor specific programs of medication or diet when it is desirable to maintain the urine as acid or alkaline. Keeping the urine at a consistently high or low pH requires frequent testing of the urinary pH.

Dipstick measurement
1. Multiple reagent strips treated with chemicals provide a spectrum of color changes from orange to green blue in the pH range of 5 to 9.
2. The dipstick is dipped into a urine specimen and the color change is compared to a standardized color chart on the bottle.

Clinical Implications

If urine pH is to be useful, it is necessary to use the pH information in conjunction with other information. For example, in renal tubular necrosis, the kidney is not able to excrete a urine that is strongly acid. Therefore, if a urine pH of 5 (quite acid) is measured, renal tubular acidosis is eliminated as a possibility.

A. *Acid urine (pH less than 7)*
   1. Found in acidosis, uncontrolled diabetes, pulmonary emphysema, diarrhea, starvation, dehydration
   2. Rarely excreted in severe alkalosis
   3. Found in respiratory diseases where CO_2 retention occurs and acidosis develops

B. *Alkaline urine* (pH more than 7)
   1. Found in urinary tract infections, pyloric obstruction, salicylate intoxications, renal tubular acidosis, and chronic renal failure
   2. Rarely excreted during severe acidosis
   3. Found in respiratory diseases involving hyperventilation and loss of CO_2 with alkalosis

Interfering Factors
1. On standing, the pH of urine specimens will become alkaline because bacteria split urea, producing ammonia.
2. Alkaline urine specimens tend to cause hemolysis of red cells and the disappearance of casts.
3. High protein diets will cause excessively acid urine (pH less than 6).
4. Ammonium chloride and mandelic acid may produce acid urines.
5. Alkaline urine after meals is a normal response to the secretions of HCl acid in gastric juices.
6. Sodium bicarbonate, potassium citrate, and acetazolamide may produce alkaline urines.

Clinical Alert
1. An accurate measurement of urinary pH can be done only on a freshly voided specimen. If the urine must be kept for any length of time before analysis, it should be refrigerated.
2. Alkaline urine occurs from vegetarian diets, citrus fruits, milk, and other dairy products.
3. Highly concentrated urine, such as that formed in hot, dry environments, is strongly acidic and may be irritating.
4. During sleep, decreased pulmonary ventilation causes respiratory acidosis, and urine becomes highly acid.
5. Chlorothiazide diuretic administration will cause an acid urine to be excreted.
6. Bacteria in urinary tract infection or bacterial contamination of the specimen will result in an alkaline urine. Bacteria in the urine will convert urea to ammonia.

Turbidity

Normal Values
Fresh urine is clear to slightly hazy.

Explanation of Test
The appearance of cloudy urine provides a warning of possible abnormality such as the presence of pus, red blood cells, or bacteria. How-

ever, excretion of cloudy urine may not be abnormal since the change in urine pH may cause precipitation within the bladder of normal urinary constituents. Alkaline urine may appear cloudy because of the presence of phosphates, and acid urine may appear cloudy because of urates.

Procedure
Observe the appearance of a fresh urine sample.

Clinical Implications
1. Pathologic urines are often turbid or cloudy, but so are many normal urines. Cloudy urine may result from precipitation of crystals due to rapid cooling of the urine.
2. Occasionally, urine turbidity may result from urinary tract infections.
3. Abnormal urines may be cloudy due to the presence of red blood cells, white blood cells, or bacteria.

Interfering Factors
1. After ingestion of food, urates or phosphates may produce cloudiness in normal urine.
2. Vaginal contamination from female patients is a common cause of turbidity.
3. "Greasy" cloudiness may be caused by large amounts of fat.
4. Many normal urines will develop a haze or turbidity after refrigeration or standing at room temperature.

Blood or Hemoglobin (Heme)

Normal Values
Negative

Explanation of Test
Blood in the urine is usually occult blood that has been hemolyzed or dissolved. Hemoglobin or red blood cells in the urine are not likely to be identified by the naked eye when there is less than one part of the blood per 1000 parts of urine.

The presence of free hemoglobin in the urine is referred to as *hemoglobinuria*. Hemoglobinuria is usually related to conditions outside the urinary tract and occurs when there is such extensive or rapid destruction (hemolysis) of circulating erythrocytes that the reticuloendothelial system cannot metabolize or store the excessive amounts of free hemoglobin.

When intact red blood cells are present in the urine, the term *hematuria* is used to indicate bleeding somewhere in the urinary tract. Usually, both red blood cells and hemoglobin mark this disorder. Therefore, hematuria can be distinguished from hemoglobinuria by a microscopic examination of the sediment from a fresh urine specimen.

The use of both urine dipstick and microscopic examination provide a complete clinical evaluation in regard to hemoglobinuria and hematuria. New dipsticks contain a lysing reagent that reads with occult blood urea and this can detect intact as well as lysed RBCs.

When urine gives a positive result for occult blood, but no red blood cells are seen in a microscopic examination of the sediment, *myoglobinuria* can be suspected. Myoglobinuria is the excretion of myoglobin, a muscle protein, into the urine as a result of (1) traumatic muscle injury such as may occur in automobile accidents, football injuries, or electric shock, (2) a muscle disorder such as an arterial occlusion to a muscle or muscular dystrophy, or (3) certain kinds of poisoning such as carbon monoxide or fish poisoning. Myoglobin has to be distinguished from free hemoglobin in the urine by chemical tests (see pg. 191).

Procedure
A. *Hemoglobin in urine—Hemoglobinuria*
   1. Chemical strips are dipped into the urine, and the color change on the dipstick is noted.
   2. The color of the strip is compared with a color chart.
   3. The color blocks indicate negative, moderate, and large amounts of hemoglobin. The striped area indicates trace, possible intact red blood cells; solid indicates possible free hemoglobin or myoglobin.
B. *Hematuria*
   1. The dipstick method allows detection of intact RBCs when greater than 10/HPF (high-powered field).
   2. To identify red blood cells, the urine is centrifuged and the sediment examined microscopically (see pg. 152).

Clinical Implications
1. *Hematuria* is found in
   (a) Lower urinary tract infection
   (b) Lupus erythematosus
   (c) Polyarteritis nodosa
   (d) Malignant hypertension
   (e) Subacute bacterial endocarditis
   (f) Glomerulonephritis
   (g) Heavy smokers
2. Usually, when blood is present in urine, protein will also be present.
3. *Hemoglobinuria* is found in
   (a) Extensive burns and crushing injuries
   (b) Transfusion reactions to incompatible blood
   (c) Febrile intoxication

(d) Chemical agents and alkaloids (poisonous mushrooms, snake venom)
(e) Malaria
(f) Irrigation of operated prostatic bed with water
(g) Hemolytic anemias
(h) Paroxysmal hemoglobinuria (Large quantities of hemoglobin appear in urine at irregular intervals.)

Clinical Alert

One of the early indications of renal disease is the appearance of blood in the urine. This does not mean that blood will be present in every voided specimen in every case of renal disease. It does mean that in most cases of renal disease, occult blood appears in the urine with a reasonable degree of frequency.

Interfering Factors
1. Drugs causing a positive result
   (a) Drugs that are toxic to the kidneys (bacitracin and amphotericin)
   (b) Drugs that cause actual bleeding (coumarin)
   (c) Drugs that cause hemolysis of RBCs (aspirin)
   (d) Drugs that may give a false-positive result include bromides, copper, iodides, and oxidizing agents.
2. High doses of ascorbic acid may give a false-negative result. (Ascorbic acid may be a preservative for antibiotics such as tetracycline or high vitamin C intake.)
3. High specific gravity or elevated protein reduces sensitivity.
4. Myoglobin—false positive.
5. Highly alkaline urine tends to cause hemolysis of red cells.

Protein (Albumin); Qualitative (24-hr.)

Normal Values
50–80 mg/24 hrs.
1–14 mg./dl. or 10–40 g./liter

Explanation of Test
Detection of protein in urine (proteinuria), combined with a microscopic examination of urinary sediment, provides the basis for differential diagnosis of renal disease.

In health, the urine contains no protein or only trace amounts of protein, which consists of albumin (one-third of normal urine protein is albumin) and globulins from the plasma. Since albumin is filtered more readily than the globulins, it is usually very abundant in pathologic conditions. Therefore, the term *albuminuria* is often used synonymously with *proteinuria*.

Normally, the glomerules prevent passage of protein from the blood to the glomular filtrate. Thus, the persistent presence of protein in the urine is the single most important indication of renal disease. Therefore, if more than a trace of protein is found in the urine, a quantitative 24-hour evaluation of protein excretion is necessitated.

Bence Jones Protein

Electrophoresis of urine or turbidimetric methods can be used to demonstrate Bence Jones protein, a specific low molecular weight protein. The dipstick method does not react very well with globulins; however, albumin reacts very well. This protein is found in

Forty percent of multiple myeloma cases

Tumor metastasis to the bone

Chronic lymphocytic leukemia

Amyloidosis

Macroglobulinemia

Clinical Alert

If the dipstick is negative for protein and one of the above conditions is suspected, the turbidimetric SSA method should be used and electrophoresis should be performed. It is especially important if the patient is older. This discrepancy also exists with high doses of penicillin and radiograph contrast media. If the dipstick is negative and subsequent tests are positive, this should be reported.

Procedure

To collect a specimen for qualitative protein
1. Collect urine in a clean container and test it as soon as possible.
2. Test the specimen by dipping a reagent strip into a well-mixed sample of urine, and compare the color changes immediately with the color charts provided.

Collecting the Specimen for Orthostatic Proteinuria

1. The patient is instructed to void at bedtime and discard the urine.
2. The next morning a urine specimen is collected immediately after the patient awakes and has assumed a standing position.

3. A second specimen is collected after the patient has been standing or walking for a period of time.

Differentiation from other types of proteinuria is done by testing for protein in two urine specimens: one collected before and one collected after the person is erect. In postural proteinuria the first specimen contains no protein, while the second is positive.

Procedure (for 24-Hour Collection)
1. A 24-hour urine container is labeled with the name of the patient, test, and the date.
2. Refrigeration or formalin preservation of the specimen is required.
3. General instructions for 24-hour urine collection are on page 122.
4. The exact start and ending of the collection are recorded on the specimen container with the patient's record (start 7:30 A.M. 2/6 and end 7:38 A.M. 2/7).

Interfering Factors
1. Because of renal vasoconstriction, functional, mild, and transitory protein in the urine is associated with
   (a) Violent exercise
   (b) Severe emotional stress
   (c) Cold baths
2. Increased protein in urine occurs
   (a) After eating large amounts of protein
   (b) In pregnancy or immediately following delivery
   (c) In newborn infants
   (d) In premenstrual state
   (e) In orthostatic proteinuria
3. False or accidental proteinuria may be present because of a mixture of pus and red blood cells in urinary tract infections and the menstrual flow.
4. False-positive results can occur from incorrect use and assessment out of the color strip test.
   (a) Prolonged dipping or allowing the strip to be held too long in the urine stream
   (b) Failing to match accurately the reactive area with the color chart
5. Alkaline urine can give a false-positive result on the color strip test due to alkaline, highly buffered urine.
6. A very dilute urine may give a falsely low protein value.
7. Drugs may cause false-positive and false-negative tests for protein.

Clinical Implications
1. Significant proteinuria indicates an abnormally high excretion of protein. Proteinuria is usually the result of increased glomerular

filtration of protein because of some kind of glomerular damage. A follow-up 24-hour urine test for protein is indicated to arrive at a specific diagnosis.

2. Continued proteinuria of any amount in an apparently healthy person usually indicates minimal renal disease.
3. In pathologic states, the level of proteinuria is rarely constant, and not every sample of urine will be abnormal in patients with disease.
4. Proteinuria occurs in the following diseases:
   (a) Nephritis
   (b) Nephrosis
   (c) Polycystic kidney
   (d) Tuberculosis and cancer of the kidney
   (e) Kidney stones
5. Proteinuria may occur in the following nonrenal diseases and conditions:
   (a) Fever
   (b) Trauma
   (c) Severe anemias and leukemia
   (d) Toxemia
   (e) Abdominal tumors
   (f) Convulsive disorders
   (g) Hyperthyroidism
   (h) Intestinal obstruction
   (i) Cardiac disease
   (j) Ascites
   (k) Liver disease
   (l) Acute infections
   (m)Poisoning from turpentine, phosphorous, mercury, sulfosalicylic acid, lead, phenol, opiates, and drug therapy
6. Large numbers of leukocytes accompanying proteinuria usually indicate infection at some level in the urinary tract. Large numbers of both leukocytes and erythrocytes usually indicate a noninfectious inflammatory disease of the glomerulus. Proteins with pyelonephritis may have as many red blood cells as white cells.
7. Proteinuria does not always accompany renal disease. Pyelonephritis, obstructions, nephrolithiasis, tumors, and congenital malformations can cause severe illness without protein leakage.
8. Proteinuria is associated with the finding of casts on the sediment examination because protein is necessary for cast formation.
9. Postural proteinuria is the excretion of protein by patients who are standing or moving in the daytime. The proteinuria is intermittent and disappears when the person lies down. Postural proteinuria occurs in 3% to 5% of healthy young adults.

Patient Preparation
1. Instruct the patient about the purpose and collection of the 24-hour specimen. Stress compliance.
2. Food and fluids are permitted. Fluids should not be forced, for a very dilute urine can give a false-negative value.

Protein Electrophoresis (PEP), Urine

Normal Values
Interpretive report

Explanation of Test
This test is done in the investigation of monoclonal gammopathies.

Procedure
1. When a urine PEP is done, a serum specimen must be submitted at the same time.
2. A fresh random or 24-hour refrigerated specimen is required.

Clinical Implications
1. Trace amounts of urine albumin and occasionally trace amounts of both kappa and lambda light chains occur in a 2 : 1 ratio. Variations in this ratio are suggestive of monoclonal gammopathy or light chain urea.
2. Free light chains are found in
   (a) Other lymphoid diseases
   (b) Renal failure
   (c) Systemic lupus erythematosus (SLE)

Sugar (Glucose)

Normal Values
Random specimen: negative
Quantitative 24-hr specimen: <0.5 g./d. or <2.78 mmol./d
                             1-15 mg./dl. or 0.06–0.83 mmol./liter

Explanation of Test
Urine glucose tests are used in (1) screening to detect diabetes, (2) confirming a diagnosis of diabetes, or (3) monitoring the effectiveness of diabetic control.

Normally, urine does not contain a sufficient amount of sugar to react with any of the popular testing methods. Glucose is always present in the glomerular filtrate, but it is reabsorbed by the proximal tubule. However, should the blood glucose level exceed the reabsorption capacity of the tubules, glucose will be spilled into the urine.

The presence of sugar in the urine (*glucosuria* or *glycosuria*), as evidenced by positive tests, is not necessarily abnormal. For example, sugar may appear in urine after a heavy meal is eaten or in conjunction with emotional stress. In addition, for some persons, a low tubular reabsorption rate may account for glycosuria occurring with normal blood glucose levels. This is a benign condition.

In the majority of cases, however, sugar in the urine is abnormal and is usually due to diabetes mellitus. Nonetheless, a positive test for urine sugar is not adequate for a diagnosis of diabetes. A single measurement of postprandial blood sugar gives more meaningful information in diabetes detection programs than does a urine sugar test. A urine sugar test accompanied by a blood sugar test gives more information than does a blood sugar test alone. Also, a postprandial urine sugar test is a more effective test for recognizing diabetes than a fasting urine sugar test.

Types of Glucose Tests

A. *Reduction tests:* Clinitest
   1. Are based on reduction of certain metal ions by glucose. When added to urine, a heat reaction takes place, resulting in precipitation and a change in color of the urine.
   2. Are considered nonspecific for glucose because the reaction can be brought about by other reducing substances in the urine.
      (a) Hypochlorite or chlorine
      (b) Other sugars, such as galactose, lactose, fructose, and maltose
B. *Enzyme tests:* Clinistix, Diastix, Tes-Tape
   1. Are based on interaction between enzymes and glucose. When dipped into urine the strip changes color according to the amount of glucose in the urine indicated by the manufacturer's color chart.
   2. All are specific for glucose.

Procedure

1. A freshly voided specimen should be used.
2. Directions on the tablet or dipstick container must be followed exactly and the color reaction compared to the closest matching color on the manufacturer's color chart. Timing must be exact.
3. Results are recorded on the patient's record.
4. If a 24-hour urine specimen should be ordered, the urine must be refrigerated or iced during collection.

Clinical Alert

1. Determine exactly what drugs a diabetic is taking and whether the metabolites of these drugs affect the urine test.
2. Do not encourage patients to drink water between the first and second voidings since diluted urine may conceal glucose in the urine.
3. Always test for ketone bodies when the urine contains glucose.
4. Be aware that test results are reported as plus (+) or percentages. Reporting results in percentages is more accurate.

Clinical Implications

1. Increased glucose in the urine is found in diabetes mellitus, brain injury, myocardial infarction, and when a lowered renal threshold (positive urine sugar and a normal blood glucose) is present. An elevated blood glucose and negative urine sugar indicate a high renal threshold.
2. A glucose tolerance test is indicated to confirm diabetes mellitus.
3. The greater the concentration of sugar in the urine, the greater the lack of control of the diabetes.

Interfering Factors

Note: Knowledge of the manufacturer's guidelines on drugs known to affect test results must be continually updated.

1. Pregnancy and lactation may cause a false positive in a Clinitest due to lactose or galactose. About 70% of normal pregnant women show a temporary glucosuria that appears to be of no clinical significance.
2. Ascorbic acid, NegGram, Keflin, creatinine in concentrated urine, streptomycin may cause a false-positive Clinitest result; usually it will be only a trace reaction.
3. Stress, excitement, testing after a heavy meal, and following the administration of IV glucose may cause false positives of all tests. Usually it is a trace reaction.
4. Ascorbic acid in very large amounts may cause a false negative in the enzyme tests.
5. False negatives may be obtained if deteriorated reagent strips have been used, or if directions are not followed exactly.
6. Large amount of ketones—false negative.

Patient Preparation

1. Instruct the patient about the purpose of the test, the method of testing, and the second voiding technique.

2. Patient voids, tests the specimen, and discards it.
3. 30 to 45 minutes later, the patient voids, if possible, and this specimen is tested. The second specimen reflects the immediate state of glucosuria more accurately than the first specimen, which may be urine that has collected in the bladder over a period of hours.

Ketone Bodies (Acetone)

Normal Values
Negative

Explanation of Test
Ketone bodies, resulting from the metabolism of fatty acid and fat, consist mainly of three substances: acetone, betahydroxybutyric acid and acetoacetic acid. The last two substances readily convert to acetone, making acetone, in essence, the main constituent being tested. However, Ames' products measure only acetoacetic acid.

In healthy individuals, ketone bodies are formed in the liver and are completely metabolized so that only negligible amounts appear in the urine. However, when carbohydrate metabolism is altered, an excessive amount of ketones is formed (acetosis) on account of fat becoming the predominant body fuel instead of carbohydrates. When the metabolic pathways of carbohydrates are disturbed, carbon fragments from fat and protein are diverted to form abnormal amounts of ketone bodies. The body's alkaline reserves thus become depleted, resulting in acidosis.

The excess production of ketones (ketonuria) in the urine is mainly associated with diabetes. Testing for ketones in the urine of diabetics may provide the clue to early diagnosis of ketoacidosis and diabetic coma.

Indications for Ketone Testing
A. *General*
   Screening for ketonuria is valuable in hospital admissions, presurgical patients, pregnant women, children, and diabetics.
B. *Glycosuria*
   Testing for ketone bodies is indicated in any patients showing greater than normal excretion of sugar.
C. *Acidosis*
   1. Ketone testing is used to judge the severity of acidosis and to follow the effects of treatment.
   2. Blood ketone measurement frequently provides a more reliable estimate of acidosis than urine testing (especially useful in emergency room situations).

D. *Diabetes*
1. Ketonuria may indicate ketoacidosis and possible diabetic coma.
2. When treatment is being switched from insulin to oral hypoglycemic agents, the development of ketonuria within 24 hours after the withdrawal of insulin usually indicates a poor response to the oral hypoglycemic agents.
3. The urine of diabetics treated with oral hypoglycemic agents should be tested regularly for glucose and ketones, since oral hypoglycemic agents, unlike insulin, do not control diabetes when acute complications such as infection develop.
E. *Pregnancy*
In pregnancy, the early detection of ketones is essential since ketoacidosis is an important factor contributing to death in the uterus.

Procedure
1. Dip the reagent strip in fresh urine, tap the strip to remove excess urine, and compare it to the color chart at the time indicated.
2. Follow the manufacturer's directions exactly.
3. Dipsticks may not be used with *blood*. Acetest tablets are used.

Clinical Implications
1. Ketosis and ketonuria may occur whenever increased amounts of fat are metabolized, carbohydrate intake is restricted, or the diet is rich in fat.
2. Ketonuria occurs in association with
   (a) Fever   (e) Starvation
   (b) Anorexia   (f) Prolonged vomiting
   (c) Diarrhea   (g) Following anesthesia
   (d) Fasting
3. In nondiabetics, ketonuria will occur frequently in acute illness. Fifteen per cent of hospitalized patients will have ketone bodies in their urine even though they do not have diabetes.
4. Children are particularly prone to developing ketonuria and ketosis.
5. Ketone bodies appear in the urine before there is any significant increase of ketone bodies in the blood.

Interfering Factors
1. Carbohydrate-free diets as well as high protein and fat will cause ketonuria.
2. Drugs that may cause a false positive
   (a) Levodopa   (e) Isopropyl alcohol
   (b) Phthalein compound   (f) Metformin
       (BSP or PSP)   (g) Paraldehyde
   (c) Ether   (h) Pyridium
   (d) Insulin   (i) Phenformin

Clinical Implications
1. A test for ketone bodies in the urine is helpful in differentiating between a diabetic coma and an insulin shock.
2. Any stressful situation that distorts the normal regulation of a diabetic can be recognized at any early point by a positive urine ketone test.
3. Urine ketones indicate caution, not a crisis situation, in either a diabetic or a nondiabetic patient.
   (a) In a diabetic patient the appearance of ketone bodies in the urine suggests that the patient is not adequately controlled, and that adjustments of either the medication or the diet should be made promptly.
   (b) In a nondiabetic, ketone bodies indicate a small amount of carbohydrate metabolism and excessive fat metabolism.

Nitrate/Bacteria

Normal Values
Negative for bacteria.

Explanation of Test
There are two methods that are used to detect bacteria in the urine during routine urinalysis: microscopic examination and clinical testing. The sediment, when examined microscopically, can reveal bacteria when present. Chemical dipstick testing is also done routinely. The nitrite area in the multiple reagent strip is calibrated so that any shade of pink color that develops within 30 seconds indicates an amount of nitrite produced by 10^5 or more organisms per ml. in the urine specimen.

Procedure
1. A first morning specimen is preferred because urine that has been in the bladder for several hours is more likely to yield a positive nitrite test than a random urine sample that may have been in the bladder only a short time. A clean catch or midstream urine is needed to avoid bacterial contamination.
2. Follow the procedure stated in the manufacturer's guidelines *exactly* to achieve reliable test results.
3. Comparison of the reacted reagent area against a white background may aid in the detection of low levels that might otherwise be missed.

Clinical Implications
1. The finding of 20 or more bacteria per high-powered field may indicate a urinary tract infection. Untreated bacteriuria can lead to very serious kidney disease.

2. The presence of only a few bacteria should be interpreted with caution and suggests a urinary tract infection that cannot be confirmed or excluded until more definitive studies, such as culture and sensitivity tests, are performed.
3. A positive result from the nitrite test is a reliable indication of significant bacteriuria and is an indication for urine culture.
4. A negative result should *never* be interpreted as indicating absence of bacteriuria because
   (a) If an overnight sample were not used, there may have been insufficient time for the conversion of nitrate to nitrite to have occurred.
   (b) Some urinary tract infections are caused by organisms that do not convert nitrate to nitrite.
   (c) Insufficient dietary nitrate present.

Interfering Factors
1. Azo dye metabolites—false positive
2. Ascorbic acid—false negative
3. High specific gravity—sensitivity reduced false negative

Leukocyte Esterase

Normal Values
Negative

Explanation of Test
There are two methods used to determine the presence of leukocytes (WBCs) in the urine: microscopic examination, and chemical testing, using the leukocyte esterase dipstick. The dipstick is calibrated so that any shade of purple that develops in 60 seconds is considered positive for five or more WBCs per high-powered field. The leukocyte esterase test detects intact leukocytes as well as lysed ones. Since this test measures the esterase activity of leukocytes, WBC casts can also be detected.

Procedure
1. A fresh random specimen is collected. A clean catch or midstream urine is needed to avoid vaginal contamination.
2. Manufacturer's directions must be followed exactly, and timing is critical for accurate results.

Interfering Factors
Vaginal discharge, trichomonas, parasites, and heavy mucus can cause false positives.

Clinical Implications
1. Normal urine gives negative results.
2. Positive results are clinically significant and indicate pyuria.

Clinical Alert

A urine sample that tests positive for both nitrate and leukocyte esterase should be cultured for pathogenic bacteria.

Bilirubin

Normal Values
Negative or 0.02 mg./dl.

Background
Bilirubin is formed in the reticuloendothelial cells of the spleen and bone marrow from the breakdown of hemoglobin and is transported to the liver. Urinary bilirubin excretion will reach significant levels in any disease process that increases the amount of conjugated bilirubin in the bloodstream (see Chemistry Studies, Chapter 6). Normally, there is a small amount of urobilinogen, not bilirubin, in the urine.

Explanation of Test
This test should be done with a routine urinalysis. It is an aid in the diagnosis of hepatitis and liver dysfunction, and it is helpful in monitoring the course of treatment. In persons exposed to toxins and certain drugs, a positive test for bilirubinuria can be an early indication of liver damage.

Bilirubin in the urine is an early sign of hepatocellular disease or intrahepatic or extrahepatic biliary obstruction and should be routinely performed in every urinalysis. Bilirubin may often appear in the urine before other signs of liver dysfunction, such as jaundice or clinical illness, are apparent.

Procedure
1. Examine the urine within 1 hour of collection because bilirubin is not stable in urine, especially when exposed to light.
2. Strip testing:
   (a) Good lighting is necessary.
   (b) A fresh urine specimen is tested with a dipstick according to the manufacturer's directions.
   (c) Close approximation to the color chart is an absolute must. Failure to make a close comparison is an important basis of failure to recognize bilirubin in urine.

(d) The results are interpreted as negative and 1 to 3+ positive or as small, moderate, and large amounts of bilirubin.
3. Tablets and test mats. When it is important to detect very small amounts of bilirubin in the urine, as in the earliest phase of viral hepatitis, Ictotest tablets are preferred since they are more sensitive. Follow the manufacturer's directions.
(a) When elevated amounts of bilirubin are present in the urine, a blue to purplish color forms. The rapidity and the intensity of the color formation and development are proportionate to the amount of bilirubin in the urine. Normal amounts of bilirubin in the urine give a negative test result.

Clinical Implications
1. Even trace amounts of bilirubin are abnormal and warrant further investigation. Normally, there is no detectable bilirubin in the urine.
2. *Increased levels* occur in
(a) Hepatitis and liver diseases due to infectious or toxic agents
(b) Obstructive biliary tract diseases
3. Urine bilirubin is negative in hemolytic disease

Interfering Factors
1. Drugs may cause false positives and false negatives.
2. Bilirubin rapidly decreases with exposure to light.

Urobilinogen (Random, Timed)

Normal Values
2-hour specimen: 0.1–1.0 Ehrlich units/2 hr.
24-hour specimen: 1–4 mg./24 hr.
Random: 0.1–1 Ehrlich unit/ml.

Explanation of Test
This is one of the most sensitive tests used to determine impaired liver function. Although it is usually a 24-hour urine test, a random specimen may be ordered.

Formed from the metabolism of hemoglobin entering the intestine in the bile, bilirubin is transformed through the action of bacteria into urobilinogen. Part of the urobilinogen formed in the intestine is excreted with the feces; another portion is absorbed into the portal bloodstream and carried to the liver where it is metabolized and excreted in the bile. Traces of urobilinogen that escape removal from the blood by the liver are carried to the kidneys and excreted in the urine, the basis of the urine urobilinogen test. Unlike bilirubin, urobilinogen is colorless.

Procedure
1. General instructions for collection of a 24-hour or 2-hour specimen are followed depending on what has been ordered.
2. The 2-hour timed collection is best done from 1:00 P.M. to 3:00 P.M. or 2:00 P.M. to 4:00 P.M. Collect without preservatives. Record total amount of urine voided.
3. If a 24-hour test is ordered, follow general instructions and check with your laboratory for specific protocols.

Clinical Alert

If any specimens are lost during the 24-hour urine collection, the test is nullified and should be restarted immediately. Notify both laboratory and physician if this occurs.

Clinical Implications
1. Urinary urobilinogen is *increased* by any condition that causes an increase in the production of bilirubin and by any disease that prevents the liver from normally removing the reabsorbed urobilinogen from the portal circulation.
   (a) Urobilinogen is *increased* whenever there is excessive destruction of red blood cells as in
      (1) Hemolytic anemias
      (2) Pernicious anemia
      (3) Malaria
   (b) Values above normal also occur in
      (1) Infectious and toxic hepatitis
      (2) Pulmonary infarct
      (3) Biliary disease
      (4) Cholangitis
      (5) Hemolytic jaundice and anemia
      (6) Chemical injury to liver due to chloroform and carbon tetrachloride poisoning
      (7) Cirrhosis
      (8) Congestive heart failure
      (9) Infectious mononucleosis
   (c) An *increased* urobilinogen level is one of the earliest signs of acute liver cell damage.
2. Urinary urobilinogen is *decreased* or absent when normal amounts of bilirubin are not excreted into the intestinal tract. This usually indicates partial or complete obstruction of the bile ducts such as may occur in
   (a) Cholelithiasis

(b) Severe inflammatory disease
(c) Cancer of the head of the pancreas
   (1) During antibiotic therapy, suppression of normal gut flora may prevent the breakdown of bilirubin to urobilinogen, leading to its absence in the urine.
   (2) Decreased values are also associated with
      (a.) Severe diarrhea
      (b.) Renal insufficiency

Interfering Factors

1. Drugs and foods such as bananas may cause urobilinogen to be increased as well as decreased. Drugs that may cause decreased urobilinogen include those that cause cholestasis and those that reduce the bacterial flora in the gastrointestinal tract (*e.g.*, chloramphenicol and other antibiotics).
2. Peak excretion is known to occur from noon to 4:00 P.M. The amount of urobilinogen in the urine is subject to diurnal variation.
3. Strongly alkaline urine will show a higher value and strongly acid urine will show a lower level.

MICROSCOPIC EXAMINATION OF SEDIMENT

Background

In health, the urine contains small numbers of cells and other formed elements from the entire length of the genitourinary tract: casts and epithelial cells from the nephron; epithelial cells from the pelvis, ureters, bladder, and urethra; mucous threads and spermatozoa from the prostate; possibly some red or white blood cells and an occasional cast.

In renal parenchymal disease, the urine usually contains increased numbers of cells and casts discharged from an organ that is otherwise accessible only by biopsy or surgery. (See the listing of elements and their significance shown on the opposite page.)

Urinary sediment provides information useful for both prognosis and diagnosis. It constitutes a direct sampling of urinary tract morphology. The urinary sediment is obtained by pouring 10 ml. of well-mixed urine into a conical tube and using a centrifuge at a specific speed for 10 minutes. The supernatant is poured off and 1 ml. of sediment is mixed in a cover slip on a slide and examined under the microscope.

The sediment collected in the urine can be broken down into cellular elements (red and white blood cells and epithelial cells), casts, crystals, and bacteria.

These may originate anywhere in the urinary tract. When casts do occur in the urine, the indication is one of tubular or glomerular disorders.

Significance of Elements Observed in the Urinary Sediment on Microscopic Examination

Formed Elements	Significance
Red cells	Bleeding anywhere in the urinary tract
Red cell cast	Glomerulitis
Hemoglobin cast	Glomerulitis or hemoglobin-uria due to intravascular hemolysis
White blood cell cast	Pyelonephritis
Oval fat body	Heavy proteinuria
Waxy cast	Severe renal damage
Broad cast (greater than 5 RBCs)	Azotemia
Many white cells	Urinary tract infection
Many granular casts	Associated with renal disease
Bacteria (fresh clean voided urine)	Urinary tract infection; confirm with culture

Crystals	
Cystine	Diagnostic for cystinuria
Calcium phosphate (amorphous phosphate)	Alkaline urine
Calcium oxalate and uric acid	May appear in normal urine as it cools
$MgNH_4PO_4$ (struvite or "triple phosphate")	Urinary tract infection

Cast width is significant in determining the site of origin and may indicate the extent of renal damage. Cast width is described as narrow (1–2 RBCs in width), medium broad (3–4 RBCs in width) and broad (5 RBCs in width). The broad cast is formed in the collecting tubule and may be of any composition. It usually indicates a marked reduction in the functional capacity of the nephron and suggests severe renal damage or "end stage" renal disease.

Clinical Alert

The microscopic findings of the urine sediment should always be correlated with the dipstick findings.

Red Cells and Red Cell Casts

Normal Values
1 or 2/LPF—low-powered field
Red blood cells: 0–1/HPF—high-powered field
Red cell casts: 0/LPF

Explanation of Test
In health, red cells are occasionally found in the urine, but the persistent findings of even small numbers of erythrocytes (RBCs) should be thoroughly investigated, since these cells come from the kidney and indicate serious renal disease.

Procedure for Urine Microscopic Examination
Urinary sediment is examined microscopically under low and high power. Casts are searched for and enumerated under low power. Red blood cells and white blood cells are searched for and counted under high power. Bacteria are reported per high-powered field (HPF): few, moderate, packed, packed solid, or 1t, 2t, 3t, 4t. Crystals and other elements are noted.

Clinical Implications
A. *Red cell casts*
   1. Casts composed largely of red blood cells are never found normally and indicate hemorrhage or desquamative conditions of the nephron.
   2. Red blood casts indicate acute inflammatory or vascular disorders in the glomerulus.
   3. They may be the only manifestation of
      (a) Acute glomerulonephritis
      (b) Renal infarction
      (c) Collagen disease
      (d) Kidney involvement in subacute bacterial endocarditis
   4. The usual finding in systemic lupus erythematosus is red blood cell casts and epithelial cell casts.
B. *Red cells*
   1. The finding of more than one or two red cells per high-powered field is an abnormal condition and can indicate
      (a) Renal or systemic disease
      (b) Trauma to the kidney
   2. Increased red cells occur in
      (a) Pyelonephritis
      (b) Lupus
      (c) Renal stones
      (d) Cystitis
      (e) Prostatitis
      (f) Tuberculosis and malignancies of the genitourinary tract
      (g) Hemophilia

3. Red cells in excess of WBCs indicate bleeding into the urinary tract as may occur in
   (a) Trauma
   (b) Tumor
   (c) Aspirin ingestion
   (d) Anticoagulative therapy
   (e) Thrombocytopenia

Clinical Alert

1. In health, red cells are occasionally found in the urine but the persistent finding of even small numbers of erythrocytes should be thoroughly investigated.
2. Rule out menstrual contamination.

Interfering Factors
1. Increased numbers of red blood cells can be found following a traumatic catheterization and passage of stones.
2. Alkaline urine hemolyzes red cells and dissolves casts.
3. Many drugs can cause increased numbers of red blood cells to appear in the urine.
4. Red cell casts may occur after very strenuous physical activity and contact sports.
5. Heavy smokers have small amounts of red blood cells in urine.

White Cells and White Cell Casts

Normal Values
WBCs: 0–4/high-powered field
WBC casts: none–negative/low-powered field

Background
Leukocytes may come from anywhere in the genitourinary tract. White cell casts always come from the kidney tubules.

Procedure
Urinary sediment is examined microscopically under high power for cells and crystals and under low power for casts.

Clinical Implications
A. *Leukocytes*
   1. Large numbers of white cells usually indicate bacterial infection in the urinary tract.
   2. If the infection is in the kidney, the white cells tend to be associ-

ated with cellular and granular casts, bacteria, epithelial cells, and relatively few red cells.
3. Call for a urine culture (see section on urine cultures in Chapter 7, Microbiological Studies)

B. *White cell casts*
1. White cell casts indicate renal parenchymal infection.
2. May be found in
   (a) Pyelonephritis—most common cause
   (b) Acute glomerulonephritis
   (c) Interstitial inflammation of the kidney
3. It is very difficult to differentiate between white blood cell casts and epithelial cell casts.
4. Because pyelonephritis may remain completely asymptomatic even though renal tissue is being progressively destroyed, careful examination (using low power) of urinary sediment for leukocyte casts is important.

Interfering Factors
Vaginal discharge can contaminate the specimen. Either a "clean-catch" specimen or a catheterized specimen should be taken to rule out contamination.

Epithelial Cells and Epithelial Casts

Normal Values
Occasional renal epithelial cell found.

Background
Renal epithelial cell casts are formed by cast-off tubular cells. Since the tubule is a living membrane, it is always replacing itself. For this reason, the finding of occasional epithelial cells or clumps is not remarkable.

Clinical Implications
The findings of many epithelial casts occur when the following diseases have damaged the tubular epithelium:

Nephrosis
Amyloidosis
Poisoning from heavy metals and other toxins
Interfering factors

Squamous epithelium is usually seen when the urine is contaminated with vaginal discharge.

Hyaline Casts

Normal Values
Occasional hyaline casts per low power are found.

Background
Hyaline casts are clear, colorless casts formed when protein (Tamm–Horsfall) within the tubules precipitates and gels. Their appearance within the urine depends on the rate of urine flow, urine pH, and the degree of proteinuria.

Procedure
Urinary sediment is examined microscopically for casts under low power.

Clinical Implications
1. Hyaline casts indicate possible damage to the glomerular capillary membrane, which is permitting leakage of proteins through the glomerular filter.
2. Hyaline casts may be a temporary phenomenon due to
   (a) Fever
   (b) Postural strain
   (c) Emotional exercise
   (d) Strenuous exercise
   (e) Palpation of the kidney
3. When large numbers of hyaline casts appear in the urine along with heavy proteinuria, fine granular casts, fatty casts, or oval fat bodies or fat droplets, nephrotic syndrome may be suggested.
4. Casts may not be found even if proteinuria is heavy because of dilute urine (1.010) or because the pH is alkaline.
5. In cylindruria, large numbers of casts may be counted but there may not be any protein in the urine.

Granular Casts

Normal Values
Occasional granular casts are found.

Background
In pathological disease, granular casts result from the disintegration of the cellular material in white and epithelial blood cells into coarse and then fine granular particles. A rare but final step in this process may be the formation of waxy casts when urine flow is reduced and renal failure progresses. Waxy casts may be cell casts, hyaline casts, or renal

failure casts. In normal subjects, granular casts probably are the result of irregular precipitation of Tamm–Horsfall protein, and the cast is precipitated the same as cell casts.

Procedure
Urinary sediment is examined microscopically under low power.

Clinical Implications
1. Acute tubular necrosis
2. Advanced glomerulonephritis
3. Pyelonephritis
4. Malignant nephrosclerosis
5. Chronic lead poisoning

Waxy Casts
Found in

1. Chronic renal disease
2. Tubular inflammation and degeneration

Oval Fat Bodies and Fatty Casts

Background
In nephrotic syndrome, fat accumulates in the tubular cells and eventually sloughs off, forming oval fat bodies (OFB). This fat is probably a cholesterol esther. Fatty casts are usually composed of individual fat droplets. The presence of fat droplets, oval fat bodies, or fatty casts is the hallmark of the nephrotic syndrome.

Clinical Implications
Fatty casts are found in chronic renal disease and indicate tubular inflammation and degeneration.

Crystals

Background
In a routine urinalysis, the presence of crystals is identified as a normal finding. The type and number of crystals vary with the pH of the urine.

Clinical Implications
A. *Normal findings*
   1. Acid urine
      (a) Urates
      (b) Uric acid
      (c) Calcium oxalate (if numerous, may indicate hypercalcemia [only in warm, freshly voided urine])

A normal subject may have large numbers of calcium oxalate crystals once the urine cools.

   2. Alkaline urine

     (a) Amorphous phosphates   (d) Triple phosphate crystal

     (b) Calcium phosphate   (Mg, NH_4, PO_4 are the

     (c) Ammonium biurate   most common)

B. *Abnormal findings*

   1. Cystine

   2. Leucine or tyrosine (indicate protein breakdown)

   3. Cholesterin/cholesterol

   4. Drug crystals (sulfonamides)

   5. Abnormal findings are associated with urinary tract infection.

Interfering Factors

Drugs may cause increased levels of crystals.

Shreds

Background

Shreds consist of a mixture of mucus, pus, and epithelial (squamous) cells and can be seen grossly.

Clinical Implications

1. When mucus predominates, the shreds float on the surface.
2. When epithelial cells predominate, the shreds occupy the mid zone.
3. When pus (WBCs) predominates, the shreds are drawn to the bottom of the specimen.
4. Other findings in urine due to contamination include microscopic yeast, trichomonas, spermatozoa, vegetable fibers, parasites, and meat fibers. They should be reported because they have clinical significance.

DRUG INVESTIGATION SPECIMENS

To screen for an unknown drug, the most valuable types of sample are first, urine, second, gastric specimen, and third, blood. Urine drug screening is the most economical approach (Table 3-1).

Indications for Toxicology Screening

1. Confirm clinical or after-death diagnosis.
2. Differentiate drug-induced disease from other causes such as trauma, metabolic, or infectious encephalopathy.
3. Identify contributing diagnoses such as ethanol, plus head trauma or amphetamines, plus underlying psychoses.
4. Test results used as basis for high-risk interventions such as hemo-

Table 3-1
Common Urine Drug Tests*†

Amphetamines	Phencyclidine
Alcohol	LSD
Barbiturates	Analgesics
Benzodiazepines	Sedatives
Cocaine	Major tranquilizers‡
Cyanide	Stimulants
Opiates	Sympathomimetics
THC	

* Many of the above drugs that are detectable in urine are not detectable in serum.
† All drugs detectable in serum are also detectable in urine, except glutethimide.
‡ Because minor tranquilizers are extensively metabolized, they are not likely to be detected in urine unless an overdose is taken.

dialysis and hemoperfusion for certain drugs, pharmacologic antagonists for cardiac drug overdose, and chelating agents for metal poisoning.

Clinical Alert

There are a number of interfering factors that can make this type of testing unreliable—all positive tests must be confirmed with unrelated methods.

Witnessed Urine Sampling for Suspected Substance Abuse

Procedure
1. The sample is witnessed by a trained individual, collected, and tagged with a numerical code.
2. The sample is placed in a plastic heat-sealed sack and marked with a notary-style seal to protect against the possibility of unnoticed tampering.
3. "A change of custody" document originates at sample collection. The person who provides the urine specimen signs the document, as does every person who handles the sample.
4. After both initial and confirmatory testing, the sample is resealed, marked, and securely stored for a minimum of 30 days.

OTHER URINARY CONSTITUENT TESTS

Chlorides (Cl); **Quantitative** (24-hr.)

Normal Values
110–250 mEq./24 hr. or 110–250 mmol./d.
Vary greatly with salt intake and perspiration.

It is rather difficult to talk about "normal" and "abnormal" ranges. The test findings have meaning only in relation to salt intake and output.

Explanation of Test
The amount of chloride excreted in the urine in a 24-hour period is an indication of the state of electrolyte balance. Chloride is most often associated with sodium and fluid change.

The measurement of urine chloride may be useful as a means of diagnosing dehydration or as a guide in adjusting fluid and electrolyte balance in postoperative patients. It also serves as a means of monitoring the effects of reduced salt diets, which are of great therapeutic importance in patients with cardiovascular disease, hypertension, liver disease, and kidney ailments.

A patient on a restricted salt intake diet will usually not excrete more than 0.6 g. per 100 ml. of NaCl in the urine, while a person on a normal salt diet would excrete 0.7 g. per 100 ml. of NaCl or more.

Procedure
1. A 24-hour urine specimen is collected.
2. The exact times to start and complete the collection are recorded on the specimen container and on the patient's record.
3. When the specimen is completed, it should be sent to the laboratory for refrigeration.

Clinical Alert
Because electrolyte and water balance are so closely related, appraise the patient's state of hydration by checking daily weight, accurate intake and output, and by observing and recording skin turgor and the appearance of the tongue and the urine.

Clinical Implications
Results are significant only when considered in relation to other data, such as state of health or illness, salt intake, and urine volume.

A. *Normal findings*
   Urinary excretion of chloride decreases to a very low level whenever the serum level is much below 100 mEq. per liter.
B. *Decreased levels*
   1. In some conditions, urinary excretion of chloride increases even when the serum level is as low as 85 mEq. per liter or less. Occur in Addison's disease when there is a deficiency of adrenal hormone that controls the excretion of sodium and chloride.
   2. Decreased levels associated with
      (a) Malabsorption syndrome   (e) Diaphoresis
      (b) Pyloric obstruction   (f) Congestive heart failure
      (c) Prolonged gastric suction (g) Emphysema
      (d) Diarrhea
C. *Increased levels*
   Associated with
   (a) Dehydration
   (b) Starvation
   (c) Salicylate toxicity
   (d) Mercurial and chlorothiazide diuretics

Interfering Factors
1. Urinary chloride concentration varies with dietary salt intake and, to some degree, with urine volume.
2. False elevations may result if the patient has taken bromides.

Patient Preparation
Instruct the patient about the purpose of the test and the method for collecting a 24-hour specimen.

Sodium (Na); Quantitative (24-hr.)

Normal Values
40–220 mEq./liter/24 hr. or 40–220 mmol./liter, diet dependent

Explanation of Test
This test measures electrolyte balance in the body by determining the amount of sodium excreted in 24 hours. It is indicated in the study of renal and adrenal disturbances and of water and acid–base imbalances.
   Sodium is a primary regulator in the body's ability to retain or excrete water and maintain acid–base balance. The body has a strong tendency to maintain a total base content; only slight changes are found even under pathologic conditions. As the main base substance in the blood, sodium helps regulate acid–base balance because of its abil-

ity to combine with chloride and bicarbonate. Sodium also helps maintain the normal balance of electrolyte composition in intracellular and extracellular fluids by acting in conjunction with potassium (sodium–potassium pump). Sodium and potassium are important factors in nerve conduction, and they influence the irritability of the muscles, nerves, and heart.

Procedure

1. A 24-hour urine container is labeled with the name of the patient, the test, and the date.
2. Urine must be refrigerated or collected in an iced container.
3. General instructions for 24-hour urine collection are followed.
4. Exact start and ending of the collection are recorded on the specimen container and the patient's record (start 7:05 A.M. 11/10; end 7:30 A.M. 11/11).
5. Send the specimen to the laboratory refrigerator when the test is completed.

Clinical Implications

Results are significant only when considered in relation to other data, such as the state of health or illness, salt, intake, and urine volume.

A. *Increased levels*
   1. Caused by
      (a) Dehydration
      (b) Starvation
      (c) Salicylate toxicity
      (d) Adrenal cortical insufficiency
      (e) Mercurial and chlorothiazide diuretics
      (f) Chronic renal failure
      (g) Diabetic acidosis

B. *Decreased levels of sodium* associated with
   (a) Malabsorption syndrome
   (b) Congestive heart failure
   (c) Pyloric obstruction
   (d) Diarrhea
   (e) Diaphoresis
   (f) Acute renal failure
   (g) Pulmonary emphysema
   (h) Aldosteronism
   (i) Cushing's disease

C. *Decreased levels*
   Often accompanied by an equivalent loss of chloride

Interfering Factors

1. Dietary salt intake
2. Altered kidney function

Patient Preparation

1. Instruct the patient about the purpose of the test, collection, and refrigeration of 24-hour urine specimen. Give a written reminder.
2. Food and fluids are permitted and encouraged.

Clinical Alert

Since electrolyte and water balance are so closely related, determine the patient's state of hydration by checking daily weight, accurate intake and output, observation and recording of skin turgor, and appearance of tongue and urine.

Potassium (K); Quantitative (24-hr.)

Normal Values
25–125 mEq./24 hr. or 25–125 mmol./liter
Varies with diet.

Explanation of Test
This test provides some insight into the electrolyte balance of the body by measuring the amount of potassium excreted in 24 hours. This measurement is useful in the study of renal and adrenal disorders and of water and acid–base imbalances. When a patient gives an obscure history in the presence of a known potassium deficit, evaluation of urinary potassium can be helpful in determining the origin of the deficit.

Potassium acts as a part of the body's buffer system; therefore, potassium balance serves a vital function in the body's overall electrolyte balance. Since the kidneys cannot conserve potassium, this balance is regulated by the kidneys' excretion of potassium through the urine.

Procedure
1. A 24-hour urine container is labeled with the name of the patient, test, and date.
2. Urine must be refrigerated or collected in an iced container.
3. General instructions for 24-hour urine collection are followed.
4. Exact start and ending of the collection are recorded on the specimen container and the patient's record (start 7:05 A.M. 11/10; end 7:30 A.M. 11/11).
5. Send the specimen to the laboratory refrigerator when the test is completed.

Clinical Implications
A. *Elevated levels*
   1. Found in:
      (a) Chronic renal failure
      (b) Diabetic and renal tubular acidosis
      (c) Dehydration

    (d) Starvation
    (e) Primary aldosteronism
    (f) Cushing's disease
    (g) Salicylate toxicity
    (h) Mercurial chlorothiazide, ammonium chloride, and Diamox diuretics

B. *Decreased levels*
  1. Associated with
    (a) Malabsorption syndrome
    (b) Diarrhea
    (c) Acute renal failure
    (d) Adrenal cortical insufficiency (can be normal or decreased)
    (e) Excessive mineralocorticoid activity (aldosterone)
       Since licorice contains a mineralocorticoid compound, people who consume large amounts of licorice may have lowered urinary potassium levels.
  2. In patients with potassium deficiency, regardless of the cause, the urine *p*H tends to fall. This fall occurs because hydrogen ions are secreted in exchange for sodium ions, inasmuch as both potassium and hydrogen are excreted by the same mechanism.

C. *Cautionary findings*
  1. In excessive vomiting or stomach suctioning, the accompanying alkalosis maintains urinary potassium excretion at levels inappropriately high for the degree of actual potassium depletion.
  2. In diabetes insipidus, urinary potassium is normal.

Interfering Factors
Vary with dietary intake.

Patient Preparation
1. Instruct the patient about the purpose of the test, collection and refrigeration of 24-hour urine specimen. Give a written reminder.
2. Food and fluids are permitted and encouraged.

Clinical Alert
1. Since electrolyte and water balance are so closely associated, determine the patient's state of hydration by checking daily weight, accurate intake and output, and by observing and recording skin turgor and appearance of the tongue and urine.
2. Observe for signs of muscle weakness, tremors, and changes in electrocardiograms. The level of potassium increase or decrease at which these symptoms become apparent varies from patient to patient.

Uric Acid; Quantitative (24-hr.)

Normal Values
250–750 mg./24 hr. on normal diet or 1.48–4.43 mmol./d.
120 mg./24 hr. on a purine-free diet or 2.48 mmol./d.
1000 mg./24 hr. on a high-purine diet or 5.90 mmol./d.

Uric acid formation occurs as a result of the metabolic breakdown of nucleic acids; purines are the principal source of this breakdown. The test is indicated in the investigation of metabolic disturbances to identify gout and diagnose kidney disease. It will also reflect the effect of uricosuric agents when these drugs are used, by indicating the total amount of uric acid excreted.

Procedure
1. A 24-hour urine container with preservative added is labeled with the name of the patient, test, and date.
2. General instructions for 24-hour urine collection are followed.
3. Exact start and ending of the collection are recorded on the specimen container and the patient's record (start 7:30 A.M. 1/3; end 7:15 A.M. 1/4).
4. Send the specimen to the laboratory when the test is completed.

Clinical Implications
A. *Increased levels* (uricosuria)
   1. Found in
      (a) Gout
      (b) Chronic myelogenous leukemia
      (c) Polycythemia vera
      (d) Liver disease
      (e) Febrile illness
      (f) Toxemias of pregnancy
      (g) Fanconi's syndrome
   2. Cytotoxic drugs to treat lymphoma and leukemia often cause greatly increased urinary uric acid levels.
   3. High uric acid concentration plus low urine pH may lead to uric acid stones in the urinary tract.
B. *Decreased levels*
   Found in kidney disease (chronic glomerulonephritis) because impaired renal function depresses uric acid excretion.

Interfering Factors
1. Many drugs, such as
   (a) Salicylates
   (b) Thiazide diuretics
   (c) Chronic alcohol ingestion

2. Radiograph contrast media can markedly increase urine acid levels.

Patient Preparation
1. Instruct the patient about the purpose of the test, collection, and refrigeration of 24-hour urine specimen. Give a written reminder.
2. Food and fluids are permitted and encouraged. In some diagnostic situations, a diet high or low in purines may be ordered during the test period.

Calcium; Quantitative (24-hr.) Sulkowitch

Normal Values
24-hour levels
100–300 mg./average diet or 2.50–7.50 mmol./d.
50–150 mg./low-calcium diet or 1.25–3.75 mmol./d.

Explanation of Test
The bulk of the calcium discharged by the body is excreted in the stool. However, there is a small quantity of calcium that is normally excreted in the urine, the amount increasing or decreasing as a result of changes in the quantity of dietary calcium ingested.

The 24-hour test is most often ordered to determine the function of the parathyroid gland, which maintains a balance between calcium and phosphorous by means of parathyroid hormone. Hyperparathyroidism is a generalized disorder of calcium, phosphate, and bone metabolism that results from an increased secretion of parathyroid hormones and an increased excretion of urinary calcium. In hypoparathyroidism, the urinary calcium is decreased.

Procedure
1. A 24-hour urine container is labeled with the name of the patient, test, and date.
2. Usually, an acid-washed bottle is required if not ordered with any other tests. Some laboratories will require a preservative or refrigeration.
3. General instructions for 24-hour urine collection are followed.
4. Exact start and ending of the collection are recorded on the specimen container and the patient's record (start 7:05 A.M. 11/10; end 7:30 A.M. 11/11).
5. Send the specimen to the laboratory refrigerator when the test is completed.

Clinical Implications
A. *Increased levels*
   1. Caused by
      (a) Hyperparathyroidism (results in constant 3+ to 4+ Sulkowitch tests)
      (b) Sarcoidosis
      (c) Primary cancers of breast and lung
      (d) Metastatic malignancies
      (e) Myeloma with bone metastasis
      (f) Wilson's disease
      (g) Renal tubular acidosis
      (h) Glucocorticoid excess
   2. Increased urinary calcium almost always accompanies elevated blood calcium levels.
   3. Calcium excretion greater than intake is always excessive, and excretion above 400 to 500 mg. per 24 hours is reliably abnormal.
   4. Increased excretion of calcium occurs whenever calcium is mobilized from the bone, as in metastatic cancer and prolonged skeletal immobilization.
   5. When calcium is excreted in increasing amounts, a potential for nephrolithiasis or nephrocalcinosis is created.
B. *Decreased levels*
   1. Caused by
      (a) Hypoparathyroidism (hypocalcemia caused by hypoparathyroidism is usually associated with a negative reaction)
      (b) Vitamin D deficiency (Vitamin D is necessary for absorption of calcium)
      (c) Malabsorption syndrome

Interfering Factors
A. *False elevated levels* are due to
   1. High sodium and magnesium intake
   2. Very high milk intake
   3. Some drugs
   4. Level higher immediately after meals
B. *False-negative levels* are due to
   1. Increased dietary phosphates
   2. Alkaline urine
   3. Some drugs

Patient Preparation
1. Instruct the patient about the purpose of the test, collection of 24-hour urine specimen. Give a written reminder.

2. Food and fluids are permitted and encouraged.
3. If the urine calcium test is done because of a metabolic disorder, the patient should eat a low-calcium diet and be on calcium medication restrictions for a 1- to 3-day period prior to collection of the specimen.
4. If the patient has a history of renal stone formation, a general diet will be prescribed.

Clinical Alert

1. Observe patients with very low urine calcium levels for signs and symptoms of tetany.
2. The first sign of calcium imbalance may be the occurrence of pathological fracture that can be related to calcium excess.
3. The Sulkowitch test can be used in an emergency especially when hypercalcemia is suspected since hypercalcemia is life-threatening. A fasting, first morning specimen is examined for turbidity. Normal is 8–12 mg./dl.; Increased is >12 mg./dl.

Magnesium; Quantitative (24-hr.)

Normal Values
6.0–10.0 mEq./24-hr. or 3.00–5.00 mmol./24-hr.

Explanation of Test
A 24-hour urine test is useful in the evaluation of renal disease and magnesium deficiency. In magnesium deficiency, urine magnesium decreases before serum magnesium.

Procedure
1. A 24-hour urine specimen is obtained in a metal-free container with no preservative.
2. See page 122 for specific instructions.

Clinical Implications
1. *Increased excretion* is associated with
   (a) Drugs such as thiazide, diuretics, ethacrynic acid, alcohol, corticosteroids, platinum therapy, and aldosterone.
   (b) Bartter's syndrome.
2. *Decreased excretion* is associated with
   (a) Renal disease
   (b) Magnesium deficiency

Oxalate; Quantitative (24-hr.)

Normal Values
Urine: 8–40 mg./24 hr. or 91–456 μmol./24 hr.

Explanation of Test
This test is of value in diagnosing systemic poisoning due to ethylene glycol poisoning, kidney stones, and primary hyperoxalurea, a genetic disorder.

Procedure
A 24-hour urine specimen is collected using hydrochloric acid as a preservative. See page 122 for specifics.

Interfering Factors
Foods such as rhubarb, strawberries, beans, beets, spinach, and tomatoes, gelatin, chocolate, cocoa, and tea, as well as calcium and ascorbic acid and some drugs increase excretion.

Clinical Implications
1. *Increased values* are associated with
   (a) Ethylene glycol poisoning
       (>150 mg./d. or >1710 μmol./d.)
   (b) Primary hyperoxaluria
       (100–600 mg./d or 1140–6840 μmol./d.
       [nephrocalcinosis])
   (c) Diabetes
   (d) Cirrhosis
   (e) B_6 deficiency
   (f) Sarcoidosis
   (g) Steatorrhea due to pancreatic insufficiency
   (h) Celiac disease
   (i) Bacterial overgrowth
   (j) Ilial resection
   (k) Jejuno-ilial shunt
   (l) Biliary tract disease
   (m) Small bowel disease
2. *Decreased values* are associated with renal failure.

Patient Preparation
Explain the purpose and procedure of the test. No foods that increase excretion are to be eaten.

Follicle-Stimulating Hormone (FSH); Luteinizing Hormone (LH)

Normal Values
FSH
Men: 4–18 IU./d.

Women: 3–10 IU./d.
Postmenopausal: 40–250 mU./d.
Midcycle peak: two times baseline
LH
Men: 13–60 IU./ml.
Women: 7.2–23.5 U./d. follicular phase
Postmenopausal: over 24 IU./d.
Midcycle peak: over three times baseline
See your laboratory for values in infants and children.

Explanation of Test

This 24-hour urine test measures the gonadotropic hormones FSH and LH and may be helpful in determining whether a gonadal insufficiency is primary or due to insufficient stimulation by the pituitary hormones. Production of these gonadotropins is believed to be under control of the pituitary gland. In women, the follicle-stimulating hormone promotes maturation of the ovarian follicle, and the maturing follicle produces estrogens. As the levels of estrogen rise, luteinizing hormones are produced. Together, FSH and LH induce ovulation. In men, the follicle-stimulating hormone produces spermatogenesis, and the luteinizing hormone stimulates the secretion of androgens and increased synthesis of testosterone. In women, LH acts on the interstitial cells, resulting in synthesis of androgens, estrogens, and progesterone.

FSH is an aid in studying various causes of hypothyroidism in females as well as endocrine dysfunction in males. In primary ovarian failure or testicular failure, FSH is increased. Measuring urine FSH and LH are of value for children with endocrine problems related to precocious puberty. Urine assays are also used to monitor ovulatory cycles of *in vitro* fertilization patients.

Procedure

1. A 24-hour urine container is labeled with the name of the patient, test, and date. The 24-hour urine collection minimizes the problems with episodic secretion spikes that occur with blood serum specimens.
2. Urine is collected either with a preservative or refrigerated only.
3. A blood sample of at least 3 ml. can also be obtained. Sometimes multiple blood specimens are necessary because of episodic release of FSH from the pituitary gland. An isolated sample may be at the peak or valley of secretion.
4. In anovulatory fertility problems, the presence or absence of a midcycle peak can be established by a series of daily blood specimens.
5. When all the urine is collected, the specimen is sent to the laboratory refrigerator.

Clinical Implications
A. *Decreased FSH levels* occur in
  1. Feminizing and masculinizing ovarian tumors when production is inhibited as a result of increased estrogen
  2. Failure of pituitary or hypothalamus
  3. Anorexia nervosa
  4. Neoplasm of testes or adrenal glands that secrete estrogens or androgens
B. *Increased FSH levels* occur in
  1. Turner's syndrome (ovarian dysgenesis). Approximately 50% of patients with primary amenorrhea have Turner's syndrome.
  2. Hypogonadism and primary gonadal failure
  3. Complete testicular feminization syndrome
  4. Precocious puberty, either idiopathic or secondary to a central nervous system lesion
  5. Klinefelter's syndrome
C. *Both FSH and LH are increased* in
  (a) Primary gonadal failure
  (b) Complete testicular feminization syndrome
  (c) Precocious puberty
D. *Decreased FSH and LH* occur in
  Failure of pituitary or hypothalamus

Patient Preparation
Instruct the patient about the purpose of the test and collection of 24-hour urine specimen. Give a written reminder.

Pregnanediol

Normal Values
This test is difficult to standardize; it varies with age, sex, and weeks of pregnancy.

Explanation of Test
This test is a measurement of ovarian and placental function. It is indicated when a deficiency of progesterone is suspected. Combined deficiency of estrogen and progesterone is evidenced by menstrual irregularities and difficulty in conceiving and maintaining a pregnancy. Specifically, it measures the hormone progesterone and its principal excreted metabolite, pregnanediol. Progesterone has its main effect in the endometrium by causing the endometrium to enter the secretory phase and become ready for implantation of the blastocyte if fertilization has occurred.

Pregnanediol excretion is high in pregnancy and low in luteal deficiency or placental failure.

Procedure
1. A 24-hour urine container is labeled with the name of the patient, test, and date.
2. Refrigeration of the specimen is required.
3. General instructions for 24-hour urine collection are followed.
4. Exact start and ending of the collection are recorded on the specimen container and the patient's record (start 7:06 A.M. 1/5; end 7:30 A.M. 1/6).
5. When all urine is collected, the specimen is sent to the laboratory refrigerator.

Clinical Implications
A. *Increased levels* are associated with
   1. Luteal cysts of ovary
   2. Arrhenoblastoma of the ovary
   3. Hyperadrenocorticism
B. *Decreased levels* are associated with
   1. Amenorrhea
   2. Threatened abortion (sometimes)
   3. Fetal death
   4. Toxemia

Patient Preparation
1. Instruct the patient about the purpose of the test and collection of 24-hour urine specimen. Give a written reminder.
2. Food and fluids are permitted.

Pregnanetriol

Normal Values
Adults: up to 2 mg./24 hr. or <5.04 umol./d.
Children: up to 1.5 mg./24 hr. or <4.46 umol./d.
Infants: up to 0.2 mg./24 hr. or up to 0.59 umol./d.

Explanation of Test
Pregnanetriol is a compound substance reflecting one segment of adrenocortical activity. Pregnanetriol should not be confused with pregnanediol, despite the similarity of name. Pregnanetriol is a precursor in adrenal corticoid synthesis and arises from 17-hydroxyprogesterone, not from progesterone.

This 24-hour urine test is done to diagnose adrenal cortical dysfunction, adrenogenital syndrome, a defect in 21-hydroxylation. The diagnosis of adrenogenital syndrome is considered in

1. Adult women who show signs and symptoms of excessive androgen production with or without hypertension

2. Craving for salt
3. Sexual precocity in boys
4. Infants who exhibit signs of failure to thrive
5. External genitalia in women (pseudohermaphroditism)

In boys, differentiation must be made between a virilizing tumor of the adrenal gland, neurogenic and constitutional types of sexual precocity, and interstitial cell tumor of the testes.

Procedure
1. A 24-hour urine container is labeled with the name of the patient, test, and date.
2. Refrigeration of the specimen is required.
3. General instructions for 24-hour urine collection are followed.
4. Exact start and ending of the collection are recorded on the specimen container and the patient's record (start 7:06 A.M. 1/5; end 7:30 A.M. 1/6).
5. When all urine is collected, the specimen is sent to the laboratory refrigerator.

Clinical Implications
Elevated pregnanetriol levels occur in
1. Congenital adrenocortical hyperplasia
2. Stein–Leventhal syndrome

Patient Preparation
1. Instruct the patient about the purpose of the test and collection of 24-hour urine specimen. Give a written reminder.
2. Food and fluids are permitted.

5-Hydroxyindoleacetic Acid (5-HIAA)
(5-Hydroxy 3, Serotonin, Indoleacetic Acid)

Normal Values
Qualitative—negative
Quantitative—2–8 mg./24 hr. or 10.4–41.6 umol./24 hr.

Explanation of Test
The qualitative random sample test may be done for screening purposes, followed by a quantitative 24-hour test if need be, or the 24-hour test may be done initially.

The urine test is conducted to diagnose a functioning carcinoid tumor, which is indicated by significant elevation of 5-hydroxyindoleacetic acid (5-HIAA), a denatured product of serotonin. Serotonin is a vasoconstricting hormone normally produced by the argentaffin cells of the GI tract. The principal function of the cells is to regulate smooth muscle contraction and peristalsis.

Procedure

1. No bananas, pineapple, tomatoes, eggplants, or avocados are to be eaten during the 24-hour test because they contain serotonin (5-hydroxyindoleacetic acid is a metabolic product of serotonin).
2. A 24-hour urine container with preservative is labeled with the name of the patient, test, and date.
3. General instructions for 24-hour urine collection are followed.
4. Exact start and ending of the collection are recorded on the specimen container and the patient's record (start 7:30 A.M., 11/17; end 7:06 A.M., 11/18).
5. Send the specimen to the laboratory refrigerator when the test is completed.

Clinical Implications

1. Levels over 100 mg. per 24 hours are indicative of large carcinoid tumor, especially when metastatic. However, this increase occurs in only 5% to 7% of patients with carcinoid tumor.
2. *Levels greater than* 10 mg. but less than 100 mg. are found in
   (a) Hemorrhage
   (b) Thrombosis
   (c) Nontropical sprue
   (d) Severe pain of sciatica or skeletal and smooth muscle spasm
   (e) Oat cell cancer of bronchus
   (f) Bronchial adenoma of carcinoid type
3. *Decreased levels* are found in
   (a) Depressive illness
   (b) Small intestinal resection
   (c) Mastocytosis
   (d) Phenylketonuria (PKU)
   (e) Hartnup's disease

Interfering Factors

A. *False positives*
   1. Bananas, pineapples, plums, walnuts, eggplants, tomatoes, and avocados may increase the 5–HIAA level, for these foods contain serotonin.
   2. There are a number of drugs that may cause false positives.
B. *False negatives*
   Specific drugs may cause false negatives (depressing 5–HIAA).

Patient Preparation

1. Instruct the patient about the purpose of the test and collection of the 24-hour urine specimen. Give a written reminder.
2. Food and water are permitted and encouraged. Foods high in serotonin content are not to be eaten during the test.

Clinical Alert

The patient should take no drugs for 72 hours before the test, if at all possible.

Vanillylmandelic Acid (VMA), (Catecholamines), (3-Methoxy-4-Hydroxymandelic Acid)

Normal Values
VMA up to 7 ug./mg./24 hr. or up to 35.4 umol./24 hr.
Catecholamines
  Epinephrine: 0–15 ug./24 hr. or 0.0–81.9 nmol./24 hr.
  Norepinephrine: 0–100 ug./24 hr. or 0–591 nmol./24 hr.
  Metanephrine: 0:25–0.8 mg./24 hr. or 1.27–4.06 umol./d.
  Dopamine: 65–400 ug./24 hr. or 424–2612 nmol./24 hr.

Explanation of Test
This 24-hour urine test of adrenal medullar function is primarily done when a person with hypertension is suspected of having pheochromocytoma, a tumor of the chromaffin cells of the adrenal medulla. (Less than 1% of hypertensive patients have pheochromocytoma.) The principal substances formed by the adrenal medulla and excreted in the urine include vanillylmandelic acid, epinephrine, norepinephrine, metanephrine, and normetanephrine. These compounds contain a catechol nucleus and an amine group and are thus referred to as *catecholamines*. The major portion of the hormones are changed into metabolites, the principal one being 3-methoxy-4-hydroxymandelic acid, or VMA.

VMA is the main urinary metabolite of the catecholamine group, having a urine concentration much greater than the other amines (10–100 times). It is also easier to detect due to simpler laboratory methods than the methods that must be used for catecholamine determination. Testing for VMA is important in pheochromocytoma since these tumors secrete excessive amounts of catecholamine, resulting in high urine levels of VMA.

Procedure
1. A 24-hour urine container with preservative is labeled with the name of the patient, test, and date.
2. General instructions for 24-hour urine collection are followed.
3. Exact start and ending of the collection are recorded on the specimen container and the patient's record (start 10:06 A.M. 1/3; end 10:15 A.M. 1/4).

4. When all the urine is collected, the specimen is sent to the laboratory refrigerator.

Clinical Implications
A. *Elevated VMA levels*
   1. High levels found in pheochromocytoma
   2. Slight to moderate elevations in
      (a) Neuroblastomas
      (b) Ganglioneuromas
      (c) Ganglioblastomas
B. *Elevated catecholamines*
   Found in

   (1) Pheochromocytoma
   (2) Neuroblastomas
   (3) Ganglioneuromas
   (4) Ganglioblastomas
   (5) Progressive muscular dystrophy
   (6) Myasthenia gravis

Interfering Factors
A. *Increased levels of VMA* are caused by
   1. Starvation. (For this reason, the test should *not* be scheduled while the patient is NPO.)
   2. Foods

      (a) Tea
      (b) Coffee
      (c) Cocoa
      (d) Vanilla
      (e) Fruit, especially bananas
      (f) Fruit juice
      (g) Chocolate
      (h) Cheese
      (i) Cider vinegar
      (j) Gelatin foods
      (k) Salad dressing
      (l) Carbonated drinks, except gingerale
      (m)Jelly and jam
      (n) Candy and mints
      (o) Cough drops
      (p) Chewing gum
      (q) Foods containing artificial flavoring or coloring
      (r) Foods containing licorice

   3. Many drugs will cause increased VMA levels.
B. *False decreased levels* of VMA are caused by
   1. Alkaline urine
   2. Uremia (causes toxicity and impaired excretion of VMA)
   3. Radiographic iodine contrast agents (For this reason, an IVP should not be scheduled prior to a VMA test.)
   4. Specific drugs
C. *Interfering factors in determining catecholamine levels*
   1. Vigorous exercise may cause increase
   2. Certain drugs may cause increase.

Patient Preparation
1. Instruct the patient about the purpose of the test and collection of the 24-hour urine specimen. Give a written reminder.

2. Explain diet and drug restrictions.
3. Diet restrictions will vary among laboratory policies, but coffee, tea, bananas, cocoa products, vanilla products, and aspirin are always excluded for 3 days (2 days prior to testing and day of the test).
4. Many laboratories require that all drugs be discontinued for 3 to 7 days before testing.
5. Rest and adequate food and fluids are encouraged, and stress is to be avoided during the test.

Patient Aftercare
Restricted foods, drugs, and activity are permitted as soon as the test is completed.

17-Ketosteroids (17-KS);
17-Hydroxycorticosteroids (17-OHCS)

Normal Values
17-Ketosteroids (17-KS)
Men: 8–20 mg./24 hr.
Women: 6–15 mg./24 hr.
17-Hydroxycorticosteroids (17-OHCS)
4–12 mg./24 hr.

Explanation of Test
These 24-hour tests of adrenal function measure the excretion of urinary steroids and are indicated in the investigation of endocrine disturbances of the adrenals and testes.
    Urinary steroids can be divided into three main groups:

17-ketosteroids (17-KS)—adrenal hormones and metabolites of testicular androgens. In men, the adrenals produce two-thirds of 17-KS, while the testes produce the remainder. In women the adrenals produce all of these hormones. In both sexes, 17-KS decline with age.
17-ketogenic steroids (17-KGS)—adrenal cortex activity
17-hydroxycorticosteroids (17-OHCS)—Porter–Silber chromogens

Procedure
1. A 24-hour urine container with preservative is labeled with the name of the patient, test, and date.
2. General instructions for 24-hour urine collection are followed.
3. Exact start and ending of the collection are recorded on the specimen container and the patient's record (start 8:06 A.M. 11/30; end 8:00 A.M. 12/1).
4. Send the specimen to the laboratory refrigerator when the test is completed.

Interfering Factors

1. Severe stress and obesity will cause increased levels of KS and OHCS.
2. KS levels are often increased in the third trimester of pregnancy.
3. Many drugs affect test outcomes.

The 17-ketosteroids are excreted in the urine as the sulfates and glucuronides of androsterone.

Dehydroepiandrosterone (DHEA)
Etiocholanalase
11-beta hydroxyandrosterone
11-beta hydroxyetiocholanolone
11-ketoandrosterone
and
11-ketoetiocholanolone

Increased 17-KS:

1. Adrenal carcinomas
2. Pregnancy
3. Premature infants
4. ACTH administration
5. Testicular interstitial cell tumors
6. Cushing's syndrome
7. Nonmalignant virilizing adrenal tumors
8. Androgenic arrhenoblastoma
9. Luteal cell ovarian tumors
10. Female pseudohermaphroditism
11. Adrenogenital syndrome associated with adrenal hyperplasia

Decreased 17-KS:

1. Addison's disease
2. Panhypopituitarism
3. Myxedema
4. Nephrosis
5. Castration or eunuchoidism in man
6. Gout
7. Chronic illness
8. Thyrotoxicosis

Increased 17-OHCS

1. Any acute illness
2. Cushing's disease
3. Adrenal adenoma
4. Carcinoma
5. Ectopic ACTH syndrome
6. Severe hypertension
7. Acromegaly
8. Thyrotoxicosis

Decreased 17-OHCS:

1. Addison's disease
2. Congenital adrenal hyperplasia
3. Hypopituitarism
4. Hypothyroidism

Patient Preparation
1. Instruct the patient about the purpose of the test and collection of 24-hour urine specimen. Give a written reminder.
2. Food and fluids are permitted and encouraged.

Porphyrins and Porphobilinogens

Normal Values
Porphobilinogens: 0–2 mg./24 hr. or negative or 0–8.8 umol./24 hr.
Porphyrins: 50–300 mg./24 hr.
DAL or ALA: 1.0–710 mg./24 hr.
Fluorescent: negative

Explanation of Test
Porphyrins are cyclic compounds formed from delta-aminolevulinic acid (DAL or ALA), which is important in the formation of hemoglobin and other hemoproteins that function as carriers of oxygen in the blood and tissues. In health, insignificant amounts of porphyrin are excreted in the urine. However, in certain conditions such a porphyria (disturbance in metabolism of porphyrin), liver disease, lead poisoning, and pellagra, there is an increased level of porphyrins, as well as DAL and ALA in the urine. Disorders in porphyrin metabolism also result in porphobilinogen.

In acute attacks of porphyria, the patient may suffer skin lesions, abdominal pain, neuropathy, and mental disturbances. The urine of patients with this disease usually has a pinkish to reddish black tinge and will become darker upon standing.

In the laboratory the urine is tested for the presence of porphyrins, porphobilinogen, and DAL or ALA. It is also given the black light screening test (porphyrins are fluorescent when exposed to black or ultraviolet light).

Procedure
1. A 24-hour clean catch urine container with preservative is labeled with the name of the patient, test, and date.
2. Refrigeration is required. The specimen is kept protected from exposure to light.
3. General instructions for 24-hour urine collection are followed.
4. Exact start and ending of the collection are recorded on the specimen container and the patient's record (start 7:05 A.M. 11/15; end 7:30 A.M. 11/16).
5. Send the specimen to the laboratory refrigerator when the test is completed.
6. Porphobilinogens are always done with the porphyrin test. Should a single, fresh-voided specimen be ordered, only a porphobilinogen

will be done. Protect specimen from light. Take specimen to laboratory immediately. The test must be performed within 60 minutes of voiding for test to be valid. If possible, obtain specimen between 10:00 A.M. and 2:00 P.M.

7. Observe and record the color of urine. If porphyrins are present, the urine may have a grossly recognizable amber red or burgundy color. It may vary from pale pink to almost black. Some patients will excrete a urine of normal color that turns dark after standing in the light.

Clinical Implications

A. *Porphyria*
   1. In the porphyrias, the urine contains increased amounts of porphyrins and porphobilinogens and may not contain increased quantities of DAL or ALA.
   2. ALA and DAL excretion is elevated in acute intermittent porphyria, an hepatic porphyria that is aggravated by alcohol, barbiturates, and other drugs affecting the liver.
B. *Lead poisoning*
   1. ALA or DAL will be present in the urine.
   2. Porphyrins may or may not be present in the urine.
C. *Other conditions with increased levels of porphyrins*
   1. Cirrhosis
   2. Infectious hepatitis
   3. Hodgkin's disease
   4. Some cancers
   5. Central nervous system disorders
   6. Heavy metal poisoning
   7. Carbon tetrachloride or benzine toxicity
   8. Vitamin deficiency
D. A number of drugs may cause false-positive tests.

Patient Preparation

1. Instruct the patient about the purpose and collection of a 24-hour urine specimen. Give a written reminder.
2. Food and fluids are permitted; alcohol and excessive fluid intake during collection should be avoided.

Clinical Alert

This test should not be ordered for patients receiving Donnatal and other barbiturate preparations. However, if intermittent porphyria is the reason for testing, the test should be done with the patient receiving these medications because these drugs may provoke an attack of porphyria.

Amylase Excretion/Clearance

Normal Values
70–275 Somogyi units/hr. or 13–51 u./hr.
1500–6000 Somogyi units/24 hr. or 277–1110 u./24 hr.

Background
Amylase is an enzyme that changes starch to sugar. It is produced in the salivary glands, pancreas, liver, and fallopian tubes and normally is excreted in small amounts in the urine. If there is an inflammation of the pancreas or salivary glands, much more of the enzyme enters the blood and more amylase is excreted in the urine.

Explanation of Test
This test of blood and urine is an indication of pancreatic function and is done to differentiate acute pancreatitis from peptic ulcer and other disorders in which amylase is increased. The timed urine and amylase test (2 hours or 24 hours) is ordered to detect inflammation of the salivary glands or pancreas, to monitor treatment of acute pancreatitis, and to recognize recurrent attacks of acute pancreatitis in persons who exhibit severe abdominal pain.

The 2-hour amylase excretion in the urine is a more sensitive test than either the serum amylase or lipase test. In patients with acute pancreatitis, the urine often shows a prolonged elevation of amylase as compared to the short-lived peak in the blood. However, urine amylase may be elevated when blood amylase is within normal range, and conversely, the blood amylase may be elevated when urine amylase is within normal range. The 24-hour level may be normal even when some of the 1- or 2-hour specimens show increased values.

Procedure
A venous blood sample of 4 ml. may be collected at the same time a random urine specimen is obtained.

1. A 1-hour, 2-hour, or 24-hour timed specimen will be ordered. A 2-hour specimen is usually collected.
2. No preservative or refrigeration is required.
3. General instructions for a timed or 24-hour urine collection are followed.
4. Exact start and ending of the collection are recorded on the specimen container and on the patient's record (start 8:06 A.M. 11/17; end 10:15 A.M. 11/17).
5. Send the specimen to the laboratory refrigerator when the test is completed.

Clinical Implications
1. Elevated levels of urine amylase are associated with acute pancreatitis, choledocholithiasis, and peptic ulcer.
2. Patients with acute pancreatitis have values about 900 units per hour during the first 2 days of the attack; it increases sooner than blood amylase. Urine amylase also stays elevated longer in acute pancreatitis.
3. Values will increase about five per unit in pancreatitis; in other disorders associated with hyperamylase, the level is less than 5%.

Patient Preparation
1. Instruct the patient about the purpose of the test and collection of the urine specimen. Give a written reminder for 2-hour or 24-hour test.
2. Encourage fluids during test if fluids are not restricted for other medical reasons.

Phenylketonuria (PKU) in Blood and Urine

Normal Values
Blood <4 mg./100 ml.
Urine: Negative dipstick; no observed color change

Explanation of Test
Routine blood and urine tests are done on newborns to detect PKU, a genetic disease that can lead to mental retardation and brain damage if untreated. This disease is characterized by a lack of the enzyme that converts phenylalanine, an amino acid, to tyrosine, which is necessary for normal metabolic function. If tyrosine accumulates in the tissues, phenylpyruvic acid, a metabolite of phenylalanine, will be produced, resulting in brain damage. Phenylalanine can be detected in the blood of an abnormal child in 4 days. Phenylpyruvic acid appears in the urine of an abnormal child about 2 to 8 weeks after birth. Current practice is to test for PKU either with a blood phenylalanine test or with a phenylpyruvic acid urine test.

Procedure (Collecting Blood Sample)
1. After the skin is cleansed with an antiseptic, the infant's heel is punctured with a sterile disposable lancet.
2. If bleeding is slow, it is helpful to hold the leg dependent for a short time before spotting the blood on the filter paper.
3. The circles on the filter paper must be filled completely. This can best be done by placing one side of the filter paper against the infant's heel and watching for the blood to appear on the front side of the paper and completely fill the circle.

Procedure (Collecting Urine Sample in Nursery or at Home)
1. The reagent strip is either dipped into a fresh sample of urine or pressed against a wet diaper.
2. After exactly 30 seconds, the strip is compared to a color chart scaled at concentrations of 0, 15, 40, and 100 mg. phenylpyruvic acid.

Clinical Implications
1. In a positive test for PKU, the blood phenylalanine is greater than 15 mg. per 100 ml. Blood tyrosine is less than 5 mg. per 100 ml. It is never increased in phenylketonuria.
2. The urine test is positive in PKU.

Interfering Factors
1. Premature infants, infants weighing less than 11 kg. (5 lbs.) may have elevated phenylalanine and tyrosine levels without having the genetic disease. This is probably a result of delayed development of appropriate enzyme activity in the liver.
2. Large amounts of ketones in urine will produce an atypical color reaction.

Instructions to Mothers
1. Inform the mother about the purpose of the test and the method of collecting the specimens.
2. Most parents would be interested in knowing that PKU (a genetic disease in which a defective gene is passed on from each parent) was first recognized about 40 years ago by a young mother of two mentally retarded children. She was aware that the urine of these children had a peculiar odor, and on the basis of this was able to have a biochemist study the urine and identify phenylpyruvic acid. About 20 years ago the first successful dietary treatment (restriction of phenylalanine as in milk) of newborn babies identified as having PKU was started, resulting in normal mental development.

Clinical Alert
1. The blood test must be performed at least 3 days after birth or after the child has had a chance to ingest protein (milk) for a period of 24 hours.
2. Urine testing is usually done at the 4 or 6 week checkup if a blood sample was not obtained.
3. PKU studies should be done on all infants 5 pounds or more before they leave the hospital.

Tubular Reabsorption Phosphate (TRP)

Normal Values
82–95% on normal diet or 0.82–0.95

Explanation of Test
This test is done to detect hyperparathyroidism. A fasting blood and a 24-hour or a 4-hour urine sample is obtained to determine the levels of phosphorus and creatinine. The results of the test are based on the ratio of creatinine clearance to phosphate clearance. TRP is a rough estimation of the level of parathyroid hormone in the blood. The test is based on the fact that excessive parathyroid hormone increases renal tubular reabsorption of phosphate. However, the test has a limited value, and a determination of increased calcium in the blood is still essential for the exact diagnosis of hyperparathyroidism.

Procedure
1. An overnight fast from food is usually necessary. Water is permitted.
2. A venous blood sample will be obtained the morning of the day the test is completed.
3. A 24-hour urine container (also used for 4-hour test) with preservatives is labeled with the name of the patient, test, and date.
4. General instructions for 24-hour or 4-hour urine collection are followed.
5. A good time to do this test is from noon to noon, although it is not necessary.
6. Exact start and ending of the collection are recorded on the specimen container and the patient's record. (12 noon, 11/17; end 12:06 P.M., 11/18).
7. Send the specimen to the laboratory refrigerator when the test is completed.

Clinical Implications
1. In hyperparathyroidism, the reabsorption of phosphate is increased.
2. The TRP is decreased in hypoparathyroidism.

Interfering Factors
False-positive results may occur in the presence of uremia, renal tubular disease, osteomalacia, and sarcoidosis.

Patient Preparation
1. Instruct the patient about the purpose of the test, collection of 24-hour or 4-hour urine specimen, overnight fast if ordered, and blood

sample. A normal or phosphate diet will be ordered. Give a written reminder.
2. If fasting is ordered, encourage the patient to drink water.

D-Xylose Absorption

Normal Values
Urine: more than 1.2 g.
Blood: 25–40 mg./100 ml. in 2 hr.

Explanation of Test
This test is an indirect measure of intestinal absorption and is used in the differential diagnosis of steatorrhea. The usual problem is the differentiation of pancreatic from enterogenous steatorrhea. When d-xylose (which is not metabolized by the body) is administered orally, blood and urine levels are checked for absorption rates. Absorption is normal in pancreatic steatorrhea but will be impaired in enterogenous steatorrhea.

Procedure
1. No food or liquids by mouth after midnight on the day of the test.
2. Have the patient void between 8:00 and 9:00 A.M. Discard urine.
3. Then give 5 g. of d-xylose orally. Dissolve 250 ml. (8 oz.) of water. Follow immediately with an additional 250 ml. of water. Note time and record on the patient's record. No further fluids or food until the test is completed.
4. Exactly 2 hours later, a venous blood sample of 3 ml. is obtained.
5. The patient must remain stationary until completion of test.
6. Save all urine voided during the test. Five hours after the test is started, have the patient void. Add this urine to collected urine, if any. Send the urine specimen to the laboratory.

Clinical Implications
Decreased levels in
Enterogenous steatorrhea
Malabsorption

Patient Preparation
Explain the purpose and procedure of the test and collection of the urine specimen.

Patient Aftercare
Provide food and fluids and allow patient to be ambulatory.

Clinical Alert

Nausea, vomiting, and diarrhea may occur as side-effects of d-xylose, especially if more than 5 g. of drug are given.

Creatinine/Creatinine Clearance

Normal Values
Men: 0.7–1.3 mg/dl or 62–115 μmol/liter
Women: 0.6–1.2 mg/dl or 53–106 μmol/liter
Men: 800–1200 mg/24 Hr. or 7.1–17.7 mmol/24 Hr.
Women: 600–1800 mg/24 Hr. or 5.3–15.9 mmol/24 Hr.

Explanation of Test
This blood and urine test is a specific measurement ordered to determine kidney function, primarily glomerular filtration. It measures the rate at which creatinine is cleared from the blood by the kidney. Clearance of a substance may be defined as the imaginary volume (ml./min.) of plasma from which the substance would have to be completely extracted in order for the kidney to excrete that amount in 1 minute.

Creatinine is a substance that, in health, is easily excreted by the kidney. Creatinine is the by-product of muscle energy metabolism and is produced at a constant rate depending on the muscle mass of the individual. Endogenous production of creatinine is constant as long as muscle mass remains constant. Since all the creatinine that is filtered in a given time interval appears in the urine, the creatinine is equivalent to the glomerular filtration rate (GFR). A disorder of kidney function prevents excretion of creatinine. More than 50 of the total kidney nephrons have to be altered to reflect change in the normal value. Creatinine is co-ordered with virtually every quantitative urine test. Creatinine is measured along with other urinary constituents to assess the accuracy of the collection and to interpret the excretion rate of specific urinary constituents.

Procedure
1. A 12-hour or 24-hour urine container is labeled with the name of the patient, test, and date.
2. Refrigeration is necessary or keep the specimen on ice.
3. General instructions for 24-hour urine collection are followed.
4. Exact start and ending of the collection are recorded on the specimen container and the patient's record (start 8:32 A.M./date; end 8:35 A.M./date).

5. Send the specimen to the laboratory refrigerator when the test is completed.
6. A venous blood sample of 7 ml. for serum creatinine is obtained the morning of the day that the 12-hour or 24-hour collection will be completed.

Clinical Implications
1. A normal clearance cannot be used as a standard for a patient who is known to have existing renal disease.
2. A decreased clearance gives a reliable indication of impaired kidney function.
3. However, a normal blood creatinine does not always indicate unimpaired renal function.

Interfering Factors
Phenacetin will cause creatinine clearance to be decreased.

Clinical Alert

A 24-hour urine test for cyclic adenosine monophosphate (cAMP) is a second order test in difficult-to-diagnose cases of primary hyperparathyroidism. Urine excretion of cAMP is compound with a measurement of glomerular filtration.

Patient Preparation
1. Instruct the patient about the purpose of the test and collection of the urine specimen. Give a written reminder.
2. Food and fluids are permitted. Encourage fluids so that voiding is easier because a large urine flow is best for greatest accuracy of the test. Avoid coffee, tea, and vigorous exercise during the test.

Cystine

Normal Values
Qualitative: Negative
Quantitative: Children under 8: 2–13 mg./24 hr.
Children over 8 and adults: 7–28 mg./hr.

Explanation of Test
These tests of urine are useful in the differential diagnosis of cystinuria, an inherited disease characterized by bladder calculi (cystine has a low solubility). In cystinosis, cystine is deposited in lung tissues. A positive test is confirmed in a 24-hour collection.

Procedure
1. A urine specimen of 20 ml. is obtained for a qualitative specimen.
2. If a 24-hour urine specimen is ordered, it is collected in a container with a preservative. Follow general procedures for collection of a 24-hour specimen.
3. Schedule before an IVP.
4. Notify the laboratory if the patient is taking penicillamine.

Clinical Implications
Values are increased in

(a) Cystinuria (up to 20 times normal) in which there is excess urinary excretion of lysine, ornithine, arginine, and cystine.
(b) Cystinosis (no excess of lysine, ornithine, or arginine).

Clinical Alert

A cystine screen can also be done. Persons with cystinuria can be put on a special diet that minimizes kidney stone formation.

1. A random urine is collected.
2. A drop of Na cyanide in 1 N NaOH is added to an acetest tablet.

Hydroxyproline

Normal Values
Total: 15–43 mg./24 hr. or 0.11–0.33 mmol./24 hr.
Free: 2–5% of total or 0.02–0.05 of total.

Explanation of Test
This study is an indication of bone reabsorption in various disorders, as well as an indication of the degree of destruction from primary or secondary bone tumors. It is an important measurement as a determinant of the severity of Paget's disease and the response to treatment. Hydroxyproline is an amino acid that is increased during periods of rapid growth, bone diseases, and some endocrine disorders. Less than 10% is normally free; almost all is peptide bound. In adults, hydroxyproline excretion reflects bone resorption, whereas alkaline phosphatase reflects bone formation.

Procedure
1. A 2-hour specimen is usually obtained after an overnight fast.
2. Notify the laboratory of the patient's age and sex.

3. A 24-hour urine specimen may also be collected in a container with preservative. Refrigerate the specimen.
4. Follow the general 24-hour collection procedure. The laboratory will record the total 24-hour volume.
5. A blood sample is the preferred method of testing in the first few months of life.

Clinical Implications
1. *Free hydroxyproline is increased* in
   (a) Hydroxyprolinemia, a hereditary autosomal recessive condition.
   (b) Familial iminoglycinuria, also inherited.
2. *Total hydroxyproline levels are increased* in
   (a) Hyperparathyroidism   (e) Osteoporosis
   (b) Paget's disease   (f) Bone tumors
   (c) Marfan syndrome   (g) Myeloma
   (d) Klinefelter's syndrome

Lysozyme

Normal Values
Blood plasma: 2.8–15.8 μg./ml.
Urine: 1.3–3.6 mg./24 hrs.

Background
Lysozyme (muramidase) in blood or urine comes from degradation of granulocytes and monocytes.

Explanation of Test
This test of blood and urine is used in the investigation of leukemia, chronic infections, and renal graft rejection.

Procedure
1. A venous blood sample of 10 ml. or a urine specimen is collected.
2. Follow general instructions for random collection or 24-hour urine collections.

Clinical Implications
1. *Levels are elevated* in
   (a) Acute myelomonocytic leukemia
   (b) Chronic granulocytic leukemia
2. *Levels may be elevated* in
   (a) Renal disorders   (d) Renal homograft rejection
   (b) Regional enteritis   (especially urine)
   (c) Chronic infections

Myoglobin

Normal Values
Urine: 0.4–4.0 μg. MB/ml.
Increases slightly with age.

Background
Myoglobin is the oxygen-binding protein of striated muscle. It resembles hemoglobin but it is unable to release oxygen except at extremely low tension. Injury to skeletal or cardiac muscle will result in release of myoglobin. It is rapidly excreted from the blood into the urine; there is no threshold level.

Explanation of Test
Urine tests are helpful in evaluating a variety of conditions, including some metabolic diseases.

Procedure
1. A urine sample of at least 1 ml. is collected.
2. The urine must test positive for hemoglobin before proceeding with the test.

Clinical Implications
A. *Increased values* are associated with
1. Myocardial infarction
2. Other muscle injury, sports, and car accidents
3. Polymyositis
4. Hereditary myoglobinuria
5. Phosphorylase deficiency
6. Unknown metabolic defects
7. Crushing injuries
8. Progressive muscle disease
9. Hyperthermia and malignant hypertension
10. Electric shock
11. Some viral illnesses

Clinical Alert
1. If large amounts of myoglobin are presented to the kidney, anuria may result from renal damage.

Pregnancy Tests

Normal Values
Negative in blood and urine

Background
From the earliest stage of development (9 days old), the placenta produces hormones, either on its own or in conjunction with the fetus. The very young placental trophoblast produces appreciable amounts of a hormone, human chorionic gonadotropin (HCG), that is excreted in the urine. HCG is not found in the urine of normal, young, nonpregnant women.

Explanation of Test
Increased urinary levels of HCG form the basis of most tests for pregnancy and for trophoblastic tumors in men. All pregnancy tests are designed to detect HCG. HCG is present in blood and urine whenever there is living chorionic/placental tissue. HCG can be further identified as alpha or beta HCG. HCG can be detected in the urine of pregnant women 26 to 36 days after the first day of the last menstrual period, or 8 to 10 days after conception. Pregnancy tests should be negative 3 to 4 days after delivery.

The tests using female rats or male frogs have been supplanted by immunologic tests that are more accurate, easier to perform, and do not require a laboratory to maintain animal facilities. New urine tests are just as sensitive as the serum tests. Quantitative analysis of HCG aids in making a differential diagnosis of a viable pregnancy versus a nonviable pregnancy, twins or multiple gestations, or developing hydatidiform mole.

Procedure (for Urine Test)
1. An early morning urine specimen is collected. The first morning specimen generally contains the greatest concentration of HCG. However, specimens collected at any time may be used, but the specific gravity must be at least 1.005.
2. A 24-hour specimen is collected for quantitative studies. Then the general procedure for collection of 24-hour urine specimens is followed.
3. Grossly bloody specimens are not acceptable; in this instance a catheterized specimen should be obtained.

Clinical Implications
1. A positive result usually indicates pregnancy. Only two-thirds of women with ectopic pregnancies will have positive pregnancy tests.
2. Positive results also occur in
   (a) Choriocarcinoma
   (b) Hydatidiform mole
   (c) Testicular tumors
   (d) Chorioepithelioma
   (e) Chorioadenoma destruens
   (f) Conditions with a high ESR such as acute salpingitis
   (g) Cancer of lung, stomach, colon, pancreas, and breast

Interfering Factors
1. *False-negative tests* and falsely low levels of HCG may be due to a dilute urine (low specific gravity) or a specimen obtained too early in pregnancy.
2. *False-positive tests* are associated with
   (a) Proteinuria
   (b) Hematuria
   (c) Presence of excess pituitary gonadotropin (HLH) as in menopausal women
   (d) Drugs
      1. Anticonvulsants
      2. Antiparkinsons
      3. Hypnotics
      4. Tranquilizers

Clinical Alert

The presence of HCG in urine should be interpreted in conjunction with other clinical and laboratory data available to the clinician.

Estrogen Fractions/Urine and Serum

Normal Values
Vary widely between women and men, pregnancy, menopausal state, and follicular, ovulatory, and luteal stage of menstrual cycle.

Explanation of Test
These measurements are useful along with gonadotropins in evaluating menstrual and fertility problems, feminization in men, estrogen-producing tumors and pregnancy. Estradiol (E_2) is the most active of endogenous estrogens. Estriol (E_3) levels in both plasma and urine rise as pregnancy advances, with significant amounts being produced in the third trimester.

Procedure
1. A venous blood sample can be obtained.
2. A 24-hour urine can be collected using a preservative.
3. General collection procedures for 24-hour specimen are followed.

Clinical Alert

1. If estriol levels are higher than expected, one of the following may be indicated
   (a) Gestation more advanced than expected
   (b) More than one fetus
   (c) Laboratory error

Clinical Implications

1. *Estrogen values are increased* in
   (a) Ovarian tumors producing estrogen
   (b) Testicular tumors
   (c) Tumors or hyperplasia of the adrenal cortex
   (d) True precocious puberty
   (e) Corpus luteum cyst
   (f) Liver cirrhosis
   (g) Stein–Leventhal syndrome
2. *Estrogen values are decreased* in
   (a) Hypofunction or dysfunction of pituitary and adrenal glands
   (b) Primary ovarian malfunction
   (c) Menopause
   (d) Anovulatory bleeding
   (e) Inadequate luteal phase
3. *Estriol values are decreased* in
   (a) Placental insufficiency
   (b) Fetal distress—an abrupt drop of 40% or more on 2 consecutive days
   (c) Fetal outcome is considered favorable if the movement is upward
   (d) Other causes of decreased estriol levels include
       (1) Anemia
       (2) Malnutrition
       (3) Pyelonephritis
       (4) Intestinal disease
       (5) Hemoglobinopathies

Patient Preparation

1. Explain the purpose and procedure of the test.
2. Address the issue of compliance. The patient must be able to adjust daily activities to accommodate to the urine collection.

Amino Acids (Total/Fractions)

Normal Values
Urine and Blood
Age dependent

Explanation of Test
This test is used as the initial screen for inborn errors of metabolism and transport when genetic abnormalities are suspected, such as mental retardation, reduced growth rates, or various other unexplained symptoms. More than 50 aminoacidopathies are now recognized.

Procedure
1. A fasting blood specimen may be obtained.
2. Urine specimens, random or 24-hour collection, preserved with boric acid are collected for the initial screening procedure.

Clinical Implications
1. *Total serum amino acids are increased* in
   (a) Diabetes with ketosis
   (b) Malabsorption
   (c) Hereditary fructose intolerance
   (d) Conditions with severe brain damage
   (e) Reye's syndrome
   (f) Acute and chronic renal failure
   (g) Eclampsia
   (h) Specific amino acidopathies
2. *Total serum amino acids are decreased* in
   (a) Adrenal cortical hyperfunction
   (b) Huntington's chorea
   (c) Phlebotomus fever
   (d) Nephritic syndrome
   (e) Rheumatoid arthritis
   (f) Hartnup disease
   (g) Fever
   (h) Malnutrition
3. *Total urine amino acids are increased* in
   (a) Viral hepatitis
   (b) Multiple myeloma
   (c) Hyperparathyroidism
   (d) Rickets (vit. D)
   (e) Osteomalacia
   (f) Hereditary fructose intolerance
   (g) Galactosemia
   (h) Cystinosis
   (i) Wilson's disease
   (j) Hartnup disease
4. *Fractions of total amino acids include*

Alanine	Anserine	Aspartic Acid
Alpha-Amino-N-Butyric Acid	Arginine	Beta-alanine
Alpha-Aminoodysic Acid	Argininosuccinic Acid	Beta-aminoisobutyric Acid
	Asparagine	Carnosine

Citrulline
Cystine
Ethanolamine
Glutamic Acid
Glutamine
Glycine
Histidine
Hydroproline
Isoleucine

Leucine
Lupine
Methionine
1-Methylhistidine
3-Methylhistidine
Ornithine
Phenylalanine
Phosphaethanol-
amine

Proline
Sarcosine
Serine
Taurine
Threonine
Tryptophan
Valine

BIBLIOGRAPHY

American Society for Medical Technology Urinalysis: An Educational Program. (Pilot project in competence assurance, sponsored by BMC-BioDynamics. Indianapolis, Publisher Research Media, 1979)

Ames Company: Factors Affecting Urine Chemistry Tests. Elkhart, IN, Ames Company, 1982

Ames Company: Modern Urine Chemistry: A Guide to the Diagnosis and Metabolic Disorders of Urinary Tract Diseases. Elkhart, IN, Ames Company, 1976

Bradley M: Urine crystals—Identification and significance. Lab Med 13(6):348–353, 1982

Chairmna, Gambino: Laboratory Testing: New and Future Procedures; An International Symposium. Tarpon Springs, FL, 1983

Davidsohn I, Henry JB: Todd–Sanford–Davidsohn Clinical Diagnosis and Management by Laboratory Methods, 17th ed. Philadelphia, WB Saunders, 1984

Free AH, Free HM: Rapid convenience urine tests: Their use and misuse. Lab Med 9(12):9–17, 1978

Free AH, Free HM: Urinalysis in Clinical Laboratory Practice. Cleveland, CRC Press, 1975

Free AH, Free HM: Urodynamics: Concepts Relating to Routine Urine Chemistry. Elkhart, IN, Ames Company, 1976

Haber HM: Urinary Sediment: A Textbook Atlas. Chicago, American Society of Clinical Pathologists, 1981

Halsted CH, Halsted JA (eds): The Laboratory in Clinical Medicine, 2nd ed. Philadelphia, WB Saunders, 1981

Inhorn SL (ed): Quality Assurance Practices for Health Laboratories. Washington, DC, American Public Health Association, 1978

Isselbacher KJ, et al (eds): Harrison's Principles of Internal Medicine, 11th ed. New York, McGraw–Hill, 1987

Jacobs DS et al: Laboratory Test Handbook with DRG Index. St. Louis, CV Mosby/Lexi–Comp, 1984

Kaplan A, Szabo LL: Clinical Chemistry: Interpretation and Techniques, 2nd ed. Philadelphia, Lea & Febiger, 1983

Leavelle DE: Medical Laboratories Handbook. Rochester, MN, Mayo Clinic, 1986

Lipo RF: Crisis: Substance Abuse in the Workplace; Solutions for Business and Industry. Oak Creek, WI, Chem–Bio Corporation, 1986

McConnell EA: Urinalysis: A common test, but never routine. Nurs 12(2):108–109, 111, 1982

Ravel R: Clinical Laboratory Medicine, 4th ed. Chicago, Year Book Medical Pub 1984

Rocom Press: Urine Under the Microscope. Nutley, NY, Rocom Press, 1975

Schumann GB: Urine Sediment Examination. Baltimore, Williams & Wilkins, 1980

Sonnenwirth AC, Jarett L (eds): Gradwohl's Clinical Laboratory Methods and Diagnosis, 8th ed. St. Louis, CV Mosby, 1980

Tietz NW: Clinical Guide to Laboratory Tests. Philadelphia, WB Saunders, 1983

Widmann FK: Goodale's Clinical Interpretation of Laboratory Tests, 9th ed. Philadelphia, FA Davis, 1983

FECAL STUDIES

Introduction: Formation and Composition of Feces

The elimination from the body of waste products of digestion is essential to health. These excreted waste products are known as *stool* or *feces*. Stool examination is often done in the evaluation of gastrointestinal disorders and results are helpful in detecting gastrointestinal bleeding and obstruction, obstructive jaundice, parasitic disease, dysentery, ulcerative colitis, and increased fat excretion.

An adult excretes 100 to 300 grams of fecal matter a day, and of this as much as 70% may be water. The feces are what remains of the 8 to 10 liters of fluid that enter the intestinal tract each day. Food and fluid taken orally, saliva, gastric secretions, pancreatic juice, and bile contribute to the formation of feces.

Feces are composed of

1. Waste residue of indigestible material such as cellulose in food eaten over the previous 4 days
2. Bile (pigments and salts); color is normally due to bile pigments that have been altered somewhat by bacterial action
3. Intestinal secretions, including mucus
4. Leukocytes that migrate from the bloodstream
5. Shed epithelial cells
6. Large numbers of bacteria that make up to one-third of total solids
7. Inorganic material (10%–20%) that is chiefly calcium and phosphates
8. Undigested or unabsorbed food (present in very small quantities)

The output of feces depends on a complex series of absorptive, secretory, and fermentative processes. Normal function of the colon involves three physiologic processes: (1) absorption of fluid and electrolytes, (2) contractions that churn the contents, expose contents to the mucosa, and transport the contents to the rectum, and (3) defecation.

The small intestine is approximately 23 feet long, and the large intestine is 4 to 5 feet long. The small intestine degrades ingested fats, proteins, and carbohydrates to absorbable units and absorbs them. Pancreatic, gastric, and biliary secretions operate in the luminal contents to prepare them for active mucosal transport. Other active substances absorbed in the small intestine include fat-soluble vitamins, iron, and calcium. Vitamin B_{12}, after combining with intrinsic factors, is absorbed in the ileum. The small intestine also absorbs as much as 9.5 liters of water and electrolytes for return to the bloodstream. Small intestine contents (chyme) begin to enter the rectum as soon as 2 to 3 hours after a meal, but the process is not complete until 6 to 9 hours after eating.

The large intestine performs less complex functions than the small intestine. The proximal or right colon absorbs most of the remaining water. Colonic absorption of water, sodium, and chloride is a passive process. Daily water excretion in the feces is only about 100 ml. The motility of the colon consists mainly of moving the luminal contents to and fro by seemingly random contractions of circular smooth muscle. More propulsive activity (peristalsis) occurs after eating. These peristaltic waves are caused by the gastrocolic and duodenocolic reflexes, which are initiated after meals and which are caused by the filling of the duodenum by food from the stomach. The muscles of the colon are innervated by the autonomic nervous system. The parasympathetic nervous system stimulates movement and the sympathetic system inhibits movement. Massive peristalsis usually occurs several times a day. Resultant distention of the rectum initiates the urge to defecate. In persons with normal motility and with a mixed dietary intake, transit time in the colon is 24 to 48 hours.

Normally evacuated feces reflect the shape and caliber of the colonic lumen. The normal consistency is somewhat plastic, neither fluid, mushy, nor hard; the usual brown color results from bacterial degradation of bile pigments; the odor is produced by indole, skatole, and butyric acid. Degradation of undigested protein produces a foul odor, as does excessive carbohydrate ingestion.

Appearance

Stool examination should include size, shape, consistency, color, odor, and presence or absence of blood, mucus, pus, tissue fragments, food residues, bacteria, or parasites. (See Chapter 7 for a discussion of microbiological analysis of feces.) The gross appearance of feces should be assessed before administration of barium, laxatives, or enemas.

Patients and health personnel may dislike examining, collecting, and delivering feces for examination. However, this natural aversion must be overcome when considering the value of a feces examination in diagnosing many clinical conditions and diseases of the GI tract and in providing information relating to the liver and pancreas.

Random Collection of Stool Specimens

Stool specimens are sometimes analyzed for diagnostic purposes. Some of the more frequently ordered tests on feces are tests for blood, bile, parasites, and parasite eggs (ova). Stool is also examined in the laboratory by *chromatographic* analysis for the presence of gallstones. The recovery of a gallstone from feces provides the only proof that a common duct stone has been dislodged and excreted. A lipid profile of gallstones will reveal the cholesterol content of stones.

1. Feces should be collected in a dry, clean, urine-free container. The entire stool should be collected and transferred to a container, us-

ing tongue blades. For best results, stool specimens should be covered and delivered to the laboratory immediately after collection. When possible, the specimen should be uncontaminated with urine or other body secretions. Depending on the examination to be performed, the specimen either should be refrigerated or kept warm. Generally, the laboratory will furnish detailed instructions as to the preserving of the feces specimen.

(a) Ova and Parasites

Warm stools are best for detecting ova and parasites. Do *not* refrigerate specimens for ova and parasites. They will not live much below body temperature. Urine also will destroy parasites.

(b) Culture for Enteric Pathogens
1. Some coliform bacilli produce antibiotic substances that destroy enteric pathogens. Refrigerate immediately.
2. A diarrheal stool will usually give good results.
3. A freshly passed stool is the choice specimen.
4. Stool specimens preferably should be collected before antibiotic therapy is initiated and as early in the course of disease as possible.
5. It is recommended that the entire passed stool be sent for examination. If mucus or blood is present, it definitely should be included with the specimen because parasites are more likely to be found in these substances. If for some reason only a small amount of stool can be used for a specimen, this amount should be suitable for examination; a stool the size of a walnut is usually adequate.
6. Do not use a stool that has been passed into the toilet bowl or that has been contaminated with barium, other radiographic media, or urine.
7. Accurately label all stool specimens with the patient's name, date, and reason for testing. Care should be taken that the outside of the container remain uncontaminated.

Interfering Factors
1. Red meat interferes with some tests and usually should be omitted from the diet for 3 days before a test for blood.
2. Stool specimens from patients receiving barium, bismuth, oil, or antibiotics are not satisfactory.
3. Bismuth from paper towels and toilet tissue interferes with tests.

Patient Preparation
1. Explain the purpose and procedure of the test.
2. Instruct the patient to defecate in a clean bedpan or large-mouthed container.
3. Instruct the patient *not to urinate* into the bedpan or collecting container.

4. Remind him that no toilet paper should be placed in the bedpan or container since it interferes with testing.
5. If the patient has diarrhea, newspaper (not paper towels, which contain bismuth) can be deposited into the toilet bowl and the diarrheal stool obtained above the water level of the toilet bowl.

   Note: This method may be used if the patient collects the stool specimen at home. Another method uses a large plastic bag attached by adhesive tape to the toilet seat. After collection, the bag can be placed in the gallon container.

Clinical Alert

Often the physician will order both ova–parasites and culture. In this case, the specimen should be divided in half—one portion refrigerated (for culture testing) and one portion kept at room temperature (for ova and parasite testing).

Consistency, Shape, Form, and Amount

Normal Values
100–200 g./day

Plastic, soft, formed; soft and bulky on a high vegetable diet; small and dry on a high meat diet; seeds and vegetable skins present (see Table 4–1).

Explanation of Test
Normally evacuated feces reflect the shape and caliber of the colonic lumen as well as the colonic motility. The bowel habits of healthy persons vary widely. For this reason, the words "diarrhea" and "constipation" have little meaning except when viewed as a change from the customary individual pattern. Detailed information is important in evaluating either abnormality.

Procedure
See "Random Collection of Stool Specimens," page 200.

Clinical Implications
1. The consistency of feces may change in various disease states.
   (a) Diarrhea mixed with mucus and red blood cells is associated with
   (1) Typhus   (4) Amebiasis
   (2) Typhoid   (5) Large bowel cancer
   (3) Cholera

Table 4-1
Normal Values in Stool Analysis

Macroscopic Examination	Normal
Amount	00–200 g./day
Color	Brown
Odor	Varies with pH of stool and depends on bacterial fermentation and putrefaction
Consistency	Plastic; not unusual to see suds and vegetable skins; soft and bulky in a high vegetable diet; small and dry in a high meat diet.
Size, shape	Formed
Gross blood	None
Mucus	None
Pus	None
Parasites	None

Microscopic Examination	Normal
Fat	Colorless, neutral fat (18%) and fatty acid crystals and soaps
Undigested food, meat fibers, starch, trypsin	None to small amount
Eggs and segments of parasites	None
Yeasts	None
Leukocytes	None

Chemical Examination	Normal
pH	Neutral or weakly alkaline
Occult blood	Negative
Urobilinogen	50 mg.–30 mg./24 hr.
Porphyrins	coproporphyrins: 200 g./24 hr. protoporphyrins: 1500 g./24 hr. uroporphyrins: 1000 g./25 hr.
Nitrogen	1–2 g./24 hr.
Bile	Negative in adults, positive in children
Trypsin	Positive in small amounts in adults; present in greater amounts in normal children
Osmolality, used with serum osmolality to calculate osmotic gap	No established normal. Useful formula is $2\times$ (serum Na + serum K) = stool osmolality $\pm$ 30 mOsm.

(b) Diarrhea mixed with mucus and white blood cells is associated with
  (1) Ulcerative colitis
  (2) Regional enteritis
  (3) Shigellosis
  (4) Salmonellosis
  (5) Intestinal tuberculosis

(c) "Pasty" stool is associated with a high fat content.
   (1) A significant increase of fat is usually detected grossly.
   (2) In obstruction of the common bile duct, the fat gives a putty-like appearance to the stool (alcoholic).
   (3) In sprue and celiac disease, the appearance of the stool often resembles aluminum paint due to fatty acid.
   (4) In cystic fibrosis, the increase of neutral fat gives a greasy, "butter stool" appearance.
(d) A bulky, frothy stool is associated with sprue and celiac disease.
2. Alterations in size or shape indicate altered motility or abnormalities in the colonic wall.
   (a) A narrow ribbonlike stool suggests the possibility of spastic bowel, rectal narrowing or stricture, decreased elasticity, or a partial obstruction.
   (b) Excessively hard stools are usually due to increased absorption of fluid as a result of prolonged contact of luminal contents with the mucosa of the colon because of delayed transit time.
   (c) A very large caliber stool indicates dilatation of the viscus.
   (d) Small, round, hard stools (scybala) accompany habitual, moderate constipation.
   (e) Severe fecal retention can produce huge impacted masses with a small amount of pasty stool as overflow.

Assessment of Diarrhea and Constipation
1. When patients complain of diarrhea and constipation it is important to obtain and record
   (a) An estimate of volume and frequency of fecal output
   (b) Consistency, blood, pus, mucus, oiliness and bad odor (obtain through direct examination)
   (c) Reduction or increase in frequency of defecation
   (d) Sensations of rectal fullness with incomplete evacuation of stools
   (e) Painful defecation due to hard stools
2. Assess the patient's emotional status. In many instances, psychological stress is the major reason for altered bowel habits.

Odor and pH

Normal Values
Characteristic odor varies with the pH of stool; normal pH is neutral or weakly alkaline.

Explanation of Test
Substances called indole and skatole, formed by intestinal putrefaction and fermentation by bacteria, are primarily responsible for the odor of

normal stools. An observation should be made about the odor of feces. The pH is dependent on bacterial fermentation and putrefaction in the bowel.

Interfering Factors
1. Carbohydrate fermentation changes the pH to acid.
2. Protein breakdown changes the pH to alkaline.

Color

Normal Values
Brown

Explanation of Test
The color of the feces should be noted, since it can provide information on pathologic conditions, organic dysfunction, bleeding, diet, and intake of drugs. An abnormality in color may aid the clinician in selecting appropriate diagnostic chemical and microbiological tests of stool.

The brown color of normal feces is probably due to stercobilin (urobilin), a bile pigment derivative, which results from the action of reducing bacteria in bilirubin and undetermined factors.

Procedure
See "Random Collection of Stool Specimens," page 200.

Clinical Implications
1. The color of feces changes in disease states.
    (a) Yellow to yellow green—severe diarrhea
    (b) Green—severe diarrhea
    (c) Black—usually the result of bleeding into the upper gastrointestinal tract
    (d) Tan or clay colored—associated with blockage of the common bile duct as well as pancreatic insufficiency, which produces a pale, greasy, acholic stool. In these instances, reduced quantities of bile pigments enter the intestine because of intrinsic hepatobiliary disease or obstruction.
    (e) Red—possible result of bleeding from the lower gastrointestinal tract
2. Grossly visible blood always indicates an abnormal state.
    (a) Blood streaked on the outer surface usually indicates hemorrhoids or anal abnormalities
    (b) Blood present in stool can also arise from abnormalities higher in the colon. If transit time is sufficiently rapid, blood from the stomach or duodenum can appear as bright or dark red in stool.

Interfering Factors
1. Stool darkens on standing.
2. Color is influenced by diet, food dyes, certain foods, and drugs.
    (a) Yellow to yellow green color occurs in the stool of breast-fed infants who lack normal intestinal flora. It also occurs in sterilization of bowel by antibiotics.
    (b) Green color occurs in diets high in chlorophyll-rich vegetables such as spinach, with the use of the drug calomel, and in antibiotic therapy.
    (c) Black or very dark brown color may be due to drugs such as iron, charcoal, and bismuth, to foods such as cherries, or to an unusually high proportion of meat in the diet.
    (d) Light-colored stool with little odor may be due to diets high in milk and low in meat.
    (e) Claylike color may be due to a diet with excessive fat intake or barium used in radiograph examinations
    (f) Red color may be due to a diet high in beets or use of drugs such as Bromsulphalein (sodium sulfobromophthalein).
    (g) Certain color changes may result from drugs.
        (1) Black—iron salts, bismuth salts, charcoal
        (2) Green—mercurous chloride, indomethacin, calomel
        (3) Green to blue—dithiazanine
        (4) Brown staining—anthraquinones
        (5) Red—phenolphthalein, pyrvinium pamoate, tetracyclines in syrup, Bromsulphalein
        (6) Yellow—santonin
        (7) Yellow to brown—senna
        (8) Light—barium
        (9) Whitish discoloration—antacids
        (10) Orange red—phenazopyridine
        (11) Pink to red to black—anticoagulants (excessive dose), salicylates causing internal bleeding

Clinical Alert

A good dietary and drug history will help to differentiate significant abnormalities from interfering factors.

Blood in Stool

Normal Values
Negative

Explanation of Test
The normal person passes 2.0–2.5 ml. of blood into the GI tract daily. Passage of more than 2.8 ml. of blood in 24 hours is an important sign of GI disease. Blood is most commonly seen when hemorrhoids and anal fissures are present. Detection of occult (hidden) blood in the stool is very useful in detecting or localizing disease of the GI tract. This test will demonstrate the presence of blood in upper GI bleeding, as in the presence of gastric ulcer. The real benefit is screening for colonic carcinoma and other sources of occult bleeding.

Procedure

Chemical Tests for Occult Blood in Stool
Tests for detecting blood in feces use substances that depend on peroxidase content as an indication of hemoglobin content to cause a color change in the stool specimen being tested. The reagent substances used differ in sensitivity. All the commercial tests have sensitivities intended to be consistent in the uses for which they are designed. The sensitivities are adjusted to detect blood loss greater than 5–10 ml./ day. Hematest is more sensitive and also has more false positives. Hemocult (guaiac) is less sensitive and also has less false positives. Tests to detect occult blood are

1. *Ortho-Tolidin (Hematest, Occultest).* Less sensitive than benzidine +Blood—1 : 20,000
2. *Guaiac (Hemoccult).* The least sensitive of the three tests. +Blood— 1 : 1,000

Clinical Implications
1. A dark red to black tarry appearance of the stool is indicative of a loss of 0.50 ml. to 0.75 ml. of blood from the upper GI tract. Smaller quantities of blood in the GI tract can produce similar stools or appear as bright red blood.
2. A stool should be considered grossly bloody only after chemical testing to prevent confusing bloody stool with coloring from diet or drugs (see section on color).
3. Blood in the stool is abnormal and should be reported and recorded.
4. Gross or occult blood in the stool may indicate chronic nonspecific ulcerative colitis, or carcinoma of the colon.
5. Stool specimens may be positive for blood in diaphragmatic hernia.
6. Occult blood may appear in the stool in diverticulitis, gastric carcinoma, and gastritis.
7. To be completely valid, the test employed must be repeated 3–6 times on different samples. The patient's diet should be free of meats, fish, and vegetable sources of peroxidase activity. Only after following this regimen can a positive series of tests be considered an indication for further evaluation of the patient.

Interfering Factors

Drugs such as salicylates, steroids, indomethacin, colchicine, iron (when used in massive therapy), and rauwolfia derivatives are associated with increased gastrointestinal blood loss in normal persons and with even more pronounced bleeding when disease is present. GI bleeding can also follow parenteral administration of these drugs.

1. Meat in the diet contains hemoglobin and myoglobin and enzymes that can give false-positive tests for up to 4 days after eating. The guaiac method does not require a meat-free diet due to lesser sensitivity, but it is recommended.
2. Vitamin C (ascorbic acid) taken in quantities greater than 500 mg. per day may cause a false-negative test for occult blood in the stool.
3. Drugs that may cause a false-positive test for occult blood include
    (a) Boric acid   (d) Iodine
    (b) Bromides   (e) Inorganic iron
    (c) Colchicine   (f) Oxidizing agents
4. The testing method must be followed exactly or the results are not reliable.
    (a) Use an aliquot from the center of the formed stool.
    (b) Time the reaction exactly.
    (c) Liquid stools may cause false negatives with filter paper methods.

Patient Preparation

1. The patient should be instructed to have a meat-free diet for at least 3 days before the test (all methods).
2. The patient can be given a 3-test Hemoccult to take home and collect a sample on three separate days.
    a. Thinly smear a small part of the feces from 2 separate areas of the stool onto the two spaces allowed.
    b. Do this for 3 days (minimum).
    c. The specimen does not have to be refrigerated.
    d. Mail or bring in the specimen card when finished.

Mucus in Stool

Normal Values

Negative

Explanation of Test

The mucosa of the colon secretes mucus in response to parasympathetic stimulation. Mucus in the stool appears in conditions of parasympathetic excitability.

Procedure

See "Random Collection of Stool Specimens," page 200.

Clinical Implications

1. Presence of recognizable mucus in a stool specimen is abnormal and should be reported and recorded.
2. Translucent gelatinous mucus clinging to the surface of formed stool occurs in
   (a) Spastic constipation   (c) Emotionally disturbed patients
   (b) Mucous colitis   (d) Excessive straining at stool
3. Bloody mucus clinging to the feces is suggestive of neoplasm or inflammation of the rectal canal.
4. In villous adenoma of the colon, copious quantities of mucus may be passed (up to 3 to 4 liters in 24 hours).
5. Mucus with pus and blood is associated with
   (a) Ulcerative colitis   (d) Acute diverticulitis ⎤
   (b) Bacillary dysentery   (e) Intestinal tuberculosis ⎦ rarely
   (c) Ulcerating cancer of
       colon

Collection of 24-, 48- and 72-Hour Stool Specimens

This test is used with testing for fat and urobilinogen.

Special Instructions for Submitting Individual Specimens

1. Collect all stool specimens for 1 to 3 days. The entire stool should be collected.
2. Label specimens as to *Day 1, Day 2, Day 3*, time of day, patient's name, and purpose of examination.
3. Submit individual specimens to the laboratory as soon as they are collected.

Special Instructions for Submitting Total Specimens

1. Obtain a 1 gallon container from the laboratory (paint cans are often supplied).
2. Save all stool and place in the container. Keep refrigerated or in a container with canned ice. Replace ice daily.
3. At the end of the collection period, return the properly labelled container to the laboratory.

Fat in Stool

Normal Values

In a normal diet, fat in stool will be up to 20% of total solids
Lipids measured as fatty acids: 24 hr:2g.–5g./24 hr.

Explanation of Test
This test is helpful in diagnosing malabsorption syndromes such as pancreatic insufficiency and Whipple's disease in which steatorrhea is a prominent feature.

Procedure
1. Collect a random stool specimen or a 72-hour specimen. If a 72-hour specimen is required, each individual stool specimen is collected and identified with the name of the patient, time, and date and sent immediately to the laboratory. Indicate the length of the collection period.
2. Follow the procedure for the collection of random or 72-hour specimens.
3. A diet of more than 60 g. of fat for 6 days prior to sampling is recommended.

Clinical Implications
1. Increases in fecal fat and fatty acids are associated with
   (a) Enteritis and pancreatic diseases when there is a lack of lipase
   (b) Surgical removal of a section of the intestine
   (c) Malabsorption syndromes
2. A stool specimen high in fat content will have a pasty appearance and can be detected by gross examination.
3. A high fat value is indicative of steatorrhea and excessive fat loss in the stool.
4. In chronic pancreatic disease, fat is more than 10 g. in 24 hours.

Interfering Factors
1. Increased neutral fat may occur under the following conditions:
   (a) With the use of rectal suppositories and oily creams applied to the perineum
   (b) With the ingestion of castor oil, mineral oil, and metamucil
   (c) With the ingestion of dietetic low calorie mayonnaise
2. Barium and bismuth interfere with test results.

Clinical Alert

Record the appearance and odor of all stools in persons suspected of having steatorrhea. The typical stool is foamy, greasy, soft, and foul smelling.

Patient Preparation
1. Explain the purpose of the test, interfering factors, and the procedure for the collection of specimens.

2. For a 72-hour stool collection, a diet containing 60 to 100 g. of fat, 100 g. of protein, and 180 g. of carbohydrate is ordered for 6 days before and during the test. Follow the procedure for the collection of 72-hour stool specimens.

An additional fecal test that can be used in the evaluation of malabsorption syndrome, pancreatic dysfunction, and gastrocolic fistula is a determination for meat fibers. There are no meat fibers in the normal stool.

Procedure for Meat Fibers
1. The patient must eat an adequate amount of red meat for 24 to 72 hours before testing.
2. Specimens obtained with a warm saline enema or Flet Phospho-Soda are acceptable. Specimens obtained with mineral oil, bismuth, or magnesium compounds cannot be used.

Urobilinogen in Stool

Normal Values
30–200 mg./100 g. of feces
130–250 Erlich units/100 g. of feces

Explanation of Test
This test is done to determine excess production of urobilinogen in the investigation of hemolytic diseases. Determination of this substance is an estimate of the total excretion of bile pigments, which are the breakdown products of hemoglobin. Increased destruction of red blood cells as in hemolytic anemia increases the amount of urobilinogen excreted. Normally, 80% to 90% of excreted bile pigment measured as fecal urobilinogen is derived from old erythrocytes that have lived 100 to 120 days.

Liver disease in general reduces the flow of bilirubin to the intestine and thereby decreases the fecal excretion of urobilinogen. In addition, complete obstruction of the bile duct reduces urobilinogen to very low levels.

Procedure
See "Random Collection of Stool Specimens," page 200. Send the specimen to the laboratory at once.

Clinical Implications
1. *Increased values* are associated with hemolytic anemias.
2. *Decreased values* are associated with
   (a) Complete biliary obstruction
   (b) Severe liver disease

(c) Oral antibiotic therapy that alters intestinal bacterial flora
(d) Decreased hemoglobin turnover as in aplastic anemia

Bile in Stool

Normal Values
Adults: negative
Children: positive

Explanation of Test
A test for bile in the stool is helpful in determining the presence and degree of biliary tract obstruction in jaundiced patients

Procedure
A random stool specimen is obtained.

Clinical Implications
1. Normally, unaltered bile is never found in feces.
2. In diarrheal stools, bile may be present.
3. Increased levels occur in hemolytic jaundice.
4. Implications closely follow urobilinogen in the stool.

Trypsin in Stool

Normal Values
Positive in small amounts in 95% of normal persons. Present in greater amounts in the stools of normal children. Trypsin is destroyed by bacteria in the GI tract in older children and adults.

Explanation of Test
This test is helpful in indicating pancreatic function and to rule in or rule out inability to split carbohydrates, protein, and fats by this pancreatic enzyme.

Procedure
1. Collect a first morning specimen and send it to the laboratory. Three separate fresh stools are usually collected.
2. In older children, a cathartic is ordered prior to obtaining a specimen.

Interfering Factors
No trypsin activity is detectable in constipated stools due to the prolonged exposure to intestinal bacteria.

Clinical Implications
Absence of trypsin is presumptive evidence of pancreatic deficiency and is usually accompanied by the absence of lipase and amylase.

Clinical Alert

Positive results for trypsin should be checked again in a week to rule out the possibility that the positive reaction might be due to the action of proteolytic bacteria of the intestines.

Leukocytes in Stool

Normal Values
Negative

Explanation of Test
Microscopic examination of the feces for white blood cells is often helpful in differentiating between bacterial dysentery or ulcerative colitis when there are increased leukocytes and the diarrhea caused by a virus or toxin such as viral gastroenteritis when WBCs are absent. Persons with localizing abscesses and fistulas communicating with the bowel lumen will also have increased leukocytes and pus in the feces. Recognizable pus is seldom seen in stools unless there is a draining rectal infection or ulcerating or fungating process.

Clinical Implications
1. Large amounts of pus accompany
   - (a) Chronic ulcerative colitis
   - (b) Chronic bacillary dysentery
   - (c) Localized abscesses
   - (d) Fistulas to sigmoid rectum or anus
2. Primary mononuclear leukocytes appear in typhoid.
3. Primary polynuclear leukocytes appear in
   - (a) Shigellosis
   - (b) Salmonellosis
   - (c) Invasive *E. coli* diarrhea
   - (d) Ulcerative colitis
4. Absence of leukocytes is associated with
   - (a) Cholera
   - (b) Nonspecific diarrhea
   - (c) Viral diarrhea
   - (d) Amebic colitis
   - (e) Noninvasive *E. coli* diarrhea
   - (f) Toxigenic bacteria—staphylococcus, *Clostridium* cholera
   - (g) Parasites—*Giardia, Entamoeba*

Procedure
See "Random Collection of Stool," page 200.

Clinical Alert

Pus in the stool is abnormal and should be reported.

Nitrogen in Stool

Normal Values
1 g.–2 g./24 hr.

Explanation of Test
This test is used along with the measurement of fecal fat in the evaluation of chronic progressive pancreatitis. In the course of this disease, as the pancreas is destroyed, amylase and lipase will revert to normal. However, very high levels of fecal fat and nitrogen will continue to be found.

Procedure
See the procedure for 48- to 72-hour stool collection (page 209).

Clinical Implications
Increased levels (more than 2.5 g./day) are associated with chronic progressive pancreatitis.

Porphyrins in Stool

Normal Values
Coproporphyrin: 200 g./24 hr.
Protoporphyrin: 1500 g./24 hr.
Uroporphyrin: 1000 g./24 hr.

Explanation of Test
Analysis of fecal porphyrins is especially helpful in the differential diagnoses of coproporphyrin, porphyria variegata, or protoporphyria. The pattern of excretion in feces and urine and accumulation within the red blood cells provide the basis for detecting and differentiating the porphyrias (see porphyrins, urine, page 180, and red cells, page 77).

Procedure
Collect a 24-hour stool specimen. See your laboratory for specific protocols. Fecal porphyrins can be qualitatively estimated by acid extraction and ultraviolet light; in erythropoietic protoporphyria, the fecal specimen may fluoresce due to high protoporphyrin levels.

Clinical Implications
1. *Increased fecal coproporphyrin* is associated with
   (a) Coproporphyria, persistently high (hereditary)
   (b) Porphyria variegata
   (c) Protoporphyria
   (d) Hemolytic anemia

2. *Increased fecal protoporphyrin* is associated with
   (a) Porphyria variegata
   (b) Protoporphyria
   (c) Acquired liver disease

BIBLIOGRAPHY

Bauer JD: Clinical Laboratory Methods, 9th ed. St. Louis, CV Mosby, 1982

Bradley GM: Fecal analysis: Much more than an unpleasant necessity. Diagn Med 3(2):64–67, 1980

Davidsohn I, Henry JB: Todd–Sanford–Davidsohn Clinical Diagnosis and Management by Laboratory Methods, 17th ed. Philadelphia, WB Saunders, 1984

Halsted C, Halsted JA (eds): The Laboratory in Clinical Medicine, 2nd ed. Philadelphia, WB Saunders, 1981

Helena Laboratories: Coloscreen Self-Test: A Technical Overview. Beaumont, TX, Helena Laboratories, 1987

Isselbacher KJ et al (eds): Harrison's Principles of Internal Medicine, 11th ed. New York, McGraw-Hill, 1987

Ravel R: Clinical Laboratory Medicine, 4th ed. Chicago, Year Book Medical Pub, 1984

Sheller MG: Stool specimens: Key to detecting intestinal invaders. RN 43(10):50–53, 1980

Sonnenwirth AC, Jarett L: Gradwohl's Clinical Laboratory Methods and Diagnosis, 8th ed. St. Louis, CV Mosby, 1980

Widmann FK: Goodale's Clinical Interpretation of Laboratory Tests, 9th ed. Philadelphia, FA Davis, 1983

CEREBROSPINAL FLUID STUDIES

Description, Formation, and Composition of Cerebrospinal Fluid

Background

Cerebrospinal fluid (CSF) is a clear, colorless liquid formed within the cavities or ventricles of the brain by the choroid plexus and diffused blood plasma. Approximately 500 ml. of the fluid are formed per day, although there are only 120 ml. to 150 ml. in the system at any one time. CSF is completely replaced about three times a day.

Circulating slowly from the ventricular system into the spaces surrounding the brain and spinal cord, CSF serves as an hydraulic shock absorber diffusing the force from a hard blow to the skull that might otherwise cause severe injury. CSF also helps to regulate intracranial pressure, which may change according to blood flow, and to transport nutrients and waste products. This fluid is believed to influence other control mechanisms such as glucose levels on the hypothalamus and hunger sensations and eating behaviors.

Most constituents of CSF are present in the same or lower concentrations as in the blood plasma, except for chloride concentrations, which are usually higher. Thus, like blood plasma, CSF contains few cells and little protein. Disease, however, can cause elements ordinarily restrained by the blood-brain barrier to enter the spinal fluid. Erythrocytes and leukocytes can enter the CSF from the rupture of blood vessels or from meningeal reaction to irritation. Bilirubin, normally not present, can be found in the spinal fluid after intracranial hemorrhage. In such cases, the arachnoid granulations and the nerve root sheaths will reabsorb the bloody fluid. Normal CSF pressure will consequently be maintained by the absorption of CSF in amounts equal to production. Blockage will cause an increase in the amount of CSF, resulting in hydrocephalus in infants or increased pressure in adults. The normal pressure of CSF is approximately 100 ml. to 200 ml. of water in the lateral decubitus position. Of the many factors that regulate the level of CSF pressure, venous pressure is the most important since the reabsorbed fluid ultimately drains into the venous system.

Despite the continuous production (about 0.3 ml./minute) and reabsorption of CSF and the exchange of substances between the CSF and the blood plasma, considerable pooling occurs in the lumbar sac. The lumbar sac at L4 to L5 is the usual site for puncture since damage to the nervous system is unlikely to occur in this area. In infants, the spinal cord is situated more caudally than in adults (L3–L4 until 9 months, when the cord ascends to L1–L2), and a low lumbar puncture should be made. The removal of CSF can give rise to a headache. This is because when fluid is withdrawn from the ventricle or subarachnoid

Table 5-1
Normal CSF Values in Adults

Volume	90 ml.–150 ml.
Clarity	Crystal clear, colorless
Pressure	50 m.–180 m. H_2O
Total cell count	0–5 WBC/μl.
	(All cells are lymphocytes; PMNs and RBCs absent)
Specific gravity	1.006–1.008
Osmolality	280–290mOsm./kg.

Clinical Tests

Glucose	45–85 mg./dl.
Protein	15–45 mg./dl. (lumbar)
	15–25 mg./dl. (cisternal)
	5–15 mg./dl. (ventricular)
Lactic acid	24 mg./dl.
Glutamine	6–15 mg./dl.
A/G ratio (albumin to globulin)	8:1
Chloride	118–132 mEq./liter
Urea nitrogen	6–16 mg./dl.
Creatinine	0.5–1.2 mg./dl.
Cholesterol	0.2–0.6 mg./dl.
Uric acid	0.5–4.5 mg./dl.
Bilirubin	0 (None)
LDH	1/10 that of serum

Electrolytes and pH

pH	7.30–7.40
Chloride	118–132 mEq./liter
Sodium	144–154 mEq./liter
Potassium	2.0–3.5 mEq./liter
CO_2 content	25–30 mEq./L. (m. mol.)
PCO_2	42–53 mm. Hg
PO_2	40–44 mm. Hg
Calcium	2.1–2.7 mEq./liter
Magnesium	2.4–mEq./liter

Syphilis

VDRL	Negative

spaces, free nerve endings along the major vessels of the inner dura are stretched—a result of the partially collapsed brain tugging on the meninges.

General Observations:
Explanation of Test
Cerebrospinal fluid is usually obtained by lumbar puncture. A lumbar puncture is done for several reasons

1. To examine the spinal fluid, as in cases of suspected meningitis and intracranial hemorrhage
2. To determine level of CSF pressure to document impairment of CSF flow or to lower the pressure by removal of a volume of fluid (Fluid removal can be dangerous; the brain stem could be dislocated.)
3. To introduce anesthetics, drugs, and radiographic contrast media

Examination of CSF
Certain observations are made every time lumbar puncture is performed (see Table 5-1):
1. General appearance, consistency, and tendency to clot are noted.
2. Pressure is measured.
3. Cell count is performed in laboratory to distinguish types of cells present; this must be done within 2 hours.
4. Protein, chloride, and sugar concentrations are determined.
5. Other clinical serologic and bacteriologic tests are done when the patient's condition warrants them (e.g., tests for aerobes and anaerobes, tuberculosis, Venereal Disease Research Laboratories [VDRL] test for syphilis, fungal studies, and colloidal gold tests).
6. There are tumor markers in CSF that are useful as supplements to CSF cystology analysis. See Table 5-2.

Table 5-2
Tumor Markers in CSF

Determination	Used in Diagnosis of:	Normal Value
Alpha-fetaprotein (AFP)	CNS dysgerminomas and meningeal carcinomatosis	<1.5 mg./ml.
Beta-glucuronidase	Possible meningeal carcinomatosis	<49 mU./liter Indeterminate 49–70 mU./liter Suspicious >70 mU./liter
Carcinoembryonic antigen (CEA)	Meningeal carcinomatosis: intradural or extradural, or brain parenchymal metastasis from adenocarcinoma. Although the assay appears to be specific for adenocarcinoma and squamous cell carcinoma, increased CEA values in CSF are not seen in all such tumors of the brain.	<0.6 mg./ml.
Human Chorionic Gonadotropin (HCG)	Adjunct in determining CNS dysgerminomas and meningeal carcinomatosis	<0.21 U./liter

Note: Blood levels should always be measured simultaneously with CSF.

Procedure for Sterile Lumbar Puncture (Spinal Tap)

1. The patient is usually placed in a side-lying position with head flexed onto the chest and knees drawn up to but not compressing the abdomen to bow the back. This position helps to increase the space between the lower lumbar vertebrae so that the spinal needle can be inserted with ease between the spinal processes. However, a sitting position (patient straddles a straight-backed chair) with head flexed to chest can be used. The patient is helped to relax with soothing words and instructed to breathe slowly and deeply with mouth open.
2. The puncture site is selected, usually between L4 and L5 or lower. There is a little bone at the L5-S interspace ("surgeon's delight") that facilitates puncture. The site is thoroughly cleansed with an antiseptic solution, and the surrounding area is draped with sterile towels. However, care should be taken so that drapes do not obscure important landmarks.
3. A local anesthetic is injected slowly into the dermis.
4. A spinal needle with stylet is inserted into the midline between the spines of the lumbar space. The needle is to enter the subarachnoid space. The patient may feel the entry ("pop") of the needle through the dura mater. Patient should then be helped to slowly straighten the legs to relieve abdominal compression.
5. The stylet is removed and a manometer is attached to the needle to record the opening CSF pressure.

    Note: If the initial pressure is normal, the Queckenstedt's test may be done. This test is not done if a central nervous system (CNS) tumor is suspected. In this test, pressure is placed on both jugular veins to temporarily occlude them and to produce an acute rise in CSF fluid. Normally, pressure rapidly returns to average levels. Total or partial spinal block is diagnosed if the lumbar pressure fails to rise when both jugular veins are compressed or if the pressure requires more than 20 seconds to fall after compression is released. Pressure reading is height dependent and sitting equals pressure in the midventricular system.

6. A specimen of CSF is removed and is usually collected in three tubes. Tubes are labeled, 1, 2, and 3 in correct order of collection. A closing pressure reading may be done, and the needle is withdrawn. In cases of increased intracranial pressure, very little fluid is withdrawn.

7. A small sterile dressing is applied to the puncture site.
8. Tubes should be correctly labeled with the proper number (1, 2, or 3), the patient's name, and date. CSF specimens must be delivered immediately to laboratory personnel. The spinal fluid should never be placed in the refrigerator provided for other specimens. Refrigeration will alter test results if bacteriological and fungal studies are done. Analysis should be started immediately. If viral studies are to be done, the specimen should be frozen.
9. Record the completion time of the procedure, the condition and reaction of the patient, the appearance of the CSF, and the pressure readings. Time specimens are sent to the laboratory.

Patient Preparation
1. Explain the purpose of the test; give a step-by-step description of the procedure.
2. Help the patient to be as relaxed as possible. Breathing slowly and deeply may help the patient to relax. Tell the patient to refrain from breath holding, straining, and talking during the procedure.

Patient Aftercare
1. The patient should lie prone (flat or horizontal) usually for 4 to 8 hours. Or the patient may lie on the abdomen to help prevent headache. Turning from side to side is permitted.
2. Women will have difficulty voiding in this position. The use of a "fracture bedpan" may help to alleviate voiding problems.
3. Fluids are encouraged to help in the prevention and relief of possible headache.
4. Observe the patient for important changes in his neurological state, such as a change in his conscious state and in his pupils. Elevated temperature, increased blood pressure, irritability, as well as numbness and tingling sensations in the lower extremities should also be assessed.
5. If headache should occur, administer ordered analgesics and encourage a longer period of bedrest.
6. Check the puncture site for leakage.

Clinical Alert
1. Extreme caution should be used in lumbar puncture when intracranial pressure is elevated, especially when papilledema or split cranial sutures are present. However, in some cases of increased intracranial pressure, such as with a comatose patient, intracranial bleeding, or suspected meningitis, the need to establish a diagnosis is absolutely essential and outweighs the danger of the procedure.

2. Other contraindications to lumbar puncture are
   (a) Suspected epidural infection
   (b) Infection or severe dermatologic disease in the lumbar area, which may result in spinal fluid infiltration and infectious complications
   (c) Severe psychiatric problems or chronic back pain in neurotics
3. If there is a sign of leakage at the puncture site, notify the physician immediately.

Pressure of CSF

Normal Values
75–150 mm. H_2O lateral decubitus
To midventricular position when sitting
This value is height dependent and will change if patient is in a horizontal or sitting posture.

Background
The pressure should be measured before any fluid is withdrawn. CSF fluid pressure is directly related to pressure in the jugular and vertebral veins that connect with the intracranial dural sinuses and the spinal dura. In conditions such as congestive heart failure and obstruction of the superior vena cava, CSF pressure is increased, but in circulatory collapse, it is decreased.

Clinical Implications
1. *Increases* in pressure can be a significant finding in
   (a) Intracranial tumors or abscess
   (b) Purulent or tuberculous meningitis
   (c) Inflammatory processes of meninges
   (d) Hypo-osmolality due to hemodialysis
   (e) Congestive heart failure
   (f) Acute observation of superior vena cava
   (g) Subarachnoid hemorrhage
   (h) Cerebral edema
2. *Decreases* in pressure can be a significant finding in
   (a) Circulatory collapse
   (b) Severe dehydration
   (c) Hyperosmolality
   (d) Leakage of spinal fluid
   (e) Complete subarachnoid block
3. *Significant variations* between opening and closing CSF pressures can be found in
   (a) Tumors or spinal blockage when there is a large pressure drop indicative of a small CSF pool.

(b) Hydrocephalus when there is a small pressure drop that is indicative of a large CSF pool.

Clinical Alert

If initial pressure is near 200 mm., only 1 to 2 ml. of fluid should be removed. Spinal cord compression or cerebellar herniation could result. See **Note** in procedure for spinal tap for Queckenstedt's test.

Interfering Factors
1. Slight elevations of pressure may occur in an anxious person who holds his breath or tenses his muscles.
2. If a person's knees are flexed too firmly against his abdomen, venous compressions will cause an elevation in pressure. This can occur in persons of normal weight and in the obese.

Color, Turbidity of CSF

Normal Value
Crystal clear and colorless, like water

Background
A slight color change may be difficult to detect, and CSF should be compared with a test tube of distilled water held against a white background. If there is no turbidity, an newspaper can be read through the tube. Inflammatory diseases, hemorrhage, tumors, and trauma bring about an elevated cell count and a corresponding change in appearance.

Clinical Implications
1. Abnormal colors (see Table 5-3)—their causes and indications:
    (a) Blood (the blood is evenly mixed in all three tubes in subarachnoid and cerebral hemorrhage). The supernate is also xanthochromic after centrifugation—at least 400 cells/μl must be present before turbidity is detected. Clear CSF fluid does not rule out intracranial hemorrhage.
    (b) Turbid fluid usually indicates increased WBCs, RBCs, or microorganisms such as yeast and bacteria.
    (c) Xanthochromia (pale to dark yellow)
        (1) Bilirubin, as in bilirubinemia (conjugated in adults; unconjugated in infants)
        (2) Yellow pigments usually signify previous bleeding, as in subarachnoid hemorrhage, from lipid red blood cells, severe

Table 5-3
Color Changes in CSF Suggestive of Disease States*

Appearance	Condition
Opalescent, slightly yellow with delicate clot	Tuberculous meningitis
Opalescent to purulent, slightly yellow with coarse clot	Acute pyogenic meningitis
Slightly yellow; may be clear or opalescent with delicate clot	Acute anterior poliomyelitis
Bloody; purulent; may be turbid	Primary amebic meningoencephalitis
Generally clear, but may be xanthochromic	Tumor of brain or cord
Xanthochromic	Toxoplasmosis

* Color and clot changes are only *very general* indications of disease states. They must not be thought of as specific indicators.

jaundice, or high protein level. The xanthochromia grading range is 1+ to 4+.
(3) Methoglobin
(4) If the CSF protein is more than 150 mg. per dl., the fluid will be slightly yellow.
(5) Bleeding into CSF is associated with a corresponding increase in protein, about 1 mg./dl. per 700 RBC/μl. Clots will form in CSF with high protein levels (fibrinogen).
(6) Carotene, as in systemic carotenemia
(7) Melanin, from meningeal melanosarcoma

Interfering Factors
1. If the blood in the specimen is due to trauma during lumbar puncture, the fluid in the third tube is usually lighter in color than tube number one and tube number two.
2. Contamination of the specimen with a skin disinfectant will cause an abnormal color.

Microscopic Examination of Cells; Total Cell Count; Differential Cell Count of CSF

Normal Values
0–5 WBC/μl or 0–5 10^6 WBC/liter (mononuclear cells; lymphocytes and monocytes)

Background
CSF is essentially free of cells. When the cells are counted, they are identified by cell type, and the percentage of cell type is compared to

the total number of white cells present. In general, inflammatory disease, hemorrhage, neoplasms, and trauma will cause an elevated cell count.

Clinical Implications

A. *White Cell Counts*

1. An increase in the number of WBCs in CSF is termed *pleocytosis*. Disease processes may lead to abrupt increases or decreases (shift to the right or left); usually there are no WBCs in CSF.

2. White cell counts above 500 usually arise from a purulent infection and are predominantly granulocytes (neutrophils).

   (a) Increases in neutrophils are associated with

   (1) Bacterial meningitis
   (2) Early viral meningitis
   (3) Early tuberculosis
   (4) Mycotic meningitis
   (5) Amebic encephalomyelitis
   (6) Early stages of meningovascular syphilis
   (7) Aseptic meningitis
   (8) Septic emboli due to bacterial endocarditis
   (9) Osteomyelitis of skull or spine
   (10) Subdural empyema
   (11) Cerebral abscess
   (12) Phlebitis of dural sinuses or cortical veins

   (b) Noninfectious causes of neutrophilia

   (1) Reaction to central nervous system hemorrhage
   (2) Reaction to repeated lumbar puncture
   (3) Injection of foreign materials into subarchnoid space such as a contrast medium or anticancer drugs
   (4) Pneumoencephalogram
   (5) Chronic granulocytic leukemia involving the central nervous system
   (6) Lumbar puncture with needle contaminated by detergent
   (7) Metastatic tumor
   (8) Infarct

Clinical Alert

Neutrophilic reaction classically suggests meningitis due to pyogenic organism.

3. White counts of 300–500 with predominately mononuclear cells are indicative of
   (a) Viral infections such as poliomyelitis and aseptic meningitis
   (b) Syphilis of CNS
   (c) Tuberculous meningitis

(d) Tumor or abscess (WBCs may also be normal in these conditions)
(e) Partially treated bacterial meningitis
(f) Multiple sclerosis (50% of cases)
(g) Encephalopathy due to drug abuse
(h) Guillain–Barré syndrome
(i) Acute disseminated encephalomyelitis
(j) Sarcoidosis of meninges
(k) Polyneuritis
(l) Periarteritis of central nervous system
4. White cell counts with 40% or more monocytes are seen after subarachnoid hemorrhage.
B. *Other Cells*
1. Malignant cells (lymphocytes or histiocytes) may be present with primary and metastatic brain tumors, especially with meningeal extension.
2. Increased numbers of plasma cells may occur in association with lymphocytic reactions.

(a) Subacute and chronic inflammatory processes
(b) Multiple sclerosis
(c) Leukoencephalitis
(d) Delayed hypersensitivity responses
(e) Subacute viral encephalitis
(f) Meningitis (tuberculous or fungal)
(g) Some brain tumors

These cells are responsible for an increase in IgG and for altered patterns in immunoelectrophoresis.
3. Macrophages are present in traumatic and ischemic cranial infarcts, tuberculous or mycotic meningitis, reaction to erythrocytes, foreign substances, or lipids in the CSF.
4. Glial, ependymal, and plexus cells may be present after surgical procedures or trauma to the central nervous system.
5. Leukemic cells appear in CSF after several remissions have been achieved by chemotherapy. Leukemic cells may appear in CSF during apparent remission and after chemotherapy has been discontinued.

Chloride in CSF

Normal Values
118–132 mmol./liter

Background
Any condition that alters the blood plasma chloride level will also affect the CSF level. Chlorides in CSF are higher (1.2–1) than in blood

plasma. The measurement of CSF chloride is most useful in the diagnosis of tuberculous meningitis.

Clinical Implications
Decreased levels are associated with

(a) Tuberculous meningitis
(b) Bacterial meningitis

Interfering Factors
1. Concurrent IV administration of chloride will invalidate test results.
2. Test values are invalidated if blood, as in a traumatic tap, is mixed with the specimen.

Glucose in CSF

Normal Values
45–85 mg./dl.

Background
The CSF glucose level varies with the blood glucose levels. CSF is usually 60% to 70% of blood glucose. A blood glucose specimen should be obtained at least 30 to 60 minutes before lumbar puncture for comparisons. Any changes in blood sugar are reflected in the CSF after 1 to 3 hours.

Explanation of Test
This measurement is helpful in determining impaired transport of glucose from plasma to CSF and increased use of glucose by the central nervous system, leukocytes, and microorganisms. As evidenced by decreased CSF glucose, accurate evaluations of CSF glucose require a relatively constant level of plasma glucose.

Clinical Implications
1. *Decreased levels* are associated with
    (a) Pyogenic, tuberculous, and fungal infections
    (b) Lymphomas with meningeal spread
    (c) Leukemia with meningeal spread
    (d) Mumps meningoencephalitis (usually normal in viral meningoencephalitis)
    (e) Hypoglycemia

    Note: *All types* of organisms consume glucose, and decreased glucose reflects bacterial activity.

2. *Increased levels* are associated with diabetes.

3. CSF glucose levels are usually normal in some viral infections of the brain and meninges and in aseptic meningitis.

Clinical Alert

1. Glucose oxidase test strips are of no clinical value for distinguishing CSF leakage from nasal or ear secretions. Diagnosis of CSF rhinorrhea and otorrhea must be made by other means such as cotton pledgets examined for radioactivity after administration of technetium-99m.
2. Panic value is less than 20 mg./dl.

Glutamine in CSF

Normal Values
6–20 mg./dl.
Reference values vary.

Background
Glutamine is synthesized in brain tissue from ammoniaic and glutamic acid. Production of glutamine provides a mechanism for removing ammonia from the central nervous system.

Explanation of Test
This measurement is used as a determination of hepatic encephalopathy and cerebrospinal fluid acidosis.

Procedure
In the laboratory, glutamine levels can be measured by a simple method that releases ammonia and is measured by a colorimetric reaction.

Clinical Implications
Increased levels are associated with

(a) Hepatic encephalopathies
(b) Reye's syndrome
(c) Hepatic coma
(d) Cirrhosis
(e) Hypercapnia

Lactic Acid in CSF

Normal Values
24 mg./dl. (reported reference intervals vary)

Background

The source of lactic acid in the cerebrospinal fluid is probably central nervous system anaerobic metabolism (see Chapter 14). Lactic acid in CSF may vary independently of the level in the blood. It appears that diffusion of lactic acid across the blood–CSF barrier is very slow.

Explanation of Test

Measurement of CSF lactate may be useful as a screening test to detect central nervous system disease and may be an aid in the differential diagnosis of bacterial meningitis versus viral meningitis if other conditions can be excluded.

Clinical Implications

Increased levels are associated with

(a) Bacterial meningitis
(b) Hypocapnia
(c) Hydrocephalus
(d) Brain abscess
(e) Cerebral ischemia
(f) Traumatic brain injury
(g) Idiopathic seizures
(h) Respiratory alkalosis
(i) Low blood pressure
(j) Low arterial Po_2
(k) Cerebral infarct
(l) Less than 50% of multiple sclerosis
(m) Cancer of central nervous system

Lactate Dehydrogenase (LD/LDH) in CSF

Normal Values

One-tenth that of serum

Background

Although many different enzymes have been measured in CSF, only lactate dehydrogenase (LDH) appears useful clinically. Sources of LDH in normal CSF include diffusion across the blood–CSF barrier, diffusion across the brain–CSF barrier, and LDH activity in cellular elements of CSF such as leukocytes, bacteria, and tumor cells. Because the brain tissue is rich in LDH, damaged central nervous system tissue can cause increased levels of LDH in the cerebrospinal fluid.

Explanation of Test

Measurement of LDH in the cerebrospinal fluid has been used for differential diagnosis of bacteria versus viral meningitis. High levels of LDH occur in about 90% of bacterial meningitis cases and in only 10% of viral meningitis cases. When high levels of LDH do occur in viral meningitis, the condition is usually associated with encephalitis and a poor prognosis. Tests of LDH isoenzymes have been used to improve the specificity of LDH measurements (see Chapter 6 for a complete description of isoenzymes).

Clinical Implications
1. Increased LDH levels are associated with
   (a) Bacterial meningitis
   (b) Viral meningitis (10% of cases)
   (c) Subarachnoid hemorrhage
   (d) Leukemia
   (e) Lymphoma
   (f) Metastatic carcinoma of the central nervous system
2. In viral meningitis, the presence of LDH 1, 2, 3 reflects a combined central nervous system lymphocytic reaction.
3. In bacterial meningitis, the LDH isoenzyme pattern reflects a granulocytic reaction with LDH 4 and 5 present.
4. High levels of LDH 1 and 2 in either viral or bacterial meningitis suggest extensive central nervous system damage and a poor prognosis.

Total Protein in CSF

Normal Values
15–45 mg./dl. (lumbar)
15–25 mg./dl. (cisternal)
 5–15 mg./dl. (ventricular)
These values are age dependent; for example, a lumbar protein may be 65 in a 65-year-old patient.

Background
CSF normally contains very little protein because the protein in blood serum is in the form of large molecules that do not cross the blood–brain barrier. However, the proportion of albumin to globulin is higher in CSF than in the blood plasma, since the albumin molecule is significantly smaller and can more easily cross the blood–brain barrier. Increased permeability of the blood–brain barrier to protein occurs in infections.

Clinical Implications
1. Moderate to marked increases in total protein levels and alterations in the ratio of albumin to globulin (A/G ratio) are caused by increased permeability of the blood–CSF barrier, obstructions in circulation of CSF, increased synthesis of protein within the central nervous system, or tissue degeneration as in Guillain–Barré syndrome and brain tumors. Increases may also be seen in
   (a) Purulent meningitis
   (b) Froin's syndrome
   (c) Tuberculous meningitis
   (d) Aseptic meningitis
   (e) Syphilis, neurosyphilis
   (f) Brain abscesses
   (g) Subarachnoid hemorrhage
   (h) Poliomyelitis
   (i) Collagen disease
   (j) Guillain–Barré syndrome

2. In most diseases, any changes in CSF cell count and protein are parallel. For example, as the CSF cell count rises, the CSF protein level also rises.
3. There is often some increase of protein level in multiple sclerosis.
4. A traumatic tap with a mixture of peripheral blood in the CSF may cause an increase in protein.
5. Decreased concentration of protein in CSF
   (a) Leakage of CSF
   (b) Removal of large volume of CSF
   (c) Increased intracranial pressure
   (d) Hyperthyroidism

Interfering Factors
1. Drugs may cause increased or decreased levels.

VDRL Test for Syphilis

Normal values negative (nonreactive). Neurosyphilis is characterized by an increase in protein, a reactive VDRL, and an increase in number of lymphocytes.

Protein Electrophoresis of CSF; Albumin and Immunoglobulin G (IgG); Multiple Sclerosis Panel

Normal Values
Albumin: 26.0 mg./dl.
Oligoclonal banding: 0–1 Band
IgG:≤8.4 mg./dl.
IgG/albumin: 0.15–3.8

Explanation of Test
This measurement of albumin and IgG using immunoelectrophoresis is becoming accepted as a method of evaluating the integrity and permeability of the blood–CSF barrier and of the synthesis of IgG within the central nervous system. The most important clinical application of CSF protein fractionation is detection and diagnosis of multiple sclerosis. Abnormalities in CSF in multiple sclerosis include an increase in total protein primarily due to IgG. The IgG protein in multiple sclerosis and other neuropathies migrate as discrete populations rather than as a homogeneous band, and these have been called *oligoclonal bands*.

Clinical Implications
1. *Increases* in IgG or IgG/albumin index occur in
   (a) Infectious disease
   (b) Subacute sclerosing leukoencephalitis
   (c) Multiple sclerosis

(d) Neurosyphilis
(e) Chronic phases of central nervous system infections
(f) Some patients with meningitis, Guillain–Barré syndrome, lupus erythematosus involving central nervous system, and other neurologic conditions
2. IgM is normally absent; it may be abnormally present in
(a) Tumors of brain and meninges
(b) Meningitis
(c) Multiple sclerosis
3. Increased levels of albumin are associated with
(a) Lesions of choroid plexus
(b) Blockage of flow of CSF
(c) Damage to blood–central nervous system
4. Increased levels of gamma globulins in the presence of normal albumin level are associated with
(a) Multiple sclerosis
(b) Neurosyphilis
(c) Subacute sclerosing panencephalitis
(d) Chronic phase of central nervous system infections
5. Oligoclonal bands are found in
(a) Multiple sclerosis
(b) Cryptococcal meningitis
(c) Idiopathic polyneuritis
(d) Neurosyphilis
(e) Chronic rubella panencephalitis
(f) Subacute sclerosing panencephalitis

Note: In order for this test to be valid, corresponding bands must not be present in the serum.

BIBLIOGRAPHY

Bauer JD: Clinical Laboratory Methods, 9th ed. St. Louis, CV Mosby, 1982
Bradbury M: The Concept of a Blood–Brain Barrier. Chichester, England, John Wiley & Sons, 1979
Davidsohn I, Henry JB: Todd–Sanford–Davidsohn Clinical Diagnosis and Management by Laboratory Methods, 17th ed. Philadelphia, WB Saunders, 1984
Fishman A: Cerebrospinal Fluid in Diseases of the Nervous System. Philadelphia, WB Saunders, 1980
Halsted CH, Halsted JA (eds): The Laboratory in Clinical Medicine, 2nd ed. Philadelphia, WB Saunders, 1981
Inhorn L (ed): Quality Assurance Practices for Health Laboratories. Washington, DC, American Public Health Association, 1978
Isselbacher J et al (eds): Harrison's Principles of Internal Medicine, 11th ed. New York, McGraw-Hill, 1987
Kaplan A, Szabo L: Clinical Chemistry: Interpretation and Techniques. Philadelphia, Lea & Febiger, 1979

Lipman T: Cerebrospinal Fluids (unpublished thesis), Med consin, 1984

McManus C, Hallsman KA: Cerebrospinal Fluid Analysis. Nursing 1982

Merritt HH: Textbook of Neurology, 6th ed. Philadelphia, Lea & Febiger,

Ravel R: Clinical Laboratory Medicine, 4th ed. Chicago, Year Book Medical Pub, 1984

Rosenthal DL: Cerebrospinal Fluids Analysis. Basel, S. Karger, 1984

Schmidt RF (ed): Fundamentals of Neurophysiology. New York, Springer-Verlag, 1978

Sonnenwirth AC, Jarett L (eds): Gradwohl's Clinical Laboratory Methods and Diagnosis, 8th ed. St. Louis, CV Mosby, 1980

Widmann FK: Goodale's Clinical Interpretation of Laboratory Tests, 9th ed. Philadelphia, FA Davis, 1983

Wolf JK: Practical Clinical Neurology. New York, Medical Examination Publishing, 1980

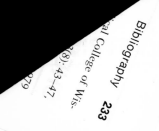

Bibliography

al College of Wis-

8): 43–47,

79

233

UDIES 6

Introduction

Blood chemistry is a means of identifying many of the body's chemical constituents found in the blood. Although the relation of the abnormal levels of these constituents to disease can be evaluated, unfortunately, very few diseases show a single abnormality in body chemistry. Thus, it is often necessary to measure several body chemicals to establish a pattern of abnormalities characteristic of a particular disease. The quantity of blood that is drawn for samples will vary, depending on the method used in testing and the available equipment.

A wide range of tests falls into the category of blood chemistry. Some can be grouped under the broad headings of enzymes, electrolytes, blood sugar, protein or protein by-products, lipids, hormones, vitamins, minerals, and drug investigation. Others have no such common denominator.

From the numerous tests included here, selected tests serve as screening devices in general patient care and help to identify target organ damage. Most of these tests constitute the patient profile that is obtained from the autoanalyzer printout shown in Figure 6-1 (A–F) (pages 238–243).

General Biochemical Profiles

Profiles are a group of various tests that screen for certain conditions. Some of the more commonly offered profiles or panels are listed in Table 6-1.

Table 6-1
Common Biochemical Profiles

Disorder	Tests Suggested
Cardiac enzymes	CPK, AST, LDH
Kidney functions and disease	UA, BUN, phosphoras, LDH, creatinine, creatinine clearance, uric acid, total protein, A/G ratio, albumin, globulins, calcium, glucose, cholesterol
Lipids	Cholesterol, triglycerides, lipoprotein electrophoresis (LDL, VLDL, HDL)
Liver function/disease	Total bilirubin, alkaline phosphatase, cholesterol, total protein, A/G ratio, albumin, globulins, AST, LDH, Australian antigen (hepatitis panel) pro time
Thyroid function	T_3, T_4, T_7, free thyroxine, cholesterol

Use of the Autoanalyzer

The use of instrumentation in a laboratory setting has made it possible to conduct a wide variety of chemical tests on a single sample of blood. Autoanalyzers such as the Ektachem 700 by Kodak; the Automated Clinical Analyzer (ACA) by Dupont; Astra by Berkman; the Sequential Multiple Analyzer by Technicon (SMAC) (see Figure 6-1, A–F) and the Multiple Sequential Screening Panel (MSSP) by Technicon can be used to process an individual specimen rapidly through a number of basic chemical analyses. The results of these tests are also recorded automatically and displayed for ease of interpretation; if an interface is available, the results can be transmitted directly to the hospital's computer.

Because of the speed of the autoanalyzer and the number of tests it can process in a short period of time, it has become a major means of screening patients. Not only does it provide a baseline for future comparisons, it also has uncovered unsuspected diseases and allowed for early diagnosis of diseases whose symptoms are either vague or absent.

Note: Normal or reference values for any chemistry determination will vary with the assay employed. For example, differences in substrates or temperature at which the assay is run will alter the "normal" range. It may be somewhat misleading to give normal ranges, for they will vary from laboratory to laboratory.

The blood chemistries usually recorded include

Total protein (TP)	Blood urea nitrogen (BUN)
Albumin	Uric acid
Calcium (Ca^{2+})	Creatinine
Inorganic phosphorus	Total bilirubin
Cholesterol	Alkaline phosphatase
Glucose	Aspartate transaminase (AST)

Various combinations of these chemical values provide insight into liver function, kidney disease, cardiovascular and pulmonary disorders, hematologic and reticuloendothelial dysfunction, and possible cancerous conditions.

Use of Multiple Laboratories

It is important to realize that, for economic reasons, it is not possible to do all the tests listed in this book in one hospital or clinic laboratory. In many cases, a number of tests are sent out to reference or commercial laboratories. A certain percentage of these tests will fall into the category of being too sophisticated or of too low a volume to obtain reliable results. This is one of the reasons why test results are not immediately available for interpretation.

(*Text continued on page 244.*)

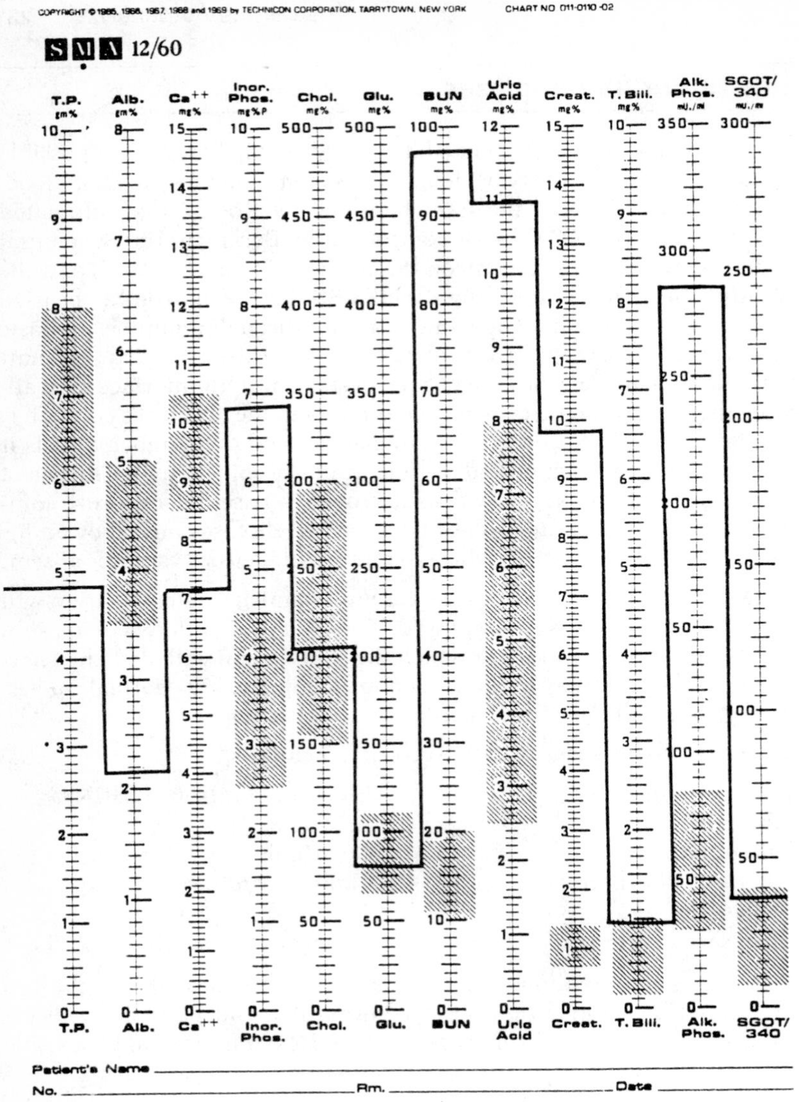

Figure 6-1 (A)

Chronic glomerulonephritis.	Alkaline phosphatase: high	Creatinine: high
Calcium: low	BUN: high	Total protein: low
Inorganic phosphorus: high	Uric acid: high	Albumin: low

Figure 6-1 (A-F)

Results of a multiparameter test provided by the Technicon SMA 12/60 System, a multichannel system that can perform 12 blood chemistry analyses simultaneously. Certain patterns of increases and decreases in blood constituents are associated with particular disease entities. The normal range for each constituent tested is indicated by a vertical shaded strip. (Used with permission of Technicon Instruments Corporation, Tarrytown, NY)

238

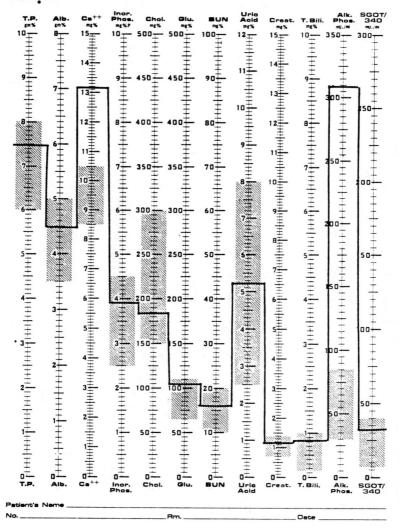

SMA 12/60

Figure 6-1 (*B*)
Metastatic carcinoma of bone.
Calcium: high
Osteoblasts: proliferate
Alkaline phosphatase: dramatically increased

(**Note:** The shaded areas represent the normal values for a given analyte.)

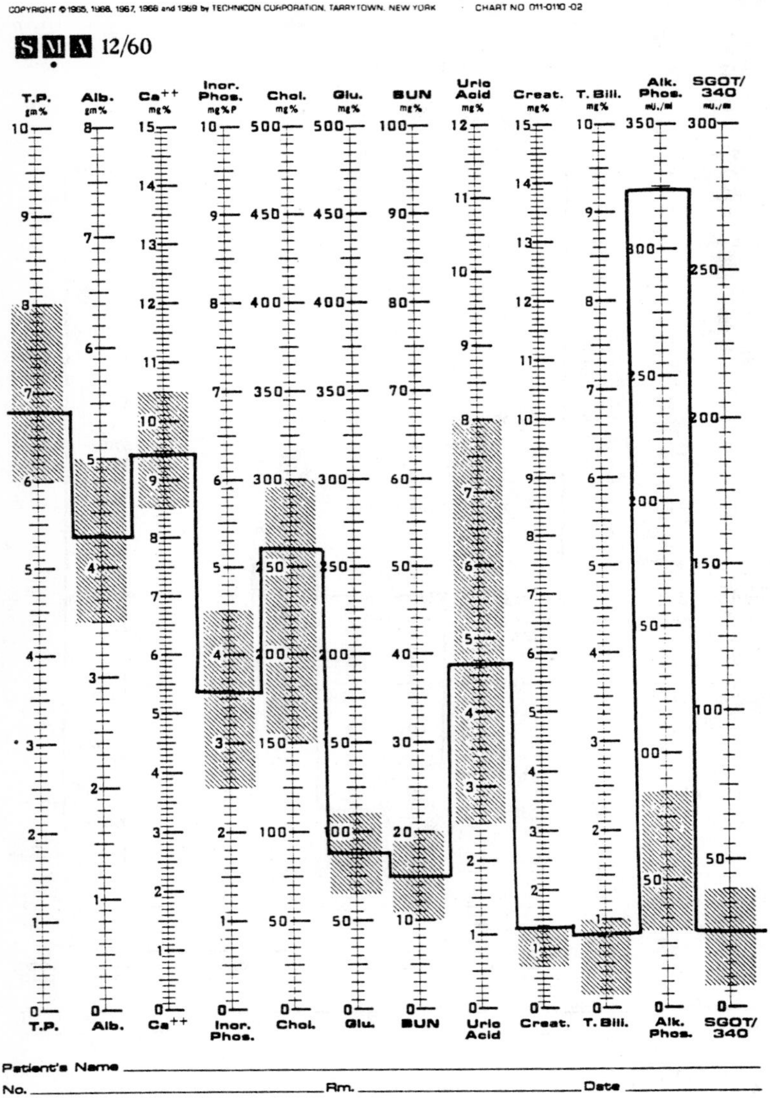

 12/60

Figure 6-1 (C)

Metastatic carcinoma of liver.
Isolated elevation of alkaline phosphatase.

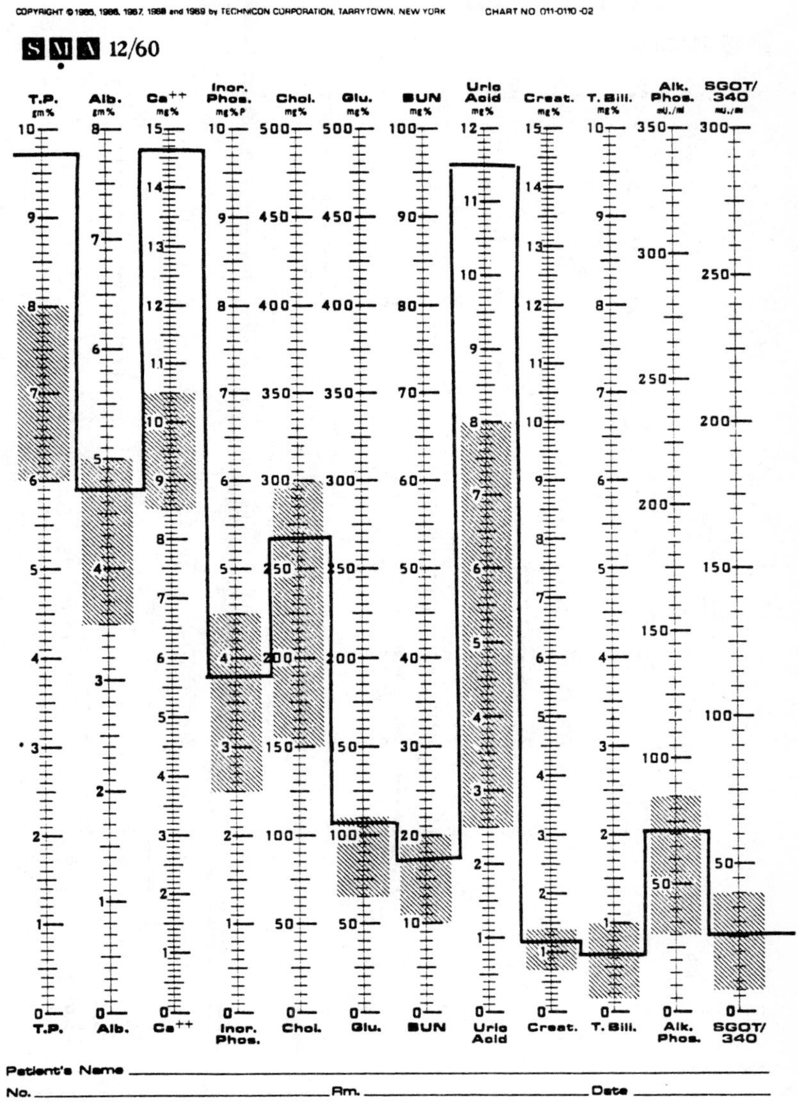

Figure 6-1 (D)
Multiple myeloma.
Calcium: elevated
Alkaline phosphatase: normal
Uric acid: elevated
Total protein: markedly elevated

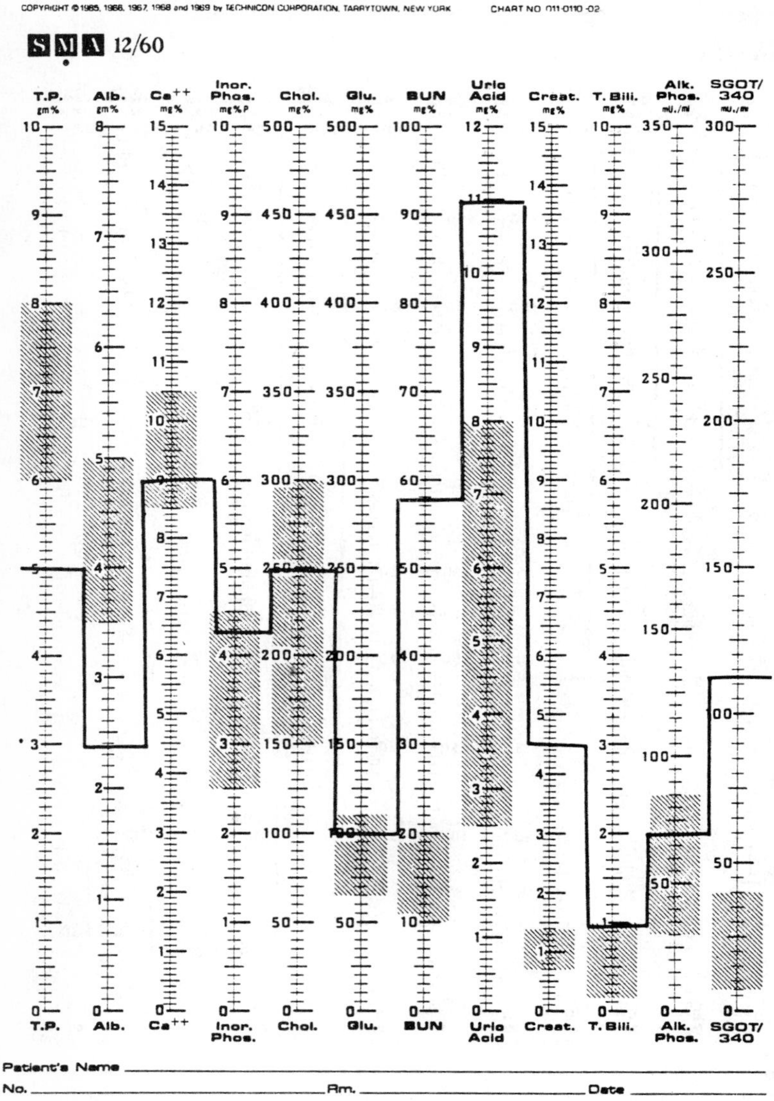

Figure 6-1 (E)
Acute eclampsia.
BUN: elevated
Uric acid: elevated
Creatinine: elevated
AST: elevated
Albumin: decreased
Total protein: decreased

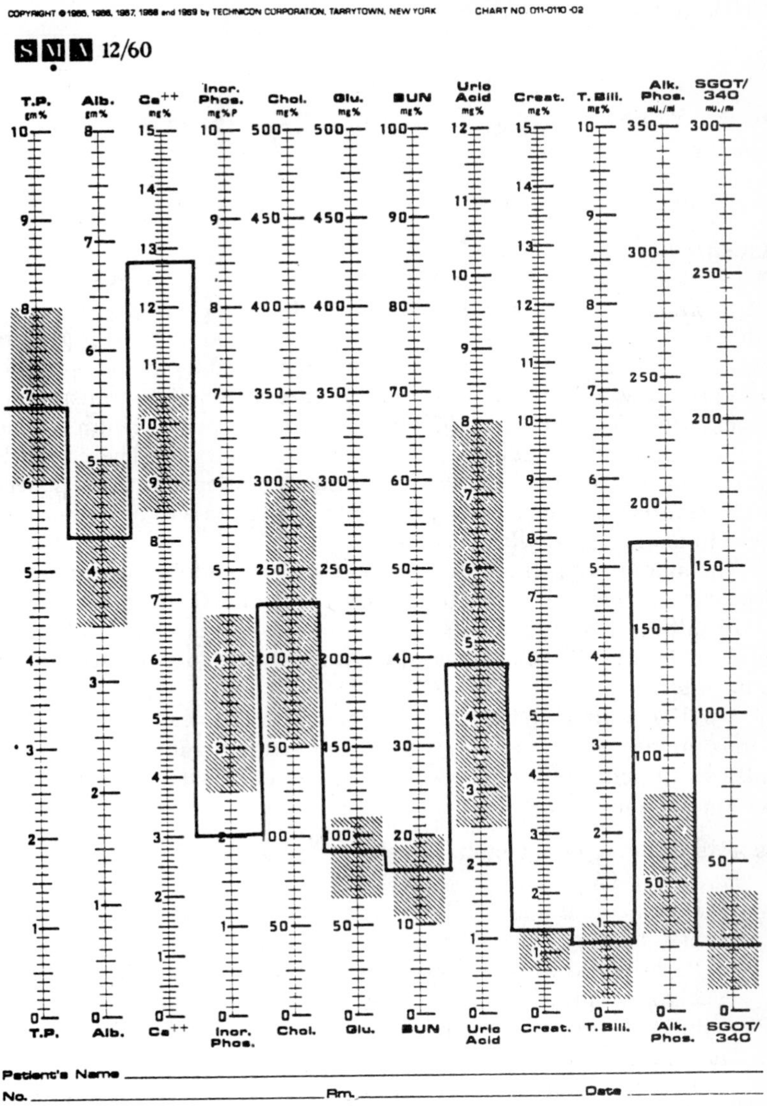

Figure 6-1 (F)
Primary hyperparathyroidism.
Calcium: elevated
Alkaline phosphatase: elevated
Inorganic phosphorus: decreased

ELECTROLYTE TESTS

Calcium (Ca^{2+})

Normal Values

Total: 8.5–10.5 mg./dl.	*Ionized:* 4.2–5.4 mg./dl.
4.5– 5.3 mEq./liter	2.1–2.6 mEq./liter
4.5– 5.3 mmol./liter	2.1–2.6 mmol./liter

Background

The bulk of body calcium (98%–99%) is stored in the skeleton and teeth, which act as huge reservoirs for maintaining the blood levels of calcium. About 50% of the blood calcium is ionized; the rest is protein-bound. However, only ionized calcium can be used by the body in such vital processes as muscular contraction, cardiac function, transmission of nerve impulses, and blood clotting. Yet the ionized calcium cannot be measured independently of the total calcium levels. Therefore, the 50% ratio is only estimated and can fluctuate depending on general acid–base balance: in acidosis, the ionized calcium will be higher than 50%; in alkalosis, it will be lower.

The amount of protein in the blood will also affect calcium levels, since 50% of the blood calcium is protein-bound. Thus, a decrease in serum albumin would result in a profound decrease in total serum calcium. However, the decrease does not alter the concentration of the ionized form.

A patient suffering from a deficiency of ionized calcium will show signs of tetany accompanied by muscular twitching and eventual convulsions (a neuromuscular response to the decreased calcium at the nerve junctions).

Factors Influencing Calcium Levels

A. *Parathyroid hormone*
   1. Blood calcium is regulated by parathyroid hormone, which exerts a direct effect on bone to release calcium into the blood.
   2. Parathyroid hormone also acts on both the intestines, increasing absorption of calcium, and the kidneys, causing calcium to be reabsorbed by the proximal tubules.
B. *Calcitonin*
   This hormone lowers blood calcium levels by increasing calcium clearance by the kidneys.
C. *Vitamin D*
   Stimulates calcium absorption by the intestines
D. *Estrogens and androgens*
   1. Estrogens increase calcium deposits in the bones. (Osteoporosis, following menopause, may respond to estrogen therapy.)
   2. Androgens—Hyperfunction of the adrenal cortex or thyroid may result in hypocalcemia and bone decalcification.

E. *Carbohydrates and lactose*
   1. Carbohydrates increase intestinal absorption of calcium.
   2. Addition of lactose to the diet increases the absorption and retention of calcium.

Explanation of Test

This test measures the concentration of total calcium in the blood and is used as a measure of parathyroid function, calcium metabolism, and in the evaluation of malignancies.

Hyperparathyroidism and cancer are the most common causes of hypercalcemia, and hypoalbuminemia is the most common cause of reduced total calcium. A test for the ionized fraction of calcium will reflect the functional states of calcium metabolism better than the total calcium.

Procedure

A venous blood sample of 5 ml. is obtained.

Clinical Implications

A. *Normal levels of total calcium* combined with other findings
   1. Normal calcium levels with overall normal findings in other tests indicate that there are no problems with calcium metabolism.
   2. Normal calcium and abnormal phophorus indicate impaired calcium absorption due to alteration of parathyroid hormone activity or secretion. In rickets, the calcium level may be normal or slightly lowered and the phosphorus level is depressed.
   3. Normal calcium and elevated BUN indicates
      (a) Possible secondary hyperparathyroidism
          Initially a lowered serum calcium results from uremia and acidosis. The lower calcium level stimulates the parathyroid to release parathyroid hormone, which acts on bone to release more calcium.
      (b) Possible primary hyperparathyroidism
          Excessive amounts of parathyroid hormone cause elevation in calcium levels, but secondary kidney disease would cause retention of phosphate and concomitant lower calcium.
   4. Normal calcium and decreased serum albumin
      This is indicative of hypercalcemia, since there should be a decrease in calcium when there is a decrease in albumin because of the 50% of serum calcium that is protein-bound.
B. *Hypercalcemia* (increased total calcium levels)
   Hypercalcemia is associated with many disorders, but its greatest clinical importance rests in its association with *cancer*, including multiple myeloma, parathyroid tumors, nonendocrine tumors producing a parathyroidlike substance, and cancers metastasizing to the bone. Increase calcium levels are caused by or associated with

 1. Hyperparathyroidism due to
    (a) Parathyroid adenoma
    (b) Hyperplasia of parathy- } Associated with hypophos-
        roid glands   phatemia
 2. Cancer
    (a) Metastatic cancers involving bone
        Cancers of lung, breast, thyroid, kidney, and testes may me-
        tastasize to bone.
    (b) Hodgkin's disease and other lymphomas
    (c) Multiple myeloma in which there is extensive bone destruc-
        tion
    (d) Lung and renal cancers may produce parathyroid hormone
        resulting in symptoms of hypercalcemia
    (e) Sarcoidosis due to increased IgG or IgA
    (f) Leukemia
 3. Addison's disease
 4. Hyperthyroidism
 5. Paget's disease of bone (also accompanied by high levels of alka-
    line phosphatase)
 6. Prolonged immobilization
 7. Bone fractures combined with bedrest
 8. Excessive intake of vitamin D
 9. Prolonged use of diuretics, thiazides
10. Respiratory acidosis
11. Milk–alkali syndrome (history of peptic ulcer could indicate
    excessive intake of milk and antacids)
C. *Hypocalcemia* (decreased total calcium levels)
   Commonly caused by or associated with
   1. Pseudohypocalcemia (hyperproteinemia)
      Actually, what looks like hypocalcemia is really a reflection of
      reduced albumin (as revealed by a serum protein electrophore-
      sis). It is the reduced protein that is responsible for the low
      calcium, since 50% of the calcium total is protein-bound.

   Note: Excessive use of IV fluids will decrease albumin levels and
   thus decrease the amount of calcium.

   2. Hypoparathyroidism (primary is very rare)
      May be due to accidental removal of parathyroid glands during
      a thyroidectomy, irradiation, hypomagnesemia, GI disorders,
      renal wasting
   3. Hyperphosphatemia
      Due to renal failure, laxatives, cytotoxic drugs
   4. Malabsorption
      Due to sprue, celiac disease, pancreatic dysfunction (fatty acids
      combine with calcium and are precipitated and excreted in the
      feces)

5. Acute pancreatitis
6. Alkalosis (calcium ions become bound to protein)
7. Osteomalacia
8. Diarrhea
9. Rickets

D. *Increased ionized calcium*
   1. Primary hyperparathyroidism
   2. Ectopic parathyroid hormone-producing tumors
   3. Excess intake of vitamin D
   4. Various malignancies

E. *Decreased ionized calcium*
   Primary hypoparathyroidism is associated with low ionized calcium level and low total calcium level.

Clinical Alert

Panic Levels
(a) <7.0 mg./dl., associated with tetany
(b) >11.0 mg./dl., suggestive of hyperparathyroidism
(c) >13.5 mg./dl., associated with hypercalcemic coma and metastatic cancer.

Rapid treatment of hypercalcemia with substance such as calcitonin solution is indicated.

Thiazide diuretics may lead to impairment of urinary calcium excretions and consequent hypercalcemia.

In patients with renal insufficiency who are undergoing dialysis, a calcium-ion exchange resin is sometimes used for hyperkalemia. The use of this resin may lead to increased calcium levels.

Increased intake of magnesium and phosphates and the excessive use of laxatives may lower the blood calcium level. This occurs because of the increased intestinal loss of calcium these elements produce.

When decreased calcium levels are due to magnesium deficiency, as in poor absorption from the bowel, the administration of magnesium will correct the calcium deficiency.

If a patient is known to have or suspected of having a *p*H abnormality, a concurrent *p*H should be requested with ionized calcium.

Interfering Factors
There are many drugs that may cause increased or decreased levels of calcium. Calcium supplements taken shortly before specimen collection will cause a falsely high value.

Chloride (Cl⁻)

Normal Values
98–106 mEq./liter
98–106 mmol./liter

Chloride, a blood electrolyte, is an anion that exists predominantly in the extracellular spaces, and in a lesser preponderance in the intravascular spaces and in the cell itself. Chemically, it exists primarily in combinations as sodium chloride or hydrochloric acid.

Chloride maintains cellular integrity through its influence on osmotic pressure. It is also significant in monitoring acid–base balance and water balance.

Chloride has the reciprocal power of increasing or decreasing in concentration whenever changes occur in the concentration of other anions. In metabolic acidosis, there is a reciprocal rise in chloride concentration when the bicarbonate concentration drops. Similarly, when aldosterone directly causes an increase in the reabsorption of sodium (which is a positive ion), the indirect effect is an increase in the absorption of chloride (the negative ion).

Chlorides are excreted with cations (positive ions) during massive diuresis from any cause and are lost from the gastrointestinal tract as a result of vomiting, diarrhea, or intestinal fistulas.

Explanation of Test
Alteration of serium chloride is seldom a primary problem. Thus, the measurement of chlorides is usually done for its inferential value and is helpful in diagnosing disorders of acid–base and water balance. Because of the relatively high concentration of chloride in the gastric juices, prolonged vomiting may lead to considerable chloride loss and lowered serum level.

Chloride is the least important electrolyte to measure in an emergency, but it is especially important to measure in the correction of hypokalemic alkalosis. If potassium is supplied without chloride, hypokalemic alkalosis may persist.

Procedure
A venous blood sample of 5 ml. is obtained.

Clinical Implications
1. Whenever the serum level is much lower than 100 mEq. per liter, the urinary excretion of chloride falls to a very low level.
2. The reason why decreased chloride levels often occur in acute infections is not clear.
3. Chloride measurements are of limited value in renal disease for the reason that plasma chloride can be maintained near normal limits even when a considerable degree of renal failure is present.

4. Decreased *chloride levels* occur in
   (a) Severe vomiting
   (b) Severe diarrhea
   (c) Ulcerative colitis
   (d) Pyloric obstruction
   (e) Severe burns
   (f) Heat exhaustion
   (g) Diabetic acidosis
   (h) Addison's disease
   (i) Fever
   (j) Acute infections such as pneumonia
   (k) Use of drugs such as mercurial and chlorothiazide diuretics
5. *Increased chloride levels* occur in
   (a) Dehydration
   (b) Cushing's syndrome
   (c) Hyperventilation
   (d) Eclampsia
   (e) Anemia
   (f) Cardiac decompensation
   (g) Some kidney disorders

Interfering Factors
1. The plasma chloride concentration of infants is usually higher than that of children and adults.
2. Many drugs may cause a change in chloride levels.

Clinical Alert

1. In IV therapy, if the solution contains 100 mEq. per liter there is ample chloride present for the correction of urine metabolic acidosis.
2. If an electrolyte disorder is suspected, daily weight and accurate fluid intake and output should be recorded.
3. Panic value for serum chloride is <70 or >120 mEq./liter; <70 or >120 mmol./liter.

Phosphate/Inorganic Phosphorus (P) (PO₄)

Normal Values

Adults: 3.0–4.5 mg./dl.	1.0–1.5 mmol./liter
Children: 4.0–7.0 mg./dl.	1.45–2.09 mmol./liter

Explanation of Test
Approximately 85% of the body's total phosphorus content is combined with calcium in the bone. The remainder is located within the cells. Most of the phosphorus in the blood exists as phosphates or esters.

Phosphate is required for generation of bony tissue and functions in the metabolism of glucose and lipids, in the maintenance of acid–base balance, and in the storage and transfer of energy from one site in the body to another. Phosphorus enters the cell with glucose and is lowered following carbohydrate ingestion. For these reasons, blood phosphate levels must be controlled within reasonably constant limits.

Phosphate levels are always evaluated in relation to calcium levels for the reason that there is an inverse relationship between the two. When calcium levels are decreased, phosphorus levels increase. When phosphorus levels decrease, calcium levels increase. An excess in serum levels of one causes the kidneys to excrete the other. Many of the causes of elevated calcium are also causes of lower phosphorus levels. As with calcium, the controlling factor is parathyroid hormone.

Procedure
A venous blood sample of 5 ml. is obtained.

Clinical Implications
A. *Hyperphosphatemia* (increased phosphorus levels)
   The most common causes of elevated blood phosphate levels are found in association with kidney dysfunction and uremia. This is because phosphate is so closely regulated by the kidneys.
   Increased phosphorus levels are associated with
   (a) Renal insufficiency and severe nephritis (accompanied by elevated BUN and creatine)
   (b) Hypoparathyroidism (accompanied by elevated phosphorus, decreased calcium, and normal renal function)
   (c) Hypocalcemia
   (d) Excessive intake of alkali (possible history of peptic ulcer)
   (e) Excessive intake of vitamin D
   (f) Fractures in the healing stage
   (g) Bone tumors
   (h) Addison's disease
   (i) Acromegaly
B. *Hypophosphatemia* (decreased phosphorus levels)
   Decreased phosphorus levels may be associated with
   (a) Hyperparathyroidism (accompanied by elevated calcium; no renal disease)
   (b) Rickets (childhood) or osteomalacia (adult)
   (c) Diabetic coma because of increased carbohydrate metabolism
   (d) Hyperinsulinism
   (e) Continuous administration of intravenous glucose in a nondiabetic patient.

Interfering Factors
1. Normally high in children
2. Falsely increased by hemolysis of blood
3. Vitamin D can be the cause of elevation; drugs can also be the cause of decreases.
4. The use of laxatives or enemas containing large amounts of sodium

phosphate will cause increased phosphorus levels. With the oral intake of the laxative, the blood level may increase as much as 5 mg. per dl. 2 to 3 hours after the dose. This increased level is only temporary (5–6 hours), but this factor should be considered when abnormal levels are seen that cannot otherwise be explained.

Clinical Alert

When phosphorus rises rapidly, calcium drops—watch for arrhythmias and muscle twitching.

Magnesium (Mg^{2+})

Normal Values
1.3–2.1 mEq./liter or 0.65–1.05 mmol./liter

Background
Since all natural foods are rich in magnesium, magnesium deficiency is rare in a normal diet. Ingestion of magnesium increases not only the amount of magnesium absorbed, but also the amount of calcium absorbed. On the other hand, a high phosphate diet suppresses both magnesium and calcium absorption.

Magnesium is required for the use of adenosine triphosphate (ADP) as a source of energy. It is therefore necessary for the action of numerous enzyme systems such as

1. Carbohydrate metabolism
2. Protein synthesis
3. Nucleic acid synthesis
4. Contraction of muscular tissue

Along with sodium, potassium, and calcium ions, magnesium also regulates neuromuscular irritability. In addition, it is needed in the clotting mechanism.

Magnesium and calcium are intimately tied together in their body functions, and deficiency of either one has a marked effect on the metabolism of the other. This is because of magnesium's importance in the absorption of calcium from the intestines and in calcium metabolism. A magnesium deficiency will result in the draft of calcium out of the bones, possibly resulting in abnormal calcification in the aorta and the kidney in the absence of a calcium pump mechanism. This condition responds to administration of magnesium salts.

Normally, 95% of the magnesium that is filtered through the glomerulus is reabsorbed in the tubule. When there is decreased kidney function, greater amounts of magnesium are retained, resulting in increased blood serum levels.

Explanation of Test
Measurement of magnesium levels is used as an index to metabolic activity in the body and to renal function.
The bulk of total magnesium in the body is concentrated in the bone, cartilage, and within the cell itself.

Procedure
A venous blood sample of 4 ml. is obtained. Avoid hemolysis.

Clinical Implications
A. *Reduced magnesium level*
   Causes of *reduced* magnesium levels include

   (a) Chronic diarrhea
   (b) Hemodialysis
   (c) Chronic renal disease
   (d) Hepatic cirrhosis
   (e) Chronic pancreatitis
   (f) Use of diuretics
   (g) Aldosteronism
   (h) Ulcerative colitis
   (i) Hyperaldosteronism
   (j) Toxemia of pregnancy
   (k) Hyperthyroidism and hypoparathyroidism
   (l) Excessive lactation
   (m) Malabsorption syndromes
   (n) Chronic alcoholism
   (o) Prolonged gastric drainage

   In magnesium deficiency states, urinary magnesium decreases before the serum does.
B. *Increased magnesium level*
   Causes of *increased* magnesium levels include
   (a) Renal failure or reduced renal function
   (b) Diabetic acidosis before treatment
   (c) Hypothyroidism
   (d) Addison's disease
   (e) Adrenalectomy
   (f) Controlled diabetes in older persons
   (g) Use of antacids containing magnesium (*e.g.*, milk of magnesia)
   (h) Dehydration
   (i) Use of thiazides
   (j) Use of ethacrynic acid

Interfering Factors
1. Prolonged salicylate therapy, lithium, and magnesium products (antacids, laxatives) will cause falsely increased magnesium levels, particularly if there is renal damage.
2. Calcium gluconate, as well as a number of other drugs, can interfere with testing methods and cause falsely decreased results.
3. Hemolysis will invalidate results because about three-fourths of the magnesium in the blood is found intracellularly in the red blood cells.

Clinical Alert

1. Treatment of diabetics in coma will often result in low plasma magnesium levels. This is because magnesium moves with potassium into the cells after insulin administration.
2. Magnesium deficiency may cause apparently unexplained hypocalcemia and hypokalemia. In these instances, patients may have neurologic and/or GI symptoms.
3. Signs of too much magnesium (which acts as a sedative) include
   (a) Lethargy, flushing, nausea, vomiting, slurred speech
   (b) Weak or absent deep tendon reflexes
   (c) ECG prolonged PR and Q–T intervals, widened QRS; bradycardia
   (d) Hypotension, drowsiness, and respiratory depression

   Treatment involves

   (a) Withholding source of magnesium excess
   (b) Promoting excretion
   (c) Giving calcium salts
   (d) Hemodialysis
4. Signs of insufficient magnesium include
   (a) Muscle tremors, twitching, tetany
   (b) Intolerance of K^+ and CA^{2+}
   (c) Hyperactive deep tendon reflexes
   (d) ECG: prolonged P–R and Q–T intervals; broad, flat T waves. PVCs, ventricular tachycardia and fibrillation
   (e) Anorexia, nausea and vomiting
   (f) Lethargy and insomnia

   Treatment:

   (a) Administer magnesium salts
   (b) Reduce auditory, mechanical, and visual stimuli
5. Panic levels for serum magnesium are <0.5 or >3.0 mEq./L; <0.5 or >3.0 mmol./Liter.

Potassium (K⁺)

Normal Values
3.5–5 mEq./liter
3.5–5.0 mmol./liter
A very narrow range of normal

Background

Potassium is the principal electrolyte (cation) of intracellular fluid, and primary buffer within the cell itself. Ninety per cent of K^+ is concentrated within the cell; only small amounts are contained in bone and blood. A kilogram of tissue such as RBC or muscle contains about 90 mEq. of K^+. Damaged cells release K^+ into the blood.

The body is adapted to efficient potassium excretion. Normally, 80% to 90% of the cells' potassium is excreted in the urine by the glomeruli of the kidneys. The remainder is excreted in sweat and in the stool. Even when no potassium is taken into the body (as in a fasting state), 40 to 50 mEq. are still excreted daily in the urine. The kidneys do not conserve potassium, and when an adequate amount of potassium is not ingested a severe deficiency will occur. Potassium balance is maintained in adults on an average dietary intake of 80 to 200 mEq. per day. The minimum daily need is about 30 mEq.; the maximum daily tolerance to an acute load is 400 mEq. The normal intake, minimal needs, and maximum tolerance for potassium are almost the same as that for sodium.

Potassium plays an important role in nerve conduction and muscle function. Moreover, it helps maintain acid–base balance and osmotic pressure. Along with calcium and magnesium, potassium controls the rate and force of contraction of the heart and thus, the cardiac output. Evidence of a potassium deficit can be noted on an electrocardiogram (ECG) by the presence of a U wave.

Potassium and sodium ions are particularly important in the renal regulation of acid–base balance because hydrogen ions are substituted for sodium and potassium ions in the renal tubule. Potassium is more important than sodium since potassium bicarbonate is the primary intracellular inorganic buffer. In potassium deficiency there is a relative deficiency of intracellular potassium bicarbonate and the pH is relatively acid. The respiratory center responds to the intracellular acidosis by lower PCO_2, through the mechanism of hyperventilation.

Concentration of potassium is greatly affected by the adrenal hormones. A potassium deficiency will cause a marked reduction in protein synthesis.

Evaluation of Test

This test is used to evaluate changes in body potassium and is helpful in diagnosing disorders of acid–base and water balance in the body. It is not an absolute value and varies with the circulatory volume and other factors. Because a totally unsuspected potassium imbalance can suddenly prove lethal, its development must be anticipated. Thus, it is important to check this value in severe cases of Addison's disease, uremic coma, intestinal obstruction, acute renal failure, gastrointestinal loss in the administration of diuretics, steroid therapy, and cardiac patients on digitalis.

Procedure
1. A venous blood sample of 5 ml. is obtained.
2. Hemolysis in obtaining the sample should be avoided; it will give falsely elevated results.
3. The sample must be delivered to the laboratory and spun at once to separate cells from serum. Potassium leaks out of the cell and will be falsely elevated after 4 hours.

Clinical Implications
A. *Hypokalemia*
   1. Values of 3.5 mEq. per liter are more commonly associated with deficiency, rather than normality.
   2. A falling trend (0.1–0.2 mEq. per day) is indicative of a developing potassium deficiency.
      (a) Most frequent cause of K$^+$ deficiency is gastrointestinal loss.
      (b) Most frequent cause of K$^+$ depletion is IV fluid administration without adequate K$^+$ supplements.
   3. *Decreased levels* (hypokalemia) are associated with
      (a) Diarrhea
      (b) Pyloric obstruction
      (c) Starvation
      (d) Malabsorption
      (e) Severe vomiting
      (f) Severe burns
      (g) Primary aldosteronism
      (h) Excessive ingestion of licorice
      (i) Renal tubular acidosis
      (j) Diuretic administration
         (1) Mercurials
         (2) Ammonium chloride
         (3) Chlorothiazides
         (4) Deamox
      (k) Other drugs
         (1) Steroids
         (2) Estrogen
      (l) Familial periodic paralysis
      (m)Liver disease with ascites
      (n) Chronic stress
      (o) Crash dieting without K$^+$
      (p) Chronic fever
B. *Hyperkalemia* (increased levels of 5.5)
   1. The most frequent causes of increased levels are
      (a) Inadequate excretion (renal failure)

(b) Cell damage as in burns, accidents, surgery, chemotherapy, disseminated intravascular coagulation (damaged cells will release potassium into the blood.)
(c) Acidosis (drives potassium out the the cells)
2. *Increased levels* are associated with
   (a) Addison's disease
   (b) Acute renal failure
      (1) Oliguria
      (2) Anuria
   (c) Selective hypoaldosteronism
   (d) Internal hemorrhage
   (e) Uncontrolled diabetes
   (f) Acidosis

Interfering Factors
1. Forearm exercise
   Opening and closing the fist ten times with a tourniquet in place results in an increase of the K^+ level by 10% to 20%.
   For this reason it is recommended that the blood sample be obtained without a tourniquet, or that the tourniquet be released after the needle has entered the vein and 2 minutes are allowed to elapse before the sample is withdrawn.
2. Drug usage
   (a) The IV use of *potassium penicillin* may cause hyperkalemia; *penicillin sodium* may cause an increased excretion of K^+.
   (b) Glucose tolerance testing or the ingestion/administration of large amounts of glucose in patients with heart disease may cause a decrease of as much as 0.4 mEq. per liter in K^+ blood levels.
   (c) There are a number of drugs that interfere with potassium levels.

Clinical Alert
1. Serum K^+ panic values are 2.5 mEq./liter or less or 6.5 mEq./liter or greater. These levels (<2.5 or >6.5 mmol/liter) may cause heart problems leading to death.
2. The most common cause of hypokalemia in patients receiving IV fluids is water and sodium chloride administration without adequate replacement for K^+ lost in urine and drainage fluids. A patient receiving IV fluids needs potassium every day. The minimum daily dose should be 40 mEq., but the optimum daily dose ranges between 60 and 120 mEq. Potas-

sium needs are greater in tissue injury, wound infection, gastric intestinal or biliary drainage. If adequate amounts of potassium are not given in IV solution (40 mEq./day) hypokalemia will develop eventually.

A 40 mEq. dose of IV potassium should be given in one or more hours, not one or more minutes. No more than 10–15 mEq. should be administered per hour, except in acute emergencies. A burning sensation felt at the site of needle insertion may indicate that the concentration is toxic and the IV should be discontinued.

3. Patients taking digitalis and diuretics should be watched closely for hypokalemia since cardiac arrhythmias can occur. Hypokalemia enhances the effect of digitalis preparations, creating the possibility of digitalis intoxication from even an average maintenance dose. Digitalis, diuretics, and hypokalemia are a potentially lethal combination.

4. The K$^+$ blood level rises 0.6 mEq. per liter for ever 0.1 decrease in blood pH.

5. Hyperkalemia can be altered by the use of hypertonic ion exchange resins orally, or by an enema (Kayexalate) to remove excess potassium.

6. If there is a massive loss of extracellular potassium, the potassium within the cells may have to support K$^+$ concentration in the blood. This process cannot be measured directly and can only be inferred from an understanding of clinical signs. Recognizing signs and symptoms of hypokalemia and hyperkalemia is very important, since many of them originate in the nervous and muscular systems and are usually nonspecific and similar.

7. *Evaluating changes in body K$^+$*

How to recognize excess K$^+$ even when the blood level is normal	How to recognize a K$^+$ deficiency or depletion even when the blood level is normal
Hyperkalemic	*Hypokalemic*
1. Record fluid intake and output.	1. Record fluid intake and output.
2. Check blood volume and venous pressure, which will give a clue to dehydration or circulatory overload.	2. Check blood volume and venous pressure, which will give a clue to circulatory overload or dehydration.

3. Identify ECG changes.
   (a) Elevated T wave heart block
   (b) Flattened P wave
   (c) Cardiac arrest may occur without any warning other than ECG changes.
4. Observe for slow pulse and oliguria.
5. Observe for neuromuscular changes.
   (a) Muscle weakness and impaired muscle function
   (b) Flaccid paralysis
   (c) Tremors, twitching preceding actual paralysis

3. Identify ECG changes.
   (a) Depressed T waves
   (b) Peaking of P waves
4. Observe for dehydration caused by severe vomiting, hyperventilation, sweating, diuresis, NG tube with gastric suction.
   Accurately record state of hydration or dehydration.
5. Observe for neuromuscular changes.
   (a) Fatigue
   (b) Muscle weakness, muscle pain, flabby muscles
   (c) Paresthesia
   (d) Hypotension and rapid pulse
   (e) Respiratory muscle weakness leading to paralysis, cyanosis, and respiratory arrest
   (f) Anorexia, nausea, vomiting, paralytic ileus
   (g) Apathy, drowsiness, irritability, tetany, coma

Clinical Alert

Be on the alert for these arrhythmias that may occur with hyperkalemia.

1. Sinus bradycardia
2. Sinus arrest
3. First-degree AV block
4. Nodal rhythm
5. Idioventricular rhythm
6. Ventricular tachycardia
7. Ventricular fibrillation
8. Ventricular arrest

Be on the alert for these arrhythmias that may occur with hypokalemia.

1. Ventricular premature beats
2. Atrial tachycardia
3. Nodal tachycardia
4. Ventricular tachycardia
5. Ventricular fibrillation

Sodium (Na⁺)

Normal Values
135–148 mmol./liter or
135–148 mEq./liter

Sodium, a blood electrolyte, is the most abundant cation (90% of the electrolyte fluid) and the chief base of the blood. Its primary functions in the body are to chemically maintain osmotic pressure and acid–base balance and to transmit nerve impulses. The body has a strong tendency to maintain a total base content, and only slight changes are found even under pathologic conditions.

Sodium concentration is under the control of the kidneys and the central nervous system acting through the endocrine system. In health, the level of sodium is kept constant within narrow limits despite wide fluctuations in dietary intake. An average dietary intake of 90 to 250 mEq. per day is enough to maintain sodium balance in adults. The minimum daily need is approximately 15 mEq.

Explanation of Test
Determinations of plasma sodium levels are useful in detecting gross changes in water and salt balance but are of little help in detecting early or subtle changes. Urinary sodium is a more sensitive indicator of altered sodium balance. Numerous factors, as listed below, determine the content and volume of urine excreted. These, in turn, determine the content and flow rate in the renal vein returning processed blood.

Mechanisms for maintaining a constant sodium level in the plasma and extracellular fluid include

1. *Renal blood flow*
   (a) Increased renal blood flow to the glomeruli will result in increased sodium and chloride excretions.
   (b) Decreased renal blood flow to the glomeruli will result in sodium and chloride retention and edema. This occurs in patients with reduced cardiac output.
2. *Carbonic anhydrase enzyme activity*
   (a) The level of activity of this system is an important factor in control of the rate of sodium excretion.

    (b) Inhibition of carbonic anhydrase enzyme activity results in increased sodium reabsorption in the tubules.

3. *Aldosterone*
    (a) Aldosterone acts on the distal tubules and also affects sodium reabsorption.
    (b) Regulation of aldosterone secretion is
        (1) Primarily by the renin–angiotensin system
        (2) Secondarily by ACTH, sodium, and potassium concentration
    (c) In primary hyperaldosteronism, sodium will be retained and hypertension will result. In exchange for sodium, potassium will often be excreted and decreased potassium may be found in this condition.

4. *Action of other steroids* whose plasma level is controlled by the anterior pituitary gland
    These steroids can cause salt and water retention. During the menstrual cycle, estrogen and progesterone cause salt and water retention before menstruation and diuresis if fertilization has not taken place.

5. *Renin enzyme secretion*
    Renin is a potent stimulus to aldosterone secretion. It regulates renal blood flow, the glomerular filtration rate, and salt and water excretion. In renal diseases excessive amounts of renin secreted into the plasma result in salt and water retention and hypertension.

6. *ADH (antidiuretic hormone, vasopressin) secretion*
    (a) ADH controls the reabsorption of water at the distal tubules of the kidney.
    (b) Secretion of this hormone is responsive to changes in extracellular fluid volume.

Procedure
A venous blood sample of 7 ml. is obtained.

Clinical Implications
A. *Hyponatremia* (decreased levels)
    1. Hyponatremia usually reflects a relative excess of body water rather than a low total body sodium.
    2. *Reduced* sodium levels (hyponatremia) are associated with
        (a) Severe burns
        (b) Severe diarrhea
        (c) Vomiting
        (d) Excessive IVs of nonelectrolyte fluids
        (e) Addison's disease (lack of adrenal steroids impairs sodium reabsorption)
        (f) Severe nephritis
        (g) Pyloric obstruction

(h) Malabsorption syndrome
(i) Diabetic acidosis
(j) Drugs
  (1) Mercurial diuretics
  (2) Chlorothiazide diuretics
(k) Edema
(l) Excessive sweating accompanied by large amounts of water by mouth
(m)Stomach suction accompanied by water or ice chips *by mouth*

B. *Hypernatremia* (increased levels)
  Increased sodium levels are uncommon, but when they do occur they are associated with
  (a) Dehydration and insufficient water intake
  (b) Conn's syndrome
  (c) Primary aldosteronism
  (d) Coma
  (e) Cushing's disease
  (f) Diabetes insipidus
  (g) Tracheobronchitis

Clinical Alert

1. IV therapy consideration
  (a) Sodium balance is maintained in adults with an average dietary intake of 90 to 250 mEq. per day. The maximum daily tolerance to an acute load is 400 mEq. per day. If a patient is given 3 liters of isotonic saline in 24 hours, he will receive 465 mEq. of sodium. This amount exceeds the average, healthy adult's tolerance level. It will take a *healthy* person 24 to 48 hours to excrete the excess sodium.
  (b) After surgery, trauma, or shock there is a decrease of extracellular fluid volume. Replacement of extracellular fluid is essential if water and electrolyte balance is to be maintained. The ideal replacement IV solution should have a sodium concentration of 140 mEq. per liter.
2. Check patients for signs of edema, hypertension.
3. Panic values are <120 or ≥155 mEq./liter or <120 or >155 mmol./liter.

Interfering Factors
There are many drugs that may cause falsely increased or decreased levels of blood sodium.

Osmolality and Water Load Test

Normal Values
275–295 mosm./kg.

Background
In health, a change in osmolality produces a sequence of physiological events that maintains homeostasis. Increased osmolality will stimulate the secretion of antidiuretic hormone (ADH) that acts on renal tubules. This results in reabsorption of water, more concentrated urine, and less concentrated serum. Low serum osmolality suppresses the release of ADH, water reabsorption is decreased, and large amounts of dilute urine are produced.

Explanation of Test
This test is used as an indication of fluid and electrolyte balance and to rule out the presence of organic acids, sugars, or ethanol. It is helpful in evaluating hydration status, seizures, liver disease, antidiuretic hormone function, liver disease, coma, and in toxicology workup.

Serum osmolality increases with dehydration and decreases with overhydration. In general, the same conditions that reduce or increase serum sodium affect the osmolality.

Procedure
A venous blood sample of at least six ml. is obtained. It is determined in the laboratory by the number (not the nature) of dissolved solute particles in solution.

Interfering Factors
1. Decreases are associated with attitude, diurnal variation with water retention at night, and some drugs.
2. Some drugs will cause increases.

Clinical Implications
1. *Increased values* (hyperosmolality) are associated with
   (a) Water restriction or loss
   (b) Brain trauma with impaired release of ADH
   (c) Hypercalcemia
   (d) Diabetes mellitus due to increased glucose
   (e) Diabetes insipidus
   (f) Cerebral lesions (often with tube feeding)
2. *Decreased values* (hypoosmolality) are associated with
   (a) Loss of sodium with diuretics and low salt diet
   (b) Addison's disease
   (c) Adrenogenital syndrome
   (d) Inappropriate secretions of ADH, as in trauma and cancer of lung
   (e) Excessive water replacement

Clinical Alert

1. Panic values are results that are <240 or >than 321. A value of 385 relates to stupor in hyperglycemia. Values of 400–420 are associated with grand mal seizures—value >420 is deadly.
2. The patient receiving intravenous fluids should have a normal osmolality. If the osmolality increases, the fluids contain relatively more electrolytes than water. If it fails, relatively more water than electrolytes is present.
3. If the ratio of serum sodium to serum osmolality falls below 0.43, the outlook is guarded. This ratio may be distorted in drug intoxication.

Water load or dilution test may be done to investigate impaired renal excretion of water.

Procedure

1. The ideal position during testing period is the recumbent position because in an upright position the response to water loading is reduced.
2. One hour before testing the patient is given 300 ml. of water to replace fluid lost during the overnight fast. This water is not counted as part of the test load.
3. The patient drinks a test load of water (calculated as 20 ml./kg. of body weight) within 30 minutes.
4. After water is consumed, all urine is collected for the next four to five hours and each voiding is checked for its amount, osmolality, and specific gravity. When the test is completed, a blood sample is obtained for osmolality and the entire volume of urine obtained is checked for osmolality.

Patient Preparation

1. Explain the purpose and procedure. The test takes 5 to 6 hours to complete.
2. No food, liquor, medications, or smoking for 8 to 10 hours before testing.
3. The patient may experience nausea, abdominal fullness, fatigue, and desire to defecate.

Clinical Alert

1. Observe for adverse reactions to water load test such as extreme abdominal discomfort, shortness of breath, or chest pain.

2. If water clearance is impaired, the water load will not induce diureses and maximum urinary dilution will not occur.
3. Accurate results may not be obtained if nausea, vomiting, or diarrhea occur or if disturbance in bladder emptying is present.

BLOOD SUGARS AND RELATED TESTS

Cortisone Glucose Tolerance

Normal Values
At 1 hr.: blood glucose 160 mg./dl.
At 2 hr.: blood glucose 140 mg./dl.
(Add an additional 18 mg./dl. at age 40 and for each decade over 40 yr.)

Explanation of Test
This is a glucose tolerance test based on the fact that cortisone increases blood glucose. The test is also known as the "steroid challenge" test because cortisone acetate is given before the standard glucose tolerance test is begun.

Indications for Test
1. When the results of the standard glucose tolerance test are doubtful, and altered carbohydrate metabolism is strongly suspected
2. In patients with suggestive signs of vascular or neurological disease
3. In persons with a strong family history of diabetes
4. In women whose pregnancies were complicated by glycosuria and delivery of large infants

Procedure
The procedure is the same as for the glucose tolerance test with the following exceptions:
1. An oral dose of cortisone acetate is given 8 hours before glucose ingestion and again 2 hours before glucose is given.
2. A venous blood sample is obtained after the second dose of cortisone.

Clinical Implications
If the 2-hour level is above 140 mg. per dl., a person is considered to be prediabetic and should be followed closely for the development of diabetes.

Interfering Factors
See "Glucose Tolerance Test."

C-Peptide

Normal Values
500–2,500 pg./ml. or ng./liter

Background
C-peptide is formed during the conversion of proinsulin to insulin in the beta cells of the pancreas. It is secreted into the blood serum in almost equal concentration with insulin. Normally, a strong correlation exists between levels of insulin and C-peptide, except possibly in obese persons and in the presence of islet cell tumors.

Explanation of Test
The measurement of C-peptide levels provides a reliable indication of beta and secretory function and insulin secretions. This determination has its most useful application in the evaluation of endogenous secretion of insulin when the presence of circulatory insulin antibodies interferes with the direct assay of insulin. This situation is most likely to occur in diabetics who have been treated with bovine/pork insulin. This test is also useful in evaluating hypoglycemic states, in identifying surreptitious injection of insulin, and in confirmation of remission of diabetes mellitus. Furthermore, monitoring following pancreatectomy for removal of cancer can provide a means of detecting the presence of residual tissue.

Procedure
A fasting venous blood sample of 1 ml. is obtained.

Clinical Implications
1. *Increased values* are associated with endogenous hyperinsulinism, in insulin-dependent diabetic persons when a high level of insulin is also present.
2. *Decreased levels* are associated with persons who have been surreptitiously injecting insulin and who have both hypoglycemia and high insulin levels.
3. *Normal levels* are found in persons who have had a remission of diabetes mellitus.

Patient Preparation
1. Explain the purpose and procedure of the test.
2. Caution the patient to fast from food for 8 to 12 hours. Water is permitted.

Glucagon

Normal Values
50–200 pg./ml. or ng./liter plasma

Glucagon response in normal person after a standard test meal of carbohydrates, fat, and protein is a gradual increase from 92 plus or minus 12 pg./ml. to a peak of 125 plus or minus 13 pg./ml.
In a glucose tolerance test, glucagon levels will significantly decline from fasting levels during the hyperglycemic first hour in normal persons.

Background
Glucagon is a peptide hormone that originates in the alpha cells of the islets of Langerhans. In the liver, this hormone promotes glucose production. This action of glucagon is opposed by that of insulin. The normal coordinated release patterns of this hormone provide a sensitive control mechanism for glucose production and storage. For example, low glucose levels result in release, whereas conditions of hyperglycemia reduce circulating glucagon levels to approximately 50% of the amount in the fasting state.

It is now believed that the kidneys play an important role in the metabolism of glucagon. Studies reveal that elevated fasting levels of glucagon in patients with renal failure return to normal following successful renal transplantation. On the other hand, renal rejection has resulted in a dramatic rise in glucagon levels several days before changes in creatinine levels.

Abnormally high levels of glucagon recede once insulin therapy begins to control diabetes, and levels slowly revert to normal in persons on maintenance doses of insulin. Also, in contrast to the normal glucagon, secretion in diabetics does not decrease following ingestion of a carbohydrate meal. However, an arginine infusion causes greatly increased glucagon secretion in normal persons.

Explanation of Test
This measurement has clinical significance in two ways. Glucagon deficiency reflects a general loss of pancreatic tissue. Compelling evidence for glucagon deficiency is the failure of glucagon levels to rise during arginine infusion. Hyperglucagonemia (increased glucagon levels) occur in diabetes, acute pancreatitis, and in situations where catecholamine secretion is greatly augmented as in pheochromocytoma and in the presence of infection.

Procedure
Five venous blood samples of 5 ml. are obtained in heparinized or EDTA containers. Special handling is required because glucagon is highly susceptible to enzymatic degradation.

Clinical Implications
1. *Increased levels* are associated with
   (a) Acute pancreatitis
   (b) Diabetes mellitus. Persons with severe diabetic ketoacidosis

are reported to have levels five times normal fasting levels despite marked hyperglycemia.
(c) Glucagonoma
(d) Uremia
(e) Infections
(f) Pheochromocytoma
2. *Reduced levels* are associated with
(a) Inflammatory disease where there is a loss of pancreatic tissue
(b) Neoplastic replacement of the pancreas
(c) Surgical removal of the pancreas

Interfering Factors
Increased levels occur in vigorous exercise and in trauma.

Patient Preparation
None necessary unless glucose tolerance testing is to be done or if arginine infusion is ordered. In this case, check with your testing laboratory for specific protocols.

Glucose; Fasting Blood Sugar (FBS)

Normal Values
Fasting serum: 70–110 mg./dl. or 3.89–6.11 mmol./liter
Fasting whole blood: 60–100 mg./dl. or 3.33–5.53 mmol./liter
Nonfasting: 85–125 mg./dl. >50 yrs. 70–115 mg./dl. <50 yrs.

Explanation of Test
The purpose of this test is to detect any disorder of glucose metabolism, mainly diabetes, and is used as an aid in diabetes management. Glucose is formed from the digestion of carbohydrates and the conversion of glycogen by the liver. Two hormones directly regulate blood glucose: glucagon and insulin. Glucagon accelerates the breakdown of glycogen in the liver, causing blood glucose to rise. Insulin increases the permeability of cellular membranes to glucose, transports glucose into cells for metabolism, and further stimulates formation of glucogen and reduces blood glucose levels. Getting insulin into the cells where metabolism takes place requires insulin and insulin receptors. Following a meal, insulin will be released by the pancreas to help the body use glucose, provided there are enough insulin receptors. Insulin binds to special receptors on the surface of target cells such as fat and muscle. This causes channels to open that allow glucose to pass into cells where it can be used to make energy. As glucose is metabolized by the cells, blood glucose falls and none passes into the urine. Other hormones that contribute to glucose metabolism are ACTH, adrenocorticosteroids, epinephrine, and thyroxine.

The test for blood sugar is used to detect disorders of metabolism that may be the result of one of several causes.

1. Inability of the beta islet cells of the pancreas to produce insulin
2. Reduced number of insulin receptors
3. Inability of the intestines to absorb glucose
4. Inability of the liver to accumulate and break down glycogen
5. The presence of increased amounts of hormones (*i.e.*, ACTH)

In most cases, any degree of elevated blood sugar (hyperglycemia) indicates diabetes. At the same time, it is important to remember that in mild cases of diabetes, the blood sugar may be within normal ranges. Therefore, in any suspected cases of diabetes, a glucose tolerance test is in order (see page 274).

While diabetes is the most readily suspected disorder in the presence of hyperglycemia, other diseases may be responsible for the elevated blood sugar and therefore should not be dismissed.

Clinical Alert

1. If a known or suspected diabetic is experiencing dizziness, weakness, or fainting, a blood sugar test must be done before any insulin is given. This is because the same symptoms may be present for both insulin reaction and high blood sugar. If there will be a delay in obtaining a blood glucose measurement, when in doubt about signs and symptoms the patient is presenting, *give glucose.*
2. Frequent determinations of blood glucose are in many situations more desirable than monitoring urine glucose. Hence, blood glucose monitoring facilitates regulation of diabetes and may increase the likelihood of achieving ideal control in Type I diabetes that approximates euglycemia.

Procedure
1. A venous blood sample of 5 ml. is drawn while the patient is in a fasting state. If the patient is a known diabetic, blood should be drawn before insulin or oral hypoglycemics are given.
2. Self-monitoring of blood glucose requires one large drop of fingertip blood and can be done using reagent strips, with or without a glucometer.

Clinical Implications
A. *Elevated blood sugar* (hyperglycemia)
   1. Diabetes
      Values over 120 mg. per dl. on several testings may indicate

diabetes mellitus. Except for diabetes, the FBS rarely exceeds 120 mg. per 100 ml.

2. Other possible conditions
   (a) Cushing's disease (increase in glucocorticoids causes increase in blood sugar)
   (b) Acute stress (such as in myocardial infarction or severe infections, such as meningitis or encephalitis)
   (c) Pheochromocytoma
   (d) Pituitary adenoma (growth hormone leads to elevated blood sugar)
   (e) Hyperthyroidism
   (f) Adenoma of pancreas (may result in production of glucagon, which counteracts insulin)
   (g) Pancreatitis
   (h) Brain trauma or brain damage
   (i) Chronic liver disease
   (j) Chronic illness
   (k) Prolonged physical inactivity
   (l) Chronic malnutrition (insufficient intake)
   (m)Potassium deficiency

B. *Lower glucose levels* (hypoglycemia)
   1. Overdose of insulin (most frequent cause)
   2. Addison's disease (hypoglycemia is accompanied by elevated potassium and decreased sodium and elevated BUN)
   3. Bacterial sepsis
   4. Islet cell carcinoma of pancreas (secretes excessive amount of insulin)
   5. Hepatic necrosis
   6. Hypothyroidism
   7. Glycogen storage disease
   8. Psychogenic causes

Interfering Factors
1. Steroids, diuretics, and many other drugs
2. Pregnancy (normally a slight elevation in glucose)
3. Anesthesia (sometimes in excess of 200 mg./dl.)
4. Overweight
5. Infections of adrenals
6. Stress

Patient Preparation
1. Since FBS is being tested, the patient must fast for 12 hours.
2. Water is permitted.

Patient Aftercare
1. The patient may eat or drink as soon as the blood sample is drawn.
2. Persons with values of 200 mg./dl. or greater should be placed on a strict I and O.

Clinical Alert

1. A confirmed fasting level (two or more tests) above 140 mg./dl. is diagnostic of diabetes mellitus. In this case, a glucose tolerance test should not be done.
2. When the value is >300 mg./dl., there will be an increased urinary output with greater chance of dehydration.
3. When glucose is <30 mg. or 1–7 mmol., brain damage is possible.
4. When glucose is >300 mg. or 16.7 mmol., coma is possible.

2-Hour Postprandial Blood Sugar (2-hr. PPBS)

Normal Values

Less than 120 mg./dl. or <6.7 mmol./liter

Explanation of Test

A *postprandial* test, a test taken *after* a meal, is an excellent screening test for diabetes. Glucose concentration in a fasting blood specimen obtained 2 hours after a meal is rarely elevated in normal persons but is significantly increased in diabetic patients. It is also used to monitor insulin therapy and to confirm diabetes in a patient with a FBS less than 120 mg./dl.

Procedure

1. For best results, the patient should be on a high carbohydrate diet 2 to 3 days before testing.
2. After an overnight fast (water is permitted), the patient eats a high carbohydrate breakfast. The meal should include orange juice, cereal with sugar, toast, and milk.
3. Two hours after the patient finishes eating breakfast, a venous blood sample of 5 ml. is obtained.
4. Record the time that breakfast is completed and notify the laboratory.

Clinical Implications

Values above 140 mg./dl. are abnormal. This figure applies only to adults under 50 years of age. The level should be raised to 160 mg./dl for those in their 60s and to as much as 180 mg./dl. for people under 60.

A. *Increased levels* occur in many stressful or serious conditions.

1. Malnutrition
2. Advanced cirrhosis of liver
3. Cushing's syndrome
4. Acromegaly
5. Hyperthyroidism
6. Pheochromocytoma

7. Lipoproteinemias
8. Myocardial or cerebral infarction
9. Some malignancies
10. Pregnancy
11. Anxiety states

B. *Decreased levels* occur in
   1. Anterior pituitary insufficiency
   2. Islet cell adenoma
   3. Steatorrhea
   4. Addison's disease

C. A 2-hour postprandial glucose greater than 200 ml./dl. is consistent with a diagnosis of diabetes mellitus.

Interfering Factors
Smoking and/or coffee drinking may raise blood glucose level.

Patient Preparation
1. Instruct the patient about the purpose and procedure of the test. The patient must fast from food overnight, at least 12 hours, and can drink water but no other liquids.
2. The patient should remain at rest during the 2-hour interval.

Patient Aftercare
After the blood sample is drawn, the patient may eat and drink normally.

Clinical Alert

1. Values of 140–200 mg./dl. indicate decreased tolerance and warrant the use of a glucose tolerance test.
2. Test results are reliable only if the patient is properly prepared.

Glycosylated Hemoglobin (HbA₁c); Glycohemoglobin (G-Hb); Diabetic Control Index

Normal Values
Results expressed as % of total hemoglobin.
Normal (nondiabetic): 4.0–7.0%
Diabetic: >7%

Background
Glycohemoglobin is one of the types of minor hemoglobins found in everyone. Hemoglobin A_1 undergoes change or glycosylation to hemoglobin A_{1a}, A_{1b}, and A_{1c} by a slow, nonenzyme process within the red blood cells during their circulating life span of 120 days. Most simply put, glycohemoglobin is blood glucose bound to hemoglobin. The red

cell, as it circulates, combines some of the glucose from the blood-stream with its own content of hemoglobin to form glycohemoglobin in a one-way reaction. The amount of glycosolated hemoglobin found and stored by the erythrocyte depends on the amount of glucose available to it over the red cell's 120-day life span. In diabetes with hyperglyce-mia, the increase in glycohemoglobin is usually caused by an increase in HbA_{1c}. The glucose concentration will increase when hyperglycemia caused by insulin deficiency develops. This glycosylation is irrevers-ible.

Explanation of Test
This test is an index of long-term glucose control. Glycosylated hemo-globin monitoring reflects the average blood sugar level for the 2- to 3-month period before the test. The more glucose the RBC is exposed to, the higher the percentage of glycosylated hemoglobin. The test pro-vides information about the success of treatment of diabetes such as adequacy of dietary or insulin therapy, allows determination of dura-tion of hyperglycemia in new cases of juvenile onset diabetes with acute ketoacidosis, provides a sensitive estimate of glucose imbalance in mild cases of diabetes, and is an evaluation of effectiveness of old and new forms of therapy such as oral hypoglycemic agents, single or multiple insulin injections, and B-cell transplantation. Test results are not affected by time of day, meal intake, exercise, just-administered diabetic drugs, emotional stress, or patient cooperation.

The measurement may be of particular value for specific groups of patients. These groups include diabetic children, diabetics in whom the renal threshold for glucose is abnormal, unstable insulin-depen-dent diabetics in whom blood sugars vary markedly from day to day, patients who do not test urine regularly for glucose, and persons who, before their scheduled appointments, will change their usual habits, dietary or otherwise, so that their metabolic control appears better than it actually is.

Procedure
A venous blood sample of at least 3 ml. is obtained.

Clinical Implications
1. Values are increased in poorly controlled and newly diagnosed dia-betes. In these instances, HbA_{1c} levels comprise 8% to 12% of the total hemoglobin.
2. With optimal insulin control, the HbA_{1c} levels return toward nor-mal.
3. A diabetic patient who has only recently come under good control may still have a high concentration of glycosylated hemoglobin. This level will decline only gradually as newly formed red blood

cells with nearly normal glycosylated hemoglobin replace older red blood cells with high concentrations of glycosylated hemoglobin.

Interfering Factors

1. Spurious results should be expected in every case of hemoglobin-opathy distinguishable from hemoglobin A by electrophoresis.
2. Decreased value in pregnancy and sickle cell anemia, increased value in thalassemia.

Clinical Alert

Confusion in interpretation of results may occur because there are two tests for determining glycosylated hemoglobin. The most specific test measures hemoglobin A_1, which includes hemoglobin A_{1a}, A_{1b} and A_{1c}. There are different expected values for each test. Keep in mind that hemoglobin A_1 is always 2% to 4% higher than A_{1c}.

Insulin

Normal Values

5–20 μU./ml. by radioimmunoassay or 35–145 pmol./liter

Background

Insulin, a hormone produced in the pancreas by the beta cells of the islets of Langerhans, regulates the metabolism of carbohydrates along with liver, adipose, muscle, and other target cells and is responsible for maintaining a constant level of blood glucose. The rate of insulin secretion is determined primarily by the level of blood glucose perfusing the pancreas and is also affected by hormonal status, the autonomic nervous system, and nutritional status.

Explanation of Test

This measurement of the insulin secretory response to glucose may be of value in establishing the diagnosis of insulinoma and in the evaluation of abnormal carbohydrate and lipid metabolism. Insulin levels are also helpful in supporting the diagnosis of diabetes in persons with borderline abnormalities of the glucose tolerance procedures. This determination is invaluable in the investigation of fasting hypoglycemic patients and may be useful in the differentiation of islet cell neoplasms.

The insulin study can be ordered in conjunction with the glucose tolerance test or in conjunction with a one-time fasting glucose.

Procedure

1. A fasting blood sample of 4 ml. is obtained.
2. If ordered in conjunction with the glucose tolerance test, blood specimens should be obtained before ingesting 100 grams of glucose and obtained again at 30, 60, and 120 minutes after glucose ingestion.

Clinical Implications

Increased values are associated with

A. Insulinoma: diagnosis of insulinoma is based on
   1. Association of hyperinsulinemia with hypoglycemia
   2. Persistent hypoglycemia along with hyperinsulinemia between 2 and 3 hours after injection of tolbutamide
   3. Failure of *C*-peptide suppression when plasma glucose is 40 mg./dl. or less. After 100 grams of glucose, normal serum insulin will rise less than 2 μU./ml. to 25 to 231 in one-half hour, 18 to 276 in 1 hour, 16 to 166 in 2 hours, and 4 to 38 in 3 hours. The results may be too variable to be of diagnostic usefulness.
B. Acromegaly
C. Cushing's syndrome

Interfering Factors

Falsely increased values are associated with food intake, obesity, and use of oral contraceptives.

Patient Preparation

1. Explain the purpose and procedure of the test.
2. The patient should be fasting overnight unless otherwise directed.
3. Water is permitted.

Standard Oral Glucose Tolerance Test (OGTT)

Normal Values

FBS: <115 mg./dl. or <64 mmol./liter
90 min.: <200 mg./dl. or <11.1 mmol./liter
2 hr.: <140 mg./dl. or <7.8 mmol./liter
3 hr.: <125 mg./dl.

All three blood values must be met to be considered normal. All urines are negative for glucose.

Explanation of Test

This timed test of blood and urine is done to rule out diabetes (see box on page 275) by determining the rate of removal of a concentrated dose of glucose from the bloodstream. In the healthy person, the insulin

---

**Type I: Insulin-Dependent
Diabetes Mellitis (IDDM)**
1. Persons who
   (a) Lack insulin
   (b) Have plentiful receptor sites
   (c) Require insulin injections
   (d) Are usually young

**Type II: Noninsulin-Dependent
Diabetes Mellitis (NIDDM)**
1. Persons who
   (a) Have insulin but whose body cells cannot use it
   (b) Have reduced number of insulin receptor sites
   (c) Are usually older, obese, and physically inactive
   (d) Require life-style change and possibly oral medication

---

response to a large oral dose of glucose is almost immediate, peaking in 30 to 60 minutes and returning to normal within 3 hours. In this instance, it can be assumed that sufficient insulin is present to allow glucose to leave the blood and enter the cells of the body.

Testing is usually done in the morning after an overnight fast. The glucose tolerance test is indicated when there is sugar in the urine or when the fasting blood sugar or 2-hour postprandial blood sugar is more than slightly elevated. The glucose tolerance test is more definite than a 2-hour postprandial blood sugar test in diagnosing hypoglycemia and malabsorption syndrome. It is also ordered in a questionable diagnosis of Cushing's syndrome or acromegaly.

Indications for Test
The glucose tolerance test rather than the 2-hour postprandial blood sugar test should be done on certain patients, particularly those with

1. Family history of diabetes
2. Obesity
3. Unexplained episodes of hypoglycemia
4. History of recurrent infections such as boils and abscesses
5. (In women) a history of delivery of large infants, stillbirths, neonatal death, premature labor, and abortions
6. Transitory glycosuria or hyperglycemia in pregnancy, surgery, trauma, stress, myocardial infarction, ACTH administration

Tolerance tests can also be performed for pentose, lactose, galactose, and D-xylose.

Procedure
This is a timed test. A 2-hour test is ordered for diabetes detection in males and nonpregnant females; a 3-hour test for pregnant women; and a 5-hour test to evaluate possible hypoglycemia.

1. A diet containing at least 150 grams of carbohydrates should be eaten for 3 days before the test.
2. Drugs that may influence the test should be discontinued for 3 days before the test.
   (a) Hormones, including oral contraceptives
   (b) Salicylates
   (c) Diuretic agents
   (d) Hypoglycemic agents
3. Insulin or oral hypoglycemics should not be given until after test is completed.
4. A sample of <7 ml. of venous blood is drawn after an overnight fast. At least three other blood samples will be obtained (dependent on physician's order and laboratory practice).
5. The patient is given a drink of a very sweet commercial preparation liquid, containing 75 g. of glucose. He is encouraged to drink it all quickly. All the solution must be taken.
6. Blood and urine samples are usually obtained at intervals of 30 minutes, 1, 2, and sometimes 3 hours after ingestion of glucose, and are tested for glucose.
7. Inclusion of the fifth hour specimens of both blood and urine is valuable in detecting hypoglycemia.

Clinical Implications
1. In Type II onset diabetes, the secretion of insulin is delayed, followed by a slightly higher than normal glucose level at 2 hours. Blood glucose is elevated until the 2-hour point.
2. In overt diabetes, there is no secretion of insulin, resulting in above normal glucose levels throughout the test.
3. In hypoglycemia, the blood glucose is below normal after the 2-hour point and up to 4 to 5 hours because of high insulin levels.
4. Tolerance tests can also be performed for pentose, lactose, galactose, and D-xylose.
5. Diagnostic criteria of 1979 National Diabetes Data Group
   (a) *Diabetic GTT*
      Fasting: <140 mg./dl.
      2hr.: >200 mg./dl.
      ½, 1, or 1½ hr.: >200 mg./dl.
   (b) *Gestational diabetes (2 or more must be met and exceeded)*
      Fasting: >105 mg./dl.
      1 hr.: >190 mg./dl.
      2 hr.: >165 mg./dl.
      3 hr.: >145 mg./dl.

(c) *Impaired GTT (all 3 must be met)*
Fasting: <140 mg./dl.
2 hr.: 140–200 mg./dl.
½, 1, or 1½ hr.: >200 mg./dl.

(d) Glucose values above the normal value concentrations, but below the criteria for diabetes or IGT, should be considered non-diagnostic for these conditions.

Interfering Factors
1. Smoking will increase the glucose level.
2. Inadequate diet (such as weight reducing diet) before testing can diminish carbohydrate tolerance and suggest a false diabetes.
3. Levels tend to increase normally in older persons; the maximum can reach 200 mg. per dl.
4. Prolonged administration of oral contraceptives will give significantly higher glucose levels in the second hour or in later blood specimens.
5. Bedrest over a lengthy period of time will influence glucose tolerance. For this reason the test should be performed on ambulatory patients, not on patients whose condition requires bedrest.
6. Infectious diseases and surgery will affect tolerance. Two weeks of recovery should be allowed before the test.
7. Certain drugs will impair glucose tolerance.
   (a) Insulin
   (b) Oral hypoglycemics
   (c) Large doses of salicylates
   (d) Thiazide diuretics
   (e) Oral contraceptives
   (f) Corticosteroids
   (g) Estrogens
   (h) Ferrous ascorbinate
   (i) Nicotinic acid
   (j) Phenothiazines
   (k) Lithium
   (l) Metapyrone
   These drugs should be discontinued, if possible, for at least 3 days before the test.

Patient Preparation
1. Instruct the patient about the purpose and procedure of the test and leave him a written reminder.
   (a) Stress a normal diet with high carbohydrates (150 g.) for 3 days preceding the test.
   (b) Fasting is required for at least 12 hours before the test and for not more than 16 hours.
   (c) Water is permitted and encouraged.
2. Determine the patient's weight and record it.
3. Collect urine and blood specimens and test for glucose, recording exact time of collection. Have the patient empty his bladder for each specimen.
   (a) No liquids can be taken other than water.
   (b) No food is to be eaten during the test periods.
   (c) No alcohol should be taken the previous evening.

    (d) Encourage the patient to stay in bed or rest quietly during the test period. Weakness or feeling faint may occur during the test, and exercise also changes glucose results.

    (e) No smoking is allowed during the test.

    (f) Coffee and unusual physical exercise should be avoided for at least 8 hours before the test.

Patient Aftercare

1. The patient may eat and drink normally as soon as the test is over.
2. Administer insulin or oral hypoglycemics to diabetics as soon as the test is completed.

Clinical Alert

1. This test is contraindicated in patients who have had a recent history of surgery, myocardial infarction, or labor and delivery, for these conditions can cause erroneous results (altered carbohydrate tolerance).
2. Record and report any reactions during the test. Weakness, faintness, and sweating may occur between the second and third hours. If this occurs, a blood sample for sugar is drawn immediately, and the test is discontinued.
3. The test should be postponed in the event of unexpected illness such as fever or gastritis or if there has been ingestion of food within 8 hours.
4. If the fasting blood sugar is over 200, the glucose tolerance test is usually not done. If it is done, the patient should be monitored very carefully for severe reaction or even coma.

Lactose Tolerance

Normal Values

Greater than a 20-mg./dl. rise in glucose and no abdominal symptoms such as pain or diarrhea

Explanation of Test

This is a glucose tolerance test to diagnose intestinal disaccharidase (lactase) deficiency.

Procedure

1. Follow instructions for the glucose tolerance test.
2. A fasting specimen is obtained and the patient is given 100 g. of lactose in 200 ml. of water.
3. Blood samples are drawn at 15, 30, 60, and 120 minutes for glucose.

Clinical Implications
A "flat" lactose tolerance finding is suspicious of a deficiency. However, this test should be followed by a monosaccharide tolerance test such as glucose galactose tolerance test.

END PRODUCTS OF METABOLISM AND OTHER TESTS
Ammonia

Normal Values
Men: 18–54 μmol./liter
Women: 12–50 μmol./liter
   There is a great deal of variation in reported values because of methods used.

Background
Ammonia, one of the end products of protein metabolism, is formed from the action of bacteria on proteins in the intestines and from hydrolysis of glutamine in the kidneys. The liver normally removes most of the ammonia from the portal vein blood flow and converts ammonia to urea. Since any appreciable level of ammonia in the blood would affect acid–base balance and brain function, an adequate mechanism for its removal is essential. The liver accomplishes this by synthesis of urea for excretion by the kidney.

Explanation of Test
Measurement of blood ammonia levels is used to evaluate metabolism as well as the progress of severe liver disease and response to treatment.

Procedure
1. A fasting venous blood sample of 3 ml. is obtained.
2. The sample is placed in an iced container and the test must be performed within 20 minutes.
3. The laboratory should be notified of all antibiotics the patient is receiving because of the possibility of these drugs lowering ammonia levels.

Clinical Implications
Increased ammonia levels occur in
1. Liver disease
2. Hepatic coma due to
   (a) Cirrhosis
   (b) Severe hepatitis
3. Severe heart failure
4. Azotemia
5. Cor pulmonale
6. Hemolytic disease of the newborn
7. Pulmonary emphysema
8. Acute bronchitis
9. Pericarditis
10. Myelocytic and lymphatic leukemia
11. Reye's syndrome

Patient Preparation
1. Instruct the patient to fast for 8 hours before the blood test.
2. Water is permitted.

Interfering Factors
1. Ammonia levels vary with protein intake.
2. Exercise may cause an increase in ammonia levels.
3. There are many drugs that may affect blood ammonia levels.

Clinical Alert

In patients with impaired liver function demonstrated by elevated ammonia levels, the blood level can be lowered by reduced protein intake and by use of antibiotics to reduce intestinal bacteria counts.

Bilirubin

Normal Values
Total bilirubin: 0.2–1.0 mg./dl. or 3.4–17.1 μmol./liter
Conjugated: 0.0–0.2 mg./dl. or 0.0–3.4 μmol./liter
Indirect unconjugated: 0.2–0.8 mg./dl. or 3.4–13.68 μmol./liter
Newborn: 1–12 mg./dl. or 17.1–205.2 μmol./liter

Background
Bilirubin, resulting from the breakdown of hemoglobin in the red blood cells, is a by-product of hemolyis (red blood cell destruction). It is produced by the reticuloendothelial system. Removed from the body by the liver, which excretes it into the bile, it gives the bile its major pigmentation.

Usually a small amount of bilirubin is found in the serum. A rise in serum levels will occur if there is an excessive destruction of red blood cells or if the liver is unable to excrete the normal amounts of bilirubin produced.

There are two forms of bilirubin in the body: (1) indirect or unconjugated bilirubin (which is protein bound), and (2) direct or conjugated bilirubin that circulates freely in the blood until it reaches the liver, where it is conjugated with glucuronide transferase and then excreted into the bile. An increase in protein-bound bilirubin (unconjugated bilirubin) is more frequently associated with increased destruction of red blood cells (hemolysis); an increase in free-flowing bilirubin is more likely seen in dysfunction or blockage of the liver.

A routine examination measures only the total bilirubin. A normal level of total bilirubin rules out any significant impairment of the excretory function of the liver or excessive hemolysis of red cells. Only when the levels are elevated will there be a call for differentiation of the bilirubin according to the conjugated and unconjugated levels.

Jaundice/Icterus
Excessive amounts of bilirubin eventually seep into the tissues, which then assume a yellow hue. The yellow color is a clinical sign of jaundice. In newborns, signs of jaundice may indicate hemolytic anemia or congenital icterus. If the bilirubin levels reach a critical point in the infant, damage to the central nervous system may occur in a condition known as *kernicterus*. Therefore, in these infants, it is the level of bilirubin that is the deciding factor in the decision to do an exchange transfusion.

Explanation of Test
The measurement of bilirubin is important in evaluating liver function, hemolytic anemias, and hyperbilirubinemia (in newborns).

Procedure
1. A venous sample of 5 ml. is obtained before the patient eats breakfast.
2. The sample must be protected from bright light.
3. Air bubbles and unnecessary shaking of the sample are to be avoided while blood is collected.
4. If the specimen cannot be examined immediately, then it should be stored in a refrigerator and in darkness.
5. In infants, blood must be collected from a heel puncture. Two full micro blood sampling tubes are collected. (In newborns, the sample size is .3 ml.)

Clinical Implications
A. *Bilirubin elevations accompanied by jaundice* may be due to hepatic, obstructive, or hemolytic causes.
   1. *Hepatocellular jaundice* results from injury or disease of the parenchymal cells of the liver and can be caused by
      (a) Viral hepatitis
      (b) Cirrhosis
      (c) Infectious mononucleosis
      (d) Reactions of certain drugs such as chlorpromazine
   2. *Obstructive jaundice* is usually the result of obstruction of the common bile or hepatic ducts due to stones or neoplasms. The obstruction produces high conjugated bilirubin levels due to bile regurgitation.
   3. *Hemolytic jaundice* is due to overproduction of bilirubin resulting from hemolytic processes that produce high levels of unconjugated bilirubin. Hemolytic jaundice can be found in

(a) Erythroblastosis fetalis
(b) Pernicious anemia
(c) Sickle cell anemia
(d) Transfusion reactions
(e) Crigler–Najjar syndrome (a severe disease that results from a genetic deficiency of a hepatic enzyme needed for the conjugation of bilirubin)

B. *Elevations of* **nonconjugate** *bilirubin levels* occur in
   1. Hemolytic anemias
   2. Trauma in the presence of a large hematoma
   3. Hemorrhagic pulmonary infarcts
   4. Crigler–Nijjar syndrome (rare)
   5. Gilbert's disease (rare)

C. *Elevated* **conjugate** *bilirubin levels* occur in
   1. Cancer of the head of the pancreas
   2. Choledocholithiasis
   3. Dubin–Johnson syndrome

D. *Elevation of* **both conjugate and nonconjugate** *levels (with the conjugate levels more elevated)* occurs in
   1. Hepatic metastasis   4. Cholestasis secondary to drugs
   2. Hepatitis   5. Cirrhosis
   3. Lymphoma

Interfering Factors
1. A 1-hour exposure of the specimen to sunlight or high intensity artificial light at room temperature will decrease the bilirubin content.
2. Contrast media 24 hours before measurement may cause an altered reaction.
3. A high fat meal may cause decreased bilirubin levels by interfering with the clinical reactions.
4. Air bubbles and shaking of the specimen may cause decreased levels.
5. Foods (carrots, yams) and drugs increase the yellow hue in the serum.

Blood Urea Nitrogen (BUN)

Normal Values
7–18 mg./dl. or 2.5–6.3 mmol./liter

Explanation of Test
Urea is formed in the liver and constitutes the major nonprotein nitrogenous end product of protein catabolism. The urea is then carried to the kidneys by the blood to be excreted in the urine.

The test for BUN, measuring the nitrogen portion of urea, is used as a gross index of glomerular function and the production and excretion of urea. Rapid protein catabolism and impairment of kidney function will result in an elevated BUN. The rate at which the BUN rises is influenced by the degree of tissue necrosis, protein catabolism, and the rate at which the kidneys excrete the urea nitrogen.

The BUN is less sensitive than creatinine clearance tests and may not be abnormal until the creatinine clearance is moderately abnormal.

Procedure

A venous blood sample of at least 5 ml. is obtained. The amount drawn depends on the method and type of equipment used.

Clinical Implications

A. *Increased* BUN
   1. The most common cause of increased BUN level is inadequate excretion due to kidney disease or urinary obstruction, frequently occurring in cases of prostate enlargement.
      (a) An increased BUN of 50 to 150 mg. per 100 ml. indicates serious impairment of renal function.
      (b) An increased BUN of 150 to 250 mg. per 100 ml. is definitive for severely impaired renal failure.
   2. *Increased BUN levels* are associated with

(a) Impaired renal function	(g) Some malignancies
(b) Shock	(h) Acute myocardial infarc-
(c) Dehydration	tion
(d) GI hemorrhage	(i) Chronic gout
(e) Infection	(j) Excessive protein intake
(f) Diabetes	or protein catabolism

   Increases of 50 mg. per 100 ml. per day in the BUN have occurred in previously healthy people who have undergone *severe crushing injuries* or are suffering from *overwhelming infection*.

B. *Decreased BUN* is associated with
   (a) Liver failure
   (b) Negative nitrogen balance as may occur in malnutrition, excessive use of IV fluids, and physiologic hydremia of pregnancy
   (c) Impaired absorption as in celiac disease
   (d) Nephrotic syndrome (occasionally)
   (e) Overhydration
      A further decreased BUN of 6 to 10 mg. per 100 ml. is possible in overhydration.

Interfering Factors

1. A combination of a low protein and a high carbohydrate diet can cause a decreased BUN level.

2. The BUN is normally lower in children and women because they have a smaller muscle mass than adult men.
3. Increased BUN values normally occur in late pregnancy and infancy because of increased use of protein.
4. Older persons may have an increased BUN when their kidneys are not able to concentrate urine adequately.
5. Decreased BUN values may occur normally earlier in pregnancy because of physiologic hydremia.
6. Many drugs may cause increased and decreased BUN levels.

Clinical Alert

1. If a patient is confused, disoriented, or has convulsions, the BUN should be checked. If the level is high, it may help to explain these signs and symptoms.
2. In patients with an elevated BUN, fluid and electrolyte regulation may be impaired.
3. Excessive IV fluids can result in lowered BUN levels.
4. Panic value of BUN is >100 mg./dl.

Cholinesterase RBC (Pseudocholinesterase)

Normal Values
5–12 μ/ml. at 37°C (or plasma thromboplastin component [PTC] as substrate)
5–12 kμ/liter
Values vary with substrate used.

Explanation of Test
The primary use of the measurement of serum cholinesterase (CHS) is to monitor the effect of muscle relaxants such as succinylcholine that are used in surgery. Patients for whom suxamethonium anesthesia is planned should be tested for the presence of atypical cholinesterase variants, which are incapable of hydrolyzing this widely used muscle relaxant. It is also used when poisoning by pesticides such as parathion or malathion is suspected. Severe insecticide poisoning causes headaches, visual distortions, nausea, vomiting, pulmonary edema, confusion, convulsions, respiratory paralysis, and coma.

Clinical Implications
Patients who are homozygous for the atypical gene that controls serum CHS activity have low levels of CHS that are not inhibited by dibu-

caine. Those persons with normal serum CHS activity show 70% to 90% inhibition by dibucaine.

1. Low or absent levels are associated with
   (a) Persons who will not be able to hydrolyze drugs such as muscle relaxants in surgery. These patients may have a prolonged period of apnea if they are given succinylcholine.
   (b) Poisoning from organic phosphate insecticides
   (c) Parenchymatous liver diseases
      (1) hepatitis
      (2) cirrhosis with jaundice
   (d) Conditions that may have decreased blood albumin, such as malnutrition, anemia, infections, skin diseases, and acute myocardial infarction.

Clinical Alert

In industrial exposure, workers should not return to work until values rise to 75% of normal. RBC cholinesterase regenerates at the rate of 1% per day. Plasma cholinesterase regenerates at the rate of 25% in 7 to 10 days.

Creatinine

Normal Values
Women: 0.6–1.2 mg./dl. or 53–106 μmol./liter
Men: 0.7–1.3 mg./dl. or 62–115 μmol./liter
Values are method dependent.

Explanation of Test
Creatinine is a by-product in the breakdown of muscle creatine phosphate resulting from energy metabolism. It is produced at a constant rate depending on the muscle mass of the person and is removed from the body by the kidneys. Production of creatinine is constant as long as muscle mass remains constant. A disorder of kidney function reduces excretion of creatinine, resulting in increased levels of blood creatinine.

The test is used to diagnose impaired renal function. It is a more specific and sensitive indicator of kidney disease than BUN, although in chronic renal disease, BUN correlates more accurately with symptoms or uremia than does the blood creatinine.

Procedure
A venous blood sample of 5 ml. is obtained.

Clinical Implications
A. *Increased creatinine levels* occur in
1. Impaired renal function
2. Chronic nephritis
3. Obstruction of the urinary tract
4. Muscle disease
    (a) Gigantism
    (b) Acromegaly
B. *Decreased creatinine levels* occur in
Muscular dystrophy

Interfering Factors
1. High levels of ascorbic acid can cause a falsely increased level.
2. Drugs that influence kidney function plus other medications can cause a change in the blood creatinine.
3. A diet high in roast meat will cause increased levels.

Clinical Alert

1. A normal blood serum creatinine does not always indicate unimpaired renal function. A normal value cannot be used as a standard for a patient who is known to have existing renal disease.
2. Panic value is 10 mg./dl. in nondialysis patients.
3. Creatinine should always be checked before giving nephrotoxic chemotherapeutics such as
    (a) Methotrexate   (d) Mithramycin
    (b) Cisplatin   (e) Semustine
    (c) Cytoxan

Sweat Test

Normal Values
Sweat Sodium Normals
Normal homozygotes: 10–40 mmol./liter
    Heterozygotes: 40–70 mmol./liter
Sweat Chlorides Normales
Normal homozygotes: 5–35 mmol./liter
    Heterozygotes: 35–60 mmol./liter

Explanation of Test
This test has become the cornerstone of diagnosis for cystic fibrosis when the outcome is taken in conjunction with clinical, radiological,

and stool tests. It is known that persistent, abnormally high concentrations of sodium and chloride appear in the secretions of eccrine sweat glands in cystic fibrosis. The abnormality is present at birth and persists throughout life. This study is based on techniques inducing sweating that is stimulated by pilocarpine iontophoresis, followed by chemical analysis to determine sodium and chloride content.

Interfering Factors

1. The sweat test does not retain its value after puberty because levels may vary over a very wide range.
2. Dehydration and edema, particularly of areas where sweat is collected, may interfere with test results.

Procedure

1. The forearm is the preferred site for stimulation of sweating, but in thin or small babies the thigh or back may be a better area to use. It may be necessary to stimulate sweating in two places to obtain enough sweat, especially in young infants. At least 100 microliters of sweat is necessary. In cold weather or if the room is cold, a warm covering should be placed over the arm or site of sweat collection.
2. Sweat is produced by transporting positive pilocarpine ions into the skin. This is commonly achieved by applying gauze pads or filter paper saturated with a measured amount of pilocarpine to the skin and attaching electrodes through which a current of 4 to 5 milliamperes is delivered at intervals for a total of 5 minutes.
3. The electrodes and pad are removed and the area is thoroughly washed with distilled water and carefully dried.
4. Successful iontophoresis is indicated by a red area about an inch in diameter that appears where the electrode was placed.
5. The skin is scrubbed thoroughly with distilled water and dried carefully. The area for sweat collection must be completely dry, free from contamination by powder or antiseptic, and the skin must be free of any area that might ooze.
6. Collection of sweat can occur by applying preweighed filter or sweat collection cups that are taped securely over the red spot. The inside surfaces of the collecting device should never be touched.
7. The paper is left on for at least 1 hour before removal and is then placed on a preweighed flask to avoid evaporation. The flask is again weighed.
8. If the cup is used, it is left on for 1 hour and then carefully removed by scraping it across the iontophoresed area. This "puddles" the sweat in the cup to reduce evaporation and to redissolve any salts left by the evaporation. Suction capillary tubes are used to take sweat out of the collection cups.

Clinical Implications

1. Children with cystic fibrosis will have sodium and chloride values above 60 mEq./liter (mmol./liter)
2. Borderline or gray-zone cases are those with values between 40 and 60 mEq./liter for both sodium and chloride and require retesting. Potassium values do not assist in differentiating these borderline cases.
3. In adolescence and adulthood, levels over 100 mEq./liter usually indicate cystic fibrosis.
4. Elevated sweat electrolytes can be associated with
   (a) Addison's disease
   (b) Congenital adrenal hyperplasia
   (c) Ectodermal dysplasia with hypoparathyroidism with sensorineural deafness
   (d) Pitressin-resistant diabetes insipidus
   (e) Glucose-6-phosphatase deficiency
   (f) Fucosidosis
   (g) Nephrotic syndrome

Clinical Alert

1. The test should always be repeated if the result, the clinical features, and the stool microscopy do not fit together.
2. The test can be used to exclude the diagnosis of cystic fibrosis in siblings of diagnosed patients.
3. There have been reports of cystic fibrosis patients with normal sweat electrolyte levels.

Patient Preparation

1. Explain the purpose and procedure of the test.
2. Inform the patient that a slight stinging sensation is usually experienced, especially in fair-skinned persons.

Uric Acid

Normal Values

Men: 3.5–7.2 mg./dl. or 0.21–0.42 mmol./liter
Women: 2.6–6.0 mg./dl. or 0.154–0.35 mmol./liter
Children: 2.0–5.5 mg./dl. or 0.12–0.32 mmol./liter

Explanation of Test

Uric acid is formed from the breakdown of nucleonic acids and is an end product of purine metabolism. In humans, a lack of the enzyme uricase allows this poorly soluble substance to accumulate in body fluids. Two-thirds of the uric acid produced daily is excreted by the kidneys while the remaining one-third exits by the stool. The basis for this test is that an overproduction of uric acids occurs in conditions in which there is excessive cell breakdown and catabolism of nucleonic acids (as in gout), excessive production and destruction of cells (as in leukemia), or an inability to excrete the substance produced (as in renal failure).

Measurement of uric acid is used most commonly in the evaluation of renal failure, gout, and leukemia. In hospitalized patients, renal failure is the most common cause of elevated uric acid levels, and gout is the least common cause. This test is also valuable in assessing the prognosis of eclampsia because of the uric acid level's ability to reflect the extent of liver damage in toxemia of pregnancy.

Procedure
A venous blood sample of 5 ml. is obtained.

Clinical Implications
A. *Elevated levels* (hyperuricemia)
   1. Increased levels of blood uric acid are associated with nitrogen retention and with increases in urea, creatinine, and other nonprotein nitrogenous substances of the blood. These findings are usually interpreted as another indication of decreased *kidney function.*
   2. Increased levels are found in *gout,* but the increase may be slight in the early stages of the disease. The amount of increase is not directly related to the severity of the disease.
   3. Other conditions associated with elevated uric acid levels
      (a) Leukemia
      (b) Acute stages of infectious diseases such as infectious mononucleosis
      (c) Lymphomas
      (d) Metastatic cancer
      (e) Severe eclampsia
      (f) Starvation
      (g) Shock
      (h) Alcoholism
      (i) Chemotherapy for cancer
      (j) Excessive radiographs
      (k) Multiple myeloma
      (l) Metabolic acidosis
      (m) Diabetic ketosis
      (n) Lead poisoning
      (o) Polycythemia
      (p) Hemaglobinopathies
B. *Decreased levels*
   Values lower than normal are not significant. However, the blood uric acid level should fall in patients who are treated with uricosuric drugs such as allopurinol, probenecid, and sulfinpyrazone.

Interfering Factors
1. Stress will cause increased levels.
2. Some drugs may cause an increase or a decrease in uric acid blood levels.

HORMONE TESTS

Androstanedione

Normal Values
Premenopausal women: 0.6–3 μg./ml.

Background
Androstanedione is one of the major androgens produced in women by the ovaries, and to a lesser extent in the adrenals. This hormone is converted to estrogens by hepatic enzymes.

Explanation of Test
This hormone measurement is helpful in the evaluation of conditions characterized by hirsutism and possible excessive ovarian androgen production.

Procedure
1. A venous blood sample of 5 ml. is obtained in the morning.
2. This specimen should be collected 1 week before or after the menstrual period.
3. Record data of the last menstrual period on the laboratory form.

Clinical Implications
Increased values are associated with
(a) Stein–Leventhal syndrome
(b) Cushing's syndrome
(c) Certain ovarian tumors
(d) Ectopic ACTH-producing tumor
(e) Late-onset congenitive adrenal hyperplasia
(f) Ovarian stromal hyperplasia

Aldosterone

Normal Values
Plasma is taken with the patient in an upright position for 4 hours and with unrestricted salt intake
Women: 5–30 ng./dl. or 0.14–0.83 nmol./liter
Men: 6–22 ng./dl. or 0.17–0.61 nmol./liter
2–3 times higher in pregnancy
Urine: >35–80 μg./d or > 97–222 mmol./d

Background
This hormone, which is derived from cholesterol, is the most potent of the mineralocorticoids. Its foremost physiologic effect is that of regulating the transport of ions across cell membranes, particularly those of the renal tubes. This hormone causes the retention of sodium and chloride and the elimination of potassium and hydrogen. The second major

effect is the maintenance of blood pressure and blood value. Minute quantities will depress the urinary and salivary sodium–to–potassium ratio primarily because of decreased sodium excretion.

The three main factors that apparently affect aldosterone levels include the renin–angiotensin system, the plasma–potassium concentration, and adrenocorticotropic hormone. The renin–angiotensin system appears to be the major mechanism that controls extracellular fluid by regulation of aldosterone secretion. Potassium loading results in increased aldosterone levels, whereas a potassium-deficient diet in the presence of aldosterone excess will result in a lowered aldosterone level. Increased concentrations of potassium in the blood plasma directly stimulate adrenal production of the hormone. ACTH may affect aldosterone production in conditions of acute stress, burns, hemorrhage, and other pathologic conditions. Under physiologic conditions, ACTH seems to have little effect on aldosterone production.

Procedure
1. A venous blood specimen of 10 ml. in heparin or EDTA is obtained. The cells must be separated from plasma immediately. The specimen should be obtained in the morning after the patient has been upright for at least 4 hours.
2. Specify and record the source of the specimen, such as from a peripheral vein, and so forth.
3. A 24-hour urine specimen is obtained.
4. It is recommended that urine be refrigerated during collection.

Explanation of Test
This test is useful in detecting primary or secondary aldosteronism. Patients with primary aldosteronism characteristically have hypertension, muscular pains and cramps, weakness, tetany, paralysis, and polyuria.

Clinical Implications
1. *Elevated levels occur in primary aldosteronism* as in
   (a) Aldosterone-producing adenoma
   (b) Adrenal cortical hyperplasia
   (c) Indeterminate hyperaldosteronism
   (d) Glucocorticoid remediable hyperaldosteronism
2. *Elevated levels also occur in secondary aldosteronism* when aldosterone output is elevated due to external stimuli or because of greater activity in the renin–angiotensin system as in
   (a) Salt depletion
   (b) Potassium loading
   (c) Large doses of ACTH
   (d) Cardiac failure
   (e) Cirrhosis of liver with ascites
   (f) Nephrotic syndrome
   (g) Bartter's syndrome
   (h) Postsurgical syndrome
   (i) Hypovolemia and hemorrhage

Interfering Factors
Values are increased in pregnancy and by posture.

Patient Preparation
1. Explain the purpose and procedure of the test.
2. Diuretic agents, progestational agents, estrogens, and licorice should be discontinued for 2 weeks before the test.
3. The patient's diet for 2 weeks before the test should be normal and include 3 g. of sodium per day.
4. Check with your laboratory for special protocols.

Antidiuretic Hormone (ADH)

Normal Values
1–5 pg./ml. or < 1.5 mg./liter

Background
The antidiuretic hormone is excreted by the posterior pituitary gland. When ADH activity is present, small volumes of concentrated urine are excreted. When ADH is absent, large amounts of diluted urine are produced.

Explanation of Test
This measurement of the level of ADH is useful in the differential diagnosis of polyuric and hyponatremic states.

Inappropriate secretion of ADH is associated with a number of abnormal findings—decreased blood sodium and chloride associated with normal blood potassium, carbon dioxide, and urea nitrogen; decreased blood osmolality; increased urine osmolality; increased ratio of urine to blood osmolality; and increased urine sodium—and it will respond to water restriction but not to administration of isotonic or hypertonic saline.

Procedure
Venous blood samples are drawn into three specimen tubes that are immediately chilled.

Clinical Implications
Increased secretion of ADH is associated with

1. Acute intermittent porphyria
2. Brain tumor
3. Pneumonia
4. Pulmonary tuberculosis
5. Systemic neoplasms

Chorionic Gonadotropin, Human
Chorionic Gonadotropin (HCG)

Normal Values
Men and nonpregnant women: 3 IU./liter or mU./ml.

Explanation of Test
This test is used as a marker in the diagnosis of testicular and tropho-blastic tumors. Serial monitoring is used to follow tumor response to surgery and chemotherapy. In this test, which uses antibodies specific to the beta subunit of human chorionic gonadotropin (HCG), luteinizing hormone (LH) can be differentiated from HCG.

Procedure
A venous blood sample of 6 ml. is obtained.

Interfering Factors
1. Lipemia
2. Hemolysis

Clinical Implications
1. Values below normal will be seen in threatened abortion and ectopic pregnancy.
2. *Increased values* are associated with
   - (a) Hydatidiform mole
   - (b) Choriocarcinoma
   - (c) Seminoma
   - (d) Ovarian and testicular teratomas
   - (e) Multiple pregnancy
   - (f) Neoplasms of stomach, pancreas, lung, colon, and liver

Cortisol (Hydrocortisone)

Normal Values
Morning: 10–25 µg./dl. or 0.28–0.70 µmol./liter
Evening: <10 µg./dl. or <0.28 µmol./liter

Background
Cortisol, compound F, is a glucocorticosteroid of the adrenal cortex and affects metabolism of proteins, carbohydrates, and lipids. Cortisol (hydrocortisone) is the most potent of the glucocorticoids and inhibits the effect of insulin. Cortisol stimulates glucogenesis by the liver and decreases the rate of glucose use by the cells. In the healthy person, the secretion rate of cortisol is higher in the early morning (6–8 A.M.) and lower in the evening (4–6 P.M.). This variation is lost in patients with Cushing's syndrome and in persons under stress.

Explanation of Test
This is a test of adrenal hormone function. Cortisol is elevated in adrenal hyperfunction and decreased in adrenal hypofunction.

Procedure
Venous blood samples of 5 ml. are obtained in the morning and evening.

Clinical Implications
Extreme elevation in the morning and no variation later in the day suggest carcinoma.

A. *Decreased levels* are expected in
   1. Liver disease
   2. Addison's disease
   3. Anterior pituitary hyposecretion
   4. Hypothyroidism
   5. Therapy with dexamethasone, prednisone, and prednisolone.
B. *Increased levels* are found in
   1. Hyperthyroidism
   2. Stress
   3. Obesity
   4. Cushing's syndrome (high upon rising but no variation later in the day)

Interfering Factors
1. Pregnancy will cause an increased value.
2. There is no normal diurnal variation in patients under stress.
3. Drugs such as spironolactone and oral contraceptives will give falsely elevated values.

Cortisol Suppression (Dexamethasone Suppression) (DST)

Normal Values
8:00 A.M.: 6–26μg./dl.
4:00 P.M.: 2–18μg./dl.
Morning following administration of dexamethasone: 5 μg./dl.

Explanation of Test
This study is a screening test for Cushing's syndrome and to identify depressed persons who are likely to respond to antidepressants or electroshock therapy. It is based on the fact that ACTH production will be suppressed in normal persons after a low dose of dexamethasone, whereas it is not in Cushing's syndrome or in some depressed persons.

Procedure
1. Venous blood samples will be obtained the day following administration of dexamethasone.
2. Late in the afternoon or at bedtime, dexamethasone tablets are administered by mouth. The dosage varies according to weight.

Interfering Factors
1. False positive tests may occur in
   (a) Pregnancy   (e) Trauma
   (b) High doses of estrogens   (f) Fever
   (c) Anorexia nervosa   (g) Dehydration
   (d) Uncontrolled diabetes   (h) Acute withdrawal from alcohol

Clinical Implications
No diurnal variation or suppression will occur in

1. Cushing's syndrome
2. Conditions of high stress
3. Depressed persons who are most likely to respond to somatic intervention
4. Failure to take dexamethasone
5. If Dilantin has been administered

Patient Preparation
1. Explain the purpose and procedure of the test.
2. All medications should be discontinued for 24 to 48 hours before the study. Especially important are Aldactone, estrogens, birth control pills, cortisol, tetracyclines, stilbestrol, and Dilantin.
3. Weigh the patient and record his weight.

Cortisol Stimulation (Cortrosyn Stimulation)

Normal Values
Rise: >7 ng./dl.
Peak: >20 ng./dl.

Explanation of Test
This study is a good test to detect adrenal insufficiency. Cortrosyn is a synthetic subunit of ACTH that exhibits the full corticosteroid stimulating effect of ACTH in normal persons. Failure to respond is an indication of adrenal insufficiency.

Procedure
1. A fasting venous blood sample of 4 ml. is obtained.
2. Cortrosyn is administered intramuscularly.
3. Additional blood specimens of 4 ml. are obtained 30 and 60 minutes after administration of Cortrosyn.

Clinical Implications
Absent or blunted response occurs in

(a) Adrenal insufficiency
(b) Hypopituitarism
(c) Prolonged steroid administration

Gastrin

Normal Values
<300 pg./ml. or <300 ng./liter
Elders: 200–800 pg./ml. or 200–800 ng./liter

Background
Gastrin is a hormone secreted by the mucosa of the pylorus of the stomach. The gastrin is absorbed into the blood and returned to the stomach where it stimulates the secretion of gastric acid. Excessive production of gastrin, then, can result in hypersecretion of gastric acid. Hydrochloric acid, one of the gastric secretions, in turn inhibits the secretion of gastrin.

Explanation of Test
Although elevated levels of gastrin are found in disorders such as pernicious anemia, measurement of serum gastrin is generally used to diagnose a stomach disorder.

Procedure
A fasting venous blood sample of at least 5 ml. is obtained.

Interfering Factors
Values will be falsely increased in nonfasting patients, diabetics taking insulin, and after gastroscopy.

Clinical Implications
Increased gastrin levels are found in

1. Stomach cancer because of significant reduction of gastric acid secretion
2. Gastric and duodenal ulcers
3. Zollinger–Ellison syndrome
4. Pernicious anemia (low secretion of hydrochloric acid results in elevated gastrin levels)
5. End-stage renal disease (gastrin is metabolized by the kidneys)
6. Elderly patients, because of reduced secretion of hydrochloric acid

Patient Preparation
1. The patient should be in a fasting state for 12 hours preceding the test.
2. Water is permitted.

Growth Hormone (hGH)

Normal Values
Men: 0–8 ng./ml. or 0–8 μg./liter
Women: 0–30 ng./ml. or 0–30 μg./liter
Children: 0–10 ng./ml. or 0–10 μg./liter

Background
Growth hormone (hGH) or somatotrophin is essential to the growth process and has an important role in the everyday metabolism of adults. It is released by the pituitary gland secondary to certain stimuli, exercise, deep sleep, hypoglycemia, and ingestion of protein. It also stimulates the production of RNA, mobilizes fatty acids from fat deposits, and is intimately connected with insulinism. If the pituitary gland secretes too little or too much in the growth phase of life, dwarfism or giantism will result. An excess of hGH during adulthood leads to acromegaly.

Explanation of Test
The test is used to confirm hypo- or hyperpituitarism so that therapy can be instituted as soon as possible. Challenge or stimulation tests are generally used to detect growth hormone deficiency.

Clinical Implication
1. Levels will rise 15 times by the second day of starvation. Levels will also rise after 2 hours of sleep.
2. Increased levels are associated with giantism and acromegaly.
3. Decreased levels are associated with dwarfism.
4. Following challenge testing to establish a diagram, the appropriate response is debatable. A response equal to or greater than 7 ng./ml. is clearly normal. Also, the suppression of growth hormone levels of 0 to 3 ng./ml. in 30 minutes to 2 hours following the ingestion of 100 g. of glucose is considered a normal response in adults. In children, a rebound-stimulated effect may be seen from 2 to 5 hours following administration of glucose.

Interfering Factors
1. *Increased levels* are associated with the use of oral contraceptives and estrogens.
2. *Decreased levels* are associated with obesity and the use of corticosteroids.

Procedure
1. A fasting venous blood sample of at least 5 ml. is obtained.
2. Check with your laboratory for specific challenge protocols for stimulation tests such as insulin-induced hypoglycemia, arginine transfusion, glucagon infusion, L-dopa, and propanolol with exercise.

Patient Preparation
1. Explain the purpose and procedure of the test.
2. Advise the patient to fast from food for 8 to 10 hours. For true baseline levels to be obtained, the patient should be free of stress and at complete rest in a quiet environment for at least 30 minutes before specimen collection. Water is permitted.

Prolactin (HPRL)

Normal Values
Premenopausal women: 2.2–19.2 mEq./liter
Postmenopausal women: 1.0–12.8 mEq./liter
Men: 1.9–11.7 mEq./liter

Background
Prolactin (HPRL) is a pituitary hormone essential for initiating and maintaining lactation. The sex difference in HPRL does not occur until puberty, when increased estrogen production results in higher prolactin levels in women. Circadian changes in HPRL concentration in adults are marked by episodic fluctuation and a sleep-induced peak in the early morning hours.

Explanation of Test
This test may be helpful in the diagnosis, management, and follow-up of a prolactin-secreting tumor in persons who have secondary amenorrhea or galactorrhea with hyperprolactinemia. It is also useful in the management of hypothalamic disease.

Procedure
A 12-hour fasting venous blood sample of at least 5 ml. is obtained. Specimens should be drawn in the morning.

Clinical Implications
Increased values are associated with

(a) Galactorrhea and/or amenorrhea
(b) Diseases of the hypothalamus and pituitary stalk
(c) Prolactin-secreting pituitary tumors
(d) Irritative chest wall lesions
(e) Ectopic production of malignant tumors
(f) Hypothyroidism
(g) Renal failure
(h) Anorexia nervosa

Interfering Factors
1. Increased values are associated with newborns, pregnancy, postpartum period, stress, exercise, sleep, and nipple stimulation.
2. Drugs may increase values.

Clinical Alert

Dopaminergic drugs inhibit prolactin secretion. Administration of L-dopa can reduce prolactin levels back to normal in galactorrhea, hyperprolactinemia, and pituitary tumor.

Parathyroid Hormone Assay; Parathyrin; Parathormone (PTH-C Terminal)

Normal Values
N-terminal: 236–630 pg./ml. as bovine PTH 230–630 ng./liter
C-terminal: 410–1760 pg./ml. as bovine PTH 410–1760 ng./liter
PTH: 20–70 μl Eq./ml. or 20–70 mL. Eq./liter

Background
PTH is a polypeptide hormone produced in the parathyroid gland, and it is one of the major factors in the regulation of calcium concentration in extracellular fluid. Three molecular forms of PTH exist: (1) intact, also called native or glandular hormone, (2) multiple N-terminal fragments, and (3) C-terminal fragments.

Explanation of Test
This test is used in studies of altered calcium metabolism and is helpful in establishing a diagnosis of hyperparathyroidism and in distinguishing nonparathyroid from parathyroid causes of hypercalcemia. A decrease in the level of ionized calcium is the primary stimulus for PTH secretions, while a rise in calcium inhibits secretions. This relationship is lost in hyperthyroidism, and PTH will be inappropriately high in relation to calcium.

The C assays tend to have higher values and are more widely accepted as better indications of hyperparathyroidism. Creatinine is usually determined with all PTH assays to determine kidney function.

Clinical Implications
1. *Increased PTH values* occur in
    (a) Chronic renal failure. This is a cause of secondary hyperparathyroidism.
    (b) Pseudohyperparathyroidism. There is a primary defect in renal tubular responsiveness to PTH (slight increase).
    (c) Vitamin D deficiency (moderate)
    (d) Malabsorption (moderate)

    (e) Rickets (moderate)
    (f) Osteomalacia (moderate)
2. *Decreased PTH values* occur in nonparathyroid hypercalcemia, as in
    (a) Use of thiazide diuretics   (e) Sarcoidosis
    (b) Mild alkali syndrome   (f) Graves' disease
    (c) Vitamin A and D intoxica-   (g) Permanent postoperative
        tion   hypoparathyroidism
    (d) Hematologic malignancies
        (some)
3. *Increased PTH-N values* occur in
    (a) Pseudohypoparathyroidism   (c) Primary hyperparathy-
    (b) Secondary hyperparathy-   roidism
        roidism
4. *Decreased PTH-N values* occur in
    (a) Hypoparathyroidism   (c) Nonparathyroid hyper-
    (b) Neoplasms   calcemia
5. *Increased PTH-C values* occurs in
    (a) Pseudohypoparathyroidism   (c) Primary hyperparathy-
    (b) Secondary hyperparathy-   roidism
        roidism   (d) Neoplasms
6. *Decreased PTH-C values* occur in
    (a) Hypoparathyroidism   (b) Nonparathyroid hyper-
         calcemia

Interfering Factors
1. Elevated blood lipids interfere with results.
2. Milk ingestion may falsely lower PTH levels.

Procedure
1. A 10-hour fasting venous blood sample of at least 6 ml. is obtained (3 ml. in two separate vials).
2. The specimen is obtained in the early morning.
3. If the patient cannot fast, notify the laboratory.

Progesterone

Normal Serum Values
Follicular phase: 0.02–0.9 ng./ml. or 0.06–2.86 nmol./liter
Luteal phase: 6–30 ng./ml. or 19.08–95.40 nmol./liter
Rises 16–24 hours before ovulation, reaches maximum 6–10 days after urinary total estrogen peak.

Explanation of Test
This test is done as part of a fertility study to confirm ovulation and in the evaluation of the function of the corpus luteum. Several samples

during the cycle are necessary. Ovarian production of progesterone is low during the follicular (first) phase of the menstrual cycle. After ovulation, progesterone levels rise for 4–5 days and then fall. During pregnancy, there is a gradual increase from the 9th to 32nd week, often to 100 times the level in the nonpregnant woman. Levels of progesterone in twin pregnancy will be higher than in a single pregnancy.

Procedure
1. A venous blood sample is obtained. The test request should include sex, day of last menstrual period, and trimester of pregnancy.
2. Urine tests can also be done.

Clinical Implications
1. *Increased levels* are associated with
   (a) Congenital adrenal hyper-
       plasia
   (b) Lipid ovarian tumor
   (c) Molar pregnancy
   (d) Chorionepithelioma of
       ovary
2. *Decreased levels* are associated with
   (a) Threatened abortion
   (b) Galactorrhea–amenorrhea
       syndrome

Somatomedin-C, Insulinlike Growth Hormone

Normal Values

Males:
  0–8 years: 4–87 ng./ml.
  9–10 years: 26–98 ng./ml.
  11–13 years: 44–207 ng./ml.
  14–16 years: 48–255 ng./ml.
  Adults: 42–110 ng./ml.

Females:
  0–8 years: 7–110 ng./ml.
  9–10 years: 39–186 ng./ml.
  11–13 years: 66–215 ng./ml.
  14–16 years: 96–256 ng./ml.
  Adults: 42–110 ng./ml.

Explanation of Test
This test is used to monitor the growth of children as well as in the diagnosis of acromegaly and hypopituitarism. Normal somatomedin results are evidence against a deficiency of growth hormone.

Procedure
Fasting (preferred) venous blood sample is obtained.

Clinical Implications
1. *Increased levels* are associated with acromegaly.
2. *Decreased levels* are associated with
   (a) Dwarfism
   (b) Hypopituitarism
   (c) Hypothyroidism
   (d) Kwashiorkor
   (e) Laron dwarfism
   (f) Cirrhosis of liver

Testosterone

Normal Values
Men: 500–860 ng./dl. or 500–860 mmol./liter
Women: 26–54 ng./dl. or 26–54 nmol./liter

Background
Testosterone is a hormone responsible for the development of male secondary sexual characteristics. This substance is synthesized mainly in the Leydig cells of the testes. It is secreted by the adrenal glands and testes in men and by the adrenal glands and ovaries in women. Excessive production induces premature puberty in men and masculinity in women. A small portion of total testosterone exists in the free or unbound state and is available for entry into cells of the target organs.

Explanation of Test
Routine testosterone measurements in men have been found useful in the assessment of hypogonadism, pituitary gonadotropin function, impotency, and cryptorchidism; these measurements are also useful in the detection of ovarian and adrenal tumors in women.

Procedure
1. Three venous blood samples of 10 ml. may be obtained from men.
2. Five venous blood samples of 10 ml. may be obtained from women. (The quantity will vary according to laboratory procedure.)
3. Indicate sex and age on the laboratory form.

Clinical Implications
1. *Decreased total testosterone levels in men* are associated with
   (a) Hypogonadism
   (b) Klinefelter's syndrome
   (c) Hypopituitarism
   (d) Orchidectomy
   (e) Estrogen therapy
2. *Increased total testosterone levels in women* are associated with
   (a) Adrenal neoplasms
   (b) Ovarian tumors, benign or malignant
   (c) Polycystic ovaries
3. *Increased free testosterone levels* are associated with
   (a) Female hirsutism
   (b) Polycystic ovaries
   (c) Virilization
4. *Decreased free testosterone levels* are associated with hypogonadism.

Interfering Factors
In adult males, an inverse correlation of free testosterone with age occurs. The upper limit of normal range generally decreases from the

age of 20 to 60 years. The lower range of free normal does not change significantly with age.

ENZYME TESTS

Acid Phosphatase

Normal Values
Men: 0.15–0.65 BLB units at 37°C or 2.5–11.7 U/liter
Women: 0.02–0.55 BLB units at 37°C or 0.3–9.2 U/liter
BLB = Bersey, Lowry, and Brock

Explanation of Test
Acid phosphatases are enzymes that are widely distributed in tissue, including the bone, liver, spleen, kidney, red blood cells, and platelets. However, their greatest importance is found in the prostrate gland where acid phosphatase activity is 100 times higher than in other tissue.

For this reason, the test of acid phosphatase levels is used to diagnose metastatic cancer of the prostate and to follow the effectiveness of treatment. It is known that elevated levels of acid phosphatase are seen in patients with prostate cancer that has metastasized beyond the capsule to other parts of the body, especially the bone. It is believed that once the carcinoma has spread, the prostate starts to release acid phosphatase, resulting in an increase in blood level. The prostatic fraction procedure specifically measures the concentration of prostatic acid phosphatase secreted by cells of the prostate gland in contrast to the total enzyme activity, which is an indirect measurement.

Acid phosphatase is also present in high concentration in seminal fluid. Tests for this enzyme may be used to investigate rape.

Procedure
A venous blood sample of 10 ml. is obtained.

Clinical Implications
1. A significantly elevated value nearly always is indicative of metastatic cancer of the prostate. If the tumor is successfully treated, this enzyme level will drop within 3 to 4 days after surgery or 3 to 4 weeks after estrogen administration.
2. Moderately elevated values also occur in the absence of prostate disease in
   (a) Paget's disease
   (b) Gaucher's disease
   (c) Hyperparathyroidism
   (d) Multiple myeloma
   (e) Any cancer that has metastasized to the bone
   (f) Hepatitis
   (g) Obstructive jaundice
   (h) Acute renal impairment
   (i) Sickle cell crisis
   (j) Excessive destruction of platelets

3. Levels are reported to be elevated in the bone marrow of patients with prostatic cancer metastatic to the bone.

Interfering Factors
1. Drugs that may cause *increased* and *decreased* levels.

Alanine Aminotransferase (ALT); Serum Glutamic-Pyruvic Transaminase (SGPT)

Normal Values
Women: 4–17 U/liter at 30°C
Men: 6–24 U/liter at 30°C

Explanation of Test
This test of enzyme levels is done primarily to diagnose liver disease. High concentratons of this enzyme occur in the liver, and relatively low concentrations are found in the heart, muscle, and kidney. These enzymes are also used to monitor the course of treatment for hepatitis, active postnecrotic cirrhosis, or the effects of drug treatment that might be toxic to the liver. This test is also used to differentiate between hemolytic jaundice and jaundice due to liver disease. In comparison to aspertate amino transferase (AST), the ALT test is more specific for liver malfunction. In addition, this enzyme is elevated in myocardial infarction.

Procedure
1. A 5 ml. sample of venous blood is obtained.
2. Hemolysis should be avoided during collection of the specimen.

Clinical Implications
A. *Increased levels* are found in
   1. Hepatocellular disease (moderate to high increase)
   2. Active cirrhosis (mild increase)
   3. Metastatic liver tumor (mild increase)
   4. Obstructive jaundice/biliary obstruction (mild to moderate increase)
   5. Infection or toxic hepatitis
   6. Liver congestion
   7. Pancreatitis (mild increase)
   8. Hepatic injury in myocardial infarction complicated by shock
B. AST/ALT *comparison*
   1. Although the AST level is always increased in acute myocardial infarction, the ALT level does not always increase proportionately.

2. The ALT is usually increased more than the AST in acute extrahepatic biliary obstruction.
3. ALT is less sensitive than AST to alcoholic liver disease.

Interfering Factors
1. Many drugs may cause falsely increased levels.
2. Salicylates may cause decreased or increased levels.

Alkaline Phosphatase (ALP)

Normal Values
25–92 U/liter (Kind & King)

Explanation of Test
Alkaline phosphatase is an enzyme originating mainly in the bone, liver, and placenta, with some activity in the kidney and intestines. It is called *alkaline* since it functions best at a pH of 9.

This enzyme test is used as a tumor marker and an index of liver and bone disease when correlated with other clinical findings. In bone disease, the enzyme rises in proportion to new bone cell production resulting from osteoblastic activity and the deposit of calcium in the bones. In liver disease, the blood level rises when excretion of this enzyme is impaired as a result of obstruction in the biliary tract.

Procedure
A venous blood sample of 10 ml. is obtained.

Clinical Implications
A. *Elevated levels*
   1. Liver disease (correlates with abnormal liver function tests)
      An elevation of alkaline phosphatase is often associated with elevated AST and elevated bilirubin.
      (a) Marked increases
         (1) Obstructive jaundice (gallstones obstructing major biliary ducts; accompany elevated bilirubin)
         (2) Space-occupying lesions of the liver such as cancer and abscesses
         (3) Hepatocellular cirrhosis
         (4) Biliary cirrhoses
         (5) Liver metastasis
      (b) Moderate increases
         (1) Hepatitis   (2) Cirrhosis of liver
   2. Bone disease
      (a) Marked increases
         (1) Paget's disease   (3) Osteitis deformans
         (2) Metastatic bone disease   (4) Osteogenic sarcoma

    (b) Moderate increases
       (1) Osteomalacia (elevated levels help differentiate between osteomalacia and osteoporosis, in which there is no elevation)
       (2) Rickets
  3. Other diseases
    (a) Hyperparathyroidism (accompanied by hypercalcemia)
    (b) Infectious mononucleosis
    (c) Leukemia
B. *Reduced levels*
  1. Hypophosphatasia (markedly reduced)
  2. Malnutrition
  3. Hypothyroidism
  4. Pernicious anemia
  5. Scurvy
  6. Milk–alkali syndrome
  7. Placental insufficiency

Interfering Factors
1. A variety of drugs produces mild to moderate elevations or decreased levels of alkaline phosphatase.
2. Young children, those experiencing rapid growth, pregnant women, as well as all women have physiologically high levels of alkaline phosphatase.
3. The level is slightly increased in older persons.
4. After IV administration of albumin there is sometimes a marked increase for several days.

Alkaline Phosphatase Isoenzymes

Normal Values
AP-1, Alpha 2: Values are reported as weak, moderate, or strong
AP-2, Beta 1: Values are reported as weak, moderate, or strong
AP-3, Beta 2: Values are reported as weak, moderate, or strong

Background
The isoenzymes of alkaline phosphatase (ALP) are produced by various tissues. AP-1, Alpha 2 is heat labile and is produced in the liver and by proliferating blood vessels. AP-2, Beta 1 is heat stable and is produced by bone anaplacental. The intestinal isoenzyme AP-3, Beta 2 is present in small quantities in Group O and B individuals. AP-1 and 2 can be partially distinguished in the laboratory by heating and urea testing. Placental alkaline phosphatase is still more stable to heat than urea.

Explanation of Test
This is done when the total alkaline phosphatase is abnormal and it is used primarily to distinguish between bone and liver origin of alkaline phosphatase.

Procedure
A venous blood sample of 5 ml. is obtained.

Clinical Implications
1. Osteoblastic bone tumors increase the bone alkaline phosphatase in the blood serum; less than 25% is thermostabile in bone disease.
2. Liver diseases such as cancer and biliary obstruction increase the liver isoenzyme; more than 25% is thermostabile in hepatic disease.
3. The intestinal isoenzyme may be increased in patients with cirrhosis.
4. The placental isoenzyme is increased in some patients with cancer (carcinoplacental antigen) and normally in pregnancy.

Aldolase (ALS)

Normal Values
1.5–12.0 μ/liter @ 37°C

Background
Aldolase is a glycolytic enzyme that catalyzes the breakdown of fructose 1,6-diphosphate into the triase phosphates. This is one of the important reactions in the intermediary glycolytic breakdown of glucose. This enzyme has a widespread distribution throughout most tissues of the body.

Explanation of Test
This test is helpful in diagnostic situations where cell destruction and necrosis or increased membrane permeability may have occurred, as in acute hepatitis, progressive muscular atrophy, myocardial infarction, and malignancy.

Procedure
A fasting venous blood sample of 5 ml. is usually obtained.

Clinical Implications
1. The *highest levels* are found in muscular dystrophy, with lesser degrees of elevation found in
    (a) Dermatomyositis
    (b) Polymyositis
    (c) Limb-girdle muscular dystrophy
2. *Normal values* are observed in
    (a) Poliomyelitis
    (b) Myasthenia gravis
    (c) Multiple sclerosis
    (d) Neurogenic muscle atrophy

3. *Normal or moderately elevated values* are found in
   (a) Chronic hepatitis   (c) Obstructive jaundice
   (b) Portal cirrhosis
4. *Increased levels* are also associated with
   (a) Gangrene   (e) Some blood dyscrasias
   (b) Prostate tumors   (f) Delirium tremens
   (c) Trichinosis   (g) Burns
   (d) Some carcinomas meta-   (h) 20% of cancer patients
       static to the liver   (more frequent with liver
                                        involvement)

Patient Preparation
Explain the purpose and procedure of the test. Advise the patient to fast from food from midnight before the specimen is obtained. Water is permitted.

Serum Angiotensin-Converting Enzyme (SACE)

Normal Values
6.1–21.1 U/liter for patients >20 years of age.

Background
Angiotensin I is produced by the action of resin on angiotensinogen. Angiotensin I-converting enzyme (CE) catalyzes the conversion of angiotensin I to the vasoactive peptide, angiotensin II. Angiotensin I is concentrated in the proximal tubules.

Explanation of Test
This test is primarily used in the study of persons with sarcoidosis to evaluate the severity and activity of the disease. Serum angiotensin-converting enzyme (SACE) levels are significantly higher in 79% of patients with active sarcoidosis. However, about 5% of the normal adult population have elevated levels.

Procedure
A venous blood sample of at least 5 ml. is obtained.

Clinical Implications
1. *Increased levels* are associated with
   (a) Sarcoidosis: SACE levels reflect the severity of the disease, with 68% positivity in stage I disease, 86% in stage II, and 92% in stage III.
   (b) Gaucher's disease
   (c) Leprosy
2. *Decreased levels* occur in many persons with the disease who are treated with prednisone.

Interfering Factors
The test should not be done on persons under age 20 because they normally have a very high level of SACE.

Amylase

Normal Values
50–150 μ/liter
0–130 IU/liter by enzymatic method

Background
Amylase is an enzyme that changes starch to sugar. It is produced in the salivary glands, pancreas, liver, and fallopian tubes. If there is an inflammation of the pancreas or salivary glands, much more of the enzyme enters the blood. Amylase levels in the urine reflect blood changes by a time-lag of 6 to 10 hours (see *Amylase Excretion/Clearance*, Chapter 3).

Explanation of Test
This test is used to diagnose and monitor treatment of acute pancreatitis and to detect inflammation of salivary glands.

Procedure
A venous blood sample of 10 ml. is obtained.

Clinical Implications
A. *Increased levels*
   1. Greatly increased in acute nonhemorrhagic pancreatitis early in the course of the disease. The increase begins in 3 to 6 hours after the onset of pain.
   2. Increases also occur in
      (a) Acute exacerbation of chronic pancreatitis
      (b) Partial gastrectomy
      (c) Obstruction of pancreatic duct
      (d) Perforated peptic ulcer
      (e) Alcohol poisoning
      (f) Mumps
      (g) Obstruction or inflammation of salivary duct or gland
      (h) Acute cholecystitis
      (i) Intestinal obstruction with strangulation
      (j) Ruptured tubal pregnancy
      (k) Ruptured aortic aneurysm
B. *Decreased levels* occur in
   1. Acute pancreatitis subsidence
   2. Hepatitis
   3. Cirrhosis of liver
   4. Toxemia of pregnancy
   5. Severe burns
   6. Severe thyrotoxicosis

Clinical Alert
1. The amylase/creatinine clearance can be used to differentiate cause if etiology is a problem.
2. Serum panic level is greater than 600 I.U./liter.

Aspartate Amino Transferase (AST) or Serum Glutamic-Oxaloacetic Transaminase (SGOT)

Normal Values
Men: 7–21 μ./liter at 30°C
Women: 6–18 μ./liter at 30°C

Explanation of Test
AST is an enzyme present in tissues of high metabolic activity. It occurs in decreasing concentration in the heart, liver, skeletal muscle, kidney, brain, pancreas, spleen, and lungs. The enzyme is released into the circulation following the injury or death of cells. Any disease that causes change in these highly metabolic tissues will result in a rise in AST. The amount of AST in the blood is directly related to the number of damaged cells and the amount of time that passes between injury to the tissue and the test. Following severe cell damage, the blood AST level will rise in 12 hours and remain elevated for about 5 days.

Procedure
A venous sample of 5 ml. is obtained. Hemolysis during the procedure should be avoided.

Clinical Implications
A. *Increased levels* occur in
   1. Myocardial infarction (MI)
      (a) In MI, the AST level may be increased 4 to 10 times the normal values.
      (b) The AST level reaches a peak in 24 hours and returns to normal by the third or fourth day. Secondary rises in AST levels suggest extension or recurrence of MI.
      (c) The AST curve in MI parallels that of Creatine Phosphokinase (CPK), page 311.
      (d) Elevated levels do not always indicate MI in suspected patients. Severe arrhythmias and severe angina can also cause elevation.
   2. Liver disease
      (a) Level is always elevated in cirrhosis of the liver.
      (b) In liver disease, the level may be 10 to 100 times the normal.
      (c) Liver diseases associated with elevated AST levels

      (1) Acute hepatitis
      (2) Active cirrhosis
      (3) Infectious mononucleosis with hepatitis
      (4) Hepatic necrosis
   3. Other diseases associated with elevated AST levels

(a) Acute pancreatitis	(g) Recent brain trauma
(b) Trauma and irradiation	with brain necrosis
of skeletal muscle	(h) Crushing injuries
(c) Acute hemolytic anemia	(i) Progressive muscular
(d) Acute renal disease	dystrophy
(e) Severe burns	
(f) Cardiac catheterization	
and angiography	

B. *Decreased levels* occur in
   1. Beriberi
   2. Uncontrolled diabetes mellitus with acidosis
   3. Liver disease occasionally may cause a decrease instead of the expected increase.

Interfering Factors
1. Slight decreases occur during pregnancy when there is abnormal metabolism of pyridoxine.
2. Many drugs can cause elevated levels.
3. Salicylates may cause falsely decreased or increased AST levels.

Clinical Alert

For diagnosis of MI, the AST levels should be done on three consecutive days because the peak is reached in 24 hours and levels are back to normal in 3 to 4 days.

Creatine Phosphokinase (CPK); Creatine Kinase (CK) and Isoenzymes

Normal Values

Men:

6–11 years	56–185 U./liter	*Isoenzymes:*
12–18 years	35–185 U./liter	MM: 100%
≥19 years	38–174 U./liter	MB: 0%
		BB: 0%

Women:

6–7 years	50–145 U./liter
8–14 years	35–145 U./liter
15–18 years	20–100 U./liter
≥19 years	96–140 U./liter

Explanation of Test

Creatine kinase (CK) is an enzyme found in high concentrations in the heart and skeletal muscles and in much smaller concentrations in the brain tissue. Since CK exists in relatively few organs, this test is used as a specific index of injury to myocardium and muscle. Thus it is important in the diagnosis of myocardial infarction and as a reliable measure of skeletal muscle diseases such as muscular dystrophy. In fact, CK levels can prove helpful in recognizing muscular dystrophy before clinical signs appear. This test is also of value in following the course of inflammatory muscle disease. The determination of CK isoenzymes may be helpful in a differential diagnosis.

CPK/CK Isoenzymes

CPK can be divided into three isoenzymes: MM or CK_3, BB or CK_1, and MB or CK_2. CK-MM is the isoenzyme that makes up almost all the circulatory enzymes in healthy persons. Skeletal muscle contains primarily MM; cardiac muscle, MM and MB; and brain tissue, GI and GU tracts, BB. Normal CK levels are virtually 100% MM isoenzyme. A slight increase in total CPK is reflected from elevated MM from central nervous system injury. The isoenzyme studies help distinguish whether the CPK originated from the heart (MB) or the skeletal muscle (MM). Thus, elevation of MM levels is an indication of skeletal muscle injury. Elevation of MB, the cardiac enzyme, provides a more definitive indication of myocardial cell damage or death than total CK alone.

CK-BB may be a useful marker for monitoring therapy in cancer of the lung, breast, and prostate.

Procedure

A blood sample of at least 5 ml. is obtained by venipuncture. If a patient has been receiving multiple injections intramuscularly (IM), this fact should be noted on the laboratory requisition.

Clinical Implications of Total CK Levels

A. Myocardial infarction (MI)
   1. Rise starts soon after an attack (about 4–6 hr.) and reaches a peak of at least several times normal within 30 hours.
   2. CK rises before and falls earlier than AST.
   3. Level returns to normal 2 to 3 days after infarction. Thus, if patient is seen within this period following an infarction, the CK levels can help determine that an infarction did occur.
   4. If the CPK rise is extensive, some clinicians believe the infarcted area is extensive and the prognosis is thus unfavorable. Others believe that subendocardial infarction causes greater increases in CPK because of easy diffusion of CPK from cell to blood.
B. Other diseases and procedures that cause increased CK levels
   1. Acute cerebrovascular disease

2. Progressive muscular dystrophy (levels may reach 300–400 times normal)
3. Dermatomyositis (involves muscle inflammation and neurons) Polymyositis
4. Delirium tremens and chronic alcoholism (an episode of acute intoxication may be accompanied by CK levels comparable to those found in MI)
5. Electric shock
6. Myxedema
7. Cardiac surgery
8. Cardiac defibrillation
9. Electromyography
10. Convulsions, cerebral infarction, ischemia, or subarachnoid hemorrhage.
11. Hypokalemia
12. Hypothyroidism (mild elevations may occur)
13. Acute psychosis
14. Central nervous system trauma
15. Pulmonary infarction or edema (rise in CK levels is unexplainable)
C. Normal values are found in myasthenia gravis and multiple sclerosis.

Clinical Implications of CK Isoenzymes

A. Elevated MM isoenzyme levels occur in
1. Muscle trauma
2. Following intramuscular injections
3. Shock
4. Postoperatively in major surgical procedures
5. MI (may remain elevated 4 or 5 days following MI)
6. Brain injury
B. Elevated MB isoenzyme levels occur in
1. Myocardial infarct (rises in 4–6 hours after MI; not demonstrable after 24–36 hours) (>5 in MI)
2. Myocardial ischemia
3. Duchenne's muscular dystrophy
4. Polymyositis
5. Significant myoglobinuria
6. Reye's syndrome
C. BB (CK_1) elevations are seen in
1. Biliary atresia
2. Some breast, small cell, lung, and prostate cancers
3. Severe shock syndrome (some)
D. After an MI, MB appears in the serum between 6 and 12 hours and remains for about 18 to 32 hours. The finding of MB in a patient

with chest pain is diagnostic of MI. In addition, if there is a negative CK-MB for 48 hours or more following a clearly defined episode under question, it is clear that the patient has not had an MI.
E. MB may also be present in the serum of some patients with some forms of muscular dystrophy. This is significant because, normally, only MM is present in serum.

Interfering Factors
1. Strenuous exercise (up to three times normal) and surgical procedures that damage skeletal muscle may cause increased levels.
2. High doses of salicylates may cause increased levels.
3. Athletes have a higher value because of greater muscle mass.
4. Multiple intramuscular injections may cause increased levels.
5. Drugs may cause increased levels.

Galactose-1-Phosphate Uridyl Transferase, Galactokinase

Normal Values
Galactose-1-Phosphate Uridyltransferase: 18.5–28.5 U./g. of hemoglobin
Galactokinase: 12.1–39.7 mu./g. of hemoglobin

Background
The enzyme galactose-1-phosphate uridyl transferase is needed in the use of galactose-1-phosphate so that it does not accumulate in the body.

Explanation of Test
This measurement is used to identify a defect in the use of galactose, which can result in widespread tissue damage and abnormalities such as cataracts, liver disease, and renal disease. This effect usually occurs in infants and children.

Procedure
A venous blood sample of at least 1 ml. is obtained.

Clinical Implications
Decreased values are associated with galactosemia, a rare genetic disorder transmitted as an autosomal recessive gene.

Clinical Alert

Parents of infants and children with positive test results should be instructed that the disease can be treated by removing galactose-containing foods, especially milk, from the diet.

Hexosaminidase; Total and A

Normal Values
Total: 10.4–23.8 U./liter
A: 56%–80% of total

Background
Hexosaminidase A is a lysosomal isoenzyme, a deficiency of which characterizes patients with Tay-Sachs disease. In the brains of affected children, there is a 100 times increase of ganglioside due to a deficiency of this enzyme.

Explanation of Test
This determination is a diagnostic test for Tay-Sachs disease and can be of help in identifying carriers among persons with no family history of Tay-Sachs. This condition is due to an autosomal recessive trait found predominantly, but not exclusively, in Ashkenazic Jews and is characterized by the appearance during infancy of psychomotor deterioration, blindness, cherry red spot on the macula, and an exaggerated extension response to sound.

Procedure
A fasting venous blood sample of at least 1 ml. is obtained.

Clinical Implications
1. The total value may be normal or decreased in this disease, but an almost total deficiency of the A component is diagnostic of Tay-Sach disease or G_{M2} gangliosidosis.
2. In a variant of Tay-Sachs disease, Sandhoff's disease, both A and B are defective, causing an absence of this enzyme.

Interfering Factors
Total values are increased in pregnancy due to the appearance of a third heat-stable enzyme.

Lactic Acid Dehydrogenase (LD, LDH)

Normal Values
Values for the normal range of LD activity in serum vary considerably, depending on the direction of the enzyme reaction, the type of method used, and the experimental parameters. For the pyruvate $\rightarrow$ lactate reaction at 30°C and at a pH of 7.4, a range of 95–200 U./liter represents the experience of most workers.

Background
Lactic acid dehydrogenase is an intracellular enzyme that is widely distributed in the tissues of the body, particularly in the kidney, heart,

skeletal muscle, brain, liver, and lungs. Increases in the reported value usually indicate cellular death and leakage of the enzyme from the cell.

Explanation of Test
Although elevated levels of LDH are nonspecific, this test is useful in confirming myocardial or pulmonary infarction when viewed in relation to other test findings. For example, LD remains elevated longer than CK in myocardial infarction (MI). It is also helpful in the differential diagnosis of muscular dystrophy and pernicious anemia. More specific findings may be found by breaking down the LDH into its five isoenzymes. (When LD values are reported or quoted, *total* LDH is meant). LDH is also valuable as a tumor marker in seminoma or germ cell testis tumor, especially when AFP and HCG are not produced in the tumor.

Procedure
1. A venous blood sample of 5 ml. is obtained.
2. Avoid hemolysis in obtaining blood sample.

Clinical Implications
A. Myocardial infarction
   The elevation of LDH that follows an MI is characterized by
   1. High levels within 12 to 24 hours of infarction (18 hr.) and 2 to 10 times normal.
   2. Elevations that may continue for 6 to 10 days (longer than SGOT or CK). For this reason, LDH determinations may be useful in the late diagnosis of MI. Elevations usually return to normal in 8 to 14 days.
B. Pulmonary infarction
   In pulmonary infarction, there is usually an increased LDH within 24 hours of the onset of pain. The pattern of normal SGOT and elevated LDH that levels 1 to 2 days after an episode of chest pain provides evidence for pulmonary infarction.
C. Conditions in general and according to degree of increase in levels
   1. *Elevated levels* of LDH are observed in a variety of conditions
      (a) Acute MI
      (b) Acute leukemia
      (c) Hemolytic anemias
      (d) Hepatic disease
      (e) Skeletal muscle necrosis
      (f) Sprue
      (g) Acute pulmonary infarction
      (h) Malignant neoplasms, extensive cancer
      (i) Acute renal infarctions and chronic renal disease
      (j) Shock with necrosis of minor organs
      (k) Myxedema
   2. The *greatest increase* (2–40 times) of LDH is seen in
      (a) Megaloblastic anemias
      (b) Extensive cancer
      (c) Shock and anoxia

3. *Moderate increase* (2–4 times) of LDH is seen in
   (a) MI
   (b) Pulmonary infarction
   (c) Granulocytic or acute leukemia
   (d) Hemolytic anemia
   (e) Infectious mononucleosis
   (f) Progressive muscular dystrophy
4. *Slight increases* occur in
   (a) Delirium tremens
   (b) Hepatitis
   (c) Obstructive jaundice
   (d) Cirrhosis
D. *Decreased LD levels* are associated with a good response to cancer therapy.
E. *Elevated urine LD levels* occur in
   1. Cancer of kidney or bladder
   2. Glomerulonephritis
   3. Malignant hypertension
   4. Lupus nephritis
   5. Acute tubular necrosis
   6. Renal transplantation and hemograft rejection
   7. Pyelonephritis (sometimes)

Interfering Factors
1. Strenuous exercise and the muscular exertion involved in childbirth will cause increased levels.
2. Skin diseases can cause falsely increased levels.
3. Hemolysis of red blood cells due to freezing, heating, or shaking the blood sample will cause falsely increased levels.
4. Some drugs may cause increased and decreased levels.

Clinical Alert

Since many diseases increase LDH levels, it is important to notify the laboratory of each disease the patient has.

Electrophoresis of LDH (LD) Isoenzymes

Normal Values
Isoenzyme normals: LD_1 17.5–28.3%
LD_2 30.4–36.4%
LD_3 19.2–24.8%
LD_4 9.6–15.6%
LD_5 5.5–12.7%

Explanation of Test
Electrophoresis or separation of LDH identifies the five isoenzymes or fractions of LDH, each with its own physical characteristics and elec-

trophoretical properties. Fractionating the LDH activity sharpens its diagnostic value since LDH is found in many organs. The LD isoenzymes are released into the bloodstream when tissue necrosis occurs. However, a complete knowledge of the clinical history is necessary to interpret properly the resulting patterns. The isoenzymes are elevated in terms of patterns established, not on the basis of the value of a single isoenzyme.

The five isoenzyme fractions of LDH show different patterns in various disorders. Abnormalities in the pattern suggest which tissues have been damaged and help to diagnose MI, pulmonary infarction, and liver disease. (This test is sensitive enough to detect increased hepatic fraction in infectious hepatitis before clinical jaundice appears.) It is in confirming the diagnosis of suspected MI that the separation of LD finds its most frequent application, especially when a second infarct occurs shortly after the first. In these cases, the ECG is already abnormal, but the isoenzyme pattern will show increased LD_1, indicating the release of more of the cardiac isoenzyme.

Procedure

A venous blood sample of 5 ml. is obtained. Avoid hemolysis.

Clinical Implications

Abnormal patterns reflect damaged tissue

1. LD_1 and LD_2 are increased in MI and in some hemolytic anemias.
2. LD_3 is increased in pulmonary infarction and extensive pneumonia.
3. LDH_5 is increased in various malignancies and liver disease but has had limited clinical use.
4. An increase in LD_2, LD_3, and LD_4 is common in malignant disease.
5. The LD pattern will be essentially the same in MI, pernicious anemia, and renal infarction. This is because red blood cells and the kidney have an isoenzyme pattern similar to that of heart muscle.
6. In most cancers, one to three of the bands (LD_2, LD_3, and LD_4) are frequently increased. A notable exception is in seminomas and dysgerminomas when LD_1 and LD_2 are increased. Frequently, an increase in LD_3 may be the first indication of the presence of cancer.

Clinical Alert

Because erythrocytes and kidney cells contain the same isoenzymes as heart muscle, patients with pernicious anemia or renal infarction may have the same serum isoenzyme patterns as those with MIs.

Lipase

Normal Values
Vary with methodology used
Using the Shihalsi/Bishop assay, the normals are 4–24 U./liter

Explanation of Test
Lipase functions in the body to change fats to fatty acid and glycerol. The major source of this enzyme is the pancreas. Therefore, lipase appears in the bloodstream following damage to the pancreas.

The test is used to diagnose pancreatitis and to differentiate pancreatitis from an acute surgical abdominal emergency. When secretions of the pancreas are blocked, the blood serum lipase levels rise.

Procedure
A venous blood sample of 5 ml. is obtained.

Clinical Implications
A. *Elevated levels in pancreatic disorders*
   1. Elevation of lipase may not occur until 24 to 36 hours after onset of illness.
   2. Elevation occurs later than amylase and persists longer than changes in blood amylase, which is also related to pancreatic disorders (up to 14 days).
   3. May be high when amylase levels are normal.
   4. Thus the lipase test is useful in late diagnosis of acute pancreatitis.
B. *Increased lipase values* are associated with
   1. Pancreatitis
   2. Obstruction of the pancreatic duct
   3. Pancreatic carcinoma
   4. Acute cholecystitis
   5. Cirrhosis
   6. Severe renal disease
   7. High intestinal obstruction
C. Usually normal in mumps

Interfering Factors
Some drugs may increase or decrease the level.

5'-Nucleotidase

Normal Values
10.6–17.5 U./liter

Background
5'-nucleotidase is an enzyme that has a wide distribution throughout the body and blood. It is known to appear in the serum in diseases of the liver.

Explanation of Test
This measurement provides supportive evidence in the diagnosis of liver disease and helps to differentiate skeletal disorders along with the investigation of alkaline phosphatase. The two tests combined may provide definitive diagnoses of Paget's disease or rickets where high levels of alkaline phosphatase accompany normal or marginally increased 5'-nucleotidase activity.

Procedure
A venous blood sample of 5 ml. is obtained.

Clinical Implications
1. *Increases* are associated with diseases of liver such as
   (a) Extrahepatic obstruction   (c) Hepatic carcinoma
   (b) Cholecystosis caused by   (d) Biliary cirrhosis
       chlorpromazine
2. Usually does not increase in skeletal disease.

Renin

Normal Values
Ages 20–39: Normal Na diet: 0.6–4.3 ng./ml./hr. or μg./liter/hr.
            Restricted NA diet: 2.9-24.0 ng./ml./hr. or μg./liter/hr.
Ages ≥40: Normal NA diet: 0.6–3.0 ng./ml./hr.
          Restricted Na diet: 2.9–10.8 ng./ml./hr.

Background
Renin is an enzyme that converts angiotensinogen to angiotensin I. Derived from the liver, angiotensinogen is an alpha-2 globulin in the serum. Angiotensin I is then converted in the lung to angiotensin II. Angiotensin II is a potent vasopressor agent responsible for hypertension of renal origin, as well as a powerful releaser of aldosterone from the adrenal cortex. Both angiotensin II and aldosterone increase blood pressure. It is known that renin levels increase when there is decreased renal perfusion pressure and when there is decreased delivery of sodium and water to the vascular pole of the glomerulus.

Relationship of Plasma Renin to Hyperaldosteronism
Increased aldosterone production associated with decreased renin and normal 17-OH corticosteroids is practically diagnostic of primary hyperaldosteronism, whether hypokalemia is present or not.

Explanation of Test

This test of renin activity is most useful in the differential diagnosis of hypertension, either essential, renal, or renovascular. In primary hyperaldosteronism, the findings will demonstrate that aldosterone secretion is exaggerated and secretion of renin is suppressed. This test is of considerable importance because the number of patients suffering from this disorder can be very substantial.

Procedure

1. A fasting venous blood sample of 10 ml. is obtained. It is important to use EDTA as the anticoagulant because it aids in preservation of any angiotensin formed before examination.
2. A second, nonfasting specimen may be ordered with exercise.

Clinical Implications

1. *Increased levels* are associated with
   - (a) Hypertension of renal origin
   - (b) Addison's disease
   - (c) Salt-losing nephropathy
   - (d) Hemorrhage
2. *Decreased levels* are associated with
   - (a) Salt-retaining steroid therapy
   - (b) Antidiuretic hormone therapy

Patient Preparation

1. Explain the purpose and procedure of the test.
2. A regular diet that contains 180 mEq./sodium and 100 mEq./potassium must be maintained for 3 days before the specimen is obtained.
3. Instruct the patient that it is necessary to be in a supine position for at least 1 hour before obtaining the specimen.
4. Drugs that interfere with testing, along with licorice, should be terminated at least 2 weeks before testing. Check with your laboratory and pharmacy.

Interfering Factors

1. Levels may vary in normal persons and will rise under influences that tend to shrink the intravascular fluid volume.
2. Values will be higher when the patient is in an upright position early in the day, in low salt diets, during pregnancy, and with drugs such as diuretics, antihypertensives, estrogen, and oral contraceptives.

Challenge Test

A challenge test has been recommended to distinguish primary from secondary hyperaldosteronism on the basis of renin levels, with the patient in both the recumbent and upright positions and after the patient has been maintained on a low salt diet. In normal persons and in those with essential hypertension, renin concentration will be increased by the reduction in volume due to sodium restriction and the upright position. In primary aldosteronism, volume depletion does not occur and renin concentration remains low.

General Procedure for Renin Stimulation Test

1. The patient should be admitted to the hospital for this test. On admission, weight is obtained and recorded.
2. A diet containing reduced sodium content (10–20 mEq./day) supplemented with potassium (10 mEq.) is given for 3 days, along with furosemide or chlorothiazide as ordered.
3. Weigh again on the third day, record, and see that the patient remains upright for 4 hours doing normal activities.
4. A venous heparinized blood sample for renin is obtained at 11 A.M. or when renin activity is usually at its maximum. Place it in ice and send it immediately to the laboratory.

Interpretation of Renin Stimulation Test

In normal persons and most hypertensive patients, the stimulation of a low salt diet, a diuretic, and upright posture will raise renin activity to very high levels and result in weight loss. However, in primary aldosteronism, the plasma level is expanded and remains so. In these patients, there is little if any weight loss and the renin level is very low or undetectable. It is important to keep in mind that a response within the normal range can occur in the presence of aldosterone.

Patient Preparation

1. Explain the purpose and procedure of the test.
2. Check with the individual laboratory for specific practices. The purpose of the preparation is to deplete the patient of sodium.

Uroporphyrinogen-1-Synthase (U1S)

Normal Values

Women: 8–16.8 nmol./liter/sec.
Men: 7.9–14.7 nmol./liter/sec.

Background

This enzyme in the red blood cells is needed to convert porphobilinogen to uroporphyrinogen. This enzyme will be diminished in any person with acute intermittent porphyria.

Explanation of Test

This measurement can be used in the detection of acute intermittent porphyria in the latent stage as well as in the confirmation of a diagnosis during an acute episode. It can most significantly be used to detect affected persons before occurrence of a first acute episode. Persons with latent acute intermittent porphyria can be identified. This is important because acute episodes of this disorder can be fatal.

Procedure
1. A fasting venous blood sample of at least 10 ml. is obtained. The specimen must be placed in wet ice at once.
2. Include the patient's hematocrit on the laboratory request.

Clinical Implications
Decreased values are associated with
1. Acute intermittent porphyria (50% below that of normal individuals)
2. Values between 6 nmol./liter/sec. and 8 nmol./liter/sec. are suggestive but indeterminate.

Patient Preparation
Advise the patient about fasting. Water is permitted.

Gamma-Glutamyl Transferase (GGT); Gamma-Glutamyl Transpeptidase (γGT); Gamma-Glutamyl Transferase (γGT)

Normal Values
Men: 6–28 U./liter at 25°C
Women: 4–18 U./liter at 25°C

Background
The enzyme γ-glutamyl transpeptidase is present mainly in the liver, kidney, prostate, and spleen. The liver is considered the source of normal serum activity, despite the fact that the kidney has the highest level of the enzyme. This enzyme is believed to function in the transport of amino acids and peptides into cells across the cell membranes and to be involved in glutathione metabolism. Men will have higher normal levels because of the large amounts found in the prostate.

Explanation of Test
This test is used to determine liver cell dysfunction and to detect alcohol-induced liver disease. It is also an efficient way to screen for the consequences of chronic alcoholism. The GGT is very sensitive to the amount of alcohol consumed by chronic drinkers. It can be used to monitor the cessation or reduction of alcohol consumption. γGT activity is elevated in all forms of liver disease. This test is much more sensitive than either the alkaline phosphatase test or the transaminase test in detecting obstructive jaundice, cholangitis, and cholecystitis.

Procedure
A venous blood sample of 10 ml. is obtained.

Clinical Implications

1. Increased γGT levels are associated with
   (a) Cholecystitis
   (b) Cholelithiasis
   (c) Cancer metastatic to the liver
   (d) Cirrhosis of the liver
   (e) Acute pancreatitis
   (f) Cancer of the bile duct
   (g) Alcoholism (occult)
   (h) Barbiturate use
   (i) Lipoid nephrosis
   (j) Obstruction to biliary tract
   (k) Hepatotoxic drugs for treatment of cancer increase levels more than the cancer itself

2. In MI, γGT is usually normal. However, if there is an increase, it occurs about the fourth day after an MI and probably implies liver damage secondary to cardiac insufficiency.

3. Values are not elevated in
   (a) Bone disorders
   (b) Pregnancy
   (c) Skeletal muscle disease
   (d) Neonatal hepatitis
   (e) Renal failure

DRUG MONITORING

Explanation of Test

Therapeutic drug monitoring is widely accepted as a reliable and practical approach to managing individual patient drug therapy. Determination of drug levels is especially important when the potential for drug toxicity is significant or when inadequate or undesirable response follows the use of a standard dose. It is an easier and more rapid estimation of dosage requirements than by observing only the drug effects themselves. For some drugs it is routinely useful (digoxin); for others it can be helpful in certain situations (antibiotics).

Drugs that can be monitored by serum levels include analgesics, tranquilizers, hypoglycemics, sedatives, antidepressants, antibiotics, anticonvulsants, antineoplastics, bronchodilators, cardiac drugs (see Tables 6-2 and 6-3), and drugs of abuse. (Urine drug testing is explained in Chapter 3, *Urine Studies.*)

Indications for Testing

1. The drug source, dose, or regimen is changed.
2. Noncompliance is suspected and patient motivation to maintain medication is poor.
3. Physiologic status is altered by factors such as weight, menstrual cycle, body water, stress, age, and thyroid function.
4. Coadministered (multiple) drugs cause synergistic or antagonistic drug reaction.

(*Text continues on page 329.*)

Table 6-2
Blood Plasma Concentration of Commonly Monitored Drugs

Drug	Therapeutic* Maintenance	Toxic† (Panic or Critical)
Acetaminophen (Tylenol)	1–30 μg./ml. or 66–199 μmol./liter	>200 μg./ml. or >1324 μmol./liter
Alcohol (Ethanol)	Driving while intoxicated: 100 mg./dl. or 10.9–21.7 mmol./liter	>400 mg./dl. >86.8 mmol./liter
Amitriptyline (Elavil)	120–250 mg./ml. or 433–903 nmol./liter	>500 mg./ml. or >1805 nmol./liter
Bromide	750–1500 μg./ml. or 9.4–18.7 nmol./liter	>1250 μg./ml. or >15.6 nmol./liter
Carbamazepine (Tegretol)	8–12 μg./ml. or 34–51 μmol./liter	>15 μg./ml. or >63 mol./liter
Chlordiazepoxide (Librium)	700–1000 ng./ml. or 2.34–3.34 μmol./liter	>5000 ng./ml. or >16.70 μmol./liter
Desopyramide (Norpace)	Variable	>7 μg./ml. or >20.7 μmol./liter
Diazepam (Valium)	100–1000 ng./ml. or 0.35–3.51 μmol./liter	>5000 ng./ml. or >17.55 μmol./liter
Digitoxin	20–35 ng./ml. or 26–46 nmol./liter	>45 ng./ml. or >59 nmol./liter

Table 6-2
Blood Plasma Concentration of Commonly Monitored Drugs (Continued)

Drug	Therapeutic* Maintenance	Toxic† (Panic or Critical)
Digoxin	CHF: 0:8–1.5 ng./ml. or 1.0–1.9 nmol./liter Arrhythmias: 1.5–2.0 ng./ml. 1.9–2.6 nmol./liter	>25 ng./ml. or >3.2 nmol./liter
Doxepin	30–150 ng./ml. or 107–537 nmol./liter	>500 ng./ml. or >1790 nmol./liter
Ethchlorvynol (Placidyl)	2–8 μg./ml. or 14–55 μmol./liter	>20 μg./ml. or >138 μmol./liter
Glutethimide (Doriden)	2–6 μg./ml. or 9–28 μmol./liter	>5 μg./ml. or >23 μmol./liter
Imipramine (Tofranil)	125–250 ng./ml. or 446–893 nmol./liter	>500 ng./ml. or >1785 nmol./liter
Lithium	0.6–1.2 mEq/liter or 0.6–1.2 mmol./liter	>2 mEq/liter or >2 mmol./liter
Lidocaine (Xylocaine)	1.5–6.0 μg./ml. or 6.4–25.6 μmol./liter	6–8 μg./ml. or 25.6–34.2 μmol./liter
Methotrexate	Variable	48 hrs. after high dose: 454 mg./ml. or 1000 mmol./liter
Methyprylon (Noludar)	8–10 μg./ml. or 45–55 μmol./liter	>50 μg./ml. or >275 μmol./liter

Drug	Therapeutic Value*	Toxic Values†
Phenobarbital	15–40 g./ml. or 65–172 mol./liter	Varies. 35–80 g./ml. or 151–345 mol./liter
Phenytoin (Dilantin)	10–20 g./ml. or 40–79 mol./liter	Varies with symptoms
Procainamide (Promestyl)	4–10 g./ml. or 17–42 mol./liter	10–12 g./ml. or 42–51 mol./liter
Primidone (Mysoline)	5–12 g./ml. or 23–35 mol./liter	15 g./ml or 69 mol./liter
Propranolol (Inderal)	50–100 ng./ml. or 193–386 nmol./liter	Not defined
Quinidine	Varies considerably	Quite variable
Salicylate	<100 µg/ml. or <724 µmol./L	begins at 100 µg/ml. or begins at 724 µmol./L
Theophylline	Bronchodilator: 8–20 µg./ml. or 44–111 µmol./liter Premature apnea: 6–13 µg./ml. or 33–72 µmol./liter	>20 µg./ml. or >111 µmol./liter
Valproic Acid (Depakene)	50–100 µg./ml. or 347–693 µmol./liter	>100 µg./ml. or >693 µmol./liter

Therapeutic value refers to expected drug concentration associated with desirable clinical effects in majority of the patient population treated.
† *Toxic values* refer to the drug concentration associated with undesirable effects or in certain cases, death.

Table 6-3
Blood Plasma Concentration of Commonly Monitored Antibiotics

Antibiotic	Peak*	Trough†
Amikacin	Therapeutic: 25–35 µg./ml. or 43–60 µml./liter Toxic: >35–40 µg./ml. or >60–80 µmol./liter	Less severe infections: 1–4 µg./ml. or Therapeutic: 1.71–6.84 µmol./liter Toxic: >10–15 µg./ml. or >17–26 µmol./liter
Ethosuximide		Therapeutic: 40–100 µg./ml. or 283–708 µmol./liter Toxic: >150 µg./ml. or >1062 µmol./liter
Gentamicin	Less severe infection: Therapeutic: 5–8 µg./ml. Toxic: >10–12 µg./ml. or 21–25 µmol./liter	Less severe: Therapeutic: <1 µg./ml. or <2.09 µ/mol./liter Toxic: >2–4 µg./mL or >4–8 µmol./liter
Kanamycin	Therapeutic: 25–35 µg./ml. or 52–72 µmol./liter Toxic: >35–40 µg./mL or 72–82 µmol./liter	Less severe: Therapeutic: 1–4 µg./mL or 2–8 µmol./liter Toxic: >10–15 µg./ml. >21–31 µmol./liter
Tobramycin	Less severe: Therapeutic: 5–8 µg./mL. or 11–17 µmol./liter Toxic: <10–12 µg./mL. or 21–26 µmol./liter	Less severe: <1 µg./ml. or Therapeutic: <2 µmol./liter Toxic: >2–4 µg./mL. or >4–9 µmol./liter

* *Peak drug level* refers to maximum drug concentration achieved following administration of a single dose. For a specific drug, both the concentration achieved and time interval between dosing and peak drug level required may vary considerably from patient to patient.
† *Trough drug level* refers to minimum drug concentration following administration of a single dose.

5. Pathology that influences drug absorption and elimination such as:
   (a) Cardiovascular dysfunction
   (b) Liver clearance
   (c) Renal clearance (urinary output and pH)
   (d) Gastrointestinal/poor absorption
   (e) Altered plasma protein binding (or change in blood proteins that carry drug)
6. Some drugs have a very small safety range (therapeutic window).

Clinical Alert

1. Reliable clinical assessment of changes in patient's condition, and knowledge of drug interaction must be used to aid in the interpretation of test results.
2. The importance of sampling time in obtaining value therapeutic drug monitoring data cannot be understated. Whatever sampling procedure is used, such as *peak* or *maximum* concentration or *trough* or *minimum drug* concentration, it is important that the same time interval between sampling and dose administration be used consistently when comparing results from serial samples on the same patient.
3. *Elimination Half-Life* refers to time required to eliminate pain from the body and reduce by one-half the drug concentration in the body after the initial distribution phase is complete. Under certain conditions, elimination half-life dates are useful in estimating how long one should wait following initiation of therapy before sampling.
4. Factors influencing drug and chemical concentrations in living patients are frequently altered significantly after death.

PROTEIN TESTS

Ceruloplasmin

Normal Values
22.9–43.1 mg./dl. or 229–431 mg./liter

Background
Ceruloplasmin is a protein that transports copper. About 95% of the copper in blood serum is normally in ceruloplasmin.

Explanation of Test
This measurement is a direct determination of copper in the blood serum. It should be determined in any person under age 30 with hepatitis, cirrhosis, hemolysis, or neurologic symptoms to attain early diagnosis and treatment of Wilson's disease.

Procedure
A venous blood sample of at least 5 ml. is obtained. Place the specimen on ice or freeze.

Interfering Factors
1. Values are increased in the first trimester of pregnancy and in consumption of estrogen or birth control pills.
2. Values are decreased in newborns.

Clinical Implications
1. *Increased values* are associated with
   (a) Rheumatoid arthritis (will   (c) Some infectious diseases
       even give the blood green-   (d) Thyrotoxicosis
       ish cast)   (e) Cancer
   (b) Biliary cirrhosis
2. *Decreased levels* are associated with
   (a) Wilson's disease (in most cases). Decreased ceruloplasmin with increased copper occurs only in Wilson's disease in normal infants less than 6 months of age.
   (b) Menkes' steely-hair disease
   (c) Severe copper deficiency that accompanies long-term hyperalimentation and parenteral nutrition
   (d) Transient deficiencies in nephrosis, sprue, and kwashiorkor

Mucoproteins (Seromucoid)

Normal Values
83–203 mg./liter
Average: 135 mg./liter

Background
Mucoproteins are amino compounds whose action in the body is undetermined. It is known that in diseases such as cancer, infections, and inflammations, there is an increase of mucoproteins in the blood. In cancer, the more widespread the condition, the greater the increase in mucoproteins.

Explanation of Test
This test has its greatest value as a guide to the successful treatment of cancer indicated by a decrease in mucoproteins and in the differential diagnosis of liver diseases.

Procedure
A venous blood sample of 10 ml. is obtained.

Clinical Implications
A. *Increased levels* are found in
   1. Cancer
   2. Rheumatoid arthritis
   3. Infections
   4. Ankylosing spondylitis
B. *Decreased levels* are found in
   1. Infectious hepatitis
   2. Infectious cirrhosis

Proteins: Albumin and Globulin; A/G Ratio

Normal Values
Total protein: 6–8 g./dl. or 60–80 g./liter
Albumin: 3.8–5.0 g./dl. or 38–50 g./liter
Globulin: 2.3–3.5 g./dl. or 23–35 g./liter
Albumin–globulin ratio (A/G): greater than one
Albumin–binding capacity (ABC): 91%–127%

Explanation of Test
Proteins and nucleic acids, the structural components of a cell, serve as biocatalysts (enzymes), regulators of metabolism (hormones), and preservers of genetic makeup (chromosomes). Amino acids are the building blocks of protein.

Much clinical information is obtained by examining and measuring proteins because of the involvement of proteins in so many functions. The three major catagories of protein are tissue or organ proteins, plasma proteins, and hemoglobin. Because of its large size, muscle mass provides the greatest amount of protein in conditions of deprivation. Tissue protein in muscle mass has the largest buffering capacity of the protein sites.

Plasma proteins serve as a source of nutrition for the body tissues and function in body buffering ability by combining with hemoglobin to exert an effect comparable to that of bicarbonate and other inorganic blood buffer systems.

Albumin and Albumin/Globulin Ratio
Albumin is a protein that is formed in the liver and that helps to maintain normal distribution of water in the body (colloidal osmotic pressure). It also helps in the transport of blood constituents such as ions, pigments, bilirubin, hormones, fatty acids, enzymes, and certain drugs. Approximately 52% to 60% of total protein is albumin, the rest is

globulin, which functions in antibody formation, and other plasma protein (fibrinogen and prothrombin) functioning in coagulation.

Although the serum globulins function mainly as immunologic agents, they also play a part in maintaining the osmotic pressure of the blood; they are less effective than the serum albumin in this role because the globulin molecule is so much larger than the albumin molecule. Normally, the capillary walls are impermeable to the plasma protein, but in certain diseases the albumin will "seep through." The larger globulins, however, remain within the bloodstream and assume the major function in maintaining osmotic pressure. Because of the globulin's inability to function as effectively as the albumin, the osmotic pressure may be below normal even though the total protein is retained at normal levels. Thus the ratio of albumin to globulin becomes an important indicator of certain disease states, although a high ratio is usually clinically insignificant.

Albumin-Binding Capacity
The ABC indicates the number of available bilirubin binding sites on albumin. The unconjugated bilirubin is carried in serum attached to albumin. Infants with elevated unconjugated bilirubin and a low ABC are more likely to develop kernicterus.

Procedure
A venous blood sample of at least 0.5 ml. is obtained.

Clinical Implications
A. *Decreased albumin levels*
   1. Severe hypoalbuminemia is often associated with edema and decreased transport function such as hypocalcemia.
   2. Decreased albumin levels are caused by many different conditions
      (a) Inadequate iron intake
      (b) Severe liver diseases
      (c) Malabsorption
      (d) Diarrhea
      (e) Eclampsia
      (f) Nephrosis
      (g) Exfoliative dermatitis
      (h) Third-degree burns
      (i) Starvation
      (j) Excessive administration of IV glucose in water
B. *Increased albumin levels* are generally not observed.
C. *Increase in total protein* (hyperproteinemia)
   1. May be due to hemoconcentration as a result of dehydration from loss of body fluid and may occur in vomiting, diarrhea, wound drainage, or poor kidney function.

    (a) Both albumin and globulins increase in the same proportions so that A/G ratio is unchanged.

    (b) This is the only instance in which an increase in albumin is found.

  2. When the total protein increases and the albumin is unchanged or slightly decreased while globulins increase, the A/G ratio falls markedly.

    Caused by

    (a) Lupus erythematosus

    (b) Rheumatoid arthritis and other collagen diseases

    (c) Chronic infections

    (d) Acute liver disease

    (e) Multiple myeloma, sarcoidosis, and other malignant tumors

D. *Decrease in total protein* (hypoproteinemia)

  1. Associated with low albumin and small change in globulin, resulting in low A/G ratio.

  2. Due to

    (a) Increased loss of albumin in urine

    (b) Decreased formation in liver

    (c) Insufficient protein intake

    (d) Severe hemorrhage when the plasma volume is replaced more rapidly than the protein level

  3. Associated conditions

    (a) Severe liver disease

    (b) Malabsorption

    (c) Nephrotic syndrome

    (d) Diarrhea

    (e) Exfoliative dermatitis

    (f) Severe burns

    (g) Dilution of excessive IV administration of glucose in water

Note: The liver is so crucial to protein metabolism that liver disease is frequently associated with alterations in proteins and disturbances of protein metabolism. For example, in undernutrition and liver disease, the albumin level may be decreased by inadequate synthesis.

E. *Decreased albumin binding capacity*
Infants below 50% should be considered for possible exchange transfusion.

Interfering Factors

1. Low levels of albumin occur normally in all trimesters of pregnancy.
2. Bromsulphalein may cause a false elevation. Therefore, a serum

protein test should not be done within 48 hours following a BSP test.
3. Drugs interfere with total protein levels.

Clinical Alert

Observe, report, and record signs and symptoms of possible accompanying edema or hypocalcemia (see tests for calcium, page 244.

LIPOPROTEIN TESTS

The lipids are fat substances and consist mainly of cholesterol, cholesterol esters, triglycerides, nonesterified fatty acids, and phospholipids. Lipoproteins are macromolecular complexes of unique plasma proteins, known as *apoproteins*, and lipids that serve in the plasma to transport otherwise insoluble lipids. The lipoproteins can be divided into groups based on density, flotation characteristics, and electrophoretic mobility. These groups are chylomicrons; beta lipoproteins (low-density lipoproteins [LDL]); prebeta lipoproteins (very-low-density lipoproteins [VLDL]); and alpha lipoproteins (very-high-density lipoproteins [HDL]). Body lipids provide energy for metabolism and serve as precursors of steroid hormones (adrenals, ovaries, and testes) and bile acids. They also play an important role in the making of cell membranes. A lipod profile will include cholesterol, triglycerides, LDL, and HDL.

Lipoprotein fractionation is the single most useful combination of procedures used to detect genetically determined disorders of lipid metabolism and to assess the risk of coronary artery disease.

Lipoprotein measurement is important in both hyper- and hypolipidemia. The different types of hyperlipidemia are classified as I, IIa, IIb, III, IV and V. In coronary heart disease and other cardiovascular disorders, two types are most important and most noted: Type II with cholesterol elevated, triglycerides slightly elevated; and Type IV with cholesterol normal, triglycerides elevated. Types of hypolipidemia are types I, II, and III, which are initially detected by low levels of cholesterol.

Clinical Alert

1. LDL and HDL have a combined function in maintaining a cellular balance of cholesterol: LDL brings cholesterol to the cell; HDL removes it. It is important to remember that high

levels of LDL are atherogenic whereas high levels of HDL are protective.
2. Therapy for hyperlipidemia should always begin with diet, and whenever possible, dieticians should supervise the patient's diet. The American Heart Association has an excellent resource that explains the diet.

Cholesterol

Normal Values
Normal values vary with age, diet, and from country to country.
An upper limit of 220 mg./dl. is desirable; as the blood level rises, the risk of atherosclerosis and heart disease increases.
Desirable range is: 140–250 mg./dl. or 3.63–6.48 mmol./liter
Cholesterol esters: 60%–75% of total cholesterol
Cholesterol to phospholipid ratio: about 1 : 1 (especially at higher levels)

Background
Cholesterol, existing in muscles, red blood cells, and cell membranes, is used by the body to form steroid hormones, bile acids, and more cell membranes. Chemically, cholesterol exists in both a free and esterized form (60%–75%) in the body. Much of the cholesterol ingested is esterized in the intestines, but since it is also esterized in the liver, cholesterol levels are frequently used as an indication of liver function. Cholesterol is transported in the blood by the low-density lipoproteins (LDL—60%–75%) and high-density lipoproteins (HDL—15%–35%).

High levels of cholesterol are associated with atherosclerosis and increased risk of coronary artery disease. There is evidence that populations consuming a smaller amount of fats in their caloric intake (by eating vegetables rather than animal fats) have a lower cholesterol level and a lower incidence of atherosclerosis and coronary disease.

Explanation of Test
The main use of cholesterol testing is to detect disorders of blood lipids to evaluate the risk potential for atherosclerosis related to coronary artery disease. Cholesterol will be elevated in the hereditary hyperlipoproteinemias. This test is also used as a secondary aid in the study of thyroid and liver function.

Measurement of the percentage of cholesterol esters is helpful in diagnosing a deficiency of the enzyme lecithin cholesterol acryl transferase (LCAT) that circulates in the blood in association with the high-density lipoproteins. In persons who are deficient in LCAT, a much smaller percentage of cholesterol is esterified. This determination can also be helpful in evaluation of the extent of metabolic disturbance caused by liver disease and pancreatic disorders.

Procedure
A fasting venous blood sample of 7 ml. is obtained.

Clinical Implications
1. *Increased levels* of cholesterol
   (a) Levels above 250 mg. per dl. are considered elevated and call for a triglyceride test.
   (b) Conditions related to elevated cholesterol
       (1) Cardiovascular disease and atherosclerosis
       (2) Type II, familial hypercholesterolemia
       (3) Obstructive jaundice (also an increase in bilirubin)
       (4) Hypothyroidism (decreased in hyperthyroidism)
       (5) Nephrosis
       (6) Xanthomatosis
       (7) Uncontrolled diabetes
       (8) Nephrotic syndrome
   (c) Free versus esterized cholesterol
       There is a markedly abnormal ratio of free to esterified cholesterol in disease of the livery biliary tract, infectious disease, and extreme cholesterolemia.
2. *Decreased levels* of cholesterol
   (a) Instances when cholesterol is not absorbed from the GI tract
       (1) Malabsorption   (5) Sepsis
       (2) Liver disease   (6) Stress
       (3) Hyperthyroidism   (7) Drug therapy such as
       (4) Anemia   antibiotics
   (b) Other conditions related to decreased cholesterol levels
       (1) Pernicious anemia   (5) Terminal stages of de-
       (2) Hemolytic jaundice   bilitating diseases such
       (3) Hyperthyroidism   as cancer
       (4) Severe infections   (6) Hypolipoproteinemias
   (c) Esterol fraction decreases in liver diseases, liver cell injury, malabsorption syndrome, and malnutrition.
3. Increased levels of cholesterol esters are associated with familial deficiency of LCAT.
4. Decreased levels of cholesterol esters are associated with liver disease. This is because persons with liver disease may have impaired formation of LCAT with a resulting deficiency of the enzyme.
5. Cholesterol ester storage disease causes accumulation of cholesterol esters in the tissues, but it has no effect on the percentage of esterified cholesterol in the blood.
6. The higher the cholesterol phospholipid ratio, the greater the possible risk of developing atherosclerosis.

Interfering Factors
1. Cholesterol is normally slightly elevated in pregnancy.
2. Estrogen decreases plasma cholesterol and oophorectomy increases it.
3. Many drugs may cause a change in the blood cholesterol levels.

Patient Preparation
1. Instruct the patient about fasting overnight for 12 hours before the test.
2. Water is permitted.
3. Before fasting, the patient should be on a normal diet for 7 days before testing.
4. No alcohol should be consumed for 24 hours before testing.
5. Lipid-lowering drugs such as estrogen, oral contraceptives, and salicylates should be withheld.

Clinical Alert
1. If the patient breaks the fast or is unable to fast, notify the laboratory.
2. Once hyperlipidemia has been definitely identified, the diet should include a decreased amount of animal fats and replacement of saturated fats with polyunsaturated fats.
3. Elevated levels should be confirmed by a repeat test.

Fatty Acid Profile of Serum Lipids

Normal Values
Linoleate: >25% of fatty acid in serum lipids
Arachidonate: >6% of fatty acids in serum lipids
Phytanate (phytanic acid): no more than 0.3% of fatty acids in serum lipids
Palmitate: 18–26% of fatty acids in serum lipids

Explanation of Test
Measurement of these specific fatty acids can be useful in monitoring nutritional status in cases of malabsorption, starvation, and long-term intravenous feedings. It is also indicated in the differential diagnosis of polyneuropathy when Refsum's disease is suspected. The enzyme that degrades phytanic acid is lacking in the rare, inherited Refsum's disease.

Procedure
A venous blood sample of at least 5 ml. of serum is obtained.

Clinical Implications

Decreased values are associated with

1. Zinc deficiency disease (lineolate and arachidonate)
2. Resum's disease with polyneuropathy (phytanate). A level of 0.8% strongly suggests Refsum's disease, but the test should be repeated for confirmation.
3. Malabsorption
4. Starvation
5. Long-term intravenous therapy

Free Fatty Acids

Normal Values

239–843 μEq./liter

Background

Free fatty acids are formed by the breakdown of lipoproteins and triglycerides. High levels of free fatty acids are usually cleaned from the blood by the liver and then converted into lipoproteins. All but 2% to 5% of blood serum fatty acids are esterified. The nonesterified or free fatty acids are protein bound. The amount of free fatty acids and triglycerides in the blood is derived from dietary sources, fat deposits, or synthesized by the body. Carbohydrates can be converted to fatty acids and then stored in fat cells as triglycerides.

Explanation of Test

This measurement of a lipid fraction is helpful in determining the metabolism of fats and carbohydrates. The ratio of fatty acid and carbohydrate use is altered in situations associated with fat breakdown such as fasting. Unusually high levels will be found in untreated diabetics. It has been shown that the response of free fatty acids to treatment occurs more rapidly than the responses of blood sugar, plasma CO_2, or excretion of ketones in the urine. The test is also used in the diagnosis of secondary hypoproteinemia. Disorders identified with excess fatty acids are usually associated with high levels of very-low-density lipoprotein.

Procedure

A fasting blood sample of 5 ml. is obtained. Serum should be separated from cells within 45 minutes of drawing and frozen at once.

Clinical Implications

Increased values are associated with

1. Uncontrolled diabetes mellitus

2. Excessive release of a lipoactive hormone such as epinephrine, norepinephrine, glucagon, thyrotropin, and adrenocorticotropin.
3. Prolonged fasting or starvation (as much as three times normal).

Interfering Factors
1. Values are increased by exercise, anxiety, lowered body temperature, and a number of drugs.
2. Values are decreased by food intake and a number of drugs.

Lipoprotein Electrophoresis

Normal Values
On 12–14 hour fasting specimen

Chylomicrons: 0
Beta or LDL: 28%–53% or 0.28– Mass fraction of total lipoprotein
.53
Pre-beta or VLDL: 3%–32% or Mass fraction of total lipoprotein
0.03–.32
Alpha or HDL: 24%–40% or Mass fraction of total lipoprotein
0.24–.40
Plasma appearance: Clear

> **Note:** Chylomicrons are proteins that are derived from dietary sources and can extend into the pre-beta area when markedly increased. The term was first applied in 1920 to the description of particles visible in lymph and plasma after the eating of fats. In hyperchylomicronemia, chylomicrons are present and represent dietary fat in transport. The standing plasma contains a cream layer over a clear layer in type I hyperlipidemia, where chylomicrons are elevated, but not in type IV, where both chylomicrons and triglycerides are elevated, causing turbidity of infranate.

High-Density Alpha-1-Fraction Lipoprotein (HDL) Cholesterol

Normal Values
Men: 30–70 mg./dl. or 30–70 g./liter
Women: 30–80 mg./dl. or 30–80 g./liter

Background
High-density lipoprotein is the cholesterol carried by the alpha lipoproteins. A high level of alpha-1-HDL is an indication of a healthy

metabolic system in a person free of liver disease or intoxication of any form. It is believed that the high-density lipoproteins serve as carriers that remove cholesterol from the peripheral tissues and transport it back to the liver for catabolism and excretion. HDL probably also inhibits cellular uptake on low-density lipoproteins. These two mechanisms help to explain how the high-density lipoproteins produce a protection in relation to the risk of coronary heart disease.

Explanation of Test
This measurement is used to assess the risk of coronary artery disease and to monitor persons with known low levels of high-density lipoproteins. It is known that low levels of HDL cholesterol are associated with increased risk for atherosclerotic disease of the coronary arteries of men and women of age 50 and older. It is also recognized that the level of HDL cholesterol can be raised in some people by increasing physical activity. Among healthy persons, those who are more physically active tend to have higher alpha-1-HDL cholesterol levels.

Procedure
A fasting venous blood sample of 5 ml. is obtained.

Clinical Implications
1. *Increased values,* especially >100 mg., are associated with a chronic liver disorder or some form of chronic intoxication.
2. *Decreased values* are associated with
   (a) Increased risk for coronary heart disease when HDL cholesterol is less than 30 mg./dl.
   (b) Inheritance and chronic physical inactivity (20–30 mg./dl.) Long distance runners have higher levels of HDL.
3. Levels can be either high or low in primary biliary cirrhosis, chronic hepatitis, or alcoholism.

Interfering Factors
1. Decreased HDL is associated with smokers.
2. Increased HDL is associated with the moderate intake of alcohol.
3. Iodine contrast substances interfere with test results.
4. Recent weight gains or losses can interfere with test results.

Patient Preparation
1. Advise the patient about the purpose of testing and that overnight fasting is required. Water is permitted.
2. If possible, all medication should be withheld for 24 to 48 hours before testing. Confer with the attending physician.
3. Ask the patient if there has been any drastic change in weight in the last few weeks before testing.

Patient Aftercare
Persons with decreased HDL can be counseled to take measures to increase levels by losing weight, cutting down on calorie consumption, eating less red meat, and taking lecithin supplements. Moderate alcohol consumption is believed by some to be a factor in increased HDL.

Very-Low-Density Lipoproteins (VLDL) and Low-Density Lipoproteins (LDL)

Normal Values
VLDL cholesterol: 25%–50% or 0.25–0.50
LDL cholesterol: 62–185 mg./dl. or 0.62 g./liter–1.85 g./liter

Background
VLDL is a major carrier of triglyceride (60%–70% triglyceride, 10%–15% cholesterol). Degradation of VLDL leads to a major source of LDL. Circulating fatty acids are vitalized by the liver to form triglycerides that are packaged with apoprotein and cholesterol and exported into the blood as very-low-density lipoproteins.

LDLs are the cholesterol-rich remnants of the lipid transport vehicle, VLDL. Since LDL has a longer half-life (3–4 days) than its precursor, VLDL, LDL is more prevalent in the blood. It is finally catabolized in the liver and possibly in nonhepatic cells as well.

Explanation of Test
This test is specifically done to determine the risk of coronary heart disease. The low-density lipoproteins are closely correlated with an increased incidence of atherosclerosis and coronary heart disease. On the other hand, a decreased incidence of coronary heart disease is seen in persons with high levels of HDL. The VLDL cholesterol concentration is expressed as a percent of total cholesterol.

Procedure
LDL is calculated using this formula

$$LDL_c = cholesterol \frac{HDL_c + triglycerides}{2}$$

Factor of 2 in the formula is derived from the molar ratio of triglyceride to cholesterol in VLDL (c = cholesterol).

Clinical Implications
1. A concentration of 0% to 24% is associated with type II hyperlipidemia.
2. A concentration of 25% to 50% is consistent with type III hyperlipidemia.

3. A concentration of 51% to 100% is consistent with type IV hyperlipidemia.

   The atherogenic index (AI) does not involve phenotyping but is a comparison of VLDL and LDL factors. It is believed that the AI correlates more closely with the predisposition of coronary heart disease than with the amount of any one of the specific lipoprotein fractions in the blood.

Triglycerides

Normal Values

Desirable level is 40–150 mg./dl. or 0.40–1.50 mmol./liter

Values are age- and diet-related. Values in the first 2 decades of life are slightly lower than those in subsequent years. Values in women are about 10 mg. per dl. lower than in men.

Background

Triglycerides are produced in the liver from glycerol and fatty acids and from triesters of these two components. Triglycerides are lipids that are normally present in the blood and are used in producing energy for the body. Excess triglycerides are stored in adipose tissue.

Explanation of Test

This test is used to evaluate patients with suspected atherosclerosis and is used as an indication of the body's ability to metabolize fat. Elevated triglycerides along with elevated cholesterol are risk factors in atherosclerotic disease. Because cholesterol and triglycerides can vary independently, measurement of both values is more meaningful than the measurement of either substance alone.

Procedure

A venous blood sample of at least 5 ml. is obtained. Notify the laboratory of the patient's age and sex.

Clinical Implications

1. *Increased triglyceride levels* are believed to be a factor in increased risk for atherosclerosis.
   (a) Increased levels occur in
       (1) Types I, IIb, III, IV, and V hyperlipoproteinemias
       (2) Liver disease
       (3) Nephrotic syndrome
       (4) Hypothyroidism
       (5) Poorly controlled diabetes
       (6) Pancreatitis
       (7) Glycogen storage disease

    (8) Myocardial infarction (Increases may last 1 year.)

    (9) Metabolic disorders related to endocrinopathies

  (b) Many of the clinical conditions that cause an increase in cholesterol levels also cause an increase in triglycerides.

    (1) Nephrotic syndrome   (3) Toxemia

    (2) Pancreatic dysfunction   (4) Hypothroidism

2. *Decreased levels* occur in malnutrition and congenital alpha–beta lipoproteinemia.

  (a) COPD   (d) Malnutrition

  (b) Brain infarction   (e) Malabsorption syndrome

  (c) Hyperthyroidism

Patient Preparation

1. Instruct the patient about fasting overnight for 12 hours before the test.
2. Water is permitted.
3. Before fasting, the patient should be on a normal diet.
4. No alcohol should be consumed for 24 hours before testing.

Interfering Factors

1. A transient increase will occur following a heavy meal or alcohol ingestion.
2. Increased values are also associated with pregnancy and oral contraceptives.

Patient Aftercare

A person with high triglyceride levels should be counseled that weight reduction, low fat diet, and an exercise program can be factors that will reduce levels.

THYROID FUNCTION TESTS

Laboratory determinations of thyroid function are useful in distinguishing patients with euthyroidism from those with hyperthyroidism or hypothyroidism (see Tests of Thyroid Function on page 344). In general, the most useful laboratory tests to confirm or exclude hyperthyroidism are total T_4, the free thyroxine index, and total T_3. The most useful tests to detect hypothyroidism are total T_4, the free thyroxine index, and thyroid-stimulating hormone (TSH). A thyrotropin-releasing hormone (TRH) stimulation test can be valuable in establishing the thyroid status in some patients with equivocal signs of thyroid dysfunction and borderline laboratory values. It should be kept in mind that values obtained for the assessment of thyroid function can be influenced by factors other than disease such as age, current illness, binding capacity of serum proteins, and some drugs.

Tests of Thyroid Function

These findings are intended only as an aid in evaluating thyroid function. In most instances, these procedures are used to confirm clinical impressions gained from history and physical examination.

Condition	T_4	T_3	FT_4	TBG	T_3UR	TSH	TRH Stimulation TSH	TRH Stimulation T_3/T_4	Antibodies
Hypothyroidism									
Primary	L	L,N	L	N	L	H	+	0	0,+
Primary with T_3Rx (euthyroid)	L	N	L	N	L,N	N (L)			0
Primary with T_4Rx (euthyroid)	N,H	N	N,H	N	N,H	N (L)			0
Secondary (pituitary)	L	L,N	L	N	L	N (L)	0	0	0
Tertiary (hypothalamic)	L	L,N	L	N	L	N (L)	+	+	0
Hyperthyroidism									
Graves' disease	H	H	H	N	H	N (I)	0	0	+
T_3 toxicosis	N	H	N	N	N	N	0	0	
Thyrotoxicosis factitia									
Due to T_3	L	H	L	N	L,N	N (L)	0	0	
Due to T_4	H	N	H	N	N,H	N (L)	0	0	
Hashimoto's thyroiditis	V	V	V	N	V	V	V		+++
Pregnancy, estrogens Excess TBG (euthyroid) hereditary	H	H	N	H	L	N			0
Androgens, steroids (high doses) Low TBG (euthyroid) hereditary	L	L	N	L	H	N			0
Nephrosis, cirrhosis	L	L	N	L	H	N	+	+	0
Diphenylhydantoin, salicylates (large doses)	L	L	N	N	H	N	+	+	0
X-ray contrast media	N	N	N	N	N	N	+	+	0

H = High; N = Normal; L = May be low; + = Responds or present; 0 = No response or absent; V = Variable
(After Bio-Science Handbook, 12th ed., p 52. Van Nuys, CA, Bio-Science Laboratories, 1979)

To understand the thyroid function tests, it is necessary to understand these basic concepts.

1. The function of the thyroid gland is to take iodine from the circulating blood, combine it with the amino acid tyrosine, and convert it to the thyroid hormones thyroxine (T_4), and triiodothyronine (T_3). Iodine comprises about two-thirds of the weight of the thyroid hormones.
2. Another function of the thyroid gland is to store T_3 and T_4 until they are released into the bloodstream under the influence of TSH from the pituitary gland.
3. Only a small amount of the hormones is not bound to protein. However, it is the free portion of the thyroid hormones that is the true determinant of the thyroid status of the patient.

Calcitonin

Normal Values
Basal
Men: ≤19 pg./ml. or ng./liter
Women: ≤14 pg./ml. or ng./liter
Calcium infusion (2.4 mg. of Ca./kg.)
Men: ≤190 pg./ml. or ng./liter
Women: ≤130 pg./ml. or ng./liter
Pentagastrin injection (0.5 μg./kg.)
Men: ≤110 pg./ml. or ng./liter
Women: ≤35 pg./ml. or ng./liter

Background
Calcitonin is a hormone secreted by the C cells or parafollicular cells of the thyroid gland. The main action of this hormone is to inhibit bone resorption by regulating the number and activity of osteoblasts. Calcitonin is secreted in direct response to high blood calcium levels and may prevent abrupt changes in calcium levels and the excessive loss of calcium.

Explanation of Test
This test is used in the differential diagnosis of cancer of the thyroid. Levels will be increased in medullary carcinoma (malignant C cell tumors), occasionally in patients with other tumors, and in some instances of renal failure.

Procedure
Two fasting specimens of 10 ml. of venous blood are obtained.

Clinical Implications
1. *Increased levels* are associated with

(a) Medullary thyroid cancers
(b) C cell hyperplasia
(c) Chronic renal failure
(d) Pernicious anemia

(e) Zollinger–Ellison syndrome
(f) Cancer of lung, breast, and pancreas

2. In a small proportion of patients who do have medullary cancer, the fasting level of calcitonin is normal. In these instances, a provocative test using calcium or pentagastrin should be followed by an abnormally large increase in calcitonin levels.

Procedure
1. A pentagastrin injection is administered. Blood samples are drawn before the injection and 1½ and 5 minutes after the injection.
2. Another method is to infuse calcium (2.4 mg./kg.) over a 4-hour period and collect blood samples before infusion and again at 3 to 4 hours.

Interfering Factors
Levels are normally *increased* in

(a) Pregnancy at term
(b) Newborns

Clinical Alert

1. Screening of families of patients with proven medullary cancer of the thyroid is recommended because the tumor has both sporadic and familial incidence.
2. Also, if the stimulus test is normal in family members, it is advisable to repeat the calcium provocative test periodically.

Patient Preparation
1. Explain the purpose and procedure of the test.
2. Advise the patient to fast from food overnight. Water is permitted.

Free Thyroxine T$_4$ (FT$_4$)

Normal Values
1–2.3 ng./dl.
For patients on Synthyroid, up to 5.0 ng./dl.

Background
Free thyroxine T$_4$ comprises a small fraction of the total thyroxine. The free T$_4$ is available to the tissues and is the metabolically active form of this hormone.

Explanation of Test
This is a measurement of that fraction (about 5%) of the circulatory thyroxine T$_4$ that exists in a free state, unbound to protein. It is commonly done to determine thyroid status, to rule out hypo- and hyperthyroidism, and to evaluate thyroid replacement therapy. This test has diagnostic value in situations where total hormone levels do not correlate with the thyrometabolic state, and there is no reason to suspect an abnormality in binding protein levels. However, it is also a useful test when there are definite or probable abnormalities in binding levels. Demonstration of the free T$_4$ provides a more accurate picture of the thyroid status in persons with abnormal TBG levels in pregnancy and in those who are receiving estrogens, hydrogens, phenytoin, and salicylates.

Procedure
A venous blood sample of at least 5 ml. is obtained. Accurate results can be obtained in as little as 0.5 ml. for pediatric cases.

Interfering Factors
1. Values are increased in infants at birth. This value rises even higher after 2 to 3 days of life.
2. Free T$_4$ levels are decreased in adolescents as compared to adults.
3. Heparin will cause falsely elevated values.

Clinical Implications
1. *Increased levels* are associated with
   (a) Graves' disease
   (b) Thyrotoxicosis due to T$_4$
2. *Decreased levels* are associated with
   (a) Primary hypothyroidism
   (b) Secondary hypothyroidism (pituitary)
   (c) Tertiary hypothyroidism (hypothalamic)
   (d) Thyrotoxicosis due to T$_3$
3. *Levels can be slightly elevated* in
   (a) Severe illness in nonthyroid disease
   (b) Cirrhosis of liver
4. *Values will be normal* in
   (a) T$_3$ toxicosis
   (b) Pregnancy and estrogen therapy
   (c) Nephrosis
   (d) Cirrhosis
   (e) Use of preceding x-ray contrast media
   (f) Use of drugs such as androgens, steroids (high doses), diphenylhydantoin, and salicylates (high doses)

Free Triiodothyronine T$_3$ (FT$_3$)

Normal Values
120–195 ng./dl. or 1.85–3.00 nmol./liter

Background
Free hormones are the best indicators of thyroid function. However, experts disagree on the selection of free T$_3$ versus the use of free T$_4$.

Explanation of Test
This is one of the determinations used in the evaluation of thyroid function and is a measure of that fraction of the circulatory triiodothyronine that exists in the free state in the blood, unbound to protein. It is done to rule out T$_3$ toxicosis, hypothyroidism, hyperthyroidism, to determine thyroid status, and to evaluate thyroid replacement therapy.

Procedure
A venous blood sample of at least 5 ml. is obtained.

Interfering Factors
Significant quantities of radioactivity in the blood of the patient can result in serious errors. For this reason, the laboratory should be informed if the patient has recently received radioactive material.

Clinical Implications
1. *Increased values* are associated with hyperthyroidism and T$_3$ toxicosis.
2. *Decreased values* are associated with hypothyroidism

Free Thyroxine T$_4$ Index (FTI)

Normal Values
5.9–10.6 (these are arbitrary units)

Explanation of Test
This index is a simple mathematical calculation used to correct the estimated total thyroxine (T$_4$) for the amount of thyroxine binding globulin (TBG) present. To perform this calculation, two results are needed: the T$_4$ value and the T$_3$ uptake ratio. The product of these two members is the FTI. The FTI is useful in the diagnosis of hyper- and hypothyroidism, especially in patients with known or suspected abnormalities in thyroxine binding protein levels. In such cases, blood levels and clinical signs may seem contradictory unless both T$_4$ and TBG are considered as interrelated parameters of thyroid status. Measurement of the free T$_4$ also gives a more accurate picture of the thyroid status

when the TBG is abnormal in pregnant women or those persons who are being treated with estrogen, androgens, phenytoin, or salicylates.

Procedure
Mathematical computation of T_3 uptake $\times$ T_4 = FTI.

Clinical Implications
Application of the equation of the FTI includes the following:

Status	TBG	T_3 Uptake	$\times$	T_4	=	FTI
Euthyroid	Normal	1.0		9.0		9.0
Euthyroid	Low	1.5		4.0		6.0
Euthyroid	High	0.6		16.0		9.6
Hypothyroid	High	0.7		4.0		2.8
Hyperthyroid	Low	1.3		13.0		16.9

Neonatal Thyrotropin-Stimulating Hormone (TSH)

Normal Values
Neonates by third day of life: under 25 milliI.U./liter

Background
Neonatal primary hypothyroidism is not only characterized by low T_4 levels in blood serum but also by elevated TSH levels.

Explanation of Test
This measurement is best used as a confirmatory test for infants with positive T_4 screens or low blood serum T_4 levels. Although TSH measurement has been suggested as the primary screening test for neonatal hypothyroidism, infants with secondary (hypothalamic or hypopituitary) hypothyroidism, which constitutes about 10% of all neonatal hypothyroid cases, would be missed in such a screening system.

Procedure
1. The skin is cleansed with an antiseptic and the infant's heel is punctured with a sterile disposable lancet.
2. If bleeding is slow, it is helpful to hold the leg dependent for a short time before spotting the blood on the filter paper.
3. The circles on the filter paper must be completely filled. This can best be done by placing one side of the filter paper against the infant's heel and watching for the blood to appear on the front side of the paper and completely fill the circle.
4. Air dry for 1 hour, fill in all requested information, and send to the laboratory immediately.

Instruction to Mother
Inform the mother about the purpose of the test and the method of collecting the specimens.

Clinical Implications
A positive test is associated with neonatal hypothyroidism.

Neonatal Thyroxine (T_4); Neonatal Screen for Hypothyroidism

Alert Limits
1–5 days: ≤4.9 µg./dl. equivalent
6–8 days: ≤4 µg./dl. equivalent
9–11 days: ≤3.5 µg./dl. equivalent
12–120 days: ≤3 µg./dl. equivalent
Alert limits are defined as T_4 values that suggest hypothyroidism. A
   follow-up TSH paper test is advised in these cases.

Background
Normal brain growth and development cannot take place without adequate thyroid hormone. Congenital hypothyroidism (cretinism) is characterized by low levels of T_4 and elevated levels of TSH.

Explanation of Test
This is a screening test of thyroxine (T_4) activity to detect neonatal hypothyroidism. It can be used in infants aged 1 to 120 days. However, specimens should be obtained after the first 24 hours of life, preferably within the first week. Thyroxine is obtained from whole blood spotted on paper using a radioimmune assay technique.

Procedure
1. The skin is cleansed with an antiseptic and the infant's heel is punctured with a sterile disposable lancet.
2. If bleeding is slow, it is helpful to hold the leg dependent for a short time before spotting the blood on the filter paper.
3. The circles on the filter paper must be completely filled. This can best be done by placing one side of the filter paper against the infant's heel and watching for the blood to appear on the front side of the paper and completely fill the circle.
4. Air dry for 1 hour, fill in all requested information, and send to the laboratory immediately.

Instructions to Mother
Inform the mother about the purpose of the test and the method of collecting the specimens.

Clinical Implications
A positive test is associated with hypothyroidism.

Clinical Alert

1. Do not interpret this test in terms of the blood serum T_4 values. This is an entirely different procedure using a different type of specimen.
2. Notify the attending physician and the mother of positive results within 24 hours.

Thyroglobulin (Tg)

Normal Values
Up to 50 ng./ml.

Background
Tg is present in normal blood and is composed of glycoprotein and the iodinated secretions of epithelial cells of the thyroid. These iodinated secretions contain both the precursors of thyroxine and triiodothyronine and these hormones themselves.

Explanation of Test
This test is helpful in the diagnosis of differentiated cancer of thyroid and hyperthyroidism. It is used to follow the course of patients with known differentiated or metastatic thyroid cancer. Levels will decrease following initial treatment, and in recurrence of metastasis, the level will again rise.

Procedure
A venous blood sample of 5 ml. is obtained.

Clinical Implications
1. *Increased levels* are associated with
   (a) Untreated and metastic differentiated thyroid cancers (elevated Tg in pleural effusions has been used as an indication of metastasis to the lungs)
   (b) Hyperthyroidism
   (c) Subacute thyroiditis (some cases)
   (d) Benign adenoma (some cases)
2. A correlation between elevated Tg levels and goiter size has been reported in nontoxic nodular growths.

Thyroid-Stimulating Hormone (TSH)

Normal Values
Adults: 0.5–6 milliI.U./liter
Neonates: under 25 milliI.U./liter by day 3 of life for both serum and
spot test

Background
The thyroid is unique among the endocrine glands because it has a
large store of hormone and a slow rate of normal turnover. Stimulation
of the thyroid gland by the thyroid-stimulating hormone (TSH), which
is produced by the anterior pituitary gland, will cause the release and
distribution of stored thyroid hormones. TSH is also influenced by the
parathyroid, which produces thyrotropin-reducing hormone. When
thyroxine and T_3 are too high, TSH secretion decreases. When thyroxine and T_3 are too low, TSH secretion increases. In primary hypothyroidism, TSH levels rise because of the low levels of thyroid hormone. If
the pituitary fails in its function, TSH is not secreted, blood levels fall,
and the thyroid becomes quiescent.

Explanation of Test
This measurement is used in the diagnosis of primary hypothyroidism
when there is thyroid gland failure due to intrinsic disease and to
differentiate primary from secondary hypothyroidism by determining
the actual circulatory level of TSH. In principle, it is the same as the
neonatal T_4 test. It is not the same measurement as the TSH stimulation test, in which the thyroid uptake of radioiodine is measured before
and after the injection of TSH.

Procedure
A venous sample of at least 1 ml. is obtained and measured by the
radioimmune assay method.

Clinical Implications
1. *Increased levels* are seen in adults and neonates with primary hypothyroidism.
2. *Decreased levels* are associated with
   (a) Hyperthyroidism
   (b) Secondary and tertiary hypothyroidism

Interfering Factors
1. Values are normally high in neonatal cord blood. There is hypersecretion of TSH in newborns up to 2 to 3 times normal. TSH returns
   to normal by 14 days of life.
2. Values are suppressed during treatment with triiodothyronine, aspirin, corticosteroids, and heparin.

3. Values are abnormally increased during drug therapy with lithium, potassium iodide, and TSH injection.

Thyrotropin-Releasing Hormone (TRH) Stimulation Test

Normal Values
TSH should increase approximately two times baseline and is usually greater in females than in males.

Background
The hypothalamus produces TRH, and the pituitary gland secretes thyrotropin-stimulating hormone (TSH) in response. Hypothalamic failure with lack of TRH leads to reduced thyroid function.

Explanation of Test
This test is done to assess the responsiveness of the anterior pituitary gland and to differentiate between the three types of hypothyroidism: primary, secondary, and tertiary. When TRH is injected, a rise in TSH indicates that the pituitary gland is functioning.

Procedure
1. A 500-μg. bolus of TRH is given intravenously.
2. Blood samples are obtained at intervals, and the TSH level is measured. The maximum response usually occurs in 20 minutes.
3. Check with your laboratory for specific procedures.

Clinical Implications
1. The TSH level shows a very slight increase or no response in hyperthyroidism.
2. In hypothyroidism, differing responses will be seen in the types of hypothyroidism.
   (a) In primary (thyroid gland failure), there is an increase of two or more times the normal response.
   (b) In secondary (anterior pituitary failure), there is no response.
   (c) In tertiary (hypothalamic failure), the TSH rises after a delay. Multiple injections of TRH may be necessary to induce the appropriate TSH response.

Thyroxine-Binding Globulin (TBG)

Normal Values
Total: 16–24 μg./dl or 160–240 μg./liter

Background
Almost all of the thyroid hormones in the blood are bound to protein. These thyroxine-binding proteins play an important role in regulating the free thyroxine FT_4. TBG is by far the most important determinant of the overall binding of T_4. For this reason, a measure of TBG is a good approximation of the thyroxine-binding function of the blood.

Explanation of Test
This measurement is useful in determining congenital excess or deficit of TBG and in confirming abnormalities of thyroxine-binding proteins suggested by the T_3 UR results. This measurement is the old T_3 test. When the TBG and T_4 are performed on the same blood sample, an accurate assessment of the state of thyroid function can be ascertained.

Procedure
A 2-ml. specimen of venous blood is obtained.

Clinical Implications
1. *The TBG level is increased* in
   (a) Hypothyroidism
   (b) Pregnancy (in some spontaneous aborters, the TBG level is not elevated)
   (c) Estrogen therapy
   (d) Oral contraceptives
   (e) Genetic and idiopathic hepatic disease
   (f) Prolonged perphenazine therapy
   (g) Acute intermittent porphyria
2. *The TBG level is decreased* in
   (a) Nephrotic syndromes
   (b) Marked hypoproteinemia
   (c) Genetic and idiopathic liver disease
   (d) Uncompensated acidosis
   (e) Acromegaly
3. *The thyroxine prealbumin (TBPA) level is decreased* in
   (a) Thyrotoxicosis
   (b) Severe illness or trauma
   (c) Surgery
   (d) Parturition

Interfering Factors
Drugs may cause both increased and decreased levels.

Thyroxine Determination by Radioimmunoassay (T_4-RIA)

Normal Values
5–12.5 μg/dl. or 50–125 μg/liter

Explanation of Test
This test measures the level of total circulatory thyroid using a radioimmunoassay procedure in the laboratory. The combination of T_4,

RIA, and T_3 uptake ratio is recommended as a screen for overall thyroid function. It will provide accurate results even if a contrast organic iodine has been used in a recent x-ray. Treatment of thyroid disorders with potassium iodide or Lugol's solution can be monitored with the use of this test.

Procedure
A venous blood sample of at least 5 ml. is obtained.

Interfering Factors
1. A lipemic specimen will cause falsely elevated results.
2. Administration of tracer doses of radioactive iodine within 48 hours before testing will interfere with the results.
3. Values normally will be increased in pregnancy and with drugs such as estrogens, antiovulatory medications, and L-thyroxine.
4. Values will be decreased with use of drugs such as androgens, anabolic steroids, salicylates (large doses), triiodothyronine, sulfonamides, phenytoin, and propranolol.

Clinical Significance
1. *Increased values* are associated with
   (a) Hyperthyroidism   (c) Early hepatitis
   (b) Acute thyroiditis   (d) Idiopathic TBG elevation
2. *Decreased values* are associated with
   (a) Hypothyroidism
   (b) Chronic thyroiditis (usually)
   (c) Nephrosis
   (d) Idiopathic TBG decreases
3. The increase in T_4 that should be associated with a normal pregnancy may not occur in the presence of estrogen inadequacy during pregnancy.
4. T_4 levels also may be normal despite signs of hyperthyroidism in cases of T_3 toxicosis.

Long-Acting Thyroid Stimulator (LATS)

Normal Values
Present in only 5% of healthy people
Some normally detectable

Background
Long-acting thyroid stimulator (LATS) is classified as a 7S gammaglobulin and does not appear to have its origin in the pituitary gland. This factor has a longer-acting effect than the thyroid-stimulating hormone (TSH) and is found in the blood of some hyperthyroid patients.

Explanation of Test
This test is very important in the evaluation of any person with thyroid disease, especially in identifying persons with malignant exophthalmos and Graves' disease.

Procedure
A venous blood sample of 5 ml. is obtained. Notify the laboratory if ^{131}I has been administered within the past 48 hours.

Clinical Implications
Increased levels are associated with

(a) Exophthalmos
(b) Persons prone to relapse of hyperthyroidism
(c) Graves' disease

Thyroxine; Total T_4

Normal Values
5–12.5 μg./dl.

Background
Thyroxine is the thyroid hormone that contains four atoms of iodine. Approximately 95% of thyroxine is bound to TBG as well as prealbumin and albumin. About 5% of the circulating T_4 is in the free or unbound portion.

Explanation of Test
T_4 is one of the thyrox panel tests used in the evaluation of thyroid function. It is a direct measurement of the concentration of total thyroxine in the blood serum. The measurement of total thyroxine (T_4) level is a good index of thyroid function when the TBG is normal. The increase in TBG levels normally seen in pregnancy and with estrogen therapy will increase the total T_4 levels. The decrease of TBG levels in persons receiving anabolic steroids, in chronic liver disease, and in nephroses will decrease the total T_4 value. This test is done commonly to rule out hyperthyroidism and hypothyroidism. The T_4 test also can be used as a guide in establishing and following maintenance doses of thyroid in the treatment of hypothyroidism. In addition, it also can be used in hyperthyroidism to follow the results of antithyroid drugs.

Procedure
A venous blood sample of at least 5 ml. is obtained. If the patient is already on thyroid treatment, it must be stopped 1 month before the test to obtain a true picture of T_4.

Interfering Factors

1. Total thyroxine levels increase during the second or third month of pregnancy as a result of increased estrogen production.
2. Values also are increased with the use of drugs such as estrogens and antiovulants.

Clinical Implications

1. *Values can be increased* in
   (a) Hyperthyroidism
   (b) Acute thyroiditis
   (c) Subacute thyroiditis
   (d) Hepatitis, early in disease (normal by 4 weeks)
2. *Values can be decreased* in
   (a) Cretinism
   (b) Myxedema
   (c) Hypothyroidism
   (d) Chronic thyroiditis (usually)
   (e) Subacute thyroiditis
   (f) Simmonds' disease
   (g) Nephrosis
   (h) Cirrhosis
   (i) Hypoproteinemia
   (j) Malnutrition

   The magnitude of decrease in values parallels the decrease in thyroid function. Therefore, lower values will occur in cretinism and myxedema than in mild hypothyroidism.
3. There is no typical androgen cancer of thyroid.
4. Values are usually normal in T₃ toxicosis.

Note: A thyroid panel usually consists of

1. Free T₃ test
2. T₃ RIA
3. Free T₄ test
4. T₄ RIA

Triiodothyronine (T₃) by Radioimmunoassay (T₃-RIA)

Normal Values

90–230 ng./dl.

Background

T₃ has three atoms of iodine as compared with four atoms in thyroxine (T₄). T₃ is more active metabolically than T₄, but its effect is shorter. There is much less T₃ than T₄ in the serum, and it is bound less firmly to thyroid-binding globulin.

Explanation of Test

The measurement of T₃ is a quantitative determination of the total triiodothyronine concentration in the blood and is the test of choice in the diagnosis of T₃ thyrotoxicosis. It is not the same as the T₃ uptake test that measures the unsaturated thyroxine binding globulin in serum. It can also be very useful in the diagnosis of hyperthyroidism. T_3 thyrotoxicosis refers to a varient of hyperthyroidism in which a thyrotoxic patient will have elevated T_3 values and normal T_4 values. It is of limited value in diagnosing hypothyroidism.

Procedure
A venous blood sample of at least 5 ml. is obtained.

Clinical Implications
1. *Increased values* are associated with
   (a) Hyperthyroidism
   (b) T_3 thyrotoxicosis
   (c) Daily dosage of 25 μg. or more of T_3
   (d) Acute thyroiditis
   (e) Idiopathic TBG elevation
   (f) Daily dosage of 300 μg. or more of T_4
2. *Decreased values* are associated with
   (a) Hypothyroidism (however, some clinically hypothyroid patients will have normal levels)
   (b) Starvation
   (c) Idiopathic TBG decrease
   (d) Acute illness

Interfering Factors
1. Values are increased in pregnancy and with the use of drugs such as estrogens and antiovulatory compounds.
2. Values are decreased in the use of drugs such as anabolic steroids, androgens, large doses of salicylates, and phenytoin.

Triiodothyronine Uptake Ratio (T_3UR, T_3UP)

Normal Values
0.8–1.30: This is a ratio between patient specimen and the standard control.
25%–35% uptake

Explanation of Test
This test is an indirect measurement of the unsaturated thyroxine-binding globulin (UTBG) in the blood. This determination is expressed in arbitrary terms and is inversely proportional to the TBG. For this reason, low T_3UR levels are indicative of situations that result in elevated levels of UTBG. For example, in hypothyroidism, when insufficient T_4 is available to produce saturation of TBG, UTBG is elevated and the T_3UR values are low. Similarly, in pregnant patients or those receiving estrogen, TBG levels are increased proportionately more than is T_4, resulting in high levels of UTBG, reflected in low T_3UR results.

Clinical Implications

1. *Increased levels* are associated with
   - (a) Hyperthyroidism
   - (b) Nephrosis
   - (c) Severe liver disease
   - (d) Metastatic malignancy
   - (e) Pulmonary insufficiency
   - (f) Thyroxine and desiccated thyroid therapy
2. *Decreased levels* are associated with
   - (a) Hypothyroidism
   - (b) Normal pregnancy
   - (c) Hyperestrogenic status
   - (d) Triiodothyronine treatment for hypothyroidism
   - (e) Propylthiouracil treatment for hyperthyroidism

Procedure

A venous blood sample of at least 2 ml. is obtained.

Interfering Factors

1. *Decreased levels* occur in normal pregnancy and when estrogens and antiovulatory drugs are used.
2. *Increased levels* occur with drugs such as dicumarol, heparin, androgens, anabolic steriods, phenytoin, and large doses of salicylates.

Clinical Alert

This test has nothing to do with the actual T$_3$ blood level in spite of its name, which is sometimes confusingly abbreviated to the T$_3$ test. It is emphasized that the T$_3$ uptake ratio and the true T$_3$ (T$_3$ by RIA) are entirely different tests. The T$_3$ uptake gives only an indirect measurement of overall binding.

BIBLIOGRAPHY

Bauer D, Ditto W: Interpretation in Therapeutic Drug Monitoring. Chicago, American Society of Pathologists, 1981

Baver JD: Clinical Laboratory Methods, 9th ed. St. Louis, CV Mosby, 1982

Berkow R (ed): Merck Manual of Diagnosis and Therapy, 14th ed. Rahway, NJ, Merck Sharp & Dohme, 1982

Cello JP: Diagnostic approaches to jaundice. Hosp Pract 17(2):49–60, 1982

Cohen JA, Pantaleo N, Shell W: A message from the heart: What isoenzymes can tell you about your cardiac patient. Nursing 12(4):46–49, 1982

Davidsohn I, Henry JB: Todd-Sanford-Davidsohn Clinical Diagnosis and Management by Laboratory Methods, 17th ed. Philadelphia, WB Saunders, 1984

Dougherty WM: Serum bilirubin. Nursing 12(11):138–139, 1982

Halsted CH, Halsted JA (eds): The Laboratory in Clinical Medicine, 2nd ed. Philadelphia, WB Saunders, 1981

Isselbacher KJ et al. (eds): Harrison's Principles of Internal Medicine, 9th ed. New York, McGraw-Hill, 1980

Jacobs, DS et al: Laboratory Test Handbook. St. Louis, CV Mosby & Lexi-Corp., 1984

Kaplan LA, Perce A: Clinical Chemistry. St. Louis, CV Mosby, 1984

Leavelle DE (ed): Mayo Medical Laboratories Handbook. Rochester, MN, Mayo Medical Laboratories, 1986

Ravel R: Clinical Laboratory Medicine, 3rd ed. Chicago, Year Book Medical Pub, 1978

Sonnenwirth AC, Jarett L (eds): Gradwohl's Clinical Laboratory Methods and Diagnosis, 8th ed. St. Louis, CV Mosby, 1980

Stark JC: BUN/creatinine: Your keys to kidney function. Nursing 10(5):33–38, 1980

Tutz NW (ed): Clinical Guide to Laboratory Tests. Philadelphia, WB Saunders, 1983

White A et al (eds): Principles of Biochemistry, 6th ed. New York, McGraw-Hill, 1978

Whittier, FC: Proteinuria: Incidental finding or tip of the iceberg? Consultant 22(2):151–156, 1982

MICROBIOLOGICAL STUDIES

7

Introduction

Diagnostic Testing and Microbial Flora

Microorganisms in diagnostic testing are known as *pathogens*. The word pathogenic is usually defined as "causing infectious disease"; however, organisms that are pathogenic at certain times may reside in or on the human body at other times without causing disease. When these organisms are indeed present without causing harm to the host, they are considered *commensals*. But once they begin to multiply excessively and cause tissue damage, they are regarded as pathogens, for they will then have the potential for increasing pathogenicity (Table 7-1).

Host Factors

Certain important factors influence the development of an infectious disease.

General health of the patient
Patient's defense mechanisms
Previous contact with the particular organism
Development of immune substances, or antibodies
Past clinical history
Type of tissue involved in the infection
Stress to the body, not necessarily of microbial origin
Age of patient
Exposure to antibiotics

Collection of Specimens

General Principles

The health-care professional is responsible for the collection of specimens used for diagnostic examinations. Since procedures vary among the testing laboratories, it is recommended that you check with your laboratory for the preferred method of obtaining the specimen, delivering the specimen to the laboratory, preserving it when necessary, and reporting the results.

Precautions

Certain routine precautions must be taken in the collection and handling of specimens. Without these precautions the patient's condition may be incorrectly diagnosed, much laboratory time wasted, and the pathogenic organisms transmitted to health-care workers and to other patients.

Table 7-1
Pathogens Detectable in Body Tissue and Fluid by Diagnostic Methods

Nasopharynx	Sputum	Feces
Beta hemolytic streptococci	*Blastomyces dermatitidis*	*Candida albicans*
Bordetella pertussis	*Bordetella pertussis*	*Campylobacter fetus*
Candida albicans	*Candida albicans*	*Clostridium botulinum*
Corynebacterium diphtheriae	*Coccidioides immitis*	*Entamoeba histolytica*
Hemophilus influenzae (large counts)	Hemolytic streptococci	*Escherichia coli* (in infants)
Meningococci	*Hemophilus influenzae*	*Mycobacterium tuberculosis*
Pneumococci (large counts)	*Histoplasma capsulatum*	*Proteus*
Staphylococcus aureus	*Klebsiella* species	*Pseudomonas* (large counts)
	Mycobacterium tuberculosis	*Salmonella*
	Yersinia pestis	*Shigella*
	Francisella tularensis	*Staphylococci*
	Pneumococci	*Vibrio cholerae*
	Staphylococcus aureus	*Vibrio comma*
		Vibrio parahaemolyticus
		Yersinia enterocolitica
		Clostridium difficile

Urine	Skin	Ear
Beta hemolytic streptococci, groups B & D	*Bacteroides* species	*Aspergillus fumigatus*
Coliform bacilli (100,000 count or more) including *Escherichia coli,* *Klebsiella,* *Enterobacter-Serratieae*	*Clostridium*	*Candida albicans* and other fungi
Enterococci *Streptococcus faecalis)*	Coliform bacilli	Coliform bacilli
Gonococci *(Neisseria gonorrhoeae)*	Fungi	Hemolytic streptococci
Klebsiella, positive and negative indole	*Proteus*	*Proteus* species
Mycobacterium tuberculosis	*Pseudomonas*	Pneumococci *(Streptococcus pneumoniae)*
Proteus species	*Staphylococcus aureus*	*Pseudomonas aeruginosa*
Pseudomonas aeruginosa	*Streptococcus pyogenes*	*Staphylococcus aureus*
Staphylococci, positive and negative coagulase		
Salmonella and *Shigella* species		
Trichomonas vaginalis		
Candida albicans and other yeasts		

(Continued)

Table 7-1
Pathogens Detectable in Body Tissue and Fluid by Diagnostic
Methods (Continued)

Cerebrospinal Fluid	Vaginal Discharge	Urethral Discharge
Acinetobacter *calcoaceticus*	*Candida albicans* *Enterococci*	*Acinetobacter* *calcoaceticus*
Bacteroides species	*Gardnerella vaginalis*	
Coliform bacilli	*Listeria monocytogenes*	*Neisseria gonorrhoeae*
Cryptococcus *neoformans*	*Neisseria gonorrhoeae* *Treponema pallidum*	*Treponema pallidum* *Trichomonas vaginalis*
Edwardsiella tarda	*Hemophilus ducreyi*	
Hemophilus influenzae	*Chlamydia trachomatis*	
Leptospira species	*Herpes simplex virus*	
Mycobacterium *tuberculosis*	*Trichomonas vaginalis*	
Neisseria meningitidis		
Pneumococci, streptococcus pneumonia		
Pseudomonas		
Staphylococci		
Streptococci		
Viruses and fungi		
Listeria mono-cytogenes		

Sources of Specimens

Microbiological specimens may be collected from many sources: blood, pus or wound exudates, urine, sputum, feces, the genital tract, cerebrospinal fluid, an eye, or an ear. During collection these general procedures should be followed:

1. Label specimens
    Specimens should be labeled with
    (a) Patient's name, age, sex, address (or hospital number or physician's name and address)
    (b) Site of specimen (*e.g.*, throat, conjunctiva)
    (c) Time of collection
    (d) Nature of studies desired
    (e) Clinical diagnosis; microorganisms suspected
    (f) Duration of illness
    (g) Patient's immune state
    (h) Previous infection
    (i) Nature of any antibiotic therapy
    (j) If in isolation, state type
    (k) Any other information the laboratory requires

2. Avoid contamination
   Collection should be as aseptic as possible. Observe the following:
   (a) Special kits may be required; for example:
      (1) For anaerobes, syringe aspiration of pus or body fluid
      (2) Use of CO_2-containing transport media for tissue specimens (rather than collection of specimens on swabs).
   (b) Use only sterile specimen containers.
   (c) Do not spill any material on the outside of the container.
   (d) Use only standard plugs to stopper tubes and bottles.
   (e) Discard plugs and caps that have come in contact with non-sterile surfaces.
3. Preserve specimens
   Prompt delivery to the laboratory is desirable; however, many specimens may be refrigerated (not frozen) for a few hours without any adverse effects. Note the following:
   (a) Urine cultures must be *refrigerated* if results of diagnostic tests are to be of value.
   (b) Cerebrospinal fluid specimens should be transported quickly to the laboratory. If this is impossible, the culture should be *incubated*, for the suspected meningococcus will not withstand refrigeration.
4. Transport of specimens
   Care and speed of transport of specimens to the laboratory is urged. The material should be transported quickly to prevent drying out of the specimen and consequent death of the microorganisms.
   (a) With anaerobic cultures, no more than 10 minutes should elapse between collection and culture.
   (b) Urine should be *refrigerated* during transport to the laboratory.
   (c) Specimens suspected of containing anaerobic bacteria should be injected into a butyl rubber-stoppered gassed-out glass tube.
   (d) Feces suspected of having *Salmonella* or *Shigella* organisms should be placed in a special transport medium such as buffered glycerol–saline if culturing will be delayed.
5. Quantity of specimens
   The quantity of specimens should be as large as possible. When only a small quantity is available, swabs should be moistened with sterile saline. This procedure is especially important in nasopharyngeal cultures.
6. Collection of specimens
   (a) Whenever possible, specimens should be collected before an antibiotic regimen is instituted.
   (b) Collection must be geared to the rise in symptoms. (The practitioner should be familiar with the clinical course of the suspected disease.)

Diagnosis of Bacterial Disease: General Observations

Bacteriological studies are done to try to determine the specific organism that is causing an infection (Table 7-2). This organism may be specific for one disease, such as *Mycobacterium tuberculosis*, the causative agent of tuberculosis, or it may be organisms such as the *Staphylococcus* species that can cause a variety of infections. Antibiotic susceptibility or sensitivity tests are also done to determine the reactions of a specific organism to antibiotics.

The questions asked in searching for bacteria as the cause of a disease process are: (1) Are bacteria responsible for this disease? and (2) Is antimicrobial therapy indicated? Most bacterial diseases follow a febrile course. From a practical standpoint, relatively soon in the evaluation of a patient with fever a diagnosis must be reached and a decision made concerning antimicrobial therapy.

Disease due to anaerobic bacteria is commonly associated with localized necrotic abscesses, each of which may yield 2 to 13 different strains of bacteria. Because of the multiple species that can be isolated, the term *polymicrobic disease* is sometimes used to refer to anaerobic bacterial diseases. Diseases caused by anaerobic bacteria are in sharp contrast to the "one organism–one disease" concept that characterizes infections such as typhoid fever, cholera, and diphtheria. The isolation and identification of different strains of anaerobic bacteria are desirable so that appropriate therapy may be given. For instance, it is important when planning therapy for patients with anaerobic disease to know that certain drugs are not an effective or appropriate treatment.

Sensitivity (Susceptibility) of Bacteria to Antimicrobial Agents

A sensitivity (susceptibility) test detects the amount of antibiotic or chemotherapeutic agent required to inhibit the growth of bacteria. Often, a sensitivity test is ordered with a culture procedure. It is used prior to selection of appropriate drugs or for the alteration of an already imposed regimen of treatment.

The most common and most useful test for antibiotic sensitivity is the disc method. A basic set of antibiotic-impregnated discs is available for routine testing against the commonly isolated microorganisms. Specific amounts of an antibiotic are inoculated with a culture of the specific bacteria to be tested. After a suitable period of incubation, sensitivity of the organisms is determined by microscopic observation of the presence or absence of growth in the antimicrobial agent and by measurement of disc zones. The diameters in millimeters are compared against standards to determine if the organism is truly sensitive or of intermediate category. The sensitive drug is preferred over the intermediate drug.

Clinical Implications

1. The term *sensitive* or *susceptible* implies that an infection caused by the strain tested, such as streptococcus, may be expected to respond favorably to the indicated antimicrobial, such as penicillin, for that type of infection and pathogen.
2. The term *intermediate* or *partially resistant* or *moderately susceptible* means that the strain tested is not inhibited completely by therapeutic concentrations of a specific drug.
3. *Indeterminant* means that the organism may be susceptible or resistant to this method of testing. Usually these organisms will be susceptible to high blood levels of antibiotics.
4. The organism is not inhibited.
5. Many physicians rely more on published reports of the antibiotics usually effective against the organism isolated than on the sensitivity report, for sensitivity is an *in vitro* (in glass) test, and the antibiotic will be working *in vivo* (in the body).

Diagnosis of Rickettsial Disease: General Observations

Rickettsiae are small, gram-negative coccobacilli that structurally resemble bacteria, but on average are only one-tenth to one-half as large. Polychromatic stains (Giemsa stain) are better than simple stains or the gram stain for demonstrating rickettsiae in cells.

Rickettsiosis is the general name given to any disease caused by rickettsiae (Table 7-3). The organisms are considered to be *obligate intracellular parasites;* that is, they cannot exist anywhere except inside the bodies of living organisms. Diseases caused by rickettsiae are transmitted by *anthropod vectors:* lice, fleas, ticks, or mites (Table 7-4). Generally, these disease entities are divided into the following groups:

1. Typhuslike fevers
2. Spotted fever
3. Scrub typhus
4. Q fever
5. Other miscellaneous groups

Signs and Symptoms

1. Fever
2. Skin rashes
3. Parasitism of blood vessels
4. Prostration
5. Stupor and coma
6. Headache
7. Ringing in the ears
8. Dizziness

(*Text continues on page 372.*)

Table 7-2
Bacterial Diseases and Their Laboratory Diagnosis

Disease	Causative Organism	Source of Specimen	Diagnostic Tests
Anthrax	*Bacillus anthracis*	Blood, sputum, sore	Blood, sputum, and skin smear and culture; specific serologic test; biopsy
Brucellosis (undulant fever)	*Brucella melitensis, Br. abortus, Br. suis*	Blood, bone marrow	Blood and bone marrow culture; skin test; specific serologic test
Bubonic plague	*Yersinia pestis*	Buboes (enlarged and inflamed lymph nodes), blood, sputum	Skin, blood, and sputum smear; culture; agglutination test
Chancre	*Hemophilus ducreyi*	Penis	Penis smear culture; biopsy; serologic test
Cholera	*Vibrio cholerae*	Feces	Stool smear and culture; skin biopsy
Chlamydia once considered virus because of small size	*Chlamydia psittaci (Psittacosis)* *Chlamydia trachomatis*	Blood, sputum, lung	Culture, smears
Diphtheria	*Corynebacterium diphtheriae*	Pharynx	Pharyngeal smear and culture; Schick test
Dysentery	*Shigella dysenteriae*	Feces	Stool culture; serologic test
Endocarditis	*Staphylococcus aureus*	Petechiae	Petechial smear
Glander's disease	*Pseudomonas mallei*	Skin sore	Skin smear and culture; serologic test
Gonorrhea	*Neisseria gonorrhoeae*	Vagina, urethra, CSF, blood, joint fluid	Smear, culture, and serologic tests
Granuloma inguinale	*Calymmatobacterium granulomatis*	Penis, groin	Smears and culture from penis and groin

Disease	Organism	Specimen	Tests
Leprosy (Hansen's disease)	*Mycobacterium leprae*	Skin scrapings	Skin smear, biopsy, histamine lepromin, serologic test
Listeriosis	*Listeria monocytogenes*	Pharynx, blood, CSF	Pharyngeal, blood, and CSF smears and culture; serologic test
Meningitis	*Neisseria meningitidis* *Angiostrongylus cantonensis*	Pharynx, CSF, blood	Pharyngeal, CSF, and blood smears and cultures
Pertussis (whooping cough)	*Bordetella pertussis*	Trachea, bronchi, nasopharynx	Cultures of swabs of trachea and nasopharynx and bronchi; serologic test
Pharyngitis	*Streptococcus pyogenes*	Pharyngeal swab, sputum	Smear of sputum and pharyngeal swab culture; antistreptolysin O (ASO) test; C-reactive protein (CRP) test; serologic test
Pneumonia	*Hemophilus influenzae, Klebsiella pneumoniae, Staphylococcus aureus, Streptococcus pneumoniae*	Pharyngeal swab, CSF, sputum, blood exudates, effusions	Smear and culture of sputum, blood, CSF, nasopharyngeal specimens, and exudates and effusions
Tetanus	*Clostridium tetani*	Wound	Wound smear and culture
Tuberculosis	*Mycobacterium tuberculosis*	Sputum, gastric washings, urine, CSF	Smear and culture of sputum; gastric washings, urine and CSF; skin biopsy; skin test
Tularemia	*Francisella tularenis*	Skin, lymph node, pharynx	Foshay skin test; serologic test
Typhoid	*Salmonella typhosa*	Blood (after first week of infection); feces (after second week of infection)	Culture and serologic test

(After Collins RD: Illustrated Manual of Laboratory Diagnosis, 2nd ed. Philadelphia, JB Lippincott, 1975)

Table 7-3
Rickettsial Diseases and Their Laboratory Diagnosis

Disease		Natural Cycle			Transmission to Man	Serologic Diagnosis	
Group and Type	Agent	Geographical Distribution	Antropod	Mammal		Weil-Felix Reaction	Complement Fixation
Typhus							
Epidemic	*Rickettsia prowazekii*	Worldwide	Body louse	Man	Infected louse feces into broken skin	Positive OX-19	
Brill's disease	*R. prowazekii*	North America, Europe	Recurrence years after original attack of epidemic typhus			Usually negative	Positive group- and type-specific
Endemic	*R. typhi*	Worldwide	Flea	Rodents	Infected flea feces into broken skin	Positive OX-19	
Spotted fever							
Rocky Mountain spotted fever	*R. rickettsii*	Western Hemisphere	Ticks	Wild rodents, dogs	Tick bite	Positive OX-19 OX-2	
North Asian tick-borne rickettsiosis	*R. sibirica*	Siberia, Mongolia	Ticks	Wild rodents	Tick bite	Positive OX-19 OX-2	Positive group- and type-specific
Boutonneuse fever	*R. conorii*	Africa, Europe, Middle East, India	Ticks	Wild rodents, dogs	Tick bite	Positive OX-19 OX-2	
Queensland tick typhus	*R. australis*	Australia	Ticks	Marsupials, wild rodents	Tick bite	Positive OX-19 OX-2	
Rickettsialpox	*R. akari*	North America, Europe	Blood-sucking mite	House mouse and other rodents	Mite bite	Negative	
Scrub typhus							
Scrub typhus	*R. tsutsugamushi*	Asia, Australia, Pacific Islands	Tromiculid mite	Wild rodents	Mite bite	Positive OX-K	Positive in about 50% of patients
Q. fever	*Coxiella burnetti*	Worldwide	Ticks	Small mammals, cattle, sheep and goats	Inhalation of dried, infected material	Negative	Positive
Trench fever	*Rochalimaea quintana*	Europe, Africa, North America	Body louse	Man	Infected louse feces into broken skin	Negative	Low titer

(After Davis BD et al: Microbiology. 3rd ed. Hagerstown, MD, Harper and Row, 1980)

Table 7-4
Modes of Transmission of the Major Rickettsial Diseases

Disease in Man	Etiologic Agent	Chain of Transmission
Epidemic typhus Endemic typhus	R. prowazekii R. typhi	. . . Man→Louse→Man→Louse . . . Rat→Rat flea→Rat→Rat flea→Rat . . . ↓ Man
Rocky Mountain Spotted Fever (boutonneuse fever, other spotted fevers	R. rickettsii	. . . Tick→Tick→Tick→Tick . . . ↓ Dog Man ↓ Tick→Man
Scrub typhus (tsutsugamushi fever)	R. tsutsugamushi	. . . Mite→Field mouse→Mite→Field mouse . . . ↓ Man
Rickettsialpox	R. akari	. . . Mite→House mouse→Mite→House mouse . . . ↓ Man
Q fever	C. burnetii	. . . Tick→Small mammal→Tick→Cattle . . . (airborne) ↓ (airborne) Man

(After Davis BD et al: Microbiology. 3rd ed. Hagerstown, MD, Harper & Row, 1980)

Note: Rickettsial diseases are often characterized by an incubation period of 10 to 14 days, with an abrupt onset of the above signs and symptoms following a history of arthropod bites.

Diagnosis of Parasitic Disease: General Observations

Many parasitic infections are asymptomatic or produce only mild symptoms. Routine blood and stool examinations will uncover many unsuspected infections (Table 7-5).

Approximately 70 species of animal parasites commonly infect the body. More than half can be detected by examination of stool specimens, since the parasites inhabit the gastrointestinal tract and its environs. Of the parasites that can be diagnosed by stool examinations, one-third are single-celled protozoa and two-thirds are multicellular worms. Only six or seven of the intestinal protozoa are important clinically, but almost all of the worms are potentially pathogenic.

Collection of Specimens
1. In general, it is not possible to identify accurately a parasite from one submitted specimen.
2. Most parasites in humans are identified from blood or feces, but organisms may also be obtained from urine, sputum, tissue fluid, and biopsies.

Clinical Alert

The number of worms harbored is the most important factor in the diagnosis of parasitic worms.

Clinical Considerations
A. General
   1. *Eosinophilia* is regarded as a definite indication of a parasitic infection. Infections with parasitic worms and protozoa may have associated eosinophilia, which varies considerably depending on the reaction of the patient.
   2. Protozoa and helminths, particularly larvae, may be found in various organs and tissues of the body, as well as in the blood.
B. According to specimen
   1. *Hepatic puncture* is useful in the diagnosis of visceral leishmaniasis. Liver biopsy may reveal toxocaral larvae and schistosomal worms and eggs.

2. *Bone marrow* may be examined in trypanosomiasis and malaria when the blood is negative. Specimens are obtained by puncturing the sternum, crest of the ilium, vertebral processes, trochanter, or tibia.
3. *Lymph nodes* may be examined for the diagnosis of trypanosomiasis, leishmaniasis, toxoplasmosis, and filariasis either by puncture or biopsy.
4. Material from *mucous membranes* and *skin* may be obtained for examination by scraping, aspirating, or biopsy. Material may be obtained from the ulcer or nodule of the sore by puncturing the indurated margin of the lesion with a sterile hypodermic needle and aspirating gently.
5. The *cerebrospinal fluid* may be examined for trypanosomes and toxoplasma.
6. *Sputum* may be examined for presence of eggs of *Paragonimus westermani* (the lung fluke). Occasionally, the larvae and the hookworm of *Strongyloides stercoralis* and *Ascaris lumbricoides* may be coughed up during their pulmonary migration. In pulmonary echinococcosis (hydatid disease), the contents of the hydatid cyst may be evacuated in the sputum.

Diagnosis of Fungal Disease: General Observations

Fungal diseases, the mycoses, are now believed to be more common than in the past because of the widespread rise of the use of antibacterial agents and immunosuppressive drugs (Table 7-6). Fungi prefer the debilitated host, the individual with impaired immunity, chronic disease, or antibiotic therapy.

Of more than 50,000 species of fungi, approximately 50 are generally recognized as being pathogenic for humans. Fungi are organisms that live in a soil enriched by decaying nitrogenous matter and are capable of maintaining a separate existence by a parasitic cycle in humans or animals. The systemic mycoses are not communicable in the usual sense of human-to-human or animal-to-animal transfer. Humans become accidental hosts by the inhalation of spores or by their introduction into the tissues through trauma. Altered susceptibility may result in fungus lesions, as in patients having debilitating disease, diabetes, or impaired immunological mechanisms resulting from steroid or antimetabolite therapy. Prolonged administration of antibiotics can result in a superinfection by a fungus.

Fungal diseases can be classified according to the type of tissues involved.

(*Text continues on page 378.*)

Table 7-5
Parasitic Diseases and Their Laboratory Diagnosis

Disease	Causative Organism	Source of Specimen	Diagnostic Tests
Amebiasis	*Entamoeba histolytica*	Stool	Stool smear, rectal biopsy, and serologic test
Ascariasis	*Ascaris lumbricoides*	Stool, sputum	Stool and sputum smear
Cestodiasis of intestine (tapeworm disease)	*Taenia saginata* *Taenia solium* *Diphyllobothrium latum*	Stool	Stool smear and Scotch tape test
Chagas' disease	*Trypanosoma cruzi*	Blood Spinal fluid	Blood and spinal fluid smear; animal inoculation
Cysticercosis	*Taenia solium* larvae		Muscle and brain cyst biopsy
Echinococcosis	*Echinococcus granulosus*	Sputum Urine	Sputum and urine smear; serologic test; Casoni skin test; liver and bone biopsy
Enterobiasis (pinworm disease)	*Enterobius vermicularis*	Stool	Scotch tape smear
Filariasis	*Wuchereria bancrofti*	Blood	Blood smear; lymph node biopsy
Hookworm disease	*Ancylostoma duodenale* *Necator americanus*	Stool	Stool smear
Kala-azar	Leishman's anemia	Liver Bone marrow Blood	Liver, bone marrow, and blood smear and culture; animal inoculation; lymph node and spleen biopsy
Malaria	*Plasmodium falciparum* *Plasmodium malariae* *Plasmodium vivax* *Plasmodium ovale*	Blood Bone marrow	Blood and bone marrow smear; serologic test; Wasserman test

Disease	Organism	Specimen	Laboratory tests
Onchocerciasis	*Onchocerca volvulus*		Skin biopsy
Paragonimiasis	*Paragonimus westernani*	Sputum	Sputum and stool smear; serologic test; skin test
Scabies	*Sarcoptes scabiei*	Stool Skin	Skin smear; serologic test; skin test
Schistosomiasis of intestine and bladder	*Schistosoma mansoni* *Schistosoma japonicum* *Schistosoma haematobium*	Stool Urine	Urine and stool smear; serologic test; skin test; rectal, bladder, and liver biopsy
Strongyloidiasis	*Strongyloides stercoralis*	Stool Duodenal aspirate	Stool and gastric smear
Toxoplasmosis	*Toxoplasma gondii*		Animal inoculation; serologic test; skin test
Trichinosis	*Trichinella spiralis*		Serologic test; skin test; muscle biopsy
Trichomoniasis	*Trichomonas vaginalis*	Vagina Bladder Urethra	Vaginal and urethral smear and culture
Trichuriasis	*Trichuris trichiura*	Stool	Stool smear
Trypanosomiasis	*Trypanosoma rhodesiense* *Trypanosoma gambiense*	Blood Spinal fluid Lymph node	Blood, spinal fluid, and lymph node smear; animal inoculation; serologic test
Visceral larva migrans	*Toxocara canis* *Toxocara cati*		Serologic test; skin test; liver biopsy

(After Collins RD: Illustrated Manual of Laboratory Diagnosis. 2nd ed. Philadelphia, JB Lippincott, 1975)

Table 7-6
Fungal Diseases and Their Laboratory Diagnosis

Disease	Causative Organism	Source of Specimen	Diagnostic Tests
Actinomycosis	*Actinomyces israelii*	Skin, subcutaneous tissue, sputum	Skin, subcutaneous tissue, and sputum culture and smear; biopsy
Blastomycosis	*Blastomyces dermatitidis*	Skin, sputum	Skin and sputum smear and culture; serologic test; skin test
Candidiasis	*Candida albicans*	Mucous membrane, sputum	Mucous membrane and sputum smear and culture
Coccidioidomycosis	*Coccidioides immitis*	Sputum	Sputum smear, culture, animal inoculation, serologic test, skin test, biopsy
Histoplasmosis	*Histoplasma capsulatum*	Sputum Urine Blood Bone marrow	Smear, culture, animal inoculation, serologic test, skin test, and biopsy
Mucormycosis	Members of the order Mucorales (*Absidia*, *Rhizopus*, and *Mucor*)	Nose Pharynx Stool CSF	Nose, pharynx, stool and CSF culture; biopsy

Disease	Organism	Specimen	Laboratory test
Nocardiosis	Nocardia asteroides, Nocardia brasiliensis	Sputum, Spinal fluid	Sputum and spinal fluid culture and smear; biopsy
Sporotrichosis	Sporothrix schenckii	Skin	Skin culture and biopsy
Torulosis	Cyptococcus neoformans	Sputum, Spinal fluid	Sputum and spinal fluid smear and culture
Tinea pedis (athlete's foot)	Epidermophytons and Candida albicans	Skin	Hair, skin, and nail scrapings for culture
Tinea capitis (ringworm of scalp)	Microsporum (any species) and Trichophyton (all except T. concentricum)	Skin	Hair, skin, and nail scrapings for culture
Tinea barbae (ringworm of the beard, barber's itch)	Trichophytons and microsporums	Skin	Hair, skin, and nail scrapings for culture
Tinea cruris (jock itch)	Epidermophytons and Candida albicans	Skin	Hair, skin, and nail scrapings for culture

(After Collins RD: Illustrated Manual of Laboratory Diagnosis, 2nd ed. Philadelphia, JB Lippincott, 1975)

1. *Dermatophytoses* includes the superficial and cutaneous mycoses such as athlete's foot, ringworm, and "jock itch." Species of microsporum, epidermophyton, and trichophyton are the causative organisms of the dermatophytoses.
2. *Subcutaneous mycoses* involve the subcutaneous tissues and muscles.
3. *Systemic mycoses* involve the deep tissues and organs and are the most serious of all three groups.

Collection of Hair and Skin Specimens
1. Cleanse the area of suspected infection with 70% alcohol to remove bacteria.
2. Scrape the area with a sterile scalpel or wooden spatula, and place the specimen in a small sterile container with a lid.
3. Hair of the infected scalp or beard should be clipped and placed in a covered sterile container.
4. Hair stubs should be plucked out with a tweezer since the fungus is usually found at the base of the hair shaft. Using a Wood's light in a darkened room will help to identify the infected hairs.

Common Diagnostic Methods
1. Direct microscopic examination of material on a slide to determine whether a fungus is actually present
2. Wood's light to determine presence of a fungus. A Wood's light is a lamp using 3,660 Angstrom units of ultraviolet rays. When used in a darkened room, infected hairs will fluoresce a bright yellow-green color.
3. The potassium hydroxide (KOH) test to determine the presence of mycelial fragments, arthrospores, spherules, and budding yeast cells involves mixing the specimen in KOH on a glass slide, covering the slip, and applying gentle heat. The slide is examined microscopically for the above fungal elements.
4. A culture is done to identify the specific type of fungus. Fungi are slow growing and are subject to overgrowth by contaminating and more rapidly growing organisms.

Types of Specimens
1. Skin
2. Nails
3. Hair
4. Ulcer scrapings
5. Pus
6. Cerebrospinal fluid
7. Urine
8. Sputum
9. Blood
10. Bone marrow
11. Stool
12. Bronchial washings
13. Biopsies

Diagnosis of Spirochetal Disease: General Observations

Spirochetes are spiral and curved bacteria. There are four genera of spiral and curved bacteria, which include a number of human pathogens. The genera are *Borrelia*, *Treponema*, *Leptospira*, and *Spirillum* (Table 7-7).

Clinical Considerations

1. *Borrelia*
   (a) *Borrelia* appears in the blood at the onset of various forms of relapsing fever. This genus is responsible for European and American relapsing fever.
   (b) *Borrelia vincentii* is the species responsible for ulcerative gingivitis (trench mouth).
2. *Treponema*
   (a) *Treponema pallidum* is the species responsible for venereal and nonvenereal syphilis in humans.
   (b) *Treponema pertenue* is the causative agent of yaws.
   (c) *Treponema carateum* causes pinta (carate).

Table 7-7
Spirochetal Diseases and Their Laboratory Diagnosis

Disease	Causative Organism	Source of Specimen	Diagnostic Tests
Pinta	*Treponema carateum*	Skin	Skin smear, serologic test
Rat-bite fever	*Spirillum minus* *Streptobacillus moniliformis*	Blood Joint fluid	Skin, blood, and joint fluid culture and serologic test
Relapsing fever	*Borrelia recurrentis*	Blood	Blood smear and culture and serologic test
Syphilis	*Treponema pallidum*	Skin	Skin smear; TPI and FTA-Ab test
Weil's disease (leptospiral jaundice)	*Leptospira icterohaemorrhagiae*	Urine, blood, CSF	Urine and blood smear; culture-muscle biopsy; serologic test
Yaws	*Treponema pertenue*	Skin	Skin smear and serologic test

(After Collins RD: Illustrated Manual of Laboratory Diagnosis, 2nd ed. Philadelphia, JB Lippincott, 1975)

3. *Leptospira*
   (a) *Leptospira* is the genus of microorganism responsible for Weil's disease (infectious jaundice), swamp fever, swineherd's disease, and canicola fever.
   (b) The organism is widely distributed in the infected person and appears in the blood early in the disease.
   (c) After 10 to 14 days the organisms are present in considerable numbers in the urine.
   (d) Patients with Weil's disease show striking antibody responses, and serologic testing is useful in diagnosis.
4. *Spirillum*
   Streptobacillus moniliformis as well as *Spirillum minus* is the species responsible for rat-bite fever. The condition occurs worldwide, is common in Japan and Asia, but uncommon in North and South America and most European countries. Cases in the USA have followed bites by laboratory rats.

Diagnosis of Viral and Mycoplasmal Disease: General Observations

Viral diseases are the most common of human infections. Once thought to be confined to the childhood years, viral infections in adults have increasingly been recognized as the cause of morbidity and death. They include infectious diseases such as hepatitis and AIDS and other sexually transmitted diseases; they are considered as possible etiologic agents in cancer, and they affect immunosuppressed patients and the elderly.

Viruses are submicroscopic, filterable, infectious organisms that exist as intracellular parasites. They are divided into two groups according to the type of nucleic acid they contain: ribonucleic acid (RNA) or deoxyribonucleic acid (DNA).

Mycoplasmas are scotobacteria without cell walls and are surrounded by a single triple-layered membrane. They are also known as *pleuropneumonia-like organisms* (PPLO).

Viruses and mycoplasmas are both small, infectious agents that are capable of passing through bacteria-retaining filters. Although smallness is the only property they have in common, viruses and mycoplasmas cause illnesses that are often indistinguishable from each other in clinical signs and symptoms, and both are found together frequently as a double infection. Thus, the serologic (antigen–antibody) procedures that are used commonly in the diagnosis of viral disease are also used for diagnosing cases of mycoplasmal infection (Table 7-8).

Table 7-8
Virus Study Procedures

Disease or Syndrome	Clinical Specimens	Suspected Viral Agents
Nervous System		
Aseptic meningitis	Stool	Enteroviruses (Cox-
Encephalitis	Throat swab	sackie, echo, polio)
Poliomyelitis	CSF	Toga virus
	(Acute and convalescent	*Herpes simplex, Vari-*
	sera)	*cella zoster,* mumps,
		measles
Respiratory		
URI	Throat washing or	Adeno-, rhino-, entero-,
	swab	myxo-, respiratory
Croup	Nasopharyngeal swab	syncytial
Bronchiolitis	(Acute and convalescent	
Influenza	sera)	
Viral pneumonia		
Infectious mono-	Serology	Epstein–Barr
nucleosis		
Exanthema and rashes		
Chickenpox	Vesicle swab	*Varicella zoster*
Zoster (shingles)	Throat swab	*Herpes simplex*
Herpes simplex	Stool	Coxsackie A
Herpangina	Urine	Measles
Measles	(Acute and convalescent	Rubella
Rubella	sera)	
Perinatal infections		
Cytomegalic inclu-	Urine	Cytomegalovirus
sion disease	Throat swab	Rubella
Rubella syndrome	CSF	*Herpes simplex*
Herpes simplex	(Acute and convalescent	
	sera)	
Gastrointestinal		
Diarrhea	Stool (For ELISA or	Rotavirus
	EM) 10–20 g as	Enterovirus
	soon after onset as	Adenovirus
	possible	Norwalk Agent
Myocarditis, peri-		
carditis,		
Pleurodynia	Stool	Coxsackie B
Epidemic myalgia	Throat swab	Echovirus
Myopericarditis	Pericardial or pleural	Cytomegalovirus
Lymphadenopathy	fluid	Other etiology
	(Acute and convalescent	
	sera)	
Eye infections	Conjunctival swab or	*Herpes simplex, adeno-*
	scraping	*varicella zoster,*
Hepatitis	Serology	vaccinia
		B, A, and Non A, Non B
		Delta virus

(After August MJ: Practical aspects of viral diagnosis. J Med Technol 2(8):502, August 1985)

Physiologically, mycoplasmas are considered generally as an intermediate disease stage between bacteria and rickettsiae. One species, *Mycoplasma pneumoniae*, is recognized as the causative agent of primary atypical pneumonia and bronchitis. Other species are suspected as possible agents in urethritis, infertility, early abortion, rheumatoid arthritis, myringitis, and erythema multiforme.

Approach to Diagnosis
1. Viral isolation in tissue culture remains the gold standard for the detection of many common viruses.
   (a) Tissue culture
   (b) Special media
   (c) Typing such as: Herpes Simplex
   (d) Identification reagents, immunofluorescence and immunoperoxidase
   (e) Electron microscope
2. Serology for antigen–antibody detection
3. The variety of available cell cultures vary greatly in sensitivity to different viruses. It is important to understand that one cell type or species may be more sensitive than another for the detection of virus in low titers. For example: Primary human monkey kidney (1 MK) can be used for adenovirus, enterovirus, herpes simplex, measles, mumps, myxovirus, pox, rubella, and varicella zoster; and human embryonic kidney (HEK) cannot be used for cytomegalovirus or myxovirus.
4. The critical first step in successful viral diagnosis is the timely and proper collection of specimens. The choice of which specimen to collect depends upon the typical signs and symptoms and the virus suspected. The improper choice and collection of specimens is one of the biggest factors in time wasted in obtaining a viral diagnosis.

Specimen Collection
1. As early as possible in the course of the illness; the first four days after symptom onset
2. Sampling
   (a) Localized infection
      (1) Direct sampling of affected site. Examples: throat swab or skin scraping
      (2) Indirect sampling. Example: If target sample is CSF in CNS infection, the indirect approach is throat swab or stool specimens for culture.
      (3) Sampling from more than one site. Example: In disseminated disease or non-specific clinical findings.
      (4) Applicators used to obtain specimens may affect successful recovery of viral agent. No wooden applicators; they are toxic to viruses, as well as chlamydia, bacteria, and mycoplasma

(5) Transporting Specimens
(a.) Keep in mind that viral specimens are unstable. Viruses rapidly lose infectivity outside of living cells.
(b.) Prompt delivery to laboratory is essential. Samples must be refrigerated and placed in a container with wet ice or cold packs for transit.
(c.) No freezing or thawing of specimens. This diminishes the quantity of viable virus.

Clinical Considerations
1. Herpes simplex virus is the virus most frequently isolated in clinical laboratories today.
2. The most common serologic request is acute viral titers (see page 444 for complete serology discussion).
3. Average waiting time for viral culture results is 3 to 4 days; more than 70% can be reported in 5 days. Rapid test results (24 hours) are accurate and available for some viruses such as cytomegalovirus (CMV).
4. Significance of viral cultures:
   (a) Positive viral culture results *diagnostic* for these sources

(1) Autopsy	(5) Other fluids
(2) Blood	(6) Cervix
(3) Biopsy	(7) Eye
(4) CSF	(8) Skin lesions

   Probably diagnostic (diagnostic if confirmed by serology)

(1) Throat	(2) Urine

   Possibly diagnostic
   Stool
   (b) In contrast to normal bacterial inhabitants of humans, viruses do not compromise flora at any site. However, bacterial or fungal contamination of specimens can occur.

Diagnosis of Sexually Transmitted Diseases: General Observations

Sexually transmitted diseases are an ever-increasing public health problem and are caused by a variety of etiologic agents (Table 7-9). Some conditions, such as chlamydia and nongonococcal urethritis (NGU), have reached epidemic proportions. Although NGU is nonreportable in the U.S.A., it is estimated that more than 2 million new cases occur each year. Manifestations of infection range from asymptomatic carriers to a spectrum of disease that includes cervicitis, conjunctivitis, endometritis, epididymitis, infertility, pharyngitis, proc-
(*Text continues on page 386.*)

Table 7-9
Sexually Transmitted Diseases and Their Laboratory Diagnoses

Disease*	Causative Agents†	Diagnosis
Chancroid	*Hemophilius ducreyi*	Gram stain of lesion or aspirate. Differential diagnosis should include syphilis and herpes culture.
Gonorrhea	*Neisseria gonorrhoeae*	Gram stain of male urethra, culture of male urethra or female cervix, rectum, or pharynx. When indicated, urogenital swab tested for direct antigen.
Granuloma inguinale (Donovanosis)	*Calymmatobacterium granulomatis* (formerly Donovania granulomatis)	Wright's or Gram stain of lesion, tissue biopsy
Hepatitis B	Hepatitis B virus (HBV)	Serologic testing HB$_e$Ag—most infectious state of disease. HB$_s$Ag: presence and persistence of infectivity and chronicity usually appear prior to symptoms.
Genital herpes	*Herpes simplex* virus (HSV) types 1 and 2	Culture from unroofed blister, scrapings examined by fluorescent microscopy or cytologic stains
Lymphogranuloma venereum (LGV)	*Chlamydia trachomates* serotypes L$_1$, L$_2$, and L$_3$	Aspirate of bubo, serologic tests of blood
Molluscum contagiosum	Molluscum contagiosum virus	Clinical appearance of lesions (pearly white, painless, umbilicated papules), microscopic exam of scrapings
Chlamydia	*Chlamydia trachomates* serotypes D–K	Cell culture, urogenital swabs for direct antigen test, or fluorescent microscopy
Candidosis (manilia)	*Candida albicans*	Culture, KOH wet mount
Pelvic inflammatory disease (PID)	*Neisseria gonorrhoeae chlamydia trachomatis*	Clinical symptoms, cervical culture, laparoscopy, or culdocentesis
Pediculosis pubis	*Phthirus pubis* (pubic or crab louse)	Adult lice or nits appear on body hairs
Scabies	*Sarcoptes scabiei*	Characteristic lesions, scrapings for microscopy
Syphilis	*Treponema pallidum*	Darkfield microscopic exam of primary and secondary lesions for *T. pallidum*. Nontreponemal reagin tests (VDRL, RPR) and specific tests (FTA–ABS, MHA–TP) are used to identify active and latent syphilis
Trichomoniasis	*Trichomonas vaginalis*	Vaginal, urethral, prostatic secretion examined microscopically in a drop of saline for motile trichomonas; culture; speculum exam reveals foamy, greenish discharge and presence of bright red dots in vaginal wall and cervix

Condition	Pathogens	Diagnosis
Nonspecific urethritis (Nongonococcal urethritis–NGU)	*Chlamydia trachomatis* (50% of cases), urea-plasma urealyticum, a human T-strain mycoplasma (*mycoplasma hominis*), *Trichomonas vaginalis*, *Candida albicans*, *Herpes simplex* virus	Failure to demonstrate *Neisseria gonorrhoeae* cell culture
Nonspecific vaginitis	*Gardnerella vaginalis*	West mount or PAP smear; fishy smell is released when specimen fluid is mixed with 10% KOH. Culture or enzyme immunoassay to RO gonorrhea
Condylomata Acuminata (venereal warts)	Human papilloma DNA Virus	Typical clinical lesion; cauliflowerlike, soft, pink growths around vulva, anus, labia, vagina, glans penis, urethra and perineum. RO syphilis.
Acquired Immune Deficiency Syndrome (AIDS)	HIV Virus	Serology
Gastrointestinal (Giardiasis Amebiasis, shigellosis, camp/bacteriosis, and anorectal infections.	Enteric infections: *Giardia lamblia* *Entamoeba histolytica* *Cryptoporidum* spp. *Shigella* spp. *Campylobacter fetus* *Strongyloides* spp. (worms)	Stool-polyvinyl alcohol fixative or formalin ethyl acetate sedimentation (FES). Same as above. Stool stain Rectal stool swab culture Rectal stool swab culture Stool (FES)
	Anorectal: *Neisseria gonorrhoeae* *Chlamydia trachomatis* *Triponema pallidum* *Herpes simplex* virus Human papilloma virus	Anal canal swab Specimen, culture Anal swab or rectal biopsy Darkfield microscopy plus serology, lesion swab, culture Signs and symptoms

* The *major* diseases are syphilis and gonorrhea.

† The pathogens causing sexually transmitted diseases span the full range of medical microbiology. The only common characteristic of these pathogens is that they may cause genital disease or may be transmitted by genital contact.

titis, lymphogranuloma venereum, salpingitis, trachoma, urethritis and, in the neonate, conjunctivitis and pneumonia.

Suggested Specimens
1. Urine
2. Semen
3. Urethral, vaginal, cervical, or oral swabs
4. Prostatic secretion
5. Tissue biopsy
6. Blood
7. Stool

Common Diagnostic Methods
1. Viral isolation in tissue cell cultures
2. Specific serologic antibody assays and syphilis detection tests
3. Cytologic techniques such as PAP and Zanck smears to demonstrate giant cells of herpes virus infection.
4. Gram's stain
5. ELISA and immunoperoxidase assay to detect causative agent
6. Monoclonal antibodies to detect and identify etiologic agent.

Clinical Considerations
1. Patients with one sexually transmitted disease are frequently infected with other sexually transmitted pathogens.
2. Asymptomatic carriage is more common than generally realized.
3. Tracing of sexual partners is very important.
4. Treatment failure may occur because the patient has been reinfected by a nontreated partner.
5. A certain subset of promiscuous male homosexuals is an important reservoir of sexually transmitted disease.

DIAGNOSTIC PROCEDURES

Six classes of laboratory tests are used in the diagnosis of infectious diseases: smears and stains, cultures, animal inoculation, tissue biopsy, serologic testing, and skin testing. Cultures and skin testing are described in detail in this chapter. Serologic testing is described in Chapter 8. A brief description of each of these procedures follows.

The Smear
A smear is a specimen for microscopic study that is prepared by spreading a small quantity of material across a glass slide. If the material is to be stained, it is generally fixed to the slide by passing the slide quickly through the flame of a Bunsen burner.

The Stain
Smears are most often observed after they have been stained. Stains are salts composed of a positive and negative ion, one of which is colored. Structures in the specimen pick up the stain, thereby making

the organism visible under the light microscope. One staining procedure, called the *negative stain*, colors the background and leaves the organisms uncolored. The gross structure of the organisms can then be seen.

Types of Stains: Bacterial stains are of two major types: *simple* and *differential*. A *simple stain* consists of a coloring agent such as gentian violet, crystal violet, carbol-fuchsin, methylene blue, or safranine. A thin smear of organisms is stained and then observed under the oil-immersion lens. A *differential stain* is one in which two chemically different stains are applied to the same smear. Organisms that are physiologically different will pick up different stains.

The *Gram stain* is the most important of all bacteriologic differential stains; it divides bacteria into two physiologic groups: gram-positive and gram-negative.

The staining procedure has four major steps: (a) staining the smear with gentian or crystal violet; (2) washing off the violet stain and flooding the smear with an iodine solution; (3) washing off the iodine solution and flooding the smear with 95% alcohol, and (4) counterstaining the smear with safranine, a red dye.

In addition to allowing for morphologic study of the bacteria under question, the Gram stain, as mentioned, divides all bacteria into two physiological groups according to their ability or inability to pick up one or both of the two stains. The two categories of bacteria (gram-positive and gram-negative) exhibit different properties, which help in their identification.

Other stains besides the Gram stain are used in examinations of bacteriologic smears. Some, such as the *acid-fast stain*, are used in identifying organisms of the genus *Mycobacterium*. Others are employed in the differentiation of certain structures such as capsules, endospores, and flagella.

Cultures

A culture is the growth of microorganisms or living tissue cells on special media conducive to the growth of this material. Cultures may be maintained in test tubes, petri dishes, dilution bottles, or any other suitable container. The container holds a food (called the *culture medium*) that is either solid, semisolid, or liquid. Each organism has its own special requirements for growth (proper combination of nutritive ingredients, temperature, and presence or absence of oxygen). The culture is prepared in accordance with its food needs. Later, it is either refrigerated or incubated according to the temperature requirements for growth.

Animal Inoculation

Animal inoculation is the means used to isolate bacteria when other means have failed. For example, when tuberculosis is suspected but smears have failed to confirm the disease, guinea pig inoculation is used. The organisms responsible for plague (*Yersinia pestis*) and tularemia (*Francisella tularensis*) may be isolated by animal inoculation. When viruses, certain spirochetes, certain fungi, and some parasites must be identified, animal inoculation is often used.

Tissue Biopsy
At times, microorganisms are isolated from small quantities of body tissue that have been surgically removed in the operating room or in the physician's office. Such tissue is removed using full aseptic technique and is transferred to a sterile container to be transported rapidly to the laboratory for analysis. Generally, the specimens are ground finely in a sterile homogenizer and plated out.

Serologic Testing
Serologic testing, which will be discussed in detail in Chapter 8, is a method for analysis of blood specimens for antigen–antibody reactions. This form of testing is generally valuable in diagnosis only late in the course of the infection. Specimens should be collected immediately after the patient has been admitted to the hospital, and again, 3 to 4 weeks after the onset of the disease.

Skin Testing
Skin testing, which will be described later in this chapter, is used to determine hypersensitivity of a person to the toxic products formed in the body by pathogens. Three types of skin tests are generally employed: scratch tests, patch tests, and intradermal tests.

BLOOD CULTURES

Background
Blood for culture is probably the single most important specimen submitted to the microbiological laboratory for examination. Blood cultures are collected whenever there is reason to suspect bacteremia or septicemia. Although a mild transitory bacteremia is a frequent finding in many infectious diseases, the persistent, continuous, or recurrent type of bacteremia is indicative of a more serious condition.

Indications for Blood Culture
1. Bacteremia
2. Septicemia
3. Unexplained postoperative shock
4. Postoperative shock following genitourinary tract manipulation
5. Unexplained fever of more than several days' duration
6. Chills and fever in patients with
   (a) Infected burns

(b) Urinary tract infections
(c) Rapidly progressing tissue infections
(d) Postoperative wound sepsis
(e) Indwelling venous or arterial catheters
7. Debilitated patients undergoing therapy with
(a) Antibiotics
(b) Corticosteroids
(c) Immunosuppressives
(d) Antimetabolites
(e) Parenteral hyperalimentation

Note: In typhoid fever and certain other diseases such as tularemia and plague, blood cultures are positive only in certain stages of the disease. Therefore, the clinician should be familiar with the clinical course of the disease, so that the most advantageous time for taking a blood sample may be known.

Procedure for Obtaining Blood Culture

Clinical Alert

In venipuncture, the potential for infecting the patient as a result of the diagnostic procedure is very high. Therefore, aseptic technique must be rigorously followed.

1. The proposed puncture site should be scrubbed with an antiseptic such as Betadine (povidone-iodine) or 70% alcohol.
2. The rubber stoppers of culture bottles should be cleansed with iodine and allowed to air dry. They should then be cleansed with 70% alcohol.
3. Venipuncture should be performed with a sterile syringe and needle, avoiding any contamination of the cleansed site.
4. Approximately 10–15 ml. of blood should be drawn in a 20 ml. syringe.
5. After the specimen is obtained, the needle on the syringe should be discarded and replaced with a second sterile needle before the sample is injected into the culture bottles.
6. If two culture bottles are to be inoculated (one anaerobic and one aerobic,) the anaerobic bottle should be inoculated first with enough blood to have a 1:10 dilution of a blood:broth mixture. Then the aerobic bottle should be inoculated aseptically to the same dilution.
7. The needle and syringe should be removed from the bottle and both

bottles should be mixed gently. To vent the aerobic bottle, a cotton plugged needle specially designed for that purpose should be used.
8. Specimens should be properly labeled with the patient's name, age, date, time, number of culture, notation of patient isolation category (if applicable), and any other information the laboratory requires.

Clinical Alert

1. Handle all blood specimens as if they are capable of transmitting disease.
2. After disinfection, *do not probe* the venipuncture site with a finger unless sterile gloves are worn or the finger has been disinfected. Probing is the greatest potential cause of contamination in blood culture.
3. The attending physician should be notified immediately about positive cultures so that appropriate treatment may be started immediately.
4. If a specimen is spilled, and the patient is in blood or body fluid isolation, far more caution must be observed than if the patient is in respiratory isolation.

Clinical Implications

A. *Negative cultures*
   If all cultures, subcultures, and Gram-stained smears are negative, the blood culture may be reported as: *No growth, aerobic or anaerobic, after 3 days' incubation. Further report to follow. Final report: No growth after 7 to 14 days' incubation.*
B. *Positive cultures*
   Pathogens most commonly found in blood cultures include the following:

1. *Bacteroides* species
2. *Brucella* species
3. Coliform bacilli
4. Filariae*
5. *Francisella tularensis*
6. *Hemophilus influenzae*
7. *Leptospira* species
8. *Listeria monocytogenes*
9. Malaria*
10. *Neisseria meningitidis*
11. Pneumococci
12. Rickettsiae*
13. *Staphylococcus aureus,*
    S. epidermidis,
    S. saprophyticus
14. *Streptococcus pyogenes*

* Culture is not the ideal method for isolating parasites. Peripheral blood smears are the usual method for detection of parasites.

15. *Salmonella* species
16. Trypanosomes*

17. Gram-negative rods *E. Coli*, Enterobactic species, klebsiella species, etc.

Interfering Factors
1. Blood cultures are subject to contamination, especially by skin bacteria. These organisms should therefore be identified in the laboratory.
2. Nonfilterable blood is usually due to the presence of abnormal proteins.

Special Situation
With patients who have already received antibacterial therapy, certain enzymes may be incorporated into the growth medium to eliminate the activity of the antibacterial agent in the blood.

URINE CULTURES

Normal Values
Negative: less than 10,000 organisms/ml. Any bacteria found are either contaminants from the skin or invading pathogens.

Clinical Alert
1. A bacterial count of less than 10,000 bacteria per ml. is not indicative of infection and possibly may be contamination. A count of 100,000 or more bacteria per ml. indicates infection.
2. Urine cultures of *E. coli* are not definitely significant unless they contain more than 100,000 organisms per ml.

Background
Urine cultures are most commonly used to diagnose a bacterial infection of the urinary tract (kidneys, ureter, bladder, and urethra). Urine is an excellent culture medium for most organisms that infect the urinary tract, grow within the urine in the body, and result in high counts in established untreated infection. The combination of pyuria (pus in the urine) and significant bacteriuria strongly suggest the diagnosis of urinary tract infection.

* Culture is not the ideal method for isolating parasites. Peripheral blood smears are the usual method for detection of parasites.

Collection of Specimens for Culture:
General Principles

1. Early morning specimens should be obtained whenever possible because bacterial counts are highest at that time.
2. A clean voided urine specimen of 3–5 ml. should be collected in a sterile container. Specimens may also be collected by catheterization, suprapubic aspiration, or directly from an indwelling catheter. Urine must not be obtained from a urine-collecting bag.

Clinical Alert

Catheterization heightens the risk of introducing infection. Whenever possible, avoid collecting urine by this method. DO NOT catheterize when merely a bacteriological specimen is needed.

3. Urine should be taken to the laboratory as soon as possible and examined immediately. When this is not possible, the urine can be refrigerated (maximum 2 hours storage time) until cultured, if necessary.
   If collected for cytomegalovirus, the urine specimen should be kept at room temperature until taken to the virus laboratory for culture. *If refrigerated, the virus will be destroyed.*
4. Two successive clean-voided or midstream specimens should be collected in order to be 95% certain that true bacteriuria is present.
5. Whenever possible, specimens should be obtained before antibiotics or other antimicrobial agents have been administered.
6. The instruction for collection of all specimens should be the responsibility of professional health personnel (nurse, physician, medical technologist). Failure to isolate a causative organism is frequently the result of faulty collection techniques that can come from misinformation about the collection procedure.
7. Proper supplies and privacy for cleansing and collection should be provided. (Sterile specimen containers and antiseptic sponges should be available.)
8. Properly instructed patients will usually cleanse their pelvis or vulva and perineum at least as well as the health attendant. However, when the patient is unable to follow the procedure, a trained person can cleanse the patient and collect the specimen.
9. The specimen should be covered and labeled with
   (a) Patient's name
   (b) Suspected clinical diagnosis
   (c) Method of collection

(d) Precise time obtained
(e) Whether forced fluids or IVs have been administered
(f) Any specific chemotherapeutic agents being administered

Procedure for Collection of Midstream or Clean-Catch Urine Specimen

Clinical Alert

Urine is an excellent culture medium, which at room temperature allows the growth of many organisms. Collection of specimens, therefore, should be as aseptic as possible. Samples should be taken immediately to the laboratory where they can be examined while still warm. If prompt analysis is not possible, the specimen must be refrigerated (2 hours maximum storage).

1. Women
   (a) Lower undergarments are to be removed.
   (b) Patient should thoroughly wash hands with soap and water and then dry them with a disposable towel.
   (c) The cap from a sterile container should be removed and placed with its outer surface down in a clean area.
   (d) The area around the urinary meatus must be cleaned from front to back with an antiseptic sponge.
   (e) With one hand, the patient should spread the labia, keeping them apart until the specimen is collected.
   (f) After cleansing, the patient voids. After the first 25 ml. has been passed into the toilet bowl, the urine is caught directly into the sterile container without stopping the stream. The patient voids until the container is almost full. The collection cup should be held in such a way that contact with the legs, vulva, or clothing is avoided. Fingers should be kept away from the rim and inner surface of the container.
2. Men
   (a) Patient washes as in (b) above.
   (b) The foreskin is completely retracted to expose the glans.
   (c) The area around the meatus is cleansed with antiseptic sponges.
   (d) Patient is to pass the first portion of urine (25 ml.) directly into the toilet bowl and then pass a portion of the remaining urine into the sterile specimen container. The patient voids until the container is almost full. The last few drops of urine should not be collected.

3. Infants and children

    In infants and young children, urine may be collected in a plastic collection apparatus. Since the collection bag touches skin surfaces and thereby picks up commensals, the specimen must be analyzed as soon as possible.

Clinical Implications

A count of 100,000 or more bacteria per ml. indicates infection. A bacterial count of less than 10,000 bacteria per ml. is not indicative of infection and possibly may be contamination. When present in significant titer, the following organisms, present in the urine, may be considered pathogenic.

1. Coliform bacilli
2. Enterococci
3. Gonococcus
4. *Klebsiella* (often)
5. *Mycobacterium tuberculosis*
6. *Proteus* species
7. *Pseudomonas aeruginosa*
8. Staphylococci, coagulase positive and coagulase negative
9. Streptococci, beta hemolytic, usually Groups B and D
10. *Trichomonas vaginalis*

Interfering Factors

1. The urine of patients who are receiving forced fluids may be sufficiently diluted to reduce the colony count below 10^5 per ml.
2. Bacterial contamination comes from sources such as
    (a) Hair from the perineum
    (b) Bacteria from beneath the prepuce in males
    (c) Bacteria from vaginal secretions from the vulva or from the distal urethra in females
    (d) Bacteria from the hands, skin, or clothing

Patient Preparation

1. Explain the purpose and procedure of the test to the patient.
2. The cleansing procedure must remove contaminating organisms from the vulva, urethral meatus, and perineal area so that bacteria found in the urine can be assumed to have come from the bladder and urethra only.

Clinical Alert

The urine studied for culture should *not* be a sample taken from a urinal or bedpan and should *not* be brought from home. The urine is to be collected directly into a sterile container that will be used for culture.

Special Situation
With suspected urinary tuberculosis, the specimen should consist of three consecutive early-morning samples that are pooled in the laboratory. Special care should be taken in washing the external genitalia to reduce contamination with commensal acid-fast *M. smegmatis.*

RESPIRATORY TRACT CULTURES

Four major types of cultures may be used to diagnose infectious diseases of the respiratory tract: (1) sputum, (2) throat swabs, (3) nasal swabs, and (4) nasopharyngeal swabs. At times, the purposes for which certain tests are ordered will overlap. Each of these cultures will be described below.

Normal Values
The following organisms may be present in the nasopharynx of apparently healthy individuals:

1. *Candida albicans*
2. Diphtheroid bacilli
3. *Hemophilus hemolyticus*
4. *Hemophilus influenzae*
5. *Branhamella catarrhalis*
6. *Staphylococcus aureus* (occasionally)
7. Staphylococci (coagulase-negative)
8. Streptococci (alpha-hemolytic)
9. Streptcococci (nonhemolytic)

Clinical Alert

1. Twenty per cent of normal adults are carriers of *Staphylococcus aureus;* 10% are carriers of Group A hemolytic streptococci.
2. A new 10-minute strep test is being used that gives results after 10 minutes instead of 24–48 hours. It shows a false negative of 5% to 10%, about the same as traditional methods. It permits rapid diagnosis and treatment.

3. Both throat and urine cultures are done to detect Epstein–Barr virus (EBV) and CMV.

Sputum

Background
Sputum is *not* material from the postnasal region and is *not* spittle or saliva. A specimen of sputum must be coughed up from deep within the bronchi.

Indications for Collection
Sputum cultures are important in the diagnosis of the following conditions:

1. Bacterial pneumonia
2. Pulmonary tuberculosis
3. Chronic bronchitis
4. Bronchiectasis
5. Suspected pulmonary mycotic infections
6. Mycoplasma pneumonia infection
7. Suspected viral pneumonia

Procedure
1. Sputum must be coughed up from the bronchi.
2. The specimen must be collected in a clear, sterile container, and the container must be capped.
3. The volume of the expectorate need not exceed 1 to 3 ml. of purulent or mucopurulent material. This quantity is sufficient for most examinations except tuberculosis testing.
4. The specimen should be examined before delivery to the laboratory to determine whether the specimen is truly sputum and not saliva. Too often the culturing of unsuitable material (saliva) results in misleading information because the true infecting agent has not been observed.

Maintenance and Delivery of Specimen
1. Specimens should not be refrigerated.
2. Specimens should be delivered to the laboratory rapidly, so that organisms are still viable.
3. All specimens should be labeled with the name of the patient, date, room number, and suspected disease.

Patient Preparation
1. The patient should be instructed that this test requires tracheo-bronchial sputum, a substance from the lungs that is brought up by a deep cough.
2. The use of superheated hypertonic saline aerosols for sputum induction is recommended when the cough is not productive. Proper decontamination of the equipment must be carried out.

Clinical Alert

In children or adults who cannot produce sputum, a laryngeal swab may be taken.

Throat Culture (Swab) (Washings)

Indications for Collection
1. Throat cultures are important in the diagnosis of the following conditions:
    (a) Streptococcal sore throat
    (b) Diphtheria
    (c) Thrush (candidal infection of the mouth)
    (d) Tonsillar infection
2. Throat cultures are useful in establishing the focus of infection in
    (a) Scarlet fever
    (b) Rheumatic fever
    (c) Acute hemorrhagic glomerulonephritis
3. Throat cultures can be used in detecting the carrier state of such organisms as
    (a) Beta hemolytic streptococcus
    (b) *Neisseria meningitidis*
    (c) *Corynebacterium diphtheriae*
    (d) *Staphylococcus aureus*

Procedure
1. The patient must be placed in a good light.
2. A sterile throat culture kit with a polyester-tipped applicator, or swab, is used.
3. A sterile container or tube of culture medium must be available.
4. With the patient's tongue depressed by a tongue blade and the throat well exposed and illuminated, the swab must be rotated firmly and gently over the back of the throat, both tonsils or fossae, and areas of inflammation, exudation, or ulceration.

(a) Care should be taken to avoid touching the tongue or lips with the swab.

(b) Since most patients will gag or cough, the collector should preferably wear a mask or stand to the side of the patient.

5. The swab is replaced in the inner tube and the ampule is crushed. The swab is then forced into the released medium. The medium is covered and the specimen is sent immediately to the laboratory.

6. If throat culture cannot be examined within 1 hour, it can be refrigerated.

Procedure for Pediatric Patients

1. Seat the patient in the adult's (parent's) lap.

2. Have the adult encircle the child's arms and chest to prevent the child from moving.

3. The collector should place one hand on the child's forehead to stabilize the head and prevent movement.

4. Proceed with the technique used for collection of the throat and nose culture.

For throat washings have the patient gargle with 5 to 10 ml of sterile saline solution and deposit it in a sterile cup. This provides more material than a throat swab and is more productive for viral isolation.

Nasal Culture (Swab)

Indications for Collection

1. Acute leukemia patients

2. Transplant recipients

3. Intermittent dialysis patients

4. Tracing epidemics

Procedure

Swab both external nares and deeper, moister recesses of the nose. Both nose and throat specimens are preferred for recovery of paramyxoviruses.

WOUND CULTURES

Normal Values

Clinical specimens taken from wounds may be expected to have any of the following microorganisms. The pathogenicity of the organisms is dependent on the quantity present.

1. *Actinomyces* species

2. *Bacteroides* species

3. *Clostridium perfringens* and other species
4. *Escherichia coli*
5. Other gram-negative enteric bacilli
6. *Mycobacterium* species
7. *Nocardia* species
8. *Pseudomonas* species
9. *Staphylococcus* species
10. *Staphylococcus epidermidis*
11. *Streptococcus faecalis*
12. *Streptococcus pyogenes*

Background
Material from infected wounds will reveal a variety of aerobic and anaerobic microorganisms. Because anaerobic microorganisms are the predominant microflora in humans and are constantly present in the upper respiratory tract, gastrointestional tract, and genitourinary tract, they are also likely to invade other parts of the body, causing severe and often fatal infections.

Clinically significant pathogens are likely to be found in the following specimens:

1. Pus from any deep wound or aspirated abscess, especially if associated with a foul odor
2. Necrotic tissue or debrided material from suspected gas gangrene tissue
3. Material from infections bordering mucous membranes
4. Drainage from postoperative wounds
5. Ascitic fluid

Procedure for Anaerobic Collection Using Aspirated Material
1. Open the collection kit; the container contains CO_2.
2. Remove the sterile syringe (sterile needle, if needed).
3. Aspirate the material; 1–3 cc is the preferred sample.

Culture Maintenance
All media must be incubated under strictly anaerobic conditions.

Procedure for Anaerobic Collection Using Swab Sets (Commonly Used Only If Unable To Aspirate Fluid or Pus).
1. Open the collection container, remove the swab and take a sample by applying the sterile swab directly to the source of the culture.
2. Insert the swab into the container. Break the swab and discard the top portion.
3. Seal the container.
4. Do not touch the swab tip or inner surface of the collection container.

5. Label the specimen with
   (a) Patient's name
   (b) Date of sample
   (c) Source of specimen
   (d) Clinical diagnosis
   (e) Isolation status
   (f) Any other pertinent information required by the laboratory
6. Take the culture in such a way that exposure to oxygen is minimized or excluded.
7. If infection from mycobacteria or fungi is suspected, exudate or tissue should be collected in place of a swab.
8. With cultures of dry wounds, swabs should be moistened in sterile saline before use.

Clinical Alert

A microscopic examination of pus and wound exudates can be very helpful in diagnosis of the pathogenic organism. Consider the following:

1. Pus from streptococcal lesions is thin and serous.
2. Pus from staphylococcal infections is gelatinous.
3. Pus from *P. aeruginosa* infections is blue-green.
4. Actinomycosis infections show "sulfur" granules.

The most useful specimens for analysis are pus or excised tissue. Dressings from discharging wounds are also acceptable. If swabs must be used, at least three swabs from one site must be submitted, and these swabs should be serum-coated. Swabs with a light smearing of pus dry out very quickly and are virtually useless.

SKIN CULTURES

Normal Values
The following organisms may be present on the skin of a healthy person. When present in low numbers, certain of these organisms may be considered normal commensals; at other times, when they multiply to excessive quantities, these same organisms may be pathogens.

1. *Clostridium* species
2. Coliform bacilli
3. Diphtheroids
4. Enterococci
5. Mycobacteria
6. *Proteus* species
7. Staphylococci
8. Streptococci
9. Yeasts and fungi

Background
The most common bacteria involved in skin infections are staphylococci, streptococci (Group A), and *Corynebacterium haemolyticum*. The common abnormal skin conditions include

1. Pyoderma
   (a) Staphylococcal impetigo characterized by bullous lesions with thin, amber, varnish-like crusts
   (b) Streptococcal impetigo characterized by thick crusts
2. Erysipelas
3. Folliculitis
4. Furuncles
5. Carbuncles
6. Secondary invasion of burns, scabies, and other skin lesions
7. Dermatophytes, especially athlete's foot, scalp and body ringworm, and "jock itch."

Procedure for Vesicular Lesions or Skin Scrapings
1. Clean the affected site with sterile saline, wipe it gently with alcohol and allow it to air dry.
2. Aspirate fluid from fresh, intact vesicles with a 25-gauge needle on a TB syringe and flush the contents into the transport medium.
3. If fluid is not present, open the vesicles and use a cotton-, rayon-, or dacron-tipped applicator to swab the base of the lesion to collect infected cells. (Exudate should be absorbed in the culturette.)
4. Place the swab directly into transport medium.
5. To make smears for stains, use a scalpel blade to scrape the base of the lesion. Being careful not to macerate the cells, spread material in a thin layer in a 1 cm circle on a slide.
6. Transport to the laboratory as rapidly as possible for viral cultures.

Clinical Alert

The most useful and common specimens for analysis are skin scrapings, nail scrapings, and hairs (see *Fungal Diseases*).

Clinical Implications
When present in significant quantities on the skin, the following organisms may be considered pathogenic and therefore indicative of an abnormal condition.

1. *Bacteroides* species
2. *Clostridium* species
3. Coliform bacilli

4. Fungi (*Sporotrichum, Actinomyces, Nocardia, Candida albicans, Trichophyton, Microsporum, Epidermophyton*)
5. *Staphylococcus aureus* (coagulase positive)
6. *Streptococcus pyogenes*

STOOL AND ANAL CULTURES AND SMEARS

Normal Values
The following organisms may be present in the stool of apparently healthy people:

1. *Candida albicans*
2. Clostridia
3. Enterococci
4. *Escherichia coli*

5. *Proteus* species
6. *Pseudomonas aeruginosa*
7. *Salmonella* species
8. Staphylococci

Clinical Alert

1. *Candida albicans* in large numbers in the stool is considered pathogenic in the presence of previous antibiotic therapy. Alterations of the normal flora by antibiotics often changes normally harmless organisms into pathogens.
2. *Cryptosporidiosis* is a cause of severe, protracted diarrhea in immunosuppressed patients.

Background
Stool cultures are commonly done to identify parasites, enteric disease organisms, and viruses in the intestinal tract. Of all specimens collected, feces are most likely to contain the greatest number and greatest variety of organisms. In a routine culture the stool is examined to rule out *Salmonella, Shigella, Campylobacter, Yersinia*, enteropathogenic *E. coli* (in the newborn), and pure cultures of staphylococcus.

A single negative stool culture should not be regarded as confirmation of noninvolvement of infectious bacteria. At least three cultures are usually done if the clinical picture of the patient suggests a bacterial involvement and if the first two cultures are negative. Moreover, after a positive diagnosis has been made, personal contacts of the patient and the convalescent patient should also have three negative stool cultures to prevent spread of infection.

Procedure for Collection
1. Feces should be collected in a dry container free of urine.
2. A freshly passed stool is the specimen of choice. The entire stool should be collected.

3. Only a small amount of stool is needed. A stool the size of a walnut is usually adequate; however, the entire passed stool should be sent for examination.
4. A diarrheal stool usually gives good results (5–10 ml).
5. Stool passed into the toilet bowl must not be used for culture.
6. No toilet paper should be placed in the bedpan or specimen container for it may contain bismuth, which interferes with laboratory tests.
7. Stool should be transferred to a container with tongue blades. The specimen should be labelled and sent immediately to the laboratory.

Clinical Alert

Fecal specimens are far superior to rectal swabs. Often rectal swabs are merely anal and provide little material of diagnostic significance.

Culture Maintenance
1. Examination should be within a few hours of collection.
2. If delays over 18 to 24 hours are suspected, the specimen should be mixed with an equal volume of buffered glycerol-saline.
3. Swabs must be examined immediately to prevent drying out of specimen.

Procedure for Taking Cellophane Tape Test
1. A tape test is indicated in cases of suspected enterobiasis (pinworms).
2. A strip of clear cellophane tape (not micropore or adhesive) is applied to the perineal region. It is then removed and spread on a slide for microscopic examination.
3. A paraffin-coated swab can be used in place of the cellophane tape test. If it is used, it is placed in a covered test tube.
4. Repeated examinations on consecutive days may be necessary.
5. The test for eggs is made preferably in the morning before the patient has defecated or bathed.
6. Test in children: In about one-third of infected children, eggs can also be obtained from beneath the fingernails. Follow the instructions on the kit provided.

Interfering Factors
Feces from patients receiving barium, bismuth, oil, or antibiotics are unsatisfactory for the identification of protozoa.

Patient Preparation for Collection of Stool Specimen
1. The patient should be instructed to defecate into a clean bedpan or a large-mouthed container.
2. The patient should be told not to defecate into the toilet bowl or to urinate into the bedpan or collecting container, since urine has a harmful effect on protozoa.
3. Toilet paper should not be placed in the bedpan or collection container.

Procedure for Taking a Rectal Swab
1. The swab is inserted gently into the rectum (to at least 3 cm) and rotated to obtain a visible amount of fecal material (Figure 7-1).
2. The swab is placed in a clean container and the cover is closed.
3. The specimen is properly labeled and sent immediately to the laboratory.

Clinical Alert
1. In the hospital, patients with diarrhea should remain in isolation until the cause of diarrhea is determined.
2. When pathogens are found in the stool, the patient usually remains isolated until the stool is formed and antibiotic therapy is completed.

CEREBROSPINAL FLUID (CSF) CULTURES AND SMEARS

Normal Values
No flora are normally present. In healthy persons the specimen may be contaminated by normal skin flora.

Pathogens Found in CSF
1. *Bacteroides* species
2. Coliform bacilli
3. *Cryptococcus* and other fungi
4. *Hemophilus influenzae* (especially in infants and children)
5. *Leptospira* species
6. *Listeria monocytogenes*
7. *Mycobacterium tuberculosis*
8. *Neisseria meningitidis*
9. Pneumococci
10. Staphylococci
11. Streptococci

Indications for Collection
1. Viral meningitis
2. Pyogenic meningitis
3. Tuberculosis meningitis
4. Chronic meningitis (due to *Cryptococcus neoformans*)

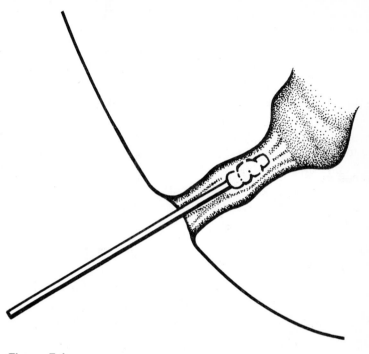

Figure 7-1
Method for obtaining the rectal culture.

Explanation of Test

Culture of bacteriological examination of cerebrospinal fluid is an essential step in the diagnosis of any case of suspected meningitis. Acute bacterial meningitis is an infection of the meninges, or membrane covering the brain and spinal cord, and is a rapidly fatal disease if untreated or if given inadequate treatment. Prompt identification of the causative agent is necessary for appropriate antibiotic therapy. Meningitis is caused by a variety of gram-positive and gram-negative microorganisms. Bacterial meningitis can also be secondary to infections in other parts of the body.

It is recommended that a smear and culture be carried out in all CSF specimens from persons with suspected meningitis, whether the fluid is clear or cloudy. (Normal cerebrospinal fluid is clear.)

In bacterial meningitis, which is caused by a variety of bacteria, the CSF shows the following characteristics:

1. Purulent (usually)
2. Increased WBC

3. Predominance of polymorphonuclear cells
4. Decreased CSF glucose

In meningitis, which is caused by tubercle bacillus, viruses, fungi, or protozoa, the CSF shows the following characteristics:

1. Nonpurulent (usually)
2. Decreased count of mononuclear white cells
3. Normal or decreased CSF glucose

In persons with suspected meningitis the fluid is generally submitted for chemical and cytological examinations, as well as for culture.

Procedure
1. The specimen must be collected under sterile conditions, sealed immediately to prevent leakage or contamination, and sent to the laboratory without delay.

Clinical Alert

It is very important that a diagnosis be made as quickly as possible. Since some organisms cannot tolerate temperature changes, it is very important that the culture be done as quickly as possible.

If a viral etiology is suspected, a portion of the fluid must be immediately frozen for subsequent attempts at isolation of the virus.

2. The specimen should be labeled with the patient's name, age, date, room number, and suspected disease. The laboratory staff should be alerted so that they can prepare to examine the specimen immediately.

Clinical Alert

The laboratory should be given adequate warning that a CSF sample will be delivered. Time is a critical factor; the cells disintegrate if the sample is kept at room temperature for more than 1 hour.

3. The attending physician should be notified as soon as results are obtained so that appropriate treatment can be started.
4. CSF specimens can be incubated after collection but can never be refrigerated.

Maintenance of Culture
1. If the specimen cannot be delivered at once to the laboratory for analysis, the container should be kept at 37°C.
2. No more than 4 hours should elapse before laboratory analysis, because of the low survival rate of the organisms causing meningitis, especially *H. influenzae* and the meningococcus.

Special Situation
In cases of suspected tuberculous meningitis, the specimen may be left standing at 37°C (98.6°F) for an hour to form the characteristic "spider web" clot. This technique is best left for later in the course of the disease, for the clot is often not found early, or it is used as a sign of the progress of chemotherapy.

Clinical Implications
Positive cultures occur in

(a) Meningitis
(b) Trauma
(c) Abscess of brain or ependyma of spine
(d) Septic thrombophlebitis of venous sinuses

CERVICAL, URETHRAL, AND ANAL CULTURES AND SMEARS FOR GONORRHEA AND OTHER SEXUALLY TRANSMITTED DISEASES

Procedure for Obtaining Cultures
A. *Female patients*
  1. *Cervical culture:* The cervix is the best site to obtain a culture specimen (Figure 7-2).
    (a) Moisten the speculum with warm water; do NOT use a lubricant.
    (b) Remove cervical mucus, preferably with a cotton ball held in a ring forceps.
    (c) Insert a sterile, cotton-tipped swab into the endocervical canal; move the swab from side to side; allow several seconds for absorption of organisms by the swab.
  2. *Anal canal culture:* This is the most likely site to be positive when a cervical culture is negative.

    Note: The anal canal specimen can be obtained after the cervical specimen without changing the patient's position and without using the anoscope.

    (a) Insert a sterile, cotton-tipped swab approximately 1 inch into the anal canal. (If the swab is inadvertently pushed into feces, use another swab to obtain the specimen.)

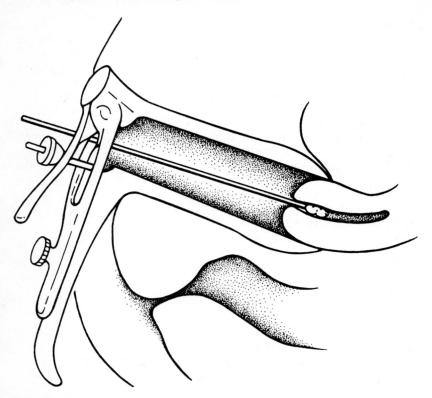

Figure 7-2
Method for obtaining the endocervical culture.

      (b) Move the swab from side to side in the anal canal to sample
          crypts; allow several seconds for absorption of organisms by
          the swab.
B. *Male patients*
    1. *Urethral culture*
       Use a sterile swab to obtain the specimen from the anterior
       urethra by gently scraping the mucosa (Figure 7-3).

Clinical Alert

If the urethral culture in males is negative, but gonorrhea is still
suspected, prostatic massage may increase the number of organisms in urethral discharge.

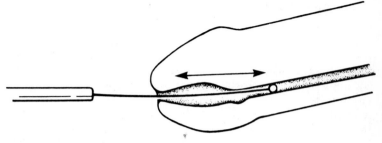

Figure 7-3
Method for obtaining the urethral culture.

2. *Anal canal culture*
   Follow the same procedure as in female patients.
C. *Both male and female patients*
   Oropharyngeal culture
   Culture specimens should also be obtained from the oropharynx
   in persons engaging in oral sex.

Clinical Alert

Repeated culturing for gonococci without detection does not exclude a diagnosis of gonorrhea.

Patient Preparation
1. The patient is to be placed in the dorsal lithotomy position and
   appropriately draped.
2. The person collecting the specimen should wear sterile, disposable
   gloves.

SKIN TESTS

Background
Skin testing is done for three major reasons: (1) to detect a person's
sensitivity to allergens such as dust and pollen, (2) to determine a
person's sensitivity to microorganisms believed to cause disease, and
(3) to determine whether a person's cell-mediated, immune function is
normal. The test that detects sensitivity to allergens will be mentioned
only briefly in this chapter. Most of the discussion will center on tests
used in the determination of sensitivity to pathogens.

In general, three types of skin tests are used

1. Scratch tests
   Scratches approximately 1 cm. long and 2.5 cm. apart are made in rows on a patient's back or forearm. Extremely small quantities of allergens are introduced into these scratches. Positive reaction: Swelling or redness at the site within 30 minutes
2. Patch tests
   A small square of gauze is impregnated with the substance in question and applied to the skin of the forearm. Positive reaction: Swollen or reddened skin at the site of the patch after a given period of time
3. Intradermal tests
   The substance that is being tested is introduced within the layers of skin by a tuberculin syringe fitted with a short-bevel 26- or 27-gauge needle. Positive reaction: Red and inflamed area at the site of the injection within a given period of time (*e.g.*, 72 hours in the Mantoux test for tuberculosis).

Skin tests revealing a hypersensitivity to a toxic product from a disease-producing agent may also indicate an immunity to the disease. Positive reactions may additionally indicate the presence of an active or inactive case of the disease under study. The following is a categorization of skin tests according to their nature and purpose:

1. Tests to determine possible susceptibility (or resistance) to infection
   Examples: Schick test (positive reaction = lack of immunity to diphtheria)
   Dick test (positive reaction = lack of immunity to scarlet fever)
2. Tests to indicate a present or past exposure with the infectious agent
   Example: Tuberculin test (positive reaction = presence of active or inactive tuberculosis)
3. Tests to show sensitivity to various types of materials to which a person may react in an exaggerated manner
   Example: Allergenic extracts such as house dust and pollen (positive reaction to sensitivity to allergen extracts)
4. Tests to detect impaired cellular immunity
   Intradermal skin testing with several common antigenic microbial substances is one way of determining whether the immune function is normal. This would be important in treating leukemias and cancer patients with chemotherapy.
   Example: PPD tuberculin skin tests, mumps virus, *Candida albicans*, skin fungi, and streptokinase–streptodornase.

(Negative reaction to any intradermal antigen is indicative of impaired immunity due to abnormal cell-mediated immune function.)

Indications for Tests
Diagnostic skin tests may be used to determine the presence of the following disease entities:

1. Blastomycosis
2. Brucellosis
3. Echinococcosis
4. Histoplasmosis
5. Lymphogranuloma venereum
6. Mumps
7. Toxoplasmosis
8. Tuberculosis
9. Tularemia

Procedure for Taking Skin Test
1. Most diagnostic skin tests come in an unopened, sterile kit. Follow the manufacturer's instructions carefully.
2. Generally, 0.1 ml. of the substance under question is injected intradermally in the volar aspect of the forearm.
3. Positive reaction: Redness or swelling of more than 1 cm. in diameter. A central area of necrosis is an even more significant finding.

Clinical Alert

Material for diagnostic skin tests may be inadvertently injected subcutaneously rather than intradermally. A subcutaneous injection will yield a false-negative result.

Procedure for Taking Patch Test
1. The skin is cleansed and allowed to dry.
2. Remove the protective cover from a specially prepared adhesive patch or gauze square impregnated with the testing substance and firmly apply it to the forearm or the interscapular region of the back.

Procedure for Taking Scratch Test
The scratch method is especially recommended in patients who give a history of extreme sensitivity.

1. The skin is cleansed with alcohol (or acetone if the patient is allergic to alcohol) and allowed to dry. Sites to be used are the forearm or the interscapular region of the back. The elbow and wrist areas are less reactive and should be avoided.

2. The skin is stretched taut, using the thumb and index finger.
3. Using a sterile lancet to puncture the epidermis, a scratch approximately 1 to 4 mm. long is made. The purpose is to raise the skin. The skin should be abraided without drawing blood. In the event that blood is drawn, the site should not be used.
4. One drop of the substance used for testing is applied to the scarification, taking care not to touch the skin with the dropper.
5. A control test should be performed for comparison purposes.

Tuberculin Skin Test (For Detection of Tuberculosis)

Normal Values
Negative or not significant

Explanation of Test
The tuberculin skin test is an intradermal test used to detect tuberculosis infection; it does not distinguish active from dormant infections. Tuberculin is a protein fraction of tubercle bacilli, and when it is introduced into the skin of a person with active or dormant tuberculosis infection, it causes a localized erythema and induration of the skin because of an accumulation of small, sensitized lymphocytes.

The tuberculin test of choice is the Mantoux test, using a needle and syringe.

Multiple puncture tests (TINE) are used for screening in asymptomatic persons.

Indications for Testing
1. Persons with signs (X-ray film abnormality) and/or symptoms (cough, hemoptysis, weight loss, etc.) suggestive of current tuberculosis disease
2. Recent contacts with known tuberculosis cases or persons suspected of having tuberculosis
3. Persons with abnormal chest roentgenograms compatible with past tuberculosis
4. Persons with medical conditions that increase the risk of tuberculosis (silicosis, gastrectomy, diabetes, immunosuppressive therapy, lymphomas, AIDS)
5. Groups at high risk of recent infection with M. tuberculosis, such as immigrants from Asia, Africa, Latin America, and Oceania; some inner city and skid row populations; personnel and long-term residents in some hospitals, nursing homes, mental institutions, and prisons

Procedure
A. Intradermal skin test
   1. P.P.D.-t is drawn up into a tuberculin syringe (follow manufacturer's directions carefully), using a ½ inch 26- or 27-gauge needle.
   2. The skin on the volar or dorsal aspect of the forearm is cleansed with alcohol and allowed to dry.
   3. The skin is stretched taut.
   4. The tuberculin syringe is held close to the skin so that the hub of the needle touches it as the needle is introduced. A discrete pale elevation of the skin—a wheal—6 mm. to 10 mm. in diameter should be produced when the prescribed amount of fluid (0.1 ml.) is accurately injected intracutaneously.

Clinical Implications
1. The larger the size of the skin reaction, the more likely it is to represent tuberculosis infection. However, a significant reaction to the skin test does not necessarily signify the presence of the disease.
2. Since a significant reaction does not distinguish between an active and a dormant infection, the stage of infection can be determined from the results of clinical bacteriologic tests of the sputum and from roentgenograms.
3. A significant reaction in a patient who is clinically ill means that active tuberculosis cannot be dismissed as a diagnostic possibility.
4. A significant reaction in healthy persons usually signifies healed tuberculosis or an infection caused by a different mycobacteria.

Clinical Alert

1. Tuberculin should never be transferred from one container to another.
2. Skin tests should be given immediately after the syringe is filled.
3. The greatest value of tuberculin skin testing is in its negative implications. This means that a negative test result in the presence of signs and symptoms of lung disease is strong evidence against active tuberculosis, in the majority of cases.
4. Bacteriologic confirmation of a presumptive diagnosis of TB must be done.
5. Incidence of TB is higher among older persons, males, non-whites, and the foreign born.
6. Typical new case: Born in 1930s, infected in 1940s, developed disease in 1980s.

7. Sixteen percent of TB is extrapulmonary.
8. Transmission of TB usually requires close, frequent, and prolonged exposure.
9. Diagnosed case of TB averages nine contacts, of which 21% are infected.

Interfering Factors

1. False-negative results may occur even in the presence of active tuberculosis and whenever sensitized T lymphocytes are temporarily depleted in the body. See Table 7-10.

Table 7-10
Potential Causes of Falsely Nonsignificant Tuberculin Test Reactions

Factors Related to the Person Being Tested
Infections:
    Viral (measles, mumps, chickenpox)
    Bacterial (typhoid fever, brucellosis, typhus, leprosy, pertussis, overwhelming tuberculosis, tuberculous pleurisy)
    Fungal (South American blastomycosis)
Live virus vaccinations (measles, mumps, polio)
Metabolic derangements (chronic renal failure)
Nutritional factors (severe protein depletion)
Diseases affecting lymphoid organs (Hodgkin's disease, lymphoma, chronic lymphocytic leukemia, sarcoidosis)
Drugs (corticosteroids and many other immunosuppressive agents)
Age (newborns, elderly patients with "waned" sensitivity)
Recent or overwhelming infection with *M. tuberculosis*
Stress (surgery, burns, mental illness, graft versus host reactions)

Factors Related to the Tuberculin Used
Improper storage (exposure to light and heat)
Improper dilutions
Chemical denaturation
Contamination
Adsorption (partially controlled by adding Tween 80)

Factors Related to the Method of Administration
Injection of too little antigen
Delayed administration after drawing into syringe
Injection too deep

Factors Related to Reading the Test and Recording Results
Inexperienced reader
Conscious or unconscious bias
Error in recording

Reading the Test Results
1. The test should be read 48 to 72 hours after infection.
2. The patient should be examined in a good light.
3. The patient should flex his forearm at the elbow.
4. The skin should be inspected for induration (hardening or thickening).
5. The examiner's finger should be rubbed lightly from the area of normal skin to the indurated zone.
6. The zone of induration should be circled with a pencil and the diameter measured in millimeters.
7. Little change in size occurs before the fifth day; however, large reactions are still evident at least seven days later.

Interpreting the Test Results
The interpretation of the test is based on the presence or absence of induration.

Negative or not significant reaction: Zone less than 5 mm. in diameter
Significant reaction: Zone 10 mm. or more in diameter

Schick Test (for Susceptibility to Diphtheria)

Normal Values
See "Clinical Implications."

Background
1. Diphtheria is a respiratory disease caused by the bacterium *Cornebacterium diphtheriae.*
2. A person who is immune to diphtheria will produce antitoxins that will circulate in his blood in significant quantities.
3. A person who is susceptible to diphtheria will lack (or have very low levels of) antitoxins, and therefore will not be able to neutralize the diphtheria toxin injected intradermally in the test.

Explanation of Test
1. The Schick test is a means for determining the presence or absence of a significant quantity of diphtheria antitoxins in the blood. The presence of these antitoxins indicates immunity to the disease.
2. If the skin test causes erythema and flaking of the skin at the site of the injection, the person tested is susceptible to diphtheria. This is a positive reaction.
3. A negative reaction, indicated by no flaking or erythema, means that under normal conditions of exposure, the person will not contract diphtheria.
4. The test gives a rough estimate of the quantity of antitoxins circulating in the blood.

Procedure

1. A 0.1 ml. quantity of purified diphtheria *toxin* (0.02 of the amount necessary to kill a guinea pig) dissolved in human serum albumin is injected intradermally on the volar surface of the forearm. A 0.1 ml. quantity of inactivated diphtheria *toxoid* is injected into the other arm as a control to rule out sensitivity to culture proteins.
2. These areas are examined at 24 and 48 hours and between the third and fourth days.

Interpreting Test Results

1. Positive test: Site of toxin injection begins to redden in 24 hours and increases and reaches a maximum size in about one week, when it will be swollen and tender and as large as 3 cm. in diameter. There is usually a small, dark red central zone that gradually turns brown and leaves a pigmented area. The area of *toxoid* injection shows no reaction.
2. Negative test: No reaction at either site

Clinical Implications

1. If a reaction occurs (*i.e.*, a positive test), the person does not have enough antibodies to neutralize the toxin and is therefore susceptible to diphtheria. The person has no immunity to diphtheria.
2. Persons who have been well immunized with four injections of diphtheria toxoid show uniformly negative reactions to the Schick test.
3. If the test is positive in a well-immunized person, this is strong evidence of the person's inability to produce antibodies.
4. A negative test means that the person has immunity to exposure to diphtheria.

Clinical Alert

1. The major significant reservoirs of diphtheria are immunized persons, particularly the elderly whose immunity has waned, and children who have not been immunized.
2. The recommended schedule for active immunization against diphtheria in normal infants and children is

2 months	18 months
4 months	4 to 6 years
6 months	

These are the ages in which a child should receive DTP, a diphtheria and tetanus toxoid combined with pertussis vaccine.

3. An adult (any person older than 16 years) requiring immunization against diphtheria would receive a combination of tetanus and diphtheria toxoids every 10 years.

Dick Test (for Susceptibility to Scarlet Fever)

Normal Values
See "Clinical Implications."

Background
1. Scarlet fever, also called *scarlatina*, is a communicable, hemolytic streptococcal infection caused by *Streptococcus pyogenes*. The condition causes generalized toxemia, a typical rash and scaling of skin, during the recovery period.
2. Occurrence of scarlet fever has been decreasing in recent years.
3. Scarlatinal or erythrogenic toxin is responsible for the rash of scarlet fever.

Explanation of Test
The Dick test is a diagnostic skin test that measures a person's susceptibility to scarlet fever. It also indicates immunity to the disease. A solution of dilute scarlatinal toxin is injected intradermally to detect antibody and to determine immunity to scarlet fever.

Procedure
1. A 0.1 ml. dilute solution of scarlet fever (Dick) toxin is injected intradermally on the volvar surface of the forearm.
2. The test area is examined within a 24-hour period.

Interpreting Test Results
1. The test should be read within 18 to 24 hours.
2. Positive reaction: Site of injection is very red and markedly swollen (3–5 cm. in diameter). Swollen area has sharply raised edges. A positive test indicates damage done by the injected toxin that has not been neutralized by antibodies present in the body.
3. Negative reaction: No more than a faint pink streak along the course of the needle.
4. Slightly positive reaction: Faint red area measuring less than 1 cm. in diameter; no swelling.

Clinical Implications
1. A positive reaction signifies that the person has insufficient circulating antitoxins to the Dick toxin and is susceptible to scarlet fe-

ver. A positive test reverts to a negative reaction following infection.
2. A negative reaction signifies that a person is relatively immune to the disease.

Clinical Alert

There are three immunologically rare but distinct toxins, which may account for second attacks of scarlet fever.

SKIN TESTS FOR ASSORTED BACTERIAL DISEASES

Brucellosis (Undulant Fever) Test

Causative Agent
Brucellosis is caused by *Brucella melitensis, Brucella abortus, and Brucella suis.*

Explanation of Test
Antigen (0.1 ml.) is injected intradermally. Two types of antigen are used.

1. A killed suspension of *Brucella* organisms
2. A protein solution, Brucellergen, derived from the organism

Interpreting Test Results
1. The test is read in 48 hours.
2. Positive reaction: Characterized by edema, redness, and induration. In infected persons, exacerbation of symptoms may accompany a local reaction. The hypersensitive patient may have both a systemic and a local reaction.

Soft Chancre Test

Causative Agent
Soft chancre is caused by *Hemophilus ducreyi.*

Explanation of Test
An antigen prepared from cultures of *Hemophilus ducreyi* or Bubo pus is injected intradermally.

Interpreting Test Results
1. The test is read in 72 hours.
2. Positive reaction: Characterized by an area of erythema of 14 mm.

or more in diameter and an area of induration of 8 mm. or more in diameter. A positive reaction may persist for weeks and indicates that the patient has had an active chancroid infection or has been injected in the past. (The skin hypersensitivity may last for many years.)

Tularemia Test

Causative Agent
Tularemia is caused by *Pasteurella tularensis.*

Explanation of Test
The Foshay antigen, which is prepared from a culture of the causative organism, is injected intradermally.

Interpreting Test Results
1. The test is read in 48 hours.
2. Positive reaction: Characterized by an area of erythema and induration. Positive reactions are known to occur during the first week of the disease.

> **Clinical Alert**
>
> Blood for agglutination tests should be drawn before the antigen is injected, since the skin-test antigen may cause false-positive agglutinins.

PARASITIC DISEASE SKIN TESTS

Echinococcosis (Hydatid Disease) Test

Causative Agent
Hydatid disease is an infection of the liver caused by hydatid cysts (larval forms) of tapeworms belonging to the genus Echinococcus.

Explanation of Test
An antigen made from infected hydatid cysts in human or dog tapeworms is injected intradermally. Usually a control material from uninfected animals is also infected.

Interpreting Test Results
1. The test is read in 15 to 20 minutes.
2. Positive reaction: Immediate erythema and swelling

Clinical Implications
1. A positive reaction is usually indicative of echinococcosis.
2. More reliable diagnostic results are obtained by complement fixation, hemagglutination, and precipitation tests.

Interfering Factors
False-positive reactions may be due to
1. Other cestode infections
2. Hypersensitivity to foreign protein in the antigen

Toxoplasmosis Test

Causative Agent
Toxoplasmosis, caused by *Toxoplasma gondii*, is a protozoan disease affecting humans. Toxoplasmosis is characterized by CNS lesions, and the condition may lead to blindness, brain damage, and ultimately, death.

Explanation of Test
An antigen from infected mice is injected intradermally, as is a control from noninfected mice.

Interpreting Test Results
1. The test is read in 24 to 48 hours.
2. Positive reaction: Area of erythema and induration more than 10 mm. in diameter.

Clinical Implications
1. A positive test indicates the presence of antibodies to *Toxoplasma gondii*.
2. A positive test gives diagnostic results similar to the Sabin–Feldman dye test, a serologic test for the diagnosis of toxoplasmosis. (The Sabin–Feldman dye test is based on the failure of living toxoplasmas, in the presence of specific antibody and accessory factor, to take up methylene blue dye.)

Trichinosis Test

Causative Agent
Trichinosis is a disease caused by eating undercooked meat containing the parasitic nematode, *Trichinella spiralis*. The condition is character-

ized by fever, colic, nausea, diarrhea, pain, stiffness, muscle swelling, eosinophilia, sweating, and insomnia.

Explanation of Test
An antigen made from material drawn from animals infected with trichinosis is injected intradermally. A control material from uninfected animals is also injected intradermally. This test is a valuable aid in the diagnosis of trichinosis, especially when only mild symptoms occur.

Interpreting Test Results
1. The test is read in 15 to 20 minutes.
2. Positive reaction: Immediate; characterized by a blanched wheal surrounded by an area of erythema

Clinical Implications
1. A positive test is usually indicative of trichinosis.
2. The skin test is not positive until about the second week of infection.

Clinical Alert

Blood for precipitins, agglutination, or complement fixation tests should be obtained before skin testing.

Interfering Factors
Up to 10% of positive reactions may be false.

VIRAL DISEASE SKIN TESTS

Frei Test (for Confirmation of Lymphogranuloma Venereum)

Causative Agent
Lymphogranuloma venereum (LGV) is an infectious venereal disease caused by a member of the genus *Chlamydia*. The condition begins with a small, ulcerative lesion of the genitals and later progresses to a systemic infection with enlargement of the regional lymph nodes. LGV may lead to chronic infection resulting in elephantiasis of genital tissues.

Explanation of Test

An antigen made from the yolk sac of infected chick embryos is injected intradermally. A control material made from normal yolk sac is also injected intradermally.

Interpreting Test Results

1. The test should be read in 48 to 72 hours.
2. Positive reaction: A raised papule 6 by 6 mm. in diameter; a reaction to the control material of 5 mm. or less
3. Negative reaction: Even in cases of apparently "negative" reactions, the test area should be examined for several days because of the frequency of delayed reactions.

Clinical Implications

The test becomes positive 1 to 6 weeks after infection begins and remains positive for the life of the patient.

Clinical Alert

Persons who are known to be allergic to eggs or chicken may react unfavorably.

Mumps Test

Causative Agent

Mumps, the common disease causing swelling and tenderness of the parotid glands, is caused by a myxovirus.

Explanation of Test

An antigen made from infected monkeys or chickens is injected intradermally, and a control material made from noninfected monkeys or chickens is also injected intradermally.

Interpreting Test Results

1. The test should be read in 48 hours.
2. Positive reaction: Erythema and a lesion larger than 10 mm. in diameter
3. Negative reaction: No erythema and a lesion less than 10 mm. in diameter

Clinical Implications

1. A positive reaction indicates resistance to the mumps virus.
2. A negative reaction indicates susceptibility to the mumps virus.

MYCOTIC INFECTION SKIN TESTS

Blastomycosis (Gilchrist's Disease) **Test**

Causative Agent
Blastomycosis, a condition characterized by cutaneous, pulmonary, and systemic lesions, is caused by organisms of the genus *Blastomyces.*

Explanation of Test
Blastomycin, an antigen, is injected intradermally. The test is reasonably specific for blastomycosis, but in practice this skin-test antigen is usually injected simultaneously with histoplasmin, coccidioiden and tuberculin.

Blastomycosis is also diagnosed by the recovery of the organism from pus, sputum, or tissue specimens.

Interpreting Test Results
1. The test should be read in 48 hours.
2. Positive reaction: Area of erythema and induration 5 by 5 mm. or greater
3. Doubtful reaction: Area of induration less than 5 mm. in diameter or erythema only
4. Negative reaction: No induration or erythema less than 5 mm. in diameter

Clinical Implications
A positive reaction may be indicative of

(a) Past infection
(b) Mild, chronic, or subacute infection
(c) Improvement in cases of serious symptomatic blastomycosis that previously had been blastomycin-negative

Coccidioidomycosis Test

Causative Agent
Coccidioidomycosis, an infectious fungus disease occurring in both an acute form and a progressive form, is caused by *Coccidioides immitis.*

Explanation of Test
Coccidioidin, an antigen prepared from culture, is injected intradermally. A skin reaction will appear 10 to 21 days after infection, and a sensitivity continues throughout life. Coccidioidomycosis can also be diagnosed by recovery of the causative organism from pus, sputum, or tissue specimens.

Interpreting Test Results
1. The test must be read in 24 to 72 hours. If an immediate reaction occurs, it is nonspecific for coccidioidomycosis and is ignored.
2. Positive reaction: Area of erythema and induration of 5 mm. or more in diameter. Reaction disappears within 24 to 72 hours.

Clinical Implications
1. The skin test becomes positive in 87% of the cases of coccidioidomycosis during the first week of clinical symptoms and in almost 100% of patients after the first week.
2. A positive reaction persists for many years, but this does not imply that active infection is present. However, when there is a positive reaction during the course of infection in which an earlier test was negative, it can indicate active infection.

Histoplasmosis Test

Causative Agent
Histoplasmosis, a systemic fungus infection of the reticuloendothelial system, is caused by the organism *Histoplasma capsulatum*.

Explanation of Test
Histoplasmin, an antigen prepared from culture, is injected intradermally. Skin reactions to histoplasmin are of relatively little diagnostic value, since anergy may provide false-negative results. Histoplasmosis is also diagnosed by identification of the causative agent in pus, sputum, or tissue specimens.

Interpreting Test Results
1. The test should be read in 24 to 48 hours. If an immediate reaction occurs, it is nonspecific for histoplasmosis and is ignored.
2. Positive reaction: Area of erythema and induration of 5 mm. or more in diameter.
3. Negative reaction: No induration; erythema less than 5 mm. in diameter.

Clinical Implications
1. A positive test indicates past or present infection.
2. Acutely ill patients may not have a positive reaction.

BIBLIOGRAPHY

August M: Practical aspects of viral laboratory diagnoses. J Med Technol 2(8):501–506, August 1985

Bailey RW: Baily and Scott's Diagnostic Microbiology, 17the ed. St. Louis, CV Mosby, 1986

Benenson AS (ed): Control of Communicable Diseases in Man, 14th ed. Washington, American Public Health Association, 1985

Berger RE (ed): Sexually transmitted diseases. Urol Clin North Am II : I, February 1984

Burrows W: Textbook of Microbiology, 22nd ed. Philadelphia, WB Saunders, 1985

Checko PJ: Guidelines for the collection, procession, and interpretation of microbiological specimens in extended care facilities. Infec Control Urol Care 5:27, 1980

Finegold S, Mertin W: Diagnostic Microbiology, 6th ed. St. Louis, CV Mosby, 1982

Halsted CH, Halsted JA (eds): The Laboratory in Clinical Medicine, 2nd ed. Philadelphia, WB Saunders, 1981

Hsiung GD: Diagnostic Virology. New Haven, Yale University Press, 1982

Isselbacher KJ et al (eds): Harrison's Principles of Internal Medicine, 11th ed. New York, McGraw–Hill, 1987

Kilbourn JP: Bacterial flora of the urinary tract. J Am Med Technol 321–332, November 1981

Koneman EW et al (eds): Color Atlas and Textbook of Microbiology, 2nd ed. Philadelphia, JB Lippincott, 1983

Sonnenwirth AC, Jarrett L: Gradwohl's Clinical Laboratory Methods and Diagnosis, 8th ed. St. Louis, CV Mosby, 1980

Washington JA II (ed): Laboratory Procedures in Clinical Microbiology. New York, Springer–Verlag, 1981

Wisconsin State Laboratory of Hygiene: Virus Study Procedures, 1985

Volk W: Essentials of Medical Microbiology, 3rd ed. Philadelphia, JB Lippincott, 1986

Youmans GP: The Biologic and Clinical Basis of Infectious Diseases, 2nd ed. Philadelphia, WB Saunders, 1980

IMMUNODIAGNOSTIC STUDIES

Introduction

Overview
Immunology is the study of antigen–antibody reactions *in vitro*. *Diagnostic immunology*, or *serodiagnostic testing*, uses serologic tests to aid in the diagnosis of infectious disease, immune disorders, allergic reactions, neoplastic disease (tumor-related antigens), and in blood grouping and typing (immunohematology.)

General Principles
1. Tests involve the study of serum proteins with immunologic action.
2. Immunologically active proteins are known as *antibodies, immunoglobulins, immunogens,* and *antigens.*
3. Patient's serum is tested to determine whether it contains antibodies against a particular antigen.
4. Common serologic methodology is based on a rise in titer of a specific antibody between the *acute phase* (beginning) of an illness and the *convalescent phase* (2–4 weeks later).
5. The formation of antibodies or autoantibodies against an antigenic challenge is identified.

Antigen–Antibody Reaction
The concepts of antigen and antibody are so interdependent that it is impossible to discuss one without the other.

1. *Antigen:* any substance that stimulates the formation of antibodies in the body and reacts with them specifically
2. *Antibody:* a substance usually appearing in the body as a result of the introduction of an antigen and which reacts specifically with that antigen

The body's antigen–antibody response is the method of natural defense against invading organisms. In autoimmune disorders the production of autoantibodies or antibodies to self occurs.

Types of Immunologic Tests
Immunologic methods demonstrate that antigen–antibody reactions have taken place. There are five or six major laboratory techniques for demonstrating this reaction. The tests described in this chapter generally fall into one of these categories.
1. *Immunofluorescence tests*
   (a) Immunofluorescent testing is based on the "sandwich" technique.
   (b) When an individual is challenged by a foreign material (antigen) the immune system responds by developing antibodies against the antigen. These antibodies are known as *immunoglobulins.*

(c) When the antibodies react with the antigens, antigen–antibody complexes are formed.

(d) The antigen–antibody complex (Ag–Ab) can be visualized in this way: a laboratory animal is challenged with human immunoglobulin. The animal recognizes this immunoglobulin as foreign and manufactures antibodies against it.

(e) Antibody molecules are treated with fluorescent dyes such as fluorescein without interfering with the molecule's function.

(f) The fluorescein-conjugated antibody (antibody plus dye) is allowed to react with the Ag–Ab complexes in (c) above. Then the resulting "sandwich" is observed under the microscope under ultraviolet light.

(g) Examples of immunofluorescent tests
   (1) Fluorescent treponemal antibody (FTA) test to diagnose syphilis
   (2) Indirect fluorescent (IFA) test to diagnose toxoplasmosis and to detect Epstein–Barr virus and antinuclear antibodies (ANA)

2. *Precipitation tests*
   (a) The reaction between a soluble antigen and its antiserum leads to a visible result in the form of precipitation.
   (b) Antigen and antibody must be mixed in a favorable ratio for a precipitate to form.
   (c) The following are examples of precipitation tests commonly used to diagnose:
      (1) CM fungal antibody test for coccidioidomycosis
      (2) Circumoral precipitin test for schistosomiasis—best done on cerebrospinal fluid
      (3) C-reactive protein, most often used to evaluate the severity and cause of many inflammatory diseases and necrotic lesions

3. *Agglutination tests*
   (a) When a particulate antigen, such as a saline suspension of red blood cells, mixes with a homologous antiserum, cells clump together and settle to the bottom of the fluid.
   (b) This type of test is relatively easy to do and is the most popular form of serologic test.
   (c) Examples
      (1) Thyroid hemagglutination test
      (2) HI or HIA test for determination of immunity for rubella
      (3) Cold agglutinins test

4. *Complement tests*
   Complement is a substance in blood serum that causes lysis when it combines with antigen-antibody complexes. There are several types of serologic tests involving complement.

(a) Complement-fixation test: A patient's serum is incubated with complement and the antigen being tested. Complement will "fix" or attach to the antigen–antibody complex if it forms. The test is commonly used to diagnose:
   (1) Histoplasmosis
   (2) Rickettsial disease
   (3) Blastomycosis
   (4) Trichinosis
   (5) Schistosomiasis
(b) Cytolysis: Cellular antigens and their antibodies in the presence of complement lead to lysis of the cell membrane.
(c) Immune adherence: Certain microorganisms adhere to nonphagocytic cells in the presence of homologous antimicrobial serum and complement.

5. *Neutralization of toxins tests*
   When exotoxins are formed, they may be neutralized by small quantities of homologous antibodies, also called antitoxins. This neutralization is tested by inoculation of laboratory animals.

6. *Enzyme-linked immunoabsorbent assay (ELISA)* used to detect rubella and hepatitis, among others.

Collection of Serum for Immunologic Tests

1. *Take two samples.* One sample should be taken at the beginning of the illness (the acute phase), and the other should be taken 3 to 4 weeks later (the convalescent phase). In general, the usefulness of the serologic tests depends on an increase in titer between the acute and the convalescent phase.

   Note: In a few serologic tests, one serum sample may be adequate since (1) presence of antibody indicates an abnormal condition, or (2) the antibody titer is unusually high. Only one sample is required in the following tests:

   (a) Antinuclear antibody   (d) Toxoplasmosis (IFA)
   (b) Heterophilic antibody titer   (e) Rubella titer
   (c) Histoplasmosis CF   (f) VDRL test

2. *Take the serologic test before skin testing.* Skin testing often induces antibody production and therefore may interfere with the results of the serologic test.

3. *Identify the sample plainly and provide appropriate clinical data.* The sample should have information on the patient's name, age, suspected diagnosis, vaccinations, therapy, and previous infections.

4. *Send samples to the laboratory before hemolysis occurs.* Hemolysis can interfere with the interpretation of the results. The presence of hemoglobin in serum can destroy complement and can interfere with the determination of complement-fixing antibodies.

Interpreting Results of Immunologic Tests
Certain factors will affect the interpretation of test results:

1. History of previous infection by the same organism
2. Previous vaccination (determine how recent it has been)
3. Anamnestic reactions caused by heterologous antigens
    (An *anamnestic reaction* is the appearance in the blood of antibodies
    after administration of an antigen to which the patient had devel-
    oped a primary immune response.)
4. Cross-reactivity
    Antibodies produced by one species of an organism frequently react
    with an entirely different species.
    Examples
    (a) Tularemia antibodies may agglutinate *Brucella* and vice versa.
    (b) Rickettsial infections may produce antibodies that react with
        Brucella.
    (c) Typhoid patients may produce antibodies to Proteus OX-19.
5. Presence of other serious conditions
    No immunologic response can be demonstrated in some persons
    having either agammaglobulinemia (inherited immune deficiency
    characterized by the lack of production of immunoglubulins) or any
    illness such as leukemia or advanced cancer that is being treated
    with immunosuppressant drugs.

Serologic vs. Microbiologic Methods
Chapter 7 provided descriptions of many microbiologic tests for diagnosing a disease entity. The best means of establishing the etiology of
an infectious disease is by isolation and confirmation of the pathogen
involved.
   Serologic methods can aid or confirm microbiologic analysis when

1. The patient is observed late in the course of the disease.
2. Antimicrobial therapy has suppressed growth of the invading or-
    ganism.
3. Culture methods were ineffective in substantiating growth of the
    suspected causative agent.

BLOOD BANKING OR IMMUNOHEMATOLOGY TESTS

These tests are done to prevent transfusion and transplant reactions, to
identify such problems as hemolytic disease of newborns, and to determine parentage. Immunohematology testing identifies highly reactive
antigens present in nucleated blood cells and their respective serum
antibodies. Each individual's blood cells demonstrate a unique combination of antigens. Almost all body fluid tissues contain ABH blood
grouplike substances. They are also found in animals, bacteria, and

432 Chapter 8: Immunodiagnostic Studies

plants. The related factors in the blood group system are inherited independently of each other according to Mendelian laws. Required testing for all donated blood and blood processing includes several determinations:

1. ABO red cell groups
2. Rh factors
3. Antibody screen
4. Hepatitis B surface antigen
5. Test for syphilis (VDRL)
6. Test for acquired immune deficiency syndrome (AIDS)

Required testing for potential whole blood recipient or packed red cells recipient includes:

1. ABO red cell group
2. Rh factor
3. Crossmatch for compatibility between donor and recipient blood

For plasma administration, no crossmatch is needed but compatible ABO typing should be done.

Platelets and granulocytes should be tested for HLA compatibility. HLA means *Histocompatibility Locus A*. These antigens are found in most tissues of the body and also on blood cells. As a result of previous transfusions or pregnancy, some patients will develop antibodies against these antigens and may have a transfusion reaction, if transfused with incompatible blood.

Blood Groups; ABO Red Cell Groups

Normal Values

Antigen Present on Red Blood Cell	Antibodies Present in Serum	Major Blood Group Designation	Distribution in U.S.	
None	Anti-A, anti-B	O (universal donor)*	O	46%
A	Anti-B	A	A	41%
B	Anti-A	B	B	9%
AB	None	AB (universal recipient)†	AB	4%

* Named *universal donor* because the person has no antigens on red blood cells and therefore is able to donate to all blood groups.

† Named *universal recipient* because the person has no antibodies in serum and therefore is able to receive blood from all blood groups.

Explanation of Test

Blood typing is a test required of all blood donors and all potential blood recipients. The main purpose of this test is to prevent the transfusion of incompatible blood products.

Human blood is grouped according to the presence or absence of specific chemical structures called *blood group antigens*. These antigens, which are found on the surface of the red blood cells, are substances capable of inducing the body to produce antibodies. Since 1900, more than 100 distinct antigens have been recognized on the red cell surface. However, compatibility of the ABO group is the foundation on which all other pretransfusion testing rests. The ABO system is now known to include several antigenic manifestations and many antibody specificities. In a strict sense, it is incorrect even to infer to the serologic findings as one system.

The red blood cell membrane is crowded with antigenically active molecules. Specific sugars, in specific linkage conformation, determine the antigenic activities called *A* and *B*. The presence of one sugar, N-acetylgalactosamine, gives the molecule A activity; a different sugar, galactose, determines B activity. The backbone molecule, without the added galactose or N-acetylgalactosamine, has antigenic activity called *H*. This H substance, as well as H gene activity, is essential to the expression of the ABO antigens. Group A contains RBCs with the A antigen; group B, with the B antigen; AB, with both A and B antigens; O cells contain neither A nor B antigens.

In general, patients are given blood of their own ABO group, for antibodies against the other blood antigens may be found in the blood serum. These antibodies are designated anti-A or anti-B, according to the antigen they act against. Under normal conditions a person's blood serum will *not* contain the antibody that is able to destroy its antigen. For example, a person with antigen A will *not* have anti-A in his serum. But he may have anti-B antibodies. Therefore, in addition to detecting antigens on red cells, it is necessary to test the patient's blood for the presence of specific antibodies to confirm ABO grouping.

Clinical Alert

To prevent a transfusion reaction, a situation that could be extremely dangerous and potentially fatal, a patient's blood group must be determined *in vitro* before any blood is administered.

Before a blood transfusion is begun, two professional persons must check the recipient's identified blood group with the donor type to be used in the transfusions. A blood group change or suppression may be induced by cancer or leukemia.

Procedure
A venous blood sample of 10 ml. is obtained.

Rh Factors; Rh Typing

Normal Values
Whites: 85% Rh-positive (*i.e.*, have the Rh antigen)
    15% Rh-negative (*i.e.*, lack the Rh antigen)
Blacks: 90% Rh-positive
    10% Rh-negative

Background
Human blood may be classified as Rh-positive or Rh-negative, depending on the presence or absence of Rh antigen on the red cell membrane. The Rh antigen, first discovered in 1939, has been extensively studied since 1943. The Rh antigen now called *Rho (D)* is, after the A and B antigen, the most important antigen in transfusion practice. Different systems of naming these antigens have been developed, and each system has its particular merits. The two nomenclatures used most frequently are given below.

Comparison of Terms Used in Rh System*

Weiner	Fisher-Race
Rh_o	D
rh'	C
rh"	E
hr'	c
hr"	e
hr	f(ce)
rh^G	G

* The term *Rh factor*, without qualification, means Rh_o
(D = Rh : 1). *Rh-positive* means RH_o (D) positive.

Explanation of Test
The Rh system is composed of antigens tested for in conjunction with the ABO group. D(Rh_o) factor is often the only factor for which testing is done. When this factor is not present, further typing is done to identify any of the less common Rh factors before the person is identified as Rh-negative. Rh-negative individuals may develop antibodies against Rh-positive antigens if they are challenged by either a transfusion of Rh-positive blood or a feto-maternal bleed from an Rh-positive fetus.

To determine the presence or absence of Rh antigen, the red blood cells are tested with anti-Dentisera. Agglutination of the cells indicates presence of antigen D. Absence of agglutination indicates absence of the antigen. There are three different ways to type blood for the Rh factor.

1. Saline tube test
2. Slide test
3. Modified tube test
   (a) Serum-suspended cells
   (b) Saline-suspended cells

Need for Rh Typing

Rh typing must be conducted because

1. The administration of Rh-positive blood to an Rh-negative person may sensitize the person to form anti-D.
2. The administration of D-positive blood to a recipient having anti-D in the serum could be fatal.
3. To identify Rho Gam (Rh immunoglobins) candidates
   (a) Rh-negative, pregnant women with Rh-positive partners may carry Rh-positive fetuses. Cells from the fetus may pass through the placenta to the mother and cause production of antibodies in the maternal blood. The maternal antibody, in turn, may pass through the placenta into the fetal circulation and cause destruction of fetal blood cells. This condition, called *hemolytic disease of the newborn* (formerly called *erythroblastosis fetalis*), may cause reactions ranging from anemia (slight or severe) to death *in utero*. This condition can be prevented if an Rh-negative woman who gives birth to an Rh-positive child is given an injection of Rh immunoglobulins (Rho Gam) shortly after delivery of an Rh-positive infant.
   (b) Rh typing must also be done in abortion patients.

Clinical Implications

1. The significance of Rh factors is based on their capacity to immunize in transfusions or pregnancies. The Rh_o (D) factor is by far the most antigenic, and the other Rh factors are much less likely to produce isoimmunization. The following general conditions must be met in immunization to Rh factors:
   (a) The blood factor must be absent in the immunized person.
   (b) The blood factor must be present in the immunizing blood.
   (c) The blood factor must be of sufficient antigenic strength.
   (d) The amount of incompatible blood must be large enough to induce antibody formation.
   Factors other than Rh_o (D) may induce formation of antibodies in Rh-positive persons, if conditions in #1 are met.
2. Antibodies for Rh' (C) are frequently found together with anti-Rh_o (D) antibodies in the Rh-negative, pregnant woman whose fetus or child was type Rh-positive and possessed both factors.
3. With exceedingly rare exceptions, Rh antibodies do not occur without preceding antigenic stimulation as in

(a) Pregnancy and abortions
(b) Blood transfusions
(c) Deliberate immunization, most commonly of repeated IV injections of blood for the purpose of harvesting a given Rh antibody.

Rh Antibody Titer Test

Normal Values
Normal is zero, no antibody

Explanation of Test
This antibody study is performed on a blood specimen to obtain the Rh-antibody level in a pregnant woman who is Rh-negative but whose partner is Rh-positive. If the Rh-negative woman is carrying an Rh-positive fetus, the antigen from the blood cells of the fetus causes antibody production in the serum of the mother. The firstborn child usually shows no ill effects, but with subsequent pregnancies the antibodies in the mother's serum increase and are sufficient to cause destruction of the red cells of the fetus (hemolytic disease of the newborn).

Procedure
A venous blood sample of 10 ml. is obtained.

Clinical Implications
If the Rh-antibody titer in the pregnant woman is greater than 1 : 64, an exchange transfusion is considered.

Crossmatch (Compatibility Test)

Normal Values
Compatibility is shown by the absence of clumping or hemolysis when serum and cells are appropriately mixed and incubated in the laboratory. (The major crossmatch is that between recipient serum and donor cells; the minor crossmatch is that between recipient cells and donor serum.)

Background
The primary purpose of the crossmatch, or compatibility test, is to prevent a transfusion reaction. The compatibility test includes the *major crossmatch* and the *minor crossmatch*. (The minor crossmatch is not usually done anymore.)

1. Major crossmatch is done to detect antibodies in the recipient's serum that may damage or destroy the cells of the proposed donor

(Table 8-1). Of the two tests, the major crossmatch is the more important.

2. Minor crossmatch is done to detect antibodies in the donor's serum capable of affecting the red blood cells of the recipient. Since donor antibodies will be greatly diluted *in vivo* by the recipient's plasma, these antibodies are considered to be of minor importance.

3. The type and screen is a group of tests performed on the blood that will determine the ABO and Rh_o (D) type as well as the presence or absence of unexpected antibodies on the recipient. The type and screen is a safe substitute for the routine one and two unit crossmatch in those operative procedures that usually do not require transfusion (*e.g.*, cholecystectomy). However, in the unlikely event that blood is needed, a major crossmatch must be performed prior to transfusion.

Explanation of Test

Crossmatching in the laboratory must be done to detect the following:

1. Different types of antibodies, such as:
    (a) High-protein medium-acting antibodies
    (b) Saline-acting antibodies
    (c) Antibodies recognizable only with the antiglobulin technique

Table 8-1
Antibodies Found in Crossmatching

Antibody	Frequency of Occurrence in Crossmatch	Description
Anti-B	Almost universal	Natural antibody-immune forms; may be hemolytic
Anti-A	Almost universal	Natural antibody-immune forms; may be hemolytic
Anti-Rh_o (D)	1 in 400	Most common immune antibody: enzyme enhanced
Anti-Rh_o' (D + C)	1 in 600	Anti-rh' (C) alone is rare; the combination of anti-C+D is frequent; enzyme enhanced
Autoantibody	1 in 2000	Acquired hemolytic anemia, lupus; occasionally specific (anti-hr'; anti-C; anti-e)
Cold agglutinin	1 in 2000	Viral pneumonitis, reacts with all cells
Anti-hr' (C)	1 in 5000	Most common immunization in Rh-positive persons
Anti-rh'' (E)	1 in 6000	Common immunization in Rh-positive persons; enzyme enhanced

(Continued)

Table 8-1
Antibodies Found in Crossmatching (Continued)

Antibody	Frequency of Occurrence in Crossmatch	Description
Anti-hr' + rh" (C + E)	1 in 6000	Combination occurs in the Rh_1Rh_1 CDe/CDe recipient, enzyme enhanced
Anti-A_1	1 in 10,000	Natural antibody may be present in A_2 and A_2B donor and recipient
Anti-K (Kell)	1 in 15,000	Potent antibody; it may occur in hemolytic disease of the newborn
Anti-(D + E)	1 in 15,000	Combination found in Rh-negative (rh) recipients (cde/cde)
anti-Le(Lewis)	1 in 20,000	Natural antibody-complex system; may be hemolytic; enzyme may enhance
Anti-Fy^a (Duffy)	1 in 20,000	Acquired by transfusion and/or pregnancy; enzyme may destroy it
Anti-P	1 in 20,000	Natural—weak—often reacts at refrigerator temperature
Anti-M	1 in 30,000	Natural—rarely immune; enzyme destroys it
Anti-(C+D+E)	1 in 30,000	Acquired antibodies in the Rh-negative person
Anti-Jk^a (Kidd)	1 in 30,000	Acquired; enzyme enhanced
Anti-rh' (C)	1 in 50,000	Acquired—rare in Rh-negative person as single antibody
Anti-hr" (e)	1 in 100,000	Acquired by transfusion and/or pregnancy in Rh_2Rh_2 (cDE/cDE) recipients
Anti-S	1 in 100,000	Natural or acquired; MN system; reacts more often with M or MC cells
Anti-rh^w_1 (C^w)	1 in 100,000	Acquired; "pure" anti-rh^w_1 (anti-C^w) in type Rh_1Rh_1 or type Rh_1rh recipient
Anti-k (Cellano)	1 in 100,000	Acquired; factor allelic to Kell
Anti-Jk^b (Kidd)	1 in 100,000	Acquired—enzyme enhanced; factor allelic to Jk^a
Anti-Fy^b (Duffy)		Acquired—enzyme may destroy; factor allelic to Fy^a
Anti-N		Natural—enzyme destroys it
Anti-Lu^a (Lutheran)		Acquired—enzyme may destroy it
Anti-hr(f)		Acquired—positive with cells of individuals having gene r or gene R^0

(After Bauer JD, et al: Bray's Clinical Laboratory Methods, 9th ed. St. Louis, CV Mosby, 1974)

Clinical Alert

Even the most carefully performed crossmatch will not detect all possible sources of incompatibility.

Procedure

A venous blood sample of 10 ml. is obtained.

Clinical Implications

1. A *transfusion reaction* will occur when incompatibile blood is transfused, specifically if antibodies in the recipient's serum would cause rapid destruction of the red blood cells of the proposed donor.
   (a) Certain antibodies, though not causing immediate red cell destruction and transfusion reaction, may nevertheless reduce the normal life span of transfused incompatible cells, necessitating subsequent transfusions.
   (b) Obviously, the patient will derive maximum benefit from red cells that survive longest in his circulation.
2. The probable benefits of each blood transfusion must be weighed against risks such as the following:
   (a) Hemolytic transfusion reactions due to infusion of incompatible blood, which can be fatal
   (b) Induction of febrile or allergic reactions
   (c) Transmission of infectious disease, especially hepatitis
   (d) Stimulation of antibody production, which could complicate later transfusion or childbearing

Clinical Alert

1. The most common cause of hemolytic transfusion reaction is the administration of blood to the wrong recipient because of improper patient identification and labeling of donor blood. The error, then, is often one of negligence.
2. Assess for *symptoms of transfusion reaction*
   a. Feeling of heat along the vein into which blood is transfused
   b. Constricting pain in chest and lumbar region of back
   c. Flushing of face
   d. Hemoglobinuria
   e. Generalized oozing of blood
   f. Bleeding from operative wounds

g. Allergic reactions such as local erythema, hives, and itching.
3. After massive blood transfusions assess for
    a. Hypocalcemia   d. Increased oxygen affinity
    b. Potassium intoxication   e. Hypothermia
    c. Increased blood ammonia   f. Hemosiderosis

Coombs' Antiglobulin Test

Normal Values
Direct Coombs' test negative, done on RBC
Indirect Coombs' test negative, done on serum

Explanation of Test
The Coombs' test is used to show the presence of antigen–antibody complexes by its direct method or it may be used to detect the presence of antibodies that react only with the aid of a potentiating medium, by its indirect method.
A. *Direct Coombs' test*
   1. Detects the presence of antigen–antibody complexes on the red blood cell membrane (*in vivo*) or red blood cell sensitization
   2. Diagnoses the following conditions:
      (a) Hemolytic disease of the newborn when the red cells of the infant are sensitized, thus exhibiting Ag–Ab complexes *in vivo*.
      (b) Acquired hemolytic anemia when the patient may have produced an antibody that coats his own cells (auto-sensitization *in vivo*).
      (c) Transfusion reaction when the patient may have received incompatible blood that has sensitized his red cells.
      (d) Red blood cell sensitization caused by drugs.
B. *Indirect Coombs' test*
   1. Detects presence of antibody in serum (*e.g.,* a major crossmatch)
   2. Reveals presence of anti-Rh antibodies in mother's blood during pregnancy
   3. Is valuable in detecting incompatibilities not found by other methods

Procedure
A venous blood sample of 10 ml. is obtained.

Clinical Implications

A. *Direct Coombs' test*
   1. Positive test in
      (a) Autoimmune hemolytic anemia (most cases)
      (b) Transfusion reaction
      (c) Patients receiving cephalothin therapy (75% of cases) and some penicillin
      (d) Also drugs such as alpha-methyldopa (Aldomet)
   2. Negative test in
      Nonautoimmune hemolytic anemias
B. *Indirect Coombs' test*
   1. Positive test in
      (a) Presence of specific antibody, usually as a result of a previous transfusion or pregnancy
      (b) Presence of a nonspecific antibody, as in cold agglutination disease and drug-induced hemolytic anemia

Interfering Factors
There are a number of drugs that may cause a positive direct Coombs' test.

Clinical Alert

Antibody identification is done when the antibody screen or direct antiglobulin tests are positive. This is a procedure by which unexpected blood group antibodies are classified. These tests are important in pretransfusion testing so that the appropriate antigen-negative blood can be selected and in the diagnosis of hemolytic disease of the newborn and autoimmune hemolytic anemia. Specimen collection includes obtaining venous blood samples of 7 ml. of whole blood with EDTA added and 20 ml. of clotted blood. Notify the laboratory of diagnosis, history of recent and past transfusions, pregnancy, and any drug therapy.

Leukoagglutinin Test

Normal Values
Negative

Background
Leukoagglutinins are antibodies that react with white blood cells and are responsible for some febrile, nonhemolytic transfusion reactions.

Patients with this type of transfusion reaction should be transfused with leukocyte-poor blood.

Explanation of Test

This study is done after a reaction occurs when compatible blood has been given. When blood containing leukoagglutinins is infused, the donor plasma contains an antibody that reacts with recipient white cells and produces an acute clinical syndrome of fever, dyspnea, cough, and pulmonary infiltrates. In severe cases, cyanosis and hypertensive episodes have also been described. Patients who have been immunized by multiple previous transfusions, during pregnancy, or during allografts often suffer from febrile, nonhemolytic transfusion reactions due to the transfused incompatible leukocytes. This type of reaction must be distinguished from hemolytic reactions before further transfusions can be safely administered.

Procedure

A venous blood sample of 10 ml. is obtained.

Clinical Implications

1. Agglutinating antibodies may appear in the donor's plasma if tested.
2. When the agglutinating antibody is in the recipient's plasma, although febrile reactions are common, no pulmonary manifestations occur when incompatible leukocytes are transfused.
3. Febrile reactions are more common in pregnant patients and those with a history of multiple transfusions.

Clinical Alert

1. Febrile reactions can be prevented by separating white cells from the donor blood before transfusion.
2. Patients whose blood contains leukoagglutinins should be notified and generally transfused with leukocyte-poor blood to avoid or reduce the chance of future febrile nonhemolytic transfusion reactions.

Platelet Antibody Detection Tests

Normal Values

PLAI: negative
ALTP: negative
PAIgG: negative

Platelet hyperlysibility: negative
Drug-dependent platelet antibodies: negative

Explanation of Test
Platelet antibody detection studies are aids to diagnosis in posttransfusion purpura, alloimmune neonatal thrombocytopenic purpura, idiopathic thrombocytopenia purpura, paroxysmal hemoglobinuria, and drug-induced immunologic thrombocytopenia.

Procedure
Ten milliliters to 30 ml. of venous blood is required for specific assays. Check with your laboratory.

Interfering Factors
Positive reactions may be produced by alloantibodies resulting from previous blood transfusions in pregnancies. Such antibodies are usually specific for HLA antigens expressed in platelets and other cells. Whenever possible, samples for platelet antibody testing should be obtained before transfusion.

Clinical Implications
1. Antiplatelet antibody, usually having anti-PLAI specificity, is detected in posttransfusion purpura.
2. A persistent or rising antibody titer in pregnancy is associated with neonatal thrombocytopenia.
3. PLAI incompatibility between mother and fetus appears to account for more than 60% of alloimmune neonatal thrombocytopenic purpura. A finding that the mother is PLAI negative and the father is PLAI positive provides presumptive evidence for the diagnosis.
4. Platelet-associated IgG antibody is present in 95% of idiopathic (autoimmune) thrombocytopenic purpura (both acute and chronic). In patients who are responding to steroid therapy or who are undergoing spontaneous remission, increased circulatory times correlate with decreased PAIgG levels.
5. The platelet hyperlysibility assay measures the sensitivity of platelets to lysis. This test is positive in paroxysmal hemoglobinuria and is specific for that diagnosis.
6. In drug-induced immunologic thrombocytopenia, antibodies reactive only in the presence of the inciting drug can be detected. Quinidine and quinine most commonly cause this type of thrombocytopenia as well as chlordiazepoxide, sulfa drugs, and diphenylhydantoin. Gold-dependent antibodies and heparin-dependent platelet IgG antibodies can be detected by direct assay. (In approximately 1% of persons receiving gold therapy, thrombocytopenia develops as a side-effect. Thrombocytopenia is a well-known side-effect of heparin, and an immune mechanism may be the cause.

Note: Platelet typing is also done. Compatibility tests of platelets assure that hemostatically effective platelets can be transfused to indicated patients as in aplastic anemia and malignant disorders. This is important because most patients transfused repeatedly with platelets from random donors become partially or totally refractory to further transfusion as a consequence of alloimmunization.

Platelet typing can also be helpful in providing additional evidence to support a diagnosis of posttransfusion purpura. Platelets are routinely typed for PLAI, HLH-A2, and PLEI. It is recognized that platelets matched for HLA antigens will generally produce satisfactory posttransfusion improvement. It has been reported that a standard platelet count performed 1 hour from the end of a transfusion of fresh platelet concentrate is a sensitive indicator of the presence or absence of clinically important antibody against HLA antigens.

Specimen requirements vary:

30 ml. of venous blood when platelet count is 50,000 to 100,000 per cu. mm.

20 ml. of venous blood when platelet count is 100,000 to 150,000 per cu. mm.

10 ml. of venous blood when platelet count is >150,000 per cu. mm.

SEROLOGIC TESTS OF INFECTIOUS DISEASES OF BACTERIAL, VIRAL, FUNGAL, AND PARASITIC ORIGIN

Bacterial

Syphilis Detection Tests

Normal Values
Nonreactive: negative

Background
Syphilis is a venereal disease caused by *Treponema pallidum,* a spirochete with closely wound coils approximately 8 to 15 microns long. The untreated disease progresses through three stages that may extend over many years.

Explanation of Tests
The major types of tests used in the diagnosis of syphilis are (1) flocculation or agglutination, (2) fluorescent antibody test (FTA), and (3) hemagglutination tests (Table 8-2).

1. *Flocculation or agglutination test*
   Flocculation reaction is a microscopic clumping of antigen and antibody. Positive results in a test of this type depend on the degree of

Table 8-2
Serologic Tests for Syphilis (STS)

Name of Test	Type/Description	Comments
FTA (fluorescent treponemal antibody)	Syphilitic serum is bound to surface of *Treponema pallidum:* antibody is made visible by using fluorescein-tagged antiserum	Fluorescent-labeled antibody against human globulin is added to serum. Spirochetes combined with antibody will fluoresce.
FTA-ABS (fluorescent treponemal antibody absorption)	Fluorescent antibody	Detects treponemal antibodies. Differentiates biologic false positives from true syphilis positives and diagnoses syphilis when definite clinical signs of syphilis are present but other tests are negative.
FTA-ABS, Igm only		Used in diagnosis of congenital syphilis; not used as screening test. A positive RPR can be confirmed with this test.
RPR (rapid plasma reagin)	Flocculation	Reagin reacts with lipid antigens; used as screening test; shows presence of reagin. More sensitive than VDRL. Patients treated for syphilis should have baseline RPR.
TPI (Treponemal pallidum immobilization)	Uses living, motile *Treponema pallidum* as antigen	Shows presence of treponemal antibody; most sensitive and specific test for syphilis. Only performed at Centers for Disease Control in Atlanta, GA.
VDRL	Flocculation	Used as a screening test. Developed in the Venereal and Research Laboratories of the U.S. Public Health Service; shows presence of reagin.
TP-MHA (micro-hemagglutination assay for *Treponema pallidum* antibodies)	Hemagglutination	Shows presence of treponemal antibody. Even more specific than an FTA-ABS.
Reiter	Complement-fixation	An antigen–antibody reagin that causes hemolysis. Detects the presence of treponemal antibody in the blood. Based on the outdated Wassermann test.

flocculant material formed in the test substance. The VDRL is an example of a flocculation test in current use. The RPR is a macroscopic agglutination test.

2. *Fluorescent antibody test*
   FTA-ABS is an example of a fluorescent antibody test in current use.
3. *Hemagglutination tests*
   The TP-MHA is an example of a hemagglutination test in current use.

Testing for Serum Antibody

During the course of the infection, two types of antibodies may form: (1) reagin, and (2) specific treponemal antibody. Different serologic tests are available to show the presence of each of these antibodies.

Tests to show reagin: VDRL and RPR
Tests to show treponemal antibody: FTA, microhemagglutination test for *T. pallidum,* and rarely used treponemal immobilization test. In general, the serologic tests for detection of treponemal antibody are used on all reactive VDRL and RPR tests or on physician request.

Interpreting Tests for Syphilis

In interpreting tests for syphilis, several factors must be considered.

1. Geographical area
2. Ability of patient to produce reagin or treponemal antibodies
3. Stage of the disease

Procedure

1. A venous blood sample is obtained (serum is used).
2. Fasting is usually *not* required.

Clinical Implications

1. These test results are considered *positive* for syphilis antibodies.
   (a) "Reactive"
   (b) "Weakly reactive"
   (c) "Borderline"
2. When the test is positive for syphilis, it is always confirmed. If none of the diseases that cause false positives are present, the diagnosis of syphilis is suggested if the history and symptoms of the patient point to the disease. A single nonreactive test *suggests* the absence of syphilis but does not *prove* it. The test requires repetition if the patient's medical history warrants it.
3. Treatment of syphilis may change both the clinical course and serological pattern of the disease. The effect of treatment during the three stages in relation to the VDRL, or any test for syphilis that shows the presence of reagin, is as follows:

(a) If the patient is treated adequately before the appearance of the primary chancre, it is probable that the VDRL will remain nonreactive (negative).

(b) If the patient is treated at the seronegative primary stage (*e.g.*, after the appearance of the chancre but before the appearance of reaction or reagin), the VDRL will remain nonreactive.

(c) If the patient is treated in the seropositive primary stage (*e.g.*, after the appearance of reaction) the VDRL usually becomes nonreactive within 6 months.

(d) If the patient is treated during the secondary stage, the VDRL will usually become nonreactive within 12 to 18 months. If the patient is treated 10 or more years after the onset of the disease, the VDRL can be expected to change little, if any. The longer the patient goes untreated, the longer it will take the VDRL to become nonreactive after adequate treatment, if it ever does.

4. A negative serological test may indicate

(a) The patient does not have syphilis.

(b) The infection is too recent to have allowed the patient to produce antibodies that give the reactions. Repeat tests should be performed 1 week, 1 month, and 3 months later to exclude syphilis in patients with typical symptoms of syphilis.

(c) The patient is temporarily nonreactive after treatment or because of other causes such as drinking of alcoholic fluids.

(d) The syphilis is in a latent or inactive phase.

(e) The patient has a faulty immunodefense mechanism.

(f) The laboratory techniques were inferior.

False-Positive Reactions

A positive reaction does not necessarily mean that the patient has syphilis. Several conditions will give a biologically false-positive (BFP) reaction for syphilis (Table 8-3). Biological false-positive reactions are by no means "false." They may reveal the presence of serious diseases other than syphilis. Little is known about the antibody or reaction concerned in the mechanism of BFP reactions. It is believed that reagin (reaction) is an antibody against tissue lipids. Lipids are presumed to be liberated from body tissue in the course of normal wear and tear, and these liberated lipids may induce the formation of antibodies within the same patient.

Interfering Factors

In tests for syphilis that detect reagin

1. Alcohol decreases the intensity of the reaction.

2. Excess chyle in the blood interferes with the reaction. For this reason, the blood sample should be drawn before a meal.

Table 8-3
Nonsyphilitic Conditions Giving Biological False
Positives (BFPs) Using VDRL and RPR Tests

Disease	Percentage (Approximate) BFPs
Malaria	100
Leprosy	60
Relapsing fever	30
Active immunization in children	20
Infectious mononucleosis	20
Lupus erythematosus	20
Lymphogranuloma venereum	20
Pneumonia, atypical	20
Rat-bite fever	20
Typhus fever	20
Vaccinia	20
Infectious hepatitis	10
Leptospirosis (Weil's disease)	10
Periarteritis nodosa	10
Trypanosomiasis	10
Chancroid	5
Chickenpox	5
Measles	5
Rheumatoid arthritis	5–7
Rheumatic fever	5–6
Scarlet fever	5
Subacute bacterial endocarditis	5
Pneumonia, pneumococcal	3–5
Tuberculosis, advanced pulmonary	3–5
Blood loss, repeated	?(low)
Common cold	?(low)
Pregnancy	?(low)

Patient Preparation
Instruct the patient not to drink alcohol for 24 hours before taking of a blood sample.

Clinical Alert

1. Sexual partners of patients with primary, secondary, or early latent syphilis should be evaluated for signs and symptoms of syphilis and should have a blood test for syphilis. Social contacts of infants with symptomatic neonatal syphilis should be examined in a similar manner.

2. After treatment, patients with early syphilis should be tested at 3-month intervals for 1 year. The reaction level declines in most patients followed for a year until little or no reaction is detected.

Lyme Disease Test

Normal values
<1:256

Explanation of Test
The test is helpful in the diagnosis of Lyme disease caused by a newly discovered spirochete, *Borrelia burgdorferi*. Ticks are the best documented vectors of the spirochete. This measurement can be used as an indication of infection or postexposure.

Procedure
A venous blood sample of 1 ml. is obtained.

Interfering Factors
1. False-positives occur in 21% of persons with high rheumatoid factors.
2. Persons with triponomal disease have considerable cross-reactivity.

Clinical Implications
1. Identification of:
   a. 50% of early Lyme disease and erythema chronica migrans
   b. 100% of patients with later complications of carditis, neuritis, arthritis, and patients in remission.

Legionnaires' Pneumophilia Antibody Test

Normal Values
Negative.

Explanation of Test
This test facilitates the diagnosis of Legionnaires' disease. This test is most supportive when serial serum samples are obtained and when used with tissue specimen testing. Serum studies are useful in evaluating epidemic disease.

Clinical Implications

1. There are more than 20 different species of Legionella and testing will be expanded to include new species as reagents become available. The test is species specific.
2. Evidence of antibody response to this disease requires a fourfold increase in titer to ≥1:128.
3. Evidence of previous infection requires a single titer of ≥1:256.
4. The most supportive evidence of recent *Legionella* infection is a fourfold rise in titer between acute (within the first week) and convalescent (three to six weeks after appearance of fever) phases.

Chlamydia Antibodies IgG Test

Normal Values
Titer ≤1:640

Background
Chlamydia have many features that bacteria have and are susceptible to antibiotic therapy. They require living cells to multiply, as do viruses. There are two species of the genus. *Chlamydia:chlamydia trachomatis* and *Chlamydia psittaci*.

Explanation of Test
This test, using paired samples, is helpful in diagnosing *Chlamydia psittaci* and lymphogranuloma venereum.

Procedure
A venous blood sample of 10 ml. is drawn.

Clinical Implications

1. A positive titer could indicate either LGV or psittacosis. Diagnosis of psittacosis should include documentation of previous contact with sick birds or employment in pet shops.
2. In females, chlamydia cause
   (a) pelvic inflammatory disease
   (b) endometriosis
   (c) salpingitis
3. In males, chlamydia cause
   (a) Reiter's syndrome
   (b) epididymitis
4. Perihepatitis (Fitz-Hugh–Curtis syndrome) has been linked with chlamydia.

Interfering Factors
Depending on geographic location, titers of ≤1:16 can be found in the general population.

Streptococcal Antibody Tests: Anti-Streptolysin O Titer (ASO), **Streptozyme**, Anti-Dnase B (ADB) (Streptodornase)

Normal Values
ASO
Adults 1:85 units
Children
Preschool 1:85 units
School age 1:170 units
Anti-Dnase B
<100 units

Background
Streptolysin "O" is a hemolytic factor produced by most strains of Group A beta-hemolytic streptococci. ASO is the specific neutralizing antibody produced after infection with these organisms. ASO appears in the serum from 1 week to 1 month after the onset of a streptococcal infection. ADB is another specific antibody formed to inhibit reactions to Group A streptococci.

Explanation of Test
ASO test is used to diagnose conditions resulting from a streptococcal infection. It is useful in the diagnosis of rheumatic fever and glomerulonephritis. This test detects antibodies to the exoenzymes of streptococcus Group A, which may develop in rheumatic fever, glomerulonephritis, bacterial endocarditis, scarlet fever, and other related conditions. Serial determinations with a rising titer over a period of weeks are more significant than a single determination.

Types of Tests
1. ASO—most widely used—will detect antistreptolysin only
2. Streptozyme will detect antibodies to multiple enzymes produced by streptococcus.
3. ADB will detect anti-Dnase B.

Procedure
1. A venous blood sample of 10 ml. (serum) is obtained and repeated 10 days later.
2. Subsequent testing is advisable two times a week for 4 to 6 weeks following a streptococcal infection.

Clinical Implications
1. The titer that is considered elevated varies, but in general a titer of greater than 166 Todd units is definitely elevated.
2. Both the ASO and ADB tests alone will be positive in 80% to 85% of

streptococcal A infections such as streptococcal pharyngitis, rheumatic fever, pyoderma, and glomerulonephritis.
3. When the two tests are run concurrently, 95% of cases of streptococcal infection can be detected.
4. A repeated low titer is good evidence that there is no active rheumatic fever. However, a high titer does not necessarily mean rheumatic fever or glomerulonephritis, yet it does indicate a focus of streptococcal infection. The deciding factors in diagnosis are clinical symptoms and other laboratory tests.
5. The production of ASO is especially high in cases of rheumatic fever and glomerulonephritis. It is characteristic for each of these conditions to show a marked increase of the ASO titer during the symptomless period preceding an attack of the illness; however ADB titers are particularly high in pyoderma.

Interfering Factors
1. An increased titer is sometimes found in healthy carriers.
2. Antibiotic therapy will suppress the streptococcal antibody response.
3. Increased beta lipoprotein levels inhibit streptolysin O, thereby giving falsely high ASO titer.

Clinical Alert

The ASO test is impractical in patients who have recently received antibiotics or who are scheduled for antibiotic therapy, since the treatment suppresses the antibody response.

Teichoic Acid Antibody Test

Normal Values
Titer of 1:2 or less
Values vary depending on laboratory methods.

Background
Gram-positive bacteria have teichoic acid as an element of cell walls.

Explanation of Test
This test is used to measure teichoic acid antibodies and is helpful in managing patient response to therapy. This antibody is found in some patients with infections caused by *Staphylococcus aureus*.

Procedure
A venous blood sample of 7 ml. is obtained.

Clinical Implications
Positive tests are associated with a greater than fourfold increase between acute and convalescent samples. Teichoic acid antibodies are associated with

1. Staphylococcal endocarditis
2. Osteomyelitis

Viral

Infectious Mononucleosis Tests: Routine; Heterophile Antibody Titer Test; Epstein–Barr Virus (EBV) Antibody Tests

Normal Values
Negative

Background
Normal serum contains heterophile antibodies. A heterophile antibody is one that is capable of reacting with an antigen that is completely unrelated to the antigen originally stimulating its formation. Infectious mononucleosis, caused by the Epstein–Barr virus (EBV), induces the formation of lymphocytes and monocytes in lymph nodes in increased numbers and in abnormal forms. It also stimulates an increase in heterophile antibody formation. Epstein–Barr virus is also known to produce a cytomegalo-viruslike lymphoproliferative disease in renal and liver transplants, in AIDS and in posttransfusion.

Explanation of Test
Monospot, Mono-test and Monostican are some of the routine diagnostic presumptive tests for infectious mononucleosis. Confirmatory tests are heterophile antibody tests and specific tests for Epstein–Barr virus.

In the laboratory, the sheep RBC is commonly used to detect heterophile antibodies in the serum of patients (not Forssman-type) with suspected infectious mononucleosis. Such patients begin developing heterophile antibodies shortly after the appearance of symptoms, usually during the first 2 weeks. When the clinical picture suggests IM with a negative heterophile antibody test, specific tests for EB can be done. A rise in the Epstein–Barr virus titer is diagnostic of IM.

IgM antibodies that are specific for the viral antigen peak (fourfold increase in 25% of patients) and disappear soon after the disease subsides, making a specific diagnosis of infectious mononucleosis possible.

EBV titers using IFA usually appear after the first week of illness, rise to 1:16 by the third week and remain for years thereafter. Three antibodies can be detected

1. Antiviral capsid antigen (VCA); most commonly used test
2. Antibody to the EBV nuclear antigen (EBNA)
3. IgG antibody to early antigen (EA)

Procedure
A venous blood sample of 5 ml. is obtained.

Clinical Implications
1. A presumptive antibody titer of 1:56 is suspicious. A titer of 1:224 or greater is diagnostic of infectious mononucleosis.
2. Positive reactions last 4 to 8 weeks after the appearance of symptoms.
3. The highest titers are usually found during the second and third week of illness, but have no relationship to the severity of the disease or its prognosis.
4. The clinical symptoms of infectious mononucleosis disappear before the abnormal blood picture disappears.
5. When interpreting the significance of the titer from the presumptive test, certain points are important:
   (a) 90% of the normal adult population have antibodies to VCA and EBA antigens.
   (b) A high incidence of elevated titers is found in infectious mononucleosis and
(1) Burkitt's lymphoma	(6) Pancreatic carcinoma
(2) Nasopharyngeal carcinoma	(7) Systemic lupus erythematosus (SLE)
(3) Hayden's disease	
(4) Lymphocytic leukemia	(8) Sarcoidosis
(5) Hepatitis A & B	(9) Izuma fever
6. The presence of IgM antibodies or of antibodies to VCA and absence of an immune response to EBNA indicate recent infection with EBV.
7. Antiviral capsid antigen (VCA). Both IgM and IgG are present during the acute state and peak during this period. Titers decline by 1 to 2 months. IgG titers decline, but present at lower levels for a few years. (Good evidence against EBV infection is the persistent absence of antibody to VCA).
8. Antibody to the EBV nuclear antigen (EBNA). This antibody is absent during the acute phase and appears weeks to months after most cases.
9. IgG antibody to early antigen EA. Most persons with infectious mononucleosis have a transient EA response. In addition, increased (1:40) EA levels occur in chronic active or reactive EBV infection. This test is also positive in nasopharyngeal carcinoma (NPC) types one and two.

Rubella Antibody Tests

Normal Values
No real normal.
Negative: not immune/no antibody detected
Positive: immune/antibody detected

Background
Rubella virus is the causative agent of German measles, a mild systemic disease characterized by fever and transient rash. It is important to identify exposure to rubella infection and susceptibility status in pregnant women, since infection in the first trimester of pregnancy is associated with congenital abnormalities, miscarriage, or stillbirth in about 3% of infected women. Rubella infection will induce IgG and IgM antibody formation.

Explanation of Test
This test is done to determine immune status and confirm rubella infection. The test is indicated in pregnancy, to identify potential carriers of rubella who may infect women of childbearing age, such as hospital employees responsible for maternal child care, and others such as teachers, dentists, nurses, physicians, and midwives.

Types of Tests
HAI, the classic test, but not state of the art; latex agglutination results within 10 minutes; EIA or ELISA (enzyme immunoassay or enzyme-linked immunoassay).

Procedure
A venous blood sample of 5 ml. is obtained.

Clinical Implications
1. Demonstration of an IgG with a fourfold rise in titer between acute and convalescent specimens and the presence of IgM antibody are indicative of a recent rubella infection.
2. Stable titers should not be interpreted as evidence of recent rubella infection.
3. In naturally acquired rubella, IgM and IgG antibodies are present, although IgM is not detectable beyond 8 weeks of onset.
4. In congenital rubella, infants' antibodies on delivery are composed of fetal IgM, fetal IgG, and fetal IgA as well as maternal IgG; mother will have only IgG.

Antibody levels in the infant that are passively acquired will decrease markedly within 2 to 3 months.

Hepatitis Tests

Normal Values
Negative for hepatitis A, hepatitis B, and non-A, non-B hepatitis and Delta Δ hepatitis.

Background
There are at least three different types of viral hepatitis: hepatitis A, hepatitis B, and non-A, non-B (NANB) hepatitis. Although these forms are clinically similar, they differ with respect to immunology, epidemiology, prognosis and prophylaxis (Figs. 8-1 and 8-2).

Hepatitis A (HA), commonly known as *infectious hepatitis,* has a characteristic incubation period of 2 to 6 weeks; onset is acute rather than insidious. It is usually transmitted through personal contact, either oral or fecal, although a parenteral mode of transmission is possible, (documented, but rare). Hepatitis A is found more frequently in children or young adults and is not associated with either development of chronic hepatitis or development of the carrier state.

In contrast, hepatitis B (HB), also called *serum hepatitis, Australian antigen hepatitis,* or *transfusion hepatitis,* may be associated with drug usage, may have a relatively longer incubation period (6 to 26 weeks), and its primary mode of transmission is parenteral. It tends to occur more often in males than in females and is a significant cause of chronic active hepatitis. It is characterized by insidious onset; approximately 10% of hepatitis B patients become carriers.

Delta hepatitis (Δ) is always associated with a coexistent hepatitis B virus infection. Common diagnosis is made by RIA or ELISA tests that detect antibody or positive tests. Although referred to in the literature, in practice it is relatively uncommon.

Non-A, non-B hepatitis (NANB) refers to viral hepatitis caused by at least two (as yet) unidentified agents that are distinct from hepatitis A and hepatitis B virus. However, one of these resembles hepatitis A and the other resembles hepatitis B.

Type 1
Epidemic non-A, non-B is similar to hepatitis A and differential diagnosis depends on exclusion of other etiologies of hepatitis, especially HA, by serologic test.

Type 2
Non-A, non-B, B-like hepatitis is also known as non-B transfusion associated hepatitis, posttransfusion non-A, non-B hepatitis, or hepatitis C. Differential diagnosis depends on exclusion of hepatitis A and B and on epidemiology.

This type of hepatitis is more common when paid blood donors are used and is the most common posttransfusion hepatitis in the USA. It

			Interpretation	Immune to further HAV infection	Potentially infectious to others for HAV
Anti-HAV	Positive	Anti-HAV/IgM Positive	Recent infection with HAV	Yes	Yes—if early in symptomatic phase
		Anti-HAV/IgM Negative	Past infection with HAV at some undetermined time*	Yes*	No—if later— 7–10 days after onset of jaundice
	Negative		Infection not due to HAV	No	No

* Anti-HAV positive result can also occur following use of IG. Passively acquired anti-HAV will provide only temporary immunity to HAV. IG does not affect the anti-HAV-IgM result.

Figure 8-1
Interpretation of hepatitis A serologic results.

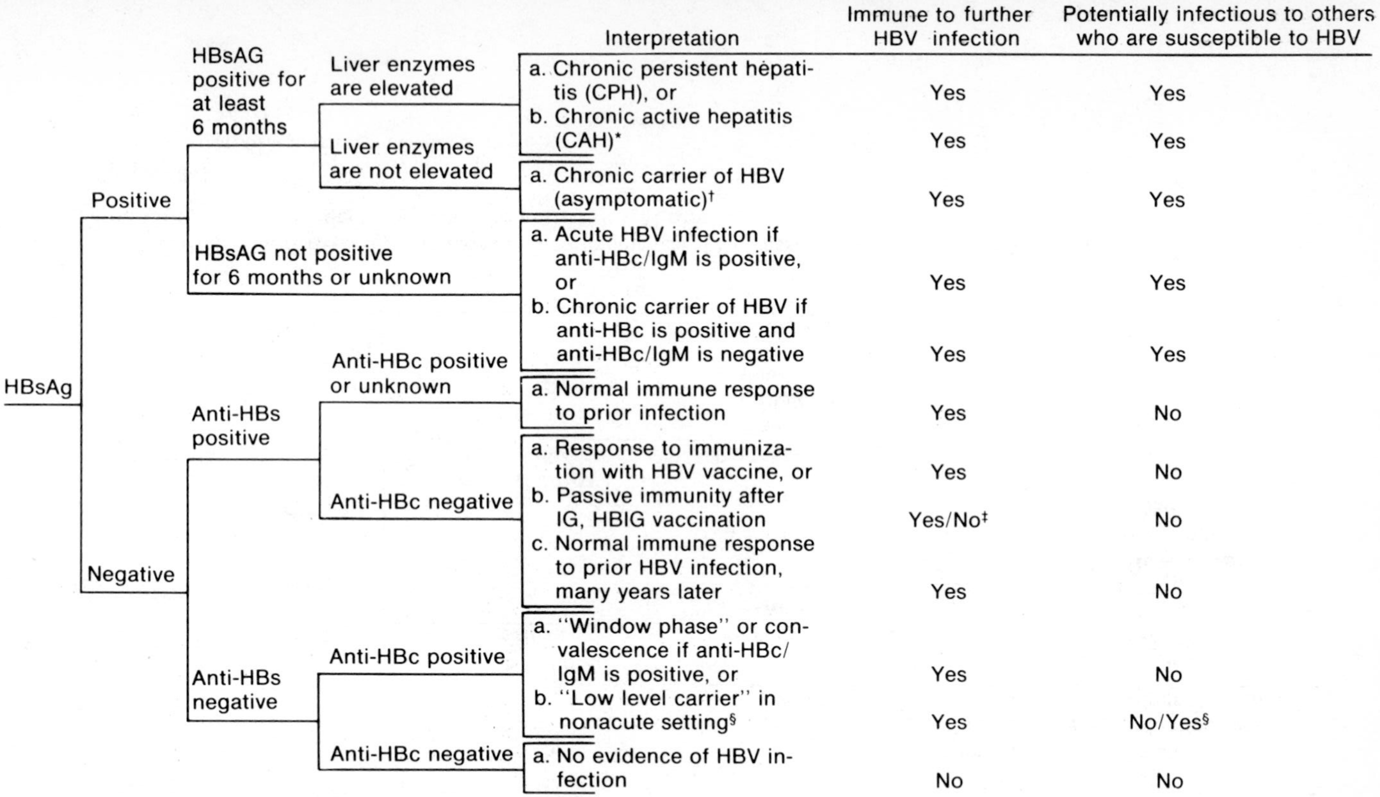

Figure 8-2
Interpretation of hepatitis B serologic results.

HBsAg				Interpretation	Immune to further HBV infection	Potentially infectious to others who are susceptible to HBV
Positive	HBsAG positive for at least 6 months	Liver enzymes are elevated		a. Chronic persistent hepatitis (CPH), or	Yes	Yes
				b. Chronic active hepatitis (CAH)*	Yes	Yes
		Liver enzymes are not elevated		a. Chronic carrier of HBV (asymptomatic)†	Yes	Yes
	HBsAG not positive for 6 months or unknown			a. Acute HBV infection if anti-HBc/IgM is positive, or	Yes	Yes
				b. Chronic carrier of HBV if anti-HBc is positive and anti-HBc/IgM is negative	Yes	Yes
Negative	Anti-HBs positive	Anti-HBc positive or unknown		a. Normal immune response to prior infection	Yes	No
		Anti-HBc negative		a. Response to immunization with HBV vaccine, or	Yes	No
				b. Passive immunity after IG, HBIG vaccination	Yes/No‡	No
				c. Normal immune response to prior HBV infection, many years later	Yes	No
	Anti-HBs negative	Anti-HBc positive		a. "Window phase" or convalescence if anti-HBc/IgM is positive, or	Yes	No
				b. "Low level carrier" in nonacute setting§	Yes	No/Yes§
		Anti-HBc negative		a. No evidence of HBV infection	No	No

* Liver biopsy is needed to make definitive diagnosis between CPH and CAH.
† HBeAg and anti-HBe testing is appropriate in this setting: HBeAg positive persons are at higher risk of transmitting disease than persons HBeAg negative and anti-HBe positive.
‡ Passive protection is of limited duration.
§ May be infectious in a transfusion setting. HBsAg level below level of detection or late convalescence with loss of anti-HBs detectability.

also causes sporadic community acquired hepatitis, accounting for 15% to 40% of cases.

Transmission is through contaminated blood or plasma derivation or by use of improperly sterilized syringe and needle. Incubation period is from 2 weeks to 6 months, but most fall within a six-to-nine week period. Prophylactic IG is used for associated needle shots.

Explanation of Test

These measurements are used in the differential diagnosis of viral hepatitis. The identification of the virus in serum will aid in determining progress, assessing probability of close contacts developing hepatitis, and help in forming a hepatitis control program.

Differentiation among the major viruses responsible for hepatitis requires the use of specific serological markers in order to characterize the infection. Specific serological markers are available for the diagnosis of hepatitis A and hepatitis B viruses, while the NANB viruses are identified by the exclusion of A and B.

By measuring just three of the seven available hepatitis markers, the viral agent causing the symptoms of acute viral hepatitis can be determined. The first of these markers is the antibody to the hepatitis A virus, IgM specific (HAV/IgM). This marker first appears between 4 weeks and 6 weeks after innoculation and indicates an acute stage of hepatitis A infection. The other two markers analyzed are the B surface antigen and B core antibody, which identify the early acute stage of a B-viral infection. The absence of these markers leads to a diagnosis of NANB infection, some other viral infection, or hepatic toxicity.

Appearance of Hepatitis Viral Markers Following Infection

Serological Marker	Time After Infection	Clinical Implications
Hepatitis A virus		
HAV-Ab/IgM	4–6 wk.	Positive for acute state, hepatitis A; develops early in disease
HAV-Ab/IgG	8–12 wk.	Indicative of previous exposure and immunity to hepatitis A
Hepatitis B virus		
HBsAg–hepatitis B surface antigen	4–12 wk.	Positive for acute stage, hepatitis B; earliest indicator of the presence of acute infection; also indicative of chronic infection
HBeAg	4–12 wk.	Positive for acute active stage with viral replication (infectivity factor), "Highly infectious"

(Continued)

Appearance of Hepatitis Viral Markers Following
Infection (Continued)

Serological Marker	Time After Infection	Clinical Implications
HBcAb, hepatitis B core antibody	6–14 wk.	Indicates past infection
HBeAb antibody	8–16 wk.	Indicates resolution of acute infection
HbsAb antibody	2–10 mo.	Indicative of previous exposure and immunity to hepatitis B, but not necessarily to other types of hepatitis; this is the marker for permanent immunity

The assessment of the hepatitis B virus involves the use of three markers that are expected to occur during the course of infection. (1) Hepatitis B surface antigen (HBsAg) is present in serum 4 weeks to 12 weeks after infection, denoting the initial acute stage of infection. (2) Shortly after the appearance of the hepatitis B surface antigen, the core antibody (HBcAb) is detectable for a period of 6 weeks to 14 weeks. (3) Finally, 2 months to 10 months after infection, hepatitis B surface antibody (HBsAb) can be detected, indicating *clinical recovery* and *immunity to the B virus.*

Procedure
A venous blood sample of 6 ml. is obtained or 2 ml. for each test.

Clinical Implications
1. HAV-Ab/IgM and HAV-Ab/IgG refer to total antibody to hepatitis A virus. They are indicators of recent acute as well as past infection and are useful in confirming previous exposure and immunity to hepatitis A.
2. If transfused, blood containing hepatitis virus markers carries a 40% to 70% risk of causing hepatitis. Transfusion of HBsAg negative blood tends to cause a clinical mild hepatitis.
   Use enteric precautions for hepatitis A.
3. Hepatitis B surface antigen (HBsAg) is found in many patients with chronic active hepatitis, whether or not acute hepatitis has occurred previously. Hepatitis B antigen is frequently found in
   (a) Patients receiving renal dialysis
   (b) Institutionalized patients with Down's syndrome
   (c) Patients receiving immunosuppressive medication (certain cases)
   (d) Lymphocytic leukemia
   (e) Hodgkin's disease
   (f) Lepromatous leprosy

A small number of seemingly healthy persons with no history of acute illness have hepatitis A and B virus in their blood serum. It may be that in these patients a very mild, subclinical infection has occurred that is more likely to produce a carrier state than an acute illness and subsequent clearing. However, normal subjects will not be positive for anti-HAV/IgM. IgM titers are only positive during the acute episode and generally become negative 4 months after exposure. The presence of HBeAg is an early indicator of acute, active hepatitis B infection representing the most infectious period. It is usually short-lived (3–6 weeks). Persistence of "e" antigen in the acute stage beyond 10 weeks is indicative of progression to chronic carrier state and probable chronic disease.

4. Presence of HBcAb is an early indicator of acute infection and a lifelong marker that represents past exposure as well as active infection in the acute/chronic period. In the absence of HBsAg and anti-HBs, this hepatitis B core antibody is an important serologic marker to identify recent infection. This situation is referred to as the "core" window. The presence of HBsAB is an indication of clinical recovery and subsequent immunity to hepatitis B virus. It generally appears 1 to 4 months following onset of symptoms, but appearance may be delayed much longer. The presence of HBeAB represents seroconversion from HBeAg to anti-HBe during the acute stage and is prognostic for resolution of infection. The presence of antibody to hepatitis B "e" antigen, along with anti-HBc, can also confirm the recent acute or convalescent stage in the absence of HBsAg and anti-HBs.

5. Use blood and body fluid precautions for hepatitis B and NANB hepatitis.

Clinical Alert

1. Apply enteric precautions (continue for 7 days after onset of jaundice) in hepatitis A. Hepatitis A is most contagious before symptoms and jaundice appear. Gowns and gloves are most useful when gross soiling with feces is anticipated or possible.

2. Apply blood and body fluid precautions for type B hepatitis, including hepatitis B antigen carrier. Precautions apply until patient is HBsAG-negative and the appearance of anti-HBs. Use caution when handling blood and blood-soiled articles. Take special care to avoid needlestick injuries. Pregnant women need special counseling. Gowns are indicated when

blood splattering is anticipated. If gastrointestinal bleeding is likely, wear gloves if touching feces. A private hospital room may be indicated if preface bleeding is likely to cause environmental contamination. Wear gloves to start an intravenous infusion or to handle blood-contaminated articles from persons suspected of having hepatitis or known to have hepatitis A.

3. No one who has had a blood transfusion should donate blood for 6 months. This is because a person who acquires hepatitis from a blood transfusion may not develop symptoms for up to 6 months. Persons with a positive test for HBsAg should never be permitted to donate blood or plasma.

4. Sexual contacts of persons with hepatitis B result in a great risk of infection with the disease. HBsAg has been found in most body fluids, including saliva, semen, and cervical secretions.

5. Until a specific diagnosis of HA is made, blood and body fluid precautions are advisable.

6. Immunization of contacts should be done as soon after exposure as possible. For HB, both HBIG (or, if unavailable, IG) and HBV vaccine should be administered within 24 hours of high use needlestick and with 14 days of last sexual contact with HBsAg-positive person. For HA, IG should be given within 2 weeks to all household and sexual contacts. In day care, to all classroom contacts. If diapered children are in the day-care center, IG should be given to all children and staff in the center.

Viral Antibody Tests

Normal Values
Negative respiratory, gastrointestinal, CNS, and exanthem virus antibodies
Negative titer: 1 : 8

Explanation of Test
These studies are done to establish the diagnosis of various viral diseases: respiratory, gastrointestinal, CNS, and exanthem, on the basis of antibody level. If a specific test for respiratory viral antibodies is or-

dered, it is done to identify influenza A and B, respiratory syncytial virus, mucoplasma, and adenovirus studies. If a CNS virus antibody test is ordered, it is done to identify infection with mumps, measles, herpes simplex, lymphocytes, choriomeningitis, or encephalitis.

Procedure
Viral studies require two venous blood specimens of 10 ml. The first specimen is obtained during the acute phase of illness, and the second or convalescent specimen is obtained 10 days later. All viral studies require blood serum. Spinal fluid can be used for CNS viral examination.

Clinical Implications
Fourfold increase in antibody titer from acute to convalescent serum should be observed (*e.g.*, 1:8 to 1:32 titer). This change in antibody level implies recent viral infection and is clinically significant.

Rabies Antibody Tests

Normal Values
Negative

Explanation of Test
Serologic testing is done for several reasons, including to diagnose rabies in animals or to determine the adequacy of antibody responses in either pre- or postexposure courses of rabies immunization. The diagnosis of rabies in humans is also confirmed by culture and histologic methods. Direct immunofluorescence to demonstrate the rabies antigen is also a reliable method and is used on brain smears and corneal scrapes. It has also been reported that the rabies antigen can be detected by examination of skin biopsies taken from the nape of the neck.

Serologic Tests Used
1. Complement fixation methods
2. Mouse neutralization
3. Indirect fluorescent antibody
4. Fluorescent focus

Procedure
A venous blood sample of 10 ml. is obtained to determine titer in persons who have received the vaccine for preexposure (*e.g.*, employees of animal shelters).

Clinical Implications

A positive response or rise in titer will appear in those who have been successfully immunized with human diploid vaccine.

Clinical Alert

1. Prevention: Preexposure vaccine (HDVC) should be given to high risk individuals such as veterinarians, wildlife personnel, personnel in quarantine kennels, and those working in special laboratories.
2. Postbite. Give Rabies Immuno Globulin (RIG) as soon as possible, regardless of interval from exposure, to neutralize in the virus wound. HDVC (Human diploid cell rabies vaccine) in 5 one-ml. I.M. doses should be given in the deltoid. The first dose is given at the same time RIG is given and then 3, 7, 14, and 28 days after the first dose.
3. The animal should be killed and tested as soon as possible. Holding for observation is not recommended.

Antibody to Human Immunodeficiency Virus (HIV); Acquired Immune Deficiency Syndrome (AIDS) Test

Normal Values

Negative: nonreactive

Explanation of Test

This ELISA test is used to screen donors and blood or blood products prior to transfusion for antibody to HIV, and is used in conjunction with other clinical information in the diagnosis of Acquired Immune Deficiency Syndrome (AIDS). The personal clinical appearance, signs and symptoms of the patient, along with decreased T-helper cells, and the presence of uncommon opportunistic infections and tumors are used, along with positive test results to make a diagnosis of AIDS. The predictive value of positive tests is dependent on the population being tested, such as the Gay population in San Francisco and the drug population in New York City. In these areas, the predictive value is high. Blood banks will have a much lower incidence of false positives.

Follow-up tests are Indirect Fluorescent Antibody (IFA) and Western Blot (WB) tests, both of which are more specific, expensive, and less likely to be false positive. However, the presence of HIV antibody *alone* is neither diagnostic of AIDS nor predictive of the development of AIDS.

Procedure
A venous blood sample is obtained.

Interfering Factors
1. False negatives can occur in the interim between the active infection and development of antibody. The virus may be present in an individual for up to 6 months before antibody is detected.
2. False positives can occur because of antibody versus goat ab-enzyme conjugate, faulty technique, and unknown factors.

Clinical Implications
1. A positive antibody result should be repeated and confirmed by other tests.
2. A positive Elisa that fails to be confirmed by IFA or Western Blot should not be considered negative, especially in the presence of symptoms and/or signs of AIDS.
3. A negative test for antibody tends to rule out AIDS as a diagnosis for high-risk group patients with illness but who do not have the characteristic opportunistic infection and/or tumor.
4. Antibody to HIV has been found on 90% to 100% of AIDS patients and the HIV or a closely related retrovirus has been isolated from one-third of AIDS patients (biopsy of tissue for Kaposi's carcinoma or cryptococcal pneumonia).
5. A positive result may occur in absolutely normal persons, due to unknown factors.
6. *The risk factors that predict the development of AIDS in infected persons are*
   (a) Increased number of T-suppression cells
   (b) Decreased number of T-helper cells
   (c) Increased level of antibody to cytomegalovirus
   (d) Reduced level of antibodies to AIDS virus (rather than expected high levels, low levels occur because the AIDS virus has killed off the portion of the immune system that helps create antibodies.)
   (e) Duration of infection. Roughly one-third of all persons infected with the AIDS virus will develop the disease within 7 years.

Clinical Alert
1. Results should not be given over telecommunication systems; no phone, no computer records.

2. Positive results in the medical record. Precautions should be taken so information cannot be released to insurance companies.
3. The physician must sign a legal form stating that the patient has been informed of the risks of testing.
4. Preventive medical uses of test include:
   (a) Determination of the capability of the person transmitting the infection, if the person is infected with the AIDS-related virus through sexual contact, shared needles, or blood transfusion.
   (b) When pregnancy is considered and one or both parties may be at risk for AIDS-related virus infection.

Patient Preparation
1. An informed consent must be signed by any person who is being tested for AIDS. The consent must accompany the specimen to the laboratory, or if the patient goes to the laboratory for the venipuncture, the consent must accompany the patient.
2. The patient must be aware of the benefits and risks of the test as well as the consequences of a positive test, such as the possibility of losing his job and not being able to get insurance.
3. The test is reported to national public health authorities when the guidelines for case definition have been met.
   (a) In the absence of the opportunistic diseases required by the current case definition, any of the following diseases will be considered indicative of AIDS if the patient has a positive serologic or virologic test for HIV:
      (1) Disseminated histoplasmosis (not confined to lungs or lymph nodes), diagnosed by culture, histology, or antigen detection
      (2) Isoporiasis, causing chronic diarrhea (over 1 month), diagnosed by histology or stool microscopy
      (3) Bronchial or pulmonary candidiasis, diagnosed by microscopy or by the presence of characteristic white plaques grossly on the bronchial mucosa (not by culture alone)
      (4) Non-Hodgkin's lymphoma of high-grade pathologic type (diffuse, undifferentiated) and of B-cell or unknown immunologic phenotype, diagnosed by biopsy
      (5) Histologically confirmed Kaposi's sarcoma in patients who are 60 years old or older when diagnosed
   (b) In the absence of the opportunistic diseases required by the current case definition, a histologically confirmed diagnosis of

chronic lymphoid interstitial pneumonitis in a child (under 13 years of age) will be considered indicative of AIDS unless test(s) for HIV are negative.

(c) Patients who have a lymphoreticular malignancy diagnosed more than 3 months after the diagnosis of an opportunistic disease used as a marker for AIDS will no longer be excluded as AIDS cases.

(d) To increase the specificity of the case definition, patients will be excluded as AIDS cases if they have a negative result on testing for serum antibody to HIV, have no other type of HIV test with a positive result, and do not have a low number of T-helper lymphocytes or a low ratio of T-helper to T-suppressor lymphocytes. In the absence of test results, patients satisfying all other criteria in the definition will continue to be included.

4. Infection control measures are the same as for hepatitis B and non-A, non-B via transfusion.

Herpes Simplex Antibodies IgG and IgM

Normal Values
Some level of antibody can be found in the normal population.

Background
Herpes simplex virus (HSV) has become quite prevalent in the past few years; it is often the most common cause of sexually transmitted disease.

Explanation of Test
This test is used to determine the infectious status of pregnant patients in their last days of gestation as the virus could be transmitted to the infant via the birth canal. The detection of HSV infections provides for quick antiviral therapy and is useful for patient counseling and epidemiological considerations.

Procedure
1. A venous blood sample is obtained.
2. Paired samples should be used to demonstrate an increase in titer.

Clinical Implications
1. The presence of IgM antibodies or a fourfold or greater increase in IgG titer is indicative of recent infection.
2. Antibodies for HSV appear approximately 4 to 6 weeks after infection, then decline, but remain at a persistent stable level. There is a crossmatching between the virus types one and two, and distinguishing one from the other may be difficult.

Fungal

Fungal Antibody Tests (Histoplasmosis, Blastomycosis, Coccidioidomycosis)

Normal Values
Negative

Background
Certain species of fungi are associated with human respiratory diseases acquired by inhalation of spores from sources such as dust, soil, and bird droppings. Serologic tests may be used for diagnosis of these conditions.

Fungal diseases may be categorized as either "superficial" or "deep." For the most part, the superficial mycoses are limited to the skin, mucous membranes, nails, and hair. The deep mycoses involve the deeper tissues and internal organs. Histoplasmosis, coccidioidomycosis, and blastomycosis are three diseases caused by the deep mycoses.

The following are brief descriptions of the fungal diseases:

1. Coccidioidomycosis (desert fever, San Joaquin fever, valley fever) is contracted from inhalation of soil or dust containing spores of *Coccidioides immitis.*
2. Blastomycosis is an infection caused by organisms of the genus *Blastomyces.*
3. Histoplasmosis is a granulomatous infection caused by *Histoplasma capsulatum.*

Explanation of Test
These tests are used to detect serum precipitin antibodies and complement-fixing antibodies present in the fungal diseases coccidioidomycosis, blastomycosis, and histoplasmosis.

Procedure
A venous blood sample of at least 7 ml. is obtained (serum is used).

Clinical Implications
Antibodies to coccidioidomycosis, blastomycosis, and histoplasmosis appear early in the disease (from the first to fourth weeks) and then disappear.

Interfering Factors
1. Antibodies against fungi may be found in the blood of apparently normal people.
2. In tests for blastomycosis, there may be cross-reactions with histoplasmosis.

Candida Antibody Test

Normal Values
Negative

Background
Candidiasis is usually caused by *Candida albicans* and affects the mucous membranes, skin, and nails. Compromised individuals are most likely to have invasive disease.

Explanation of Test
Identifying this antibody is helpful when the diagnosis of systemic candidiasis cannot be shown by culture or tissue sample. Clinical symptomology must be present for the test to be useful.

Procedure
A venous blood sample of 7 ml. is drawn.

Clinical Implications
1. A titer greater than 1:8 in latex agglutination is indicative of systemic infection.
2. A fourfold rise in titer of paired blood samples 10–14 days apart indicates acute infection.
3. Patients on long-term intravenous therapy commonly have disseminated infection by *Candida albicans*.
4. Vulvovaginal candidiasis, common in late pregnancy, can transmit candidiasis to the infant via the birth canal.

Interfering Factors
1. Approximately 25% of the normal population tests positive.
2. Cross-reaction can occur with LA testing in cases involving cryptococcosis and tuberculosis.
3. Positive results can be obtained with mucocutaneous candidiasis or severe vaginitis.

Aspergillus Antibody Test

Normal Values
Negative

Background
The aspergilli, especially *A. fumigatus, A. flavus,* and *A. niger,* are associated with pulmonary infections and invasive fatal disease in immunosuppressed patients. Manifestations of infection with aspergillus include allergic bronchopulmonary disease, mycetoma of the lung,

endophthalmitis, and disseminated disease involving the brain, kidney, heart, and bone.

Explanation of Test
This test is used to detect antibodies present in aspergillosis infections.

Procedure
A venous blood sample of at least 2 ml. is obtained.

Clinical Implications
Positive tests are associated with

1. Pulmonary infection in compromised patients
2. Infection of prosthetic heart valves with aspergillus
3. If the serum exhibits one to four bands, aspergillosis is strongly suggested. The presence of weak bands suggests early disease or hypersensitivity pneumonitis.

Cryptococcus Antibody Test

Normal Values
Negative

Background
Cryptococcus neoformans, a yeastlike fungus, causes an infection that is thought to be acquired by inhalation into the lungs. The organism has been isolated from several sites in nature, especially weathered pigeon droppings. Knowledge of unusual exposure by affected patients is not recognized. Symptoms include fever, headache, dizziness, ataxia, somnolence, and, occasionally, cough.

Explanation of Test
This test is used to detect antibodies present in cryptococcus infections. It appears that 50% of patients have a predisposing condition, such as lymphoma, sarcoidosis, or steroid therapy. Infection with *C. neoformans* has long been known to be associated with Hodgkin's disease and other malignant lymphomas. Infection with *C. neoformans* in conjunction with malignancy occurs to such a degree that some researchers have raised a question of an etiologic relationship between the two diseases.

Procedure
A venous blood sample of 1 ml. or 2 ml. of spinal fluid is obtained.

Clinical Implications
Positive tests are associated with infections of the lower respiratory tract by inhalation of aerosols containing *C. neoformans* cells disseminated by the fecal droppings of pigeons.

Parasitic

Toxoplasmosis (TPM) Antibody Tests; Indirect Fluorescent Antibody (IFA) Tests

Normal Values
Normals:
Titer <1:16: no previous infection (*except* for ocular infection)
Titer 1:16–1:256: prevalent in general population
Titer >1:256: suggests recent infection
Titer >1:1,024: indicates active infection
Rising titer of greatest significance

Background
Toxoplasmosis is a disease caused by the sporozoal parasite *Toxoplasma gondii*. It may be a severe generalized disease or a granulomatous disease of the CNS. The condition may be either congenital or postnatal, and is found in man as well as domestic (cats) and wild animals. Humans may acquire infection by ingestion of inadequately cooked meat or other contaminated material.

Congenital toxoplasmosis may lead to fetal death. Symptoms of subacute infection may also appear shortly after birth or months and even years later. Complications of congenital toxoplasmosis include hydrocephaly, microcephaly, convulsions, and chronic retinitis.

It is believed that one-quarter to one-half of the adult population is asymptomatically infected with toxoplasmosis. The Centers for Disease Control therefore recommend that physicians consider serologic testing of their pregnant patients for detection of this disease.

Explanation of Test
The IFA test helps to differentiate toxoplamosis from infectious mononucleosis. Antibodies appear in one to two weeks and peak at six to eight months. It is also a valuable screening test for latent toxoplasmosis.

Procedure
A venous blood sample of 5 ml. is obtained (serum is tested).

Clinical Implications
The IFA test may be considered positive under any of the following conditions:

1. The titer is 1:256 or higher; recent exposure or current infection
2. Any titer in a newborn infant
3. Titer of 1:1,024 or greater is significant and may reflect active disease
4. Titer of 1:16 or less may be seen in ocular toxoplasmosis.

Amebiasis (*Entamoeba histolytica*) Antibody Detection

Normal Values
Negative

Explanation of Test
Entamoeba histolytica, the causative agent of amebiasis, is a pathogenic parasite found in the intestine. The *E. histolytica* test is used to detect the presence or absence of specific serum antibodies to this parasite. The usual definitive method of diagnosis of amebiasis is stool examination. However, the absence of detectable organisms in the stool does not necessarily rule out the disease, because antibiotic therapy, oil enemas, and barium make a stool identification impossible.

Types of Tests
1. Indirect hemagglutination
2. Latex agglutination
3. Counterimmunoelectrophoresis

Procedure
A venous blood sample of 5 ml. is obtained (serum is tested).

Clinical Implications
1. Indirect hemagglutination—positive 1:128 and greater—indicates active or recent infection.
2. A positive test may reflect only past, not current, infections.
3. Positive results occur in
   (a) Amebic liver abscess
   (b) Amebic dysentery
4. In persons currently infected, titer range from 1:256–1:2048.
5. Titer of 1:32 or less generally exclude pressure of disease.

Mixed

TORCH Test

Normal Values
Negative

Background
TORCH is an acronym that stands for *Toxoplasma*, rubella, cytomegalovirus, syphilis, and herpes simplex. These etiological agents are frequently implicated in congenital or neonatal infections that are not clinically apparent and may result in serious impairment of the central nervous system. Congenital infection can be confirmed serologically by

the demonstration of specific IgM-associated antibodies in the infant blood.

Explanation of Test
These measurements are performed on both mother and newborn infant to test for exposure to agents involved in congenital infection of the newborn. The test is used in the differential diagnosis of acute, congenital, and intrapartum infections caused by *Toxoplasma gondii,* rubella virus, cytomegalovirus, syphilis, and herpes virus disorders. The presence of IgA or IgM in newborns reflects actual fetal production. High levels of IgM at birth indicate fetal response to an antigen. In this instance an intrauterine infection should be ruled out. TORCH is more useful in excluding a possible infection than proving etiology.

Procedure
A venous or cord blood sample of 3 ml. is obtained.

Clinical Implications
1. Persistence of rubella antibody in an infant beyond 6 months is highly suggestive of congenital infection. Congenital rubella is characterized by neurosensory deafness, heart anomalies, cataracts, growth retardation, and encephalitic symptoms.
2. Diagnosis of toxoplasmosis is established by sequential examination, rather than by a single positive test. Sequential examination reveals rising antibody titers, changing titers, and conversion of serologic tests from negative to positive. A titer of 1:256 suggests recent infections. About one-third of infants who acquire infection *in utero* will show signs of cerebral calcifications and choroidoretinitis at birth. The remainder of infected infants will be born asymptomatic.
3. A marked and persistent rise in complement-fixing antibody titer over time is consistent with rubella in infants before 6 months of age.
4. Presence of antibodies in CSF, with signs of herpetic encephalitis and the persistence of antibody levels in herpes virus type 2 in a newborn showing no obvious external lesions is consistent with a diagnosis of herpes simplex.

Cold Agglutinins (Acute and Convalescent Studies)

Normal Values
Normal: ≤1:16

Background
Cold agglutinins are complete antibodies that cause the agglutination of the patient's own red blood cells at temperatures in the range of 0 to

10°C. These antibodies, with maximum activity, at temperatures below 37°C are termed *cold* and are found in the blood of normal persons in small amounts.

Explanation of Test
The test is used most commonly to diagnose primary atypical pneumonia caused by *Mycoplasma pneumoniae*, and in certain hemolytic anemias (cold agglutination disease). Diagnosis depends on the demonstration of a fourfold or higher increase in antibody titers between an acute blood serum sample taken as early as possible in the course of the infection and a blood serum sample taken in convalescence. The titer is high in convalescence.

Clinical Alert

In cases of suspected primary atypical pneumonia, there is a titer rise 8 to 10 days after onset, a peak in titer 12 to 25 days after onset, and a decrease in titer 30 days after onset. Up to 90% of those with severe illness will have a positive titer.

Clinical Implications
1. High titers are commonly associated with the following conditions:
   (a) Atypical pneumonia
       (1) Mycoplasma pneumonia
       (2) Influenza A and B
   (b) Congenital syphilis
   (c) Severe hemolytic anemia of cold variety—paroxysmal cold hemoglobinurias
   (d) Cirrhosis
   (e) Lymphatic leukemia
   (f) Malaria
   (g) Peripheral vascular disease
   (h) Cold hemagglutinin disease
2. In patients with a titer in the tens of thousands, agglutination of red blood cells may occur within their blood vessels after exposure to cold, causing such conditions as the following:
   (a) Frostbite
   (b) Focal gangrene
   (c) Raynaud's syndrome
   (d) Anemia
3. More important than any single high titer is the rise in titer during the course of illness. The titer will usually decrease by the fourth to sixth week after onset of illness.

4. Chronically increased titers are associated with
   (a) Hemolytic anemia
   (b) Cold hemoglobinemia
   (c) Severe Raynaud's phenomenon (sometimes leading to gangrene in cold weather)
   (d) Cold agglutinin disease
   (e) Cirrhosis
   (f) Lymphatic leukemia
   (g) Congenital syphilis
5. Transient increases in titers are associated with
   (a) Mycoplasma atypical pneumonia
   (b) Infectious mononucleosis
   (c) Mumps
   (d) Orchitis
   (e) Trypanosomiasis

Clinical Alert

Specimens should be collected at 37°C and then transported to the laboratory submerged in water at 37°C. When this procedure is not possible, the specimen should be warmed for 30 minutes to 37°C before the serum is separated from the cells.

Since cold agglutinins will attach themselves to the red blood cells and therefore will not be present in the serum for testing, these precautions are taken.

Interfering Factors
1. A high titer of cold agglutinins can interfere with typing and cross-matching.
2. High titers sometimes appear spontaneously in older persons. The high antibody titer may persist for years.
3. Antibiotic therapy may interfere with the development of cold agglutinins.

TESTS FOR AUTOIMMUNE DISEASES AND DISORDERS OF THE IMMUNE SYSTEM AND NONSPECIFIC STUDIES OF IMMUNE FUNCTION

Protein Electrophoresis

The principle of electrophoresis is based on the fact that a charged particle placed in an electrical field will migrate toward one of the electrodes of the field depending on (1) the electrical charge on the particle; (2) the size of the particle; (3) the strength of the electrical field; and (4) the nature of the medium used to support the particle during the migration process. Typically, though not exclusively, the use of electrophoretic techniques enjoys its greatest current applicability in the separation of proteins.

Proteins are large molecules composed of amino acids. Amino acids are molecules capable of existing either as positively or negatively charged particles, depending on the pH of the solution in which they reside. Because of their ability to exist as positive ions in acidic solutions and negative ions in basic solutions, amino acids are said to be amphoteric. For all practical purposes, the amphoteric characteristics of proteins can be considered to be very similar to those of the amino acids of which they are composed. Amino acids or proteins have one other feature that contributes to their unique properties as ampholytes: there is a pH value at which the number of positive charges and negative charges on the molecule balance each other. This point, called the *isoelectric point,* is such that if a protein is placed in a solution at the pH of its isoelectric point, that protein has no net charge and, thus, will not migrate in an electrical field. The higher the pH value above the isoelectric point, the greater the net negative charge on the protein and the further it will migrate toward the positive electrode when placed in a direct current electrical field. On the other hand, the lower the pH of the solution below the isoelectric point of the protein, the greater the net positive charge on the protein and the further it will migrate toward the negative electrode when placed into a direct current electrical field.

Proteins can be separated into five factors by standard electrophoretic techniques: albumin, and alpha 1, alpha 2, beta, and gamma globulins. High-resolution buffers allow separation into 10 to 12 serum components. Abnormalities are encountered in a variety of disease states (Fig. 8-3).

Description of Factors: Alpha 1, Alpha 2, Beta, and Gamma Globulins

The alpha 1 globulins are
Alpha 1 lipoprotein: transports lipids, fat-soluble vitamins, and hormones
Alpha 1 antitrypsin: inhibits trypsin and chymotrypsin; acute phase reactant; subject to genetic control
Alpha-acid glycoprotein: inactivates progesterone; acute phase reactant
Thyroxine-binding globulin: binds thyroxine

Alpha 2 globulins include
Alpha 2 macroglobulin: inhibitor of plasmin and trypsin; growth-factor activity; binds insulin

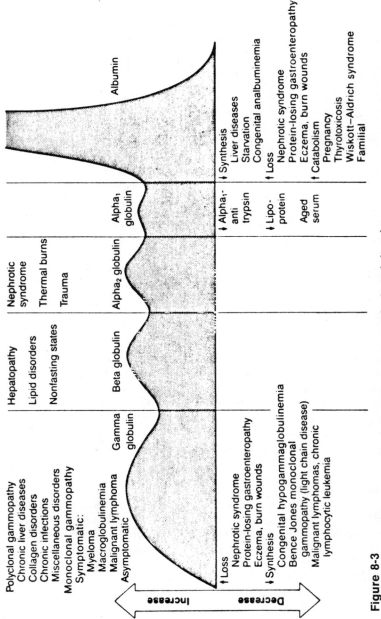

Figure 8-3

Correlation of serum protein electrophoresis patterns with clinical disorders. (After Ritzmann SE, Daniels JC: Serum protein electrophoresis. In Race GJ [ed]: Tice's Practice of Medicine, Vol 2. New York, Harper & Row, 1974)

The following labels appear in the figure:

Albumin

Alpha₁ globulin
Alpha₂ globulin
Beta globulin
Gamma globulin

Increase

Gamma globulin:
Polyclonal gammopathy
  Chronic liver diseases
  Collagen disorders
  Chronic infections
  Miscellaneous disorders
Monoclonal gammopathy
  Symptomatic:
    Myeloma
    Macroglobulinemia
    Malignant lymphoma
  Asymptomatic

Beta globulin:
Hepatopathy
Lipid disorders
Nonfasting states

Alpha₂ globulin:
Nephrotic syndrome
Thermal burns
Trauma

Decrease

Gamma globulin:
↑ Loss
  Nephrotic syndrome
  Protein-losing gastroenteropathy
  Eczema, burn wounds
↓ Synthesis
  Congenital hypogammaglobulinemia
  Bence Jones monoclonal
    gammopathy (light chain disease)
  Malignant lymphomas, chronic
    lymphocytic leukemia

Alpha₁ globulin:
↓ Alpha₁-anti trypsin

Beta globulin:
↓ Lipo-protein
Aged serum

Albumin:
↓ Synthesis
  Liver diseases
  Starvation
  Congenital analbuminemia
↓ Loss
  Nephrotic syndrome
  Protein-losing gastroenteropathy
  Eczema, burn wounds
↑ Catabolism
  Pregnancy
  Thyrotoxicosis
  Wiskott–Aldrich syndrome
  Familial

Alpha 2 lipoprotein: transports lipids, particularly triglycerides
Haptoglobin: binds hemoglobin; prevents loss of iron from body; acute-phase reactant
Ceruloplasmin: oxidase activity; has role in metabolism of copper
Cholinesterase: hydrolyzes acetylcholine
Prothrombin: essential factor in blood coagulation system
Alpha-HS glycoprotein: unknown
Zn-alpha 2 glycoprotein: unknown
G-globulin: unknown; occurs in multiple molecular forms

Beta globulins include
Beta lipoprotein: transports lipids, lipid-soluble vitamins and hormones
Transferrin: transports iron; defense against certain infectious agents
Hemopexin: binds heme
Plasminogen: lysis of fibrin in blood clots
Complement: activity involves a large number of proteins that contribute to the natural phagocytic property of blood
Beta$_2$-glycoprotein: unknown
Fibrinogen: essential factor in blood coagulation system

Gamma globulins include
Immunoglobulin G: Antibody functions against viruses, bacterial toxins, Rh antibodies, nuclear antibodies, anti-insulin, and ragweed antibodies
Immunoglobulin A (serum): Antibodies such as antibacterial agglutinins, antinuclear and anti-insulin antibodies; is the predominant immunoglobulin in body fluids and secretions
Immunoglobulin M: Antibodies such as the ABO isoagglutinins, cold agglutinins, antibodies to gram-negative bacteria, Wasserman antibody, antithyroglobin and others
Immunoglobulin D: antibody function unknown
Immunoglobulin E: antibody function unknown

Explanation of Test
Measurements are done to identify various disorders such as dysproteinemias, hypogammaglobulinemias, and some inflammatory states. The correlation of specific electrophoretic patterns with certain disorders is helpful in identifying certain clinical diseases.

Clinical Implications
1. Decreased alpha 1 antitrypsin is associated with juvenile pulmonary emphysema.
2. Increased alpha 1 acid glycoprotein is associated with chronic inflammatory, degenerative, and some malignant diseases.

3. Increased alpha 2 globulins are associated with altered vascular permeability as in nephrotic syndrome and acute inflammatory diseases. Most other increases are due to either haptoglobin, alpha 2 macroglobulin, or both.
4. Rarely are there increases or decreases in the beta globulins without the alteration being related to some disorder in the gamma globulin function.
5. Increases of gamma globulins are associated with antibodies in which one or more of the immunoglobulins are elevated. Decreases may be seen in genetic deficiencies of immunoglobulin production or immunosuppression.

Clinical Alert

1. Rarely is any single type of electrophoretic analysis used by itself to determine any of the gammopathies. It is necessary to use immunoelectrophoresis, bone marrow studies, and clinical findings to verify the data.
2. The plasma cell labeling index test is helpful in the evaluation and treatment of monoclonal gammopathies by differentiating stable from active disease. Treatment of monoclonal gammopathies is dependent upon proper classification. Prompt identification and treatment is required for patients with overt multiple myeloma (MM) to decrease morbidity and mortality rates. However, patients with monoclonal gammopathy of undetermined significance (MGUS) and smoldering multiple myeloma (SMM) must avoid immediate treatment as their diseases are nonprogressive.

Immunoelectrophoresis; Quantitative AGM Test for Immunoglobulins IgG, IgA, and IgM

Normal Values
The following values refer to the serum concentrations of immunoglobulins:

IgG—565–1765 mg./dl. or 5.65–17.65 g./liter
IgA—90–450 mg./dl. (25D) or 0.9–4.50 g./liter (25D)
IgM—60–280 mg./dl. (25D) or 600–2800 mg./liter (25D)
IgD—very small amount
IgE—small amount

These values are age-dependent.

Background

Immunoglobulin is a general term for *antibody*. Five classes of immunoglobulins—IgG, IgA, IgM, IgD, and IgE—have been isolated in humans. Each of the immunoglobulins bears a structural similarity to the other antibody molecules. The basic functions of immunoglobulins are to neutralize toxic substances (antigens) entering the body, to allow for phagocytosis, and to kill microbial organisms.

A brief description of three major immunoglobulins and their properties follows:

IgG
1. Major immunoglobulin of blood; 4 subclasses
2. Accounts for 85% of total human immunoglobulin
3. Occurs as a secondary response after IgM
4. Possesses antibody activity against viruses, some bacteria, fungi, and toxins
5. The only immunoglobulin that crosses the placenta

IgA
1. Main immunoglobulin; exists in 2 forms, serum and secretary; in secretary forms in most secretions such as colostrum, saliva, tears, and secretions of gastrointestinal tract and bronchial tract
2. Mostly present in secretory of IgA_1 with lesser levels in serum IgA_2
3. Accounts for 10% to 15% of total human immunoglobulin
4. Protects the mucous membranes in the respiratory and GI tract as first line defense against invasion by microorganisms at point of entrance
5. Does not cross the placenta and is therefore absent in infants
6. Persons with IgA deficiency are predisposed to autoimmune diseases and can develop antibody to IgA with possible anaphylaxis occurring if transferred

IgM
1. Constitutes 5% to 10% of total human immunoglobulin
2. First antibody to appear after antigens enter the body
3. Possesses antibody activity against gram-negative organisms and rheumatoid factors
4. Forms the natural antibodies such as the ABO blood group
5. Is a powerful activator of complement
6. Does not pass across the placenta and is therefore usually absent in the newborn, but it is observed approximately 5 days after birth

Explanation of Test

This test measures the levels of three classes of immunoglobulins (IgG, IgA, and IgM) in the blood. It is difficult to identify these immunoglobulins by conventional electrophoresis, and this test constitutes a special method of differentiation.

Procedure
1. A venous blood sample of 10 ml. is usually obtained.
2. Check with the individual laboratory requiring the sample. Quantities needed may vary from laboratory to laboratory.

Clinical Implications
A. *IgG*
  1. Increases in
      (a) Chronic granulomatous infections
      (b) Infections of all types
      (c) Hyperimmunization
      (d) Liver disease
      (e) Malnutrition (severe)
      (f) Dysproteinemia
      (g) Disease associated with hypersensitivity granulomas, dermatologic disorders, and IgG myeloma
      (h) Rheumatoid arthritis
  2. Decreases in
      (a) Agammaglobulinemia
      (b) Lymphoid aplasia
      (c) Selective IgG, IgA deficiency
      (d) IgA myeloma
      (e) Bence Jones proteinemia
      (f) Chronic lymphoblastic leukemia
B. *IgD*
  1. Biologic functions of these antibodies are still relatively unknown.
  2. Only small amounts are present in the blood but more than IgE
  3. Increases in
      (a) Chronic infections
      (b) Connective tissue disorders
      (c) Certain liver diseases
      (d) IgD myeloma
  4. Decreases in many hereditary and acquired deficiency syndromes
C. *IgE*
  1. Possesses antibody activity for hypersensitivity reactions and presence may be a protection against parasitic worms
  2. Increases in
      (a) Atopic skin diseases such as eczema
      (b) Hay fever
      (c) Asthma
      (d) Anaphylactic shock
      (e) E-myeloma
  3. Only very small amounts are present in the blood

4. Decreases in
    (a) Congenital agammaglobulinemia
    (b) Hypogammaglobulinemia due to faulty metabolism or synthesis of immunoglobulins
D. *IgA*
  1. Increases in
    (a) Chronic, nonalcoholic liver diseases, especially primary biliary cirrhosis (PBC). PBC is a progressive disease most commonly seen in women in the second half of their reproductive period.
    (b) Obstructive jaundice
    (c) Wide range of conditions that affect mucosal surfaces
    (d) Asparaginase treatment
    (e) Exercise
    (f) Alcoholism
    (g) Subacute and chronic infections
  2. Elevated levels of IgA in patients with carcinoma are associated with the presence of hepatic metastases.
  3. Decreased levels of IgA are seen in patients with
    (a) Ataxia-telangiectasia
    (b) Chronic sinopulmonary disease
    (c) Congenital deficit
    (d) Late pregnancy
    (e) Prolonged exposure to benzene
    (f) Abstinence from alcohol after a period of one year
    (g) Drugs and dextrin immunosuppressive therapy
    (h) Protein-losing gastroenteropathies
    (i) Immunologic deficiency states
E. *IgM*
  1. Increases (in adults) in
    (a) Waldenström's macroglobulinemia
    (b) Trypanosomiasis
    (c) Actinomycosis
    (d) Carrión's disease (bartonellosis)
    (e) Malaria
    (f) Infectious mononucleosis
    (g) Lupus erythematosus
    (h) Rheumatoid arthritis
    (i) Dysgammaglobulinemia (certain cases)

Note: In the newborn, a level of IgM above 20 ng./dl. is an indication of *in utero* stimulation of the immune system and stimulation by the rubella virus, the cytomegalovirus, syphilis, or toxoplasmosis.

2. Decreases in
    (a) Agammaglobulinemia
    (b) Lymphoproliferative disorders (certain cases)
    (c) Lymphoid aplasia
    (d) IgG and IgA myeloma
    (e) Dysgammaglobulinemia
    (f) Chronic lymphoblastic leukemia

Total Hemolytic Complement (CH50)

Normal Values
75–160 μ./ml. or 75–kU/ml.

Background
Complement (C) is a complex cascade system in which inactive proteins become active and interact in a sequential system very much like the clotting system. The complement system is very important as part of the body's defense mechanism against infection. Activation of complement results in cell lysis, release of histamine from mast cells and platelets, increased vascular permeability, contraction of smooth muscle, and chemotaxis of leukocytes. These inactive proteins make up about 10% of the globulins in normal blood serum. The complement system is also interrelated with the coagulation, fibrinolytic, and kinin systems. Complement is critical during infection in its capacity to mediate the inflammatory response. The action of complement is not always beneficial, however. The potent reactions mediated by this complex system are not always normally contained. In the presence of gram-negative bacteremia, the complement can escape its built-in control mechanisms, causing severe damage to the body in the process. It is not clear how this happens, but it is known that complement abnormalities develop before shock occurs.

Explanation of Test
This test is used as a screen for certain autoimmune diseases and is a prognostic aid in the successful treatment of others. Measurement of complement activity is used to estimate the extent of immune complex formation, and should detect all inborn and most acquired C deficiencies. Serial measurements are valuable in monitoring the course of disease and treatment in systemic lupus erythematosus, rheumatoid arthritis, and glomerulonephritis. It is a useful adjunct to specific tests for rheumatoid factor and systemic lupus erythematosus when immune complexes appear to be the primary mediators of tissue injury.

Procedure
A venous blood sample of 10 ml. is obtained. A joint fluid specimen of at least 1 ml. can also be collected in a tube with no additives and brought immediately to the laboratory.

> **Clinical Alert**
> Complement deteriorates rapidly at room temperature and serum or fluid samples should be brought to the laboratory as soon as possible.

Clinical Implications
1. *Increased values* are associated with most inflammatory responses.
   (a) Pyogenic infections
   (b) Acute gout
   (c) Myocardial infarction
   (d) Nonspecific polyarthritis
   (e) Diabetes, especially if associated with proliferative retinopathy (usually normal in diabetic nephropathy)
   (f) Ulcerative colitis
2. *Decreased values* are associated with
   (a) Specific deficiency of a complement component
       (1) Hereditary defect of an important C protein. C2-deficient patients may have autoimmune disorders such as lupus erythematosus, and C1q deficiency may cause agammaglobulinemia.
       (2) Lack of one of the inhibitors of the complement system such as occurs in hereditary angioedema
   (b) Complement consumption by activation of an alternative pathway as in certain infectious diseases, which can cause complement exhaustion or decrease
       (1) Gram-negative septicemia
       (2) Acute glomerulonephritis
       (3) Subacute bacterial endocarditis
   (c) Complement consumption due to activation of proteolytic enzymes and tissue damage as in
       (1) Systemic lupus erythematosus
       (2) Acute glomerulonephritis
       (3) Serum sickness
       (4) Acute vasculitis
       (5) Severe rheumatoid arthritis
       (6) Membranoproliferative glomerulonephritis
       (7) Hepatitis
       (8) Cryoglobulinemia

C3 Complement Component

Normal Values
141.2 ± 14.9 mg./dl. or 1.412 ± 0.149 g./liter
Values vary depending on laboratory methods.

Background
C3 is one of the components of the complement system in the activation pathway and, along with other components of the complement system, may be used up in the complex cascade of reactions that occur in some antigen–antibody formations. C3 is synthesized in many tissues such as liver, macrophage, fibroblast, lymphoid cells, and skin.

Explanation of Test
This test is ordered when it is suspected that individual complement component concentrations are abnormally reduced. This is one of three tests frequently ordered; Clq and C4 are the other two. Of these three, C3 is the most commonly requested component of complement. It has been shown that there is a good correlation between most forms of nephritis, the degree of severity of nephritis, and C3 levels. This is particularly true with acute poststreptococcal nephritis and for patients with systemic lupus erythematosus and nephritis. C3 may be nonspecifically elevated in acute phase reactions and occasionally nonspecifically depressed in liver disease. Most active diseases with immune complex formation are associated with moderate to marked C3 levels.

Procedure
A venous blood sample of at least 2 ml. is obtained.

Clinical Implications
Decreased levels are associated with

1. Severe recurrent bacterial infections due to C3 homozygous deficiency
2. Absence of C3b inactivator factor
3. Acute glomerulonephritis
4. Immune complex disease
5. Active systemic lupus erythematosus
6. Membranoproliferative glomerulonephritis
7. Autoimmune hemolytic anemia
8. Occasional drug reactions
9. Nephritic rheumatoid arthritis
10. Disseminated intravascular coagulation (DIC) disorder

Increased levels indicate remission of disease.

Interfering Factors
Increases occur gradually, up to 50 years in both men and women and decrease in the 70s in men.

> **Clinical Alert**
>
> Patients with low C3 levels are in danger of shock and death.

C4 Complement Component

Normal Values
Males: 12–72 mg./dl.
Females: 13–75 mg./dl.
Values vary depending on laboratory methods.

Background
C4 is another of the components of the complement system in the cascade activation pathway. C4 may be bypassed in the alternate complement pathway when immune complexes are not involved, or it may be used up in the very complicated series of reactions that follow many antigen–antibody reactions. C4 is synthesized in lung and bone.

Explanation of Test
This is one of the follow-up tests done when there is a suspicion that total complement levels are abnormally decreased, as in rheumatoid disease investigation. This value is a determination of only one of the components of the complement system. The other tests are C1q and C3.

Procedure
A venous blood sample of at least 2 ml. is obtained.

Clinical Implications
Decreased levels are associated with

1. Acute systemic lupus erythematosus
2. Early glomerulonephritis
3. Immune complex disease
4. Cryoglobulinemia
5. Inborn C4 deficiency

Increased levels are associated with a variety of malignancies.

C'1 Esterase Inhibitor (C'1 INH)

Normal Values
16.6–33.0 mg./dl.

Background

C'1 esterase inhibitor of the activated first component of the complement system is an antigen; lack of this antigen causes the esterase level to rise during an attack of hereditary angioneurotic edema (HAE). The primary function of this inhibitor is to act as a regulatory brake on the complement activation process.

Explanation of Test

This determination is an important tool in diagnosing HAE. This disorder is caused by a low concentration of C'1 esterase inhibitor or by an abnormal structure of the protein. Affected persons are apparently heterozygous for the condition. It is important to differentiate persons with HAE from those suffering from the more prevalent, less serious, allergic and nonfamilial angioneurotic edema.

Procedure

A venous blood sample of at least 1 ml. is obtained.

Clinical Implications

Decreased values are associated with HAE, a genetic disease characterized by acute edema of subcutaneous tissue, gastrointestinal tract, or upper respiratory tract.

Clinical Alert

Prednisolone and transfusions of fresh frozen plasma have been successfully used to treat HAE.

T and B Cell Lymphocyte Surface Markers; T-Helper/T-Suppressor Ratio

---

Normal Values

T and B Surface Markers
Percentage T cells: 60.1%–88.1%
Percentage T-Helper cells: 34%–67%
Percentage T-Suppressor cells: 10%–41.9%
Percentage B cells: 3%–8%
Absolute Counts
Lymphocytes: 0.66–4.60 thou/μliter
T cells: 644–2,201 cells/μliter
B cells: 82–392 cells/μliter
Helper cells: 493–1,191 cells/μliter
Suppressor T cells: 182–785 cells/μliter

Lymphocyte Ratio
T_H/T_S Ratio >1.0

Background

Lymphocytes can be divided into two categories, T and B cells, according to their primary function within the immune system. In the body, T and B cells work together to help provide protection against infective agents, foreign tissue, and oncogenic agents, and they play a vital role in regulating self-destruction or autoimmunity.

The majority of circulating lymphocytes are T cells having a life span of months to years. B cells comprise 10% to 30% of the lymphocytes and have a life span measured in days.

A. *B cells (antibody)*
   1. Are considered "bursa or bone marrow dependent," and are responsible for humoral immunity (in which antibodies are present in the serum).
B. *T cells (cellular)*
   1. Are thymus derived and are responsible for cellular immunity.
   2. T cells are further divided into T-helper cells and T-suppressor cells.

Explanation of Test

This test is done to evaluate the immune system by identifying the specific cells involved in the immune response. A number of disease states are characterized by abnormalities in the number and percent of T-helper, T-suppressor and B lymphocytes. In situations such as these, measurement of T and B lymphocytes can be a valuable diagnostic aid in the classification of lymphocytic leukemia, lymphoma, and immunodeficiency diseases, including AIDS, in the assessment of immunocompetence in chronic infections, viral versus immune hepatitis, in the diagnosis and treatment of autoimmune disorders, and in the monitoring of patients following chemotherapy, radiotherapy, or surgery.

Procedure

A venous blood sample of 20 ml. is obtained. The sample must not be refrigerated or frozen.

Clinical Implications

1. B cell decrease is associated with
   (a) *Primary*
      (1) Transient hypogammaglobulinemia of infancy
      (2) X-linked hypogammaglobulinemia
      (3) Selective deficiency of IgG, IgA, IgM
   (b) *Secondary*
      (1) Lymphomas

(2) Nephrotic syndrome
(3) Multiple myeloma
2. T cell decrease:
   (a) *Primary*
      (1) DeGeorge's syndrome
      (2) Nezelof's syndrome
   (b) *Secondary*
      (1) Hodgkin's or other malignant disease
      (2) Acute viral infection such as measles (transient decrease)
3. Combined B and T cell decrease:
   (a) *Primary*
      (1) Autosomal or sex-linked recessive cause
      (2) Wiskott-Aldrich syndrome
      (3) Immunodeficiency with ataxia and telangiectasis
   (b) *Secondary*
      (1) Radiation   (2) Aging
4. T cells increase in Graves' disease and B cells increase in active lupus erythematosus and chronic lymphocytic leukemia.
5. Standard immunosuppressive and cytotoxic drug therapy usually decreases lymphocyte totals.
6. In AIDS, the T_4/T_5 ratio decreases (<1) due to a loss of T-helper lymphocytes.

Lymphocytotoxic Antibody Screen

Normal Values
Negative

Explanation of Test
This test is done to detect antibodies that will prevent rejection of renal transplant.

Procedure
A venous blood sample is obtained.

Clinical Implications
1. Positive results are reported as percentage reactivity and are indicative in the recipient of a renal transplant of preformed antibodies against donor antigens.

Thyroid Antibody Tests

Normal Values
1:100 in both thyroglobulin and microsomal components

Background

Antibodies to thyroid gland components have been found in a variety of thyroid disorders. There are a number of autoantibodies involved, including one reaction against thyroglobulin, another against the microsomal component of thyroid epithelial cells, and it has been suggested that the long-acting thyroid stimulator (LATS) may also be an autoantibody.

Thyroid antibodies are seldom found in serum of normal patients. However, 5% to 10% of the normal population may exhibit low titers of the thyroid antibodies with no symptoms of disease. The incidence is higher in women and increases with age. The presence of thyroid antibodies may also be indicative of previous autoimmune disorders. Patients with low thyroid antibody titers should be tested periodically, since the presence of the antibody may be an early sign of autoimmune disease.

In active cases of thyroid autoimmune disease and in some cases of thyrotoxicosis, moderate (1:1600) to high (1:25,600) antibody titers may be observed. The detection of a very high (greater than 1:25,600) antibody titers in a patient with a firm, hard, fast-growing, symmetrical goiter strongly suggests Hashimoto's goiter.

The presence and concentration of these antibodies in the circulation and their serological detection can play a great role in evaluation and treatment of such disease states. Tests for thyroid autoantibodies are recommended in the differential diagnosis of patients with Hashimoto's disease (chronic thyroiditis) and Graves' disease (hyperthyroidism). They are also associated with primary myxedema, nontoxic goiter, carcinoma of the thyroid, de Quervain's disease, juvenile lymphocytic thyroiditis, Sjögren's syndrome, pernicious anemia, Addison's disease, myasthenia gravis, and diabetes mellitus.

Explanation of Test

These studies detect thyroid antibodies that are elevated in certain thyroid diseases such as Hashimoto's disease. When tests for both thyroglobulin antibodies and thyroid microsomal antibodies are done in combination, the specificity for detection of thyroid autoimmune antibodies is greatly increased and is more sensitive than a single test used for detection.

Procedure

A venous blood sample of 10 ml. is obtained.

Clinical Implications

1. High titers of both antibodies are found in
   (a) Hashimoto's disease (hypothyroid)
   (b) Lymphadenoid goiter

2. Combination high titers are not found in
   (a) Nontoxic goiter
   (b) Thyroid cancer
   (c) de Quervain's subacute thyroiditis

Antithyroglobulin Antibody Test

Normal Values
Titer: <1:100

Background
In certain destructive diseases of the thyroid, intact thyroglobulin may be released from the thyroid gland, stimulating antibody formation. These antibodies may be responsible for further destruction of this gland.

Explanation of Test
This test is used in the differential diagnosis of thyroid diseases such as Hashimoto's thyroiditis and cancer of the thyroid.

Procedure
A venous blood sample of at least 2 ml. is obtained.

Clinical Implications
1. Increased antithyroglobulin antibodies are associated with
   (a) Hashimoto's thyroiditis—80% of patients
   (b) Active cases of thyroid autoimmune diseases and thyrotoxicosis (sometimes). High levels of 1:1600 to 1:25,600 will be detected.
   (c) A titer in the millions strongly suggests Hashimoto's disease
   (d) Occasionally found in
      (1) Myxedema
      (2) Granulomatous thyroiditis
      (3) Nontoxic nodular goiter
      (4) Thyroid carcinoma
   (e) Other autoimmune diseases such as
      (1) Sjögren's syndrome
      (2) Systemic lupus erythematosus
      (3) Rheumatoid arthritis
      (4) Autoimmune hemolytic anemia
2. Low titers may be associated with pediatric Hashimoto's disease.

Interfering Factors
About 10% of the population may have low titers of thyroid antibodies with no incidence of disease.

Antimicrosomal Antibody Test

Normal Values
Titer: <1:100
Present in only 5% to 10% of healthy persons

Background
Microsomes are normally present within the cytoplasm of epithelial cells surrounding the thyroid follicle. Microsomes can escape from the follicular cells. Once free, they act as antigens giving rise to specific antibodies with cytotoxic effects on these follicular cells.

Explanation of Test
This measurement is very specific for the detection of thyroid microsomal antibodies, which are present in approximately 80% of persons with Hashimoto's thyroiditis.

Procedure
A venous blood sample of at least 2 ml. is obtained.

Clinical Implications
Positive reactions are associated with

1. Hashimoto's thyroiditis in 80% of cases
2. Juvenile lymphocytic thyroiditis in 90% of cases
3. Myxedema
4. Granulomatosis thyroiditis
5. Nontoxic nodular goiter
6. Thyroid cancer in 20% of cases
7. Nonthyroid diseases such as
   (a) Sjögren's syndrome
   (b) Systemic lupus erythematosus
   (c) Rheumatoid arthritis
   (d) Autoimmune hemolytic anemia

Raji Cell Assay

Normal Values
Negative

Background
Raji cells are lymphoblastoid cells that have receptors for complement for IgG.

Explanation of Test
This test, done to detect circulating immune complexes, is helpful in determining the mechanics of autoimmune disease. This assay for immune complexes is done using the Raji lymphoblastoid cell line.

Procedure

A venous blood sample of 10 ml. is obtained.

Clinical Implications

1. Immune complexes that can be detected using this method include those found in
   (a) Microbial infections   (d) Disseminated malignancy
   (b) Viral infections   (e) Autoimmune disorders
   (c) Parasitic infections   (f) Drug reactions
2. Other disorders include
   (a) Cryoglobulinemia   (e) Ulcerative colitis
   (b) Celiac disease   (f) Cirrhosis
   (c) Dermatitis herpetiformis   (g) Sickle cell anemia
   (d) Crohn's disease

Sjögren's Antibody Test

Normal Values

Negative for SS-A and SS-B antibodies

Explanation of Test

The purpose of this measurement is to detect SS-A and SS-B antibodies that are produced in Sjögren's syndrome. This syndrome may manifest itself with symptoms that are similar to those of connective tissue disorders such as rheumatoid arthritis, systemic lupus erythematosus, or progressive systemic sclerosis. However, no immunologic test is diagnostic for Sjögren's syndrome.

Procedure

A venous blood sample of 10 ml. is obtained.

Clinical Implications

1. SS-B antibodies are associated with primary Sjögren's disease, an immunologic abnormality associated with decreased secretion of exocrine glands. Fifty per cent of these patients will have rheumatoid arthritis.
2. SS-A antibodies may be found in Sjögren's syndrome alone or in Sjögren's syndrome associated with systemic lupus erythematosus.
3. Persons with both Sjögren's syndrome and rheumatoid arthritis have neither anti-SS-A nor anti-SS-B antibodies. These patients tend to develop antibodies against the Epstein–Barr virus associated with rheumatoid arthritis nuclear antigen (RANA).
4. Autoantibodies against salivary duct antigens have been detected in 50% of cases.

Anti-Smooth Muscle Antibody (ASMA) Test

Normal Values
Normal or negative: 1:20 or less

Background
This autoantibody is associated with liver and bile duct autoimmune diseases. Apparently, these disorders are not caused by any organism or external agent; the immune response itself is believed responsible.

Explanation of Test
This measurement is helpful in differentiating chronic active hepatitis and primary biliary cirrhosis from other liver diseases in which anti-smooth muscle antibodies (ASMA) are seldom present, such as systemic lupus erythematosus.

Procedure
A venous blood sample of at least 2 ml. is obtained.

Clinical Implications
1. ASMA are found in
   (a) Chronic active hepatitis, a progressive disease of unknown etiology found predominantly in young women and having factors characteristic of both acute and chronic hepatitis (80% of patients). If this disease is associated with a positive antinuclear antibody test, the disease is often called *lupoid hepatitis*.
   (b) Biliary cirrhosis
2. When ASMA are found in acute diseases such as viral infections and infectious mononucleosis, they are frequently of the IgM class.
3. When ASMA are found in chronic hepatitis, the antibodies are of the IgG class.
4. These antibodies are seldom present in
   (a) Extrahepatic biliary obstruction
   (b) Drug-induced liver disease
   (c) Viral hepatitis
   (d) Hepatoma
5. More than 20% of patients with intrinsic asthma have ASMA.

Antimitochondrial Antibody (AMA) Test

Normal Values
Negative at 1:5 dilution

Background
Antimitochondrial antibody (AMA) is non-organ and non-species specific and is directed against a lipoprotein in the inner mitochondrial

membrane. AMAs are predominantly of the IgG class; however, they have not been proven directly to cause liver cell or bile duct destruction.

Explanation of Test
This measurement is an important aid in the diagnosis of primary biliary cirrhosis (PBC). PBC is a progressive disease most commonly seen in women in the second half of their reproductive period. These antibodies are also associated with autoantibodies and with autoimmune disease.

Clinical Implications
1. A titer of 1:160 or greater is present in 79% to 94% of patients with primary biliary cirrhosis.
2. High titers are also associated with
   (a) Long-standing hepatic obstruction
   (b) Chronic hepatitis
   (c) Cryptogenic cirrhosis
3. No titer is found in extrahepatic jaundice
4. Increased titer is occasionally found in
   (a) Systemic lupus erythematosus
   (b) Rheumatoid arthritis
   (c) Thyroid disease
   (d) Pernicious anemia
   (e) Idiopathic Addison's disease

Interfering Factors
1. These antibodies are found in persons using oxyphenisatin.
2. These antibodies may occasionally be found in healthy middle-aged persons (fewer than 1%).

Antiparietal Cell Antibody (APA) Test

Normal Values
None detected

Background
The disruption of normal intrinsic factor production or function due to autoimmune processes can lead to pernicious anemia. Antibodies to two antigens of the gastric parietal cell, antiparietal cell antibodies (APAs), and intrinsic factor antibodies are found in pernicious anemia.

Explanation of Test
This measurement is helpful in diagnosing chronic gastric disease and differentiating autoimmune pernicious anemia from other megaloblastic anemias. Persons with other anemias will not have detectable APAs.

Procedure
A venous blood sample of at least 2 ml. is obtained.

Clinical Implications
1. APAs are associated with
   (a) Autoimmune pernicious anemia
   (b) Asymptomatic or presymptomatic gastritis in apparently normal adults
2. Rarely present in
   (a) Gastric ulcer
   (b) Gastric cancer
   (c) Association with antinuclear antibodies

Interfering Factors
In normal children there is a 2% incidence of APA and up to a 10% to 20% incidence in the elderly.

Antiglomerular Basement Membrane Antibody (AGBM) Test

Normal Values
Negative

Background
Antibodies specific for renal structural components such as the glomerular basement membrane of the kidney can bind to respective tissue-fixed antigens, producing an immune response.

Explanation of Test
This test is primarily used in the differential diagnosis of glomerular nephritis induced by antiglomerular basement membrane antibodies (AGBMs) from other types of glomerular nephritis. AGBMs cause about 5% of glomerular nephritis, and about two-thirds of these patients may also develop pulmonary hemorrhage (Goodpasture's syndrome).

Procedure
A venous blood sample of 5 ml. is obtained.

Clinical Implications
AGBM antibodies are detected in

1. Anti-GBM glomerular nephritis
2. Tubulointerstitial nephritis
3. Anti-GBM Goodpasture's syndrome

Acetylcholine Receptor Antibody (ACLR) Test

Normal Values
Negative or ≤ 0.03 nmol./liter

Background
Acetylcholine receptor antibodies (ACLRs) appear in myasthenia gravis, and it is believed that this disease involves destruction by the muscle cells of acetylcholine receptors bound by antibody at the skeletal muscle motor endplate.

Explanation of Test
This test is considered by many authorities to be diagnostic for myasthenia gravis in patients with symptoms. It is also helpful in managing patient response to immunosuppressive therapy.

Procedure
A venous blood sample of at least 2 ml. is obtained. Notify the laboratory if any immunosuppressive drugs have been given.

Clinical Implications
1. ACLR antibodies are found in approximately 90% of persons with myasthenia gravis and confirm the autoimmune nature of the disease.
2. Patients who have only eye symptoms tend to have lower titers than those with generalized symptoms.

Interfering Factors
False-positive binding occurs in amyotrophic lateral sclerosis patients who have been treated with snake venom.

Allergic Antibody or Hypersensitivity Studies for IgE; RAST

Normal Values
Negative: no detectable specific IgE antibody

Background
A large number of substances have been found to have allergic potential. Measurable allergen-specific antibodies can be identified only by radioallergosorbent tests (RAST). It is recommended that the patient's serum first be screened with a selected panel of six allergens and then followed, if appropriate, by an extended panel of additional allergens. Please check with the laboratory for an up-to-date listing because additional antigens are continually being added. (More than 100 from these categories: grasses, trees, molds, venoms, weeds, animal danders, foods, house dust, mites, antibiotics, and insects.)

Explanation of Test
The purpose of this study is to test for reaction to certain respiratory and food allergy stimulants. RAST tests measure the increase and

quantity of allergen-specific immunoglobulin-E antibodies. These measurements are used in persons, especially children, with extrinsic asthma, hay fever, and atopic eczema and are an accurate and convenient alternative to skin testing. Although more expensive, they do not cause hypersensitivity reactions.

Procedure
A venous blood sample of 4 to 10 ml. is obtained for each group of six RAST tests.

Clinical Complications
1. Detection of an allergen-specific IgE antibody indicates immediate hypersensitivity to an allergen.
2. A positive RAST is diagnostic of allergy to a particular allergen or allergens, irrespective of the level of total IgE.
3. A positive test is more than 400% of the control.

Thermoproteins

Thermoproteins are plasma or urinary proteins that exhibit abnormal activity at temperatures above or below 37°. Three types of thermoproteins are cryoglobulins (see below), pyroglobulins (page 499), and Bence Jones protein (page 139). Thermoproteins are usually found in association with systemic disorders such as multiple myeloma, Waldenström's macroglobulinemia, proliferative lymphoreticular disorders, connective tissue diseases, chronic infections, and essential thermoproteinemia. Clinically, the spectrum of disorders ranges from asymptomatic disorders to life-threatening illnesses.

Cryoglobulin Test

Normal Values
Negative

Background
Cryoimmunoglobulins are protein complexes that undergo reversible precipitation at low temperatures and redissolve upon warming in the body or in the laboratory.

Explanation of Test
This test is helpful in providing additional diagnostic information in the identification of certain disorders such as malignant B-cell diseases, collagen disorders, acute and chronic infections, and primary cryoglobulinemia in persons with cold hypersensitivity.

Procedure
A venous blood sample of 10 ml. is obtained. Keep the specimen at 37°C until the cells are separated.

Clinical Implications
Cryoglobulins are associated with

1. Multiple myeloma
2. Chronic lymphocytic leukemia
3. Waldenström's macroglobulinemia
4. Lymphosarcoma (possibly)
5. Rheumatoid arthritis
6. Sjögren's syndrome
7. Systemic lupus erythematosus
8. Polyarteritis nodosa
9. Syphilis
10. Kola-azar
11. Leprosy
12. Subacute endocarditis
13. Infectious mononucleosis
14. Cytomegalovirus disease
15. Sarcoidosis
16. Poststreptococcal glomerulonephritis
17. Cirrhosis of liver
18. Hemolytic anemia
19. Essential cryoglobulinemia
20. Ulcerative colitis

Pyroglobulin Test

Normal Values
Negative

Background
Pyroglobulins are abnormal proteins that present in some instances of monoclonal gammopathies. These proteins precipitate or gel when blood serum is heated to 56°C.

Explanation of Test
The determination of this thermoprotein is one of the diagnostic measures used in identifying monoclonal gammopathies. The monoclonal peak (M peak) is produced by a single family of clones of abnormal plasma cells.

Procedure
A venous blood sample of 10 ml. is obtained.

Clinical Implications
Pyroglobulins may be associated with

1. Myeloma
2. Lymphoma
3. Polycythemia vera
4. Systemic lupus erythematosus

Ribonucleoprotein (RNP) Antibody Test

Normal Values
Negative

Explanation of Test
This determination to detect autoantibodies to ribonucleoprotein is helpful in the differential diagnosis of systemic rheumatic disease and is a useful follow-up test for collagen vascular autoimmune disorders.

Procedure
A venous blood sample of 10 ml. is obtained.

Clinical Implications
1. These antibodies are associated with a wide variety of rheumatic disorders.
   (a) Systemic lupus erythematosus   (c) Sjögren's syndrome
   (b) Progressive systemic sclerosis   (d) Discoid lupus
2. A high level of RNP antibodies is an outstanding feature of mixed connective tissue disease (MCTD). Other types of antinuclear antibody (ANA) are not seen.

Antihistone Antibody Test

Normal Values
Negative

Explanation of Test
This is a follow-up test used in the differential diagnosis of collagen vascular autoimmune diseases. Histones are a group of basic proteins in the nucleus that contain high concentrations of lysine and arginine. These substances are released into surrounding tissues by death and autolysis of cells. They have direct antimicrobial activity.

Procedure
A venous blood sample of 10 ml. is obtained.

Clinical Implications
Antibodies to nuclear histones appear to be present infrequently in patients with systemic lupus erythematosus but, when present, they are found in large concentrations.

Anti-Smith (Sm) Antibody Test

Normal Values
Negative

Explanation of Test
This test is highly diagnostic of systemic lupus erythematosus and is a follow-up for collagen vascular autoimmune disease. The Smith antigen is a glycoprotein and a nonhistone acidic nuclear protein.

Procedure
A venous blood sample of 10 ml. is obtained.

Clinical Implications
Antibodies to the Sm antigen occur in systemic lupus erythematosus and are a specific marker for the disease.

Antiscleroderma (Scl-70) Antibody Test

Normal Values
Negative

Explanation of Test
This is a follow-up test for collagen vascular autoimmune disease. This test is highly diagnostic for scleroderma. The Scl-70 antibody is rarely present in other rheumatic diseases such as mixed connective tissue disease, systemic lupus erythematosus, rheumatoid arthritis, and Sjögren's syndrome.

Procedure
A venous blood sample of 10 ml. is obtained.

Clinical Implications
The appearance of Scl-70 antibody is known as a marker for scleroderma or progressive systemic scleroses (PSS).

Human Leukocyte Antigen (HLA) Test

Normal Values
Normals are not applicable.

Background
The major histocompatibility antigens of man belong to the HLA system, are present on all nucleated cells, and can be detected most easily on lymphocytes. Each antigen is produced under genetic control by a gene that shares a locus on the chromosome with another gene, one paternal and one maternal (two alleles). More than 27 antigens have been identified. The HLA complex, located in the short arm of chromosome number six, is a major histocompatibility complex in man and controls many important immune functions.

Explanation of Test
This test is done to determine the leukocyte antigens that are present on the surface of human cells. When transplantation is contemplated, HLA typing is used to identify the degree of histocompatibility between a donor and the recipient. By matching donors and potential recipients who have compatible lymphocytes and similar HLA types, it is possible to prolong transplant survival and reduce the likelihood of rejection episodes. This test is also used as an aid in diagnosing certain rheumatoid diseases, particularly ankylosing spondylitis. HLA-B27, one of the HLA antigens, is found in 90% of patients with this disease. The presence of a certain HLA antigen may be associated with an increased susceptibility to a specific disease, but it does not mandate the development of that disease in the patient. However, 8% of North American Caucasians are HLA-B27 positive, and these people have a 120 times greater risk of developing ankylosing spondylitis than those who are HLA-B27 negative.

Procedure
A heparinized venous blood sample of 10 to 24 ml. is obtained. The HLA type is determined by testing the patient's lymphocytes against a panel of defined HLA antiserums directed against the currently recognized HLA antigens. When viable human lymphocytes are incubated with a known HLA cytotoxic antibody, an antigen antibody complex will be formed on a cell surface. The addition of serum containing complement kills the cells, which are then recognized as possessing a defined HLA antigen.
A venous blood sample of at least 10 ml. is obtained.

Clinical Implications
1. Association between particular HLA antigens and various disease states include
   (a) Ankylosing spondylitis: HLA-B27 (found in 88% of patients with this disorder)
   (b) Multiple sclerosis: HLA-B27 + Dw2 + A3 + B18
   (c) Myasthenia gravis: HLA-B8
   (d) Psoriasis: HLA-A13 + B17
   (e) Reiter's syndrome: B27
   (f) Juvenile insulin-dependent diabetes:Bw15 + B8
   (g) Acute anterior uveitis: B27
   (h) Graves' disease: B27
   (i) Juvenile rheumatoid arthritis: B27
   (j) Celiac disease: B8
   (k) Dermatitis herpetiformis: B8
   (l) Autoimmune chronic active hepatitis: B8
2. Four groups of cell surface antigens, HLA-A, HLA-B, HLA-C, and HLA-D, appear to constitute the strongest barriers to tissue transplantation.

3. If a putative father presents a phenotype (2 haplotypes, one from father and one from mother) with no haplotype or antigen pair identical to one of the child's, he is excluded as the father. If one of the putative father's haplotypes is the same as one of the child's, he may be the father. The chances of his being properly identified as the father increases with the rarity of the haplotype in the population. If the haplotype is a very common one in the population, the possibility increases that another male with the same haplotype may be the father. Knowing the incidence of haplotype in the population, the probability can be calculated that the nonexcluded man is the father with the degree of certainty diminishing as the incidence of the haplotype increases in the population.

Clinical Alert

HLA testing is best used as an adjunct to diagnosis and should not be regarded as diagnostic by itself.

Terminal Deoxynucleotidyl Transferase (TDT) Test

Normal Values
<1%
Positive in bone marrow; negative in peripheral blood or lymph nodes

Background
TDT is an intracellular protein characteristic of certain primitive lymphocytes in the normal thymus and bone marrow. It is believed by some that TDT cells make a special form of DNA, as yet undetected, that plays an important role in the diversification of B and T cells in the immune system.

Explanation of Test
This analysis is a useful tool in the differential diagnosis of leukemia. High levels of TDT are found in some lymphoblastic leukemias and lymphomas. This study may also be helpful in determining prognosis and early diagnosis of relapse. Although no single marker has been found to diagnose acute leukemia, this test is looked upon very favorably by many.

Procedure
A venous blood sample of 10 ml. is obtained.

Clinical Implications
Increased TDT cells are associated with

1. Lymphoblastic lymphoma
2. Acute lymphoblastic leukemia

Rheumatoid Factor (RA Factor)

Normal Values
Negative (<1:20)

Background
The blood of many persons with rheumatoid arthritis contains a macroglobulin type of antibody that has been called *rheumatoid factor* (RF). Rheumatoid factor has the property of an antibody. There is some evidence indicating that rheumatoid factors are antigammaglobulin antibodies; however, until a specific antigen eliciting the production of RF is discovered, the exact nature of RF can only be speculated. Even more uncertain is the role that RF plays in rheumatoid arthritis. Although RF may cause or perpetuate the destructive changes associated with rheumatoid arthritis, it may be incidental to these changes or may even serve some beneficial purpose. Rheumatoid factor is not limited to blood from patients with rheumatoid arthritis but may sometimes be found in serum from patients with a variety of other diseases. However, the incidence and titers of rheumatoid factors are higher in patients with rheumatoid arthritis than in patients with other diseases. It has been proposed that the antiglobulins in rheumatoid arthritis result from chronic stimulation by an unknown antigen, perhaps microbial in origin.

Explanation of Test
This is a specific test for rheumatoid arthritis and is both a qualitative and quantitative determination of the rheumatoid factor in the blood serum. Rheumatoid arthritis is essentially a clinical diagnosis, and seven of the following criteria must be met, one of which is this blood test.

1. Morning stiffness for at least 6 weeks
2. Pain on motion or tenderness in at least one joint for at least 6 weeks
3. Swelling in at least one joint for at least 6 weeks
4. Swelling in at least one other joint for at least 6 weeks
5. Symmetrical joint swelling with simultaneous involvement of the same joint on both sides of the body
6. Subcutaneous nodules
7. X-ray changes including bony decalcification
8. Positive blood test for rheumatoid factor
9. Poor mucin precipitate from synovial fluid

10. Characteristic histologic changes in synovium
11. Characteristic histologic changes in nodules

Procedure
A venous blood sample of 10 ml. is obtained.

Clinical Implications
1. When a patient with a positive test improves, the test will remain positive, except in a small number of patients whose titers were initially low.
2. A positive RA factor test often supports a tentative diagnosis of early rheumatoid arthritis (*e.g.*, in a young adult in whom a distinction must be made between RA and rheumatic fever) and may lend credence to a diagnosis of inactive rheumatoid arthritis in a patient with a compatible history but only a mild deformity and no obvious synovitis at the time of examination.
3. High titers occur in a variety of diseases other than rheumatoid arthritis, including lupus erythematosus, endocarditis, tuberculosis, syphilis, sarcoidosis, cancer, viral infections, diseases affecting the liver, lung, or kidney, Sjögren's syndrome, and in patients with skin and renal allografts.

Interfering Factors
The titer is normally higher in older patients and when multiple vaccinations and transfusions have been administered.

Antinuclear Antibody (ANA); Anti-DNA Antibody Tests

Normal Values
Negative

Background
Antinuclear antibodies are gamma globulins that react to specific antigens when mixed in the laboratory. These detectable antinuclear antibodies usually belong to more than one immunoglobulin classification. Such antibodies (anti-DNP, anti-DNA, extractable antibody) are produced in response to the nuclear part of white blood cells.

Explanation of Test
This test is used to detect the presence of antinucleoprotein factors associated with certain autoimmune diseases. A particular pattern is associated with systemic lupus erythematosus; another antibody pattern correlates with scleroderma, Raynaud's disease, Sjögren's syndrome, hepatitis, and tuberculosis. The antinative DNA test is done to specifically identify or differentiate native DNA antibodies from other non-native DNA antinuclear antibodies.

Procedure
A venous blood sample of 10 ml. is obtained.

Clinical Implications
1. A test is positive at a titer of 1:10 or 1:20, depending on the laboratory.
2. Appearance of a positive result does not necessarily indicate a disease process because antinuclear antibodies are present in some apparently normal persons.
3. Some positive reactions have been reported to be related to patients with connective tissue disease or to persons who may develop such a disease at a later time.
4. Positive tests are associated with
   (a) Systemic lupus erythematosus
   (b) Rheumatoid arthritis
   (c) Chronic hepatitis
   (d) Periarteritis nodosa
   (e) Dermatomyositis
   (f) Scleroderma
   (g) Atypical pneumonia
   (h) Tuberculosis
   (i) Anaplastic carcinomas or lymphomas
   (j) Raynaud's disease
   (k) Sjögren's syndrome
   (l) Mixed connective tissue disease
5. A negative test for total antinuclear antibody is strong evidence against the diagnosis of systemic lupus erythematosus.

Interfering Factors
1. There are a number of drugs that may cause positive tests for antinuclear antibodies.
2. Positive antibody patterns are also seen in the blood of
   (a) Elderly patients (certain cases)
   (b) Normal adults (small numbers)

Immunologic Specificity of Antinuclear Antibodies

Types of Antibodies	Diseases in Which Antibodies Are Seen
Antibodies to DNA 1. React *only* with double-stranded DNA[19,20]	Characteristic of systemic lupus erythematosus; few cases reported
2. React with both double- and single-stranded DNA	High levels in systemic lupus erythematosus; lower levels in other rheumatic diseases
3. React only with single-stranded DNA	Rheumatic, nonrheumatic diseases
Deoxynucleoprotein soluble form (sNP)	LE cell antibody in systemic lupus erythematosus, drug-induced LE
Histone	Infrequent; present in low titer in systemic lupus erythematosus
Sm[1]	Highly diagnostic of systemic lupus erythematosus

(Continued)

Immunologic Specificity of Antinuclear Antibodies (Continued)

Types of Antibodies	Diseases in Which Antibodies Are Seen
RNP	High levels in mixed connective tissue disease (MCTD); lower levels in other rheumatic diseases
Scl-1	Highly diagnostic of scleroderma
SS-A	High prevalence in Sjögren's syndrome sicca complex; lower prevalence in other rheumatic diseases
SS-B	High prevalence in Sjögren's syndrome sicca complex; lower prevalence in other rheumatic diseases
RAP	Present in rheumatoid arthritis (RA) and Sjögren's syndrome with RA
PM	High prevalence in polyositis
Nucleolar	High prevalence in progressive systemic sclerosis, Sjögren's syndrome

Follow-up Tests for Positive ANA and Anti-DNA
1. Ribonuclear protein antibody (anti-RNP)
2. Extractable nuclear antigen (ENA) includes RNP and Smith
3. Anti-double-stranded DNA
4. Anti-SSA, also known as RO
5. Anti-SSB, also known as LA
6. Anticentromere, also known as Crest antibody
7. Antiscleroderma Scl-70
8. Antihistone antibody

Lupus Erythematosus (LE) Test

Normal Values
Negative

Background
LE cells are neutrophils that contain in their cytoplasm large masses of depolymerized DNA from the nuclei of polymorphonuclear leukocytes. The LE factor is present in the gamma globulin fraction of the serum protein of many patients with lupus erythematosus. The LE factor has the characteristics of an antinuclear (altered nucleus) antibody.

Explanation of Test
This test is ordered to diagnose lupus erythematosus. LE cells are produced on incubation of normal neutrophils with the serum of affected patients. The test is usually repeated on 3 consecutive days for thorough testing.

Procedure
A venous blood sample of 5 to 10 ml. is obtained.

Clinical Implications
1. The test is positive in 75% to 80% of patients with lupus erythematosus.
2. Positive results are associated with
   (a) Rheumatoid arthritis
   (b) Scleroderma
   (c) Blood-sensitivity reactions
   (d) Hepatitis (certain types)
3. A positive LE test should show frequent LE cells and bodies accompanied by rosettes. *Rosette cells* are rosette-shaped neutrophils grouped around a mass of nuclear protein; they are thought to be pre-LE cells.

Interfering Factors
There are many drugs that may cause positive test for LE cells.

Anti-Insulin Antibody Test

Normal Values
None, or less than 0.3% binding of beef and pork insulin by patient's serum

Background
Diabetics may form antibodies to the insulin they are given. For this reason, larger doses are required, since the insulin is not available for glucose depressant function when insulin is partially complexed with the antibodies. These insulin antibodies are immunoglobulins called *anti-insulin AB* and act as insulin-transporting proteins. The most common type of anti-insulin AB is IgG, but it is found in all five classes of immunoglobulins in insulin-treated patients. These immunoglobulins, especially IgE, may be responsible for allergic manifestations; IgM may cause insulin resistance.

Explanation of Test
This insulin–antibody level is helpful in determining the most appropriate therapeutic agent in diabetic patients and the cause of allergic manifestations. It is also used to identify insulin resistance, a state in which the daily insulin requirement exceeds 200 units for more than 2 days and may be associated with elevated anti-insulin antibody titers and insulin-binding capacity.

Procedure
A venous blood sample of at least 2 ml. is obtained.

Clinical Implications
Elevations are associated with insulin resistance and allergic manifestations to insulin.

Antimyocardial Antibody Test

Normal Values
None detected

Background
The role of antimyocardial antibodies in cardiac disorders is not clearly established, but there appears to be a significant association between the presence of these antibodies and heart disease. The antibodies are found following cardiac surgery and myocardial infarction and may precede clinical evidence of myocardial injury.

Explanation of Test
This test may be valuable in the differential diagnosis of coronary heart disease and in detecting minimal myocardial damage when the results of other tests are inconclusive.

Procedure
A venous blood sample of 5 ml. is obtained.

Clinical Implications
These antibodies are present

1. Following cardiac surgery
2. In myocardial infarction; less frequently in coronary insufficiency without infarction
3. In rheumatic fever
4. In chronic rheumatic diseases
5. In streptococcal infections

Antisperm Antibody Test

Normal Values
Negative or 1:32

Background
The mechanism by which antisperm antibodies reduce male fertility is related neither to orchitis nor oligospermia. The majority of infertile men have blocking of the efferent ducts in the testes, and a physical explanation thus exists for reduced sperm counts. It is likely that, as in vasectomy, reabsorption of sperm from blocked ducts results in the formation of autoantibodies to sperm.

510 Chapter 8: Immunodiagnostic Studies

Explanation of Test
This test to detect sperm antibodies is done in investigations of infertility. It is known that antibodies directed toward various sperm antigens can result in reduced fertility in men. However, the precise nature of the immune response against sperm antigens and the particular type of antibody responsible is unknown.

Procedure
A venous blood sample of 10 ml. is obtained.

Clinical Implications
Antisperm antibodies are associated with

1. Blocked efferent ducts in the testes
2. Vasectomy. Antibodies and probable cellular immunity to sperm develop in most men as a result of the interaction of sperm antigens with the immune system.
3. In some studies in women, approximately 75% of women with primary infertility had sperm agglutinins. However, 11% to 15% of pregnant women also had the same sperm antibody titers.

> **Clinical Alert**
>
> The potential adverse consequences of an immune response to sperm include possible systemic effects in other organ systems and possible interference with fertility after reversal of vasectomy.

Transferrin Test; Total Iron-Binding Capacity (TIBC) and Iron

Normal Values
Iron-binding capacity: 250–450 mg./dl.
Iron: 42–135 mg./dl.

Background
Transferrin, a protein and beta globulin, regulates iron absorption and transport in the body. Transferrin (also called *siderophilin*) is believed to contribute in some nonspecific manner to the body's defense against bacterial infection. Serum iron refers to transferrin-bound iron. Iron-binding capacity reflects the transferrin content of the serum. Serum iron will be highest in the morning and lowest at night.

Explanation of Test
In the laboratory, the quantity of transferrin is measured by the amount of iron with which it can bind. This ability is referred to as the "total iron-binding capacity." In conditions where the body is deficient in iron, as in pregnancy and iron-deficiency anemia, the TIBC is increased. When the body has an excess of iron, the TIBC is decreased, as in chronic inflammatory states.

Procedure
A venous blood sample of 10 ml. is obtained.

Clinical Implications
1. *Increased levels* are caused by
   (a) Inadequate dietary iron
   (b) Iron-deficiency anemia due to hemorrhage
   (c) Acute hepatitis
   (d) Polycythemia
   (e) Oral contraceptives
2. *Decreased levels* are caused by
   (a) Pernicious anemia   (e) Cancer
   (b) Thalassemia   (f) Hepatic disease
   (c) Sickle cell anemia   (g) Uremia
   (d) Chronic infection   (h) Rheumatoid arthritis

Interfering Factors
1. Transferrin is elevated in
   (a) Children 2½ to 10 years of age
   (b) Pregnant women during the third trimester
2. Drugs that may cause increased iron-binding capacity include
   (a) Chloramphenicol
   (b) Fluorides

C-Reactive Protein (CRP) Test

Normal Values
Trace amounts

Background
During the course of an inflammatory process—whether due to infection or to tissue destruction—an abnormal specific protein, CRP, appears in the blood. This protein is virtually absent from the serum of healthy persons. CRP appears rapidly in the blood in response to many injurious stimuli. Almost any disease that brings about an inflammatory condition of any tissue will result in quantities of CRP being

present in the blood and body fluids (*e.g.*, peritoneal fluid and synovial fluid).

CRP is thought to be synthesized mainly in the liver and is found in large amounts in inflammatory body fluids such as peritoneal, pleural, pericardial, and synovial. It is considered to be a transport protein for certain polysaccharides. From recent studies, it appears that a major function of CRP in health and disease involves its ability to interact with the complement system.

Explanation of Test
The CRP is an antigen–antibody reaction test that is a nonspecific method for evaluating the severity and course of inflammatory diseases and those conditions in which there is tissue necrosis, such as myocardial infarction, malignancies, and rheumatoid arthritis. The presence of C-reactive protein in the blood serum can be detected 18 to 24 hours after the onset of tissue damage. This is a useful test in following the progress of rheumatic fever under treatment and in the interpretation of the sedimentation rate. It is also valuable in monitoring the surgical wound healing process, especially in internal incisions, burn patients, and kidney transplant care.

Procedure
A venous blood sample of 10 ml. is obtained.

Clinical Implications
1. Any titer is significant, whether 1:2 or 1:64.
2. Any positive reaction indicates the presence of an active inflammation, but not the cause of the process. The results of the test must be used in association with clinical judgment.
3. The test is positive with the following conditions:
   (a) Rheumatic fever
   (b) Rheumatoid arthritis
      Note: The test becomes negative with successful treatment, indicating that the inflammatory reaction has disappeared, even when the sedimentation rate continues.
   (c) Lupus erythematosus (disseminated)
   (d) Myocardial infarction
   (e) Malignancy (active, widespread)
   (f) Bacterial and viral infections (acute)
   (g) After surgery with no complications, will decline by fourth postoperative day.
4. Demonstration of the presence of CRP has added significance over and above the finding of an elevated erythrocyte sedimentation rate (ESR), which may be influenced by changed physiological states unassociated with any actual tissue damage such as
   (a) In the absence of inflammation
   (b) In anemia, because of a decreased number of red blood cells

(c) In pregnancy, because of increased fibrinogen
(d) In multiple myeloma and other instances of hyperglobulinemia
(e) In nephrosis, because of loss of albumin and increase of globulin
5. CRP tends to increase before rises in antibody titer and ERR. Levels of CRP tend to decrease sooner than ESR levels.

Patient Preparation
1. Instruct the patient to fast for 8 to 12 hours before test if laboratory requires fasting. (Check the policy of the laboratory being used.)
2. Water is permitted.

Alpha₁-Antitrypsin (AAT) Test

Normal Values
Average normal: 159–400 mg./dl.

Background
Alpha₁-antitrypsin is a protein produced by the liver. It is believed that this protein inhibits protease released into body fluids by dying cells. Deficiency of this protein is associated with pulmonary emphysema and liver disease. Human blood serum is known to contain at least three inhibitors of protease, two of which are best known as alpha₁-antitrypsin and alpha₂-macroglobulin. Total antitrypsin levels in blood are composed of approximately 90% alpha₁-antitrypsin and 10% alpha₂-macroglobulins.

Explanation of Test
This test is a nonspecific method of diagnosing inflammation, severe infection, and necrosis. This measurement is important in the diagnosis of respiratory disease and cirrhosis of the liver because of the direct relation this protein has been shown to have in pulmonary and other metabolic disorders. It appears that pulmonary problems such as emphysema may be brought about by the inability of antitrypsin-deficient persons to ward off the action of endoproteases. Those who are deficient in AAT develop emphysema at a much earlier age than other emphysema patients.

Procedure
1. A venous blood sample of 5 ml. is obtained.
2. Fasting is required if the patient has elevated cholesterol or triglyceride levels.

Clinical Implications
1. The following should facilitate an adequate interpretation of levels of alpha₁-antitrypsin:
   (a) High levels: generally found in normal persons

(*Text continues on page 516.*)

Table 8-4
Tumor Markers

Tumor markers are substances produced and secreted by tumor cells found in serum of persons with cancer. This table includes tumor-related antigens as well as enzymes and hormones.

Name of Test Clinical Marker in Current Use and Selected Normal Values	Type of Cancer in Which Tumor Marker May be Found	Conditions Other Than Cancer That Are Associated With Abnormal Values
1. *Carcinoembryonic antigen (CEA).* 0–2.5 ng./ml. CEA is an antigen present in embryonic tissue. This antigen is designated "carcinoembryonic" because of its initial isolation from endodermally derived adenocarcinoma and fetal gastrointestinal tissue. It is believed that as a cancer disrupts normal tissue, CEA enters the vascular system in larger amounts than normal.	1. Colon, lung, metastatic breast, pancreas, stomach, prostate, ovary, bladder, limbs, neuroblastoma, leukemia, osteogenic carcinoma	1. Hepatic cirrhosis, uremia, pancreatitis, colorectal, polypoidosis, peptic ulcer disease, ulcerative colitis, regional enteritis.
2. *Alpha-fetoprotein (AFP).* <10 ng./ml.; pregnancy: upper levels of normal. AFP is a fetal globulin produced by the embryonic liver and secreted into the blood during normal gestation. AFP disappears from the blood soon after birth and is not detectable in normal persons thereafter. As neoplastic transformation occurs, it is possible that AFP enters the vascular system when normal tissue is disrupted.	2. Liver, testicular germ cell	2. Fetal distress, neural tube defects, hepatitis, primary biliary cirrhosis
3. *Chorionic gonadotropin (HcG).* glycoprotein secreted by placenta	3. Choriocarcinoma, testicular trophoblast; germ cell testicular sominomatous testicular cancer may cause slight elevation of HcG but never increases AFP	3. A variety of benign diseases with enhanced cellular proliferation

Tumor Marker	Associated Malignancy	Benign Conditions
4. *Calcitonin (CT).* Malignant C-cell tumors often produce increased calcitronin levels.	4. Thyroid, lung, or breast, pancreas	4. Z–E syndrome, pernicious anemia, chronic renal failure, pseudohypoparathyroidism, apudomas, alcoholic cirrhosis.
5. *Prostatic acid phosphatase (PAP).* Increased PAP values are probably due to increased metabolism and catabolism of cancer cells.	5. Prostate leukemia	5. Osteoporosis, renal osteopathy, hepatic cirrhosis, pulmonary embolism
6. *Acute lymphocytic leukemia antigen (CALLA).* Human lymphocyte surface markers.	6. Leukemia	6. Liver disease (may be due to major role liver has in chemical excretion of circulating glycoproteins)

Promising New Clinical Markers

Tumor Marker	Associated Malignancy	Benign Conditions
7. *Colorectal carcinoma antigens (CA 19-9).* 37 μ./ml.; lower in cancer.	7. Pancreas, colon	7. Mesothelial cell proliferation such as pelvic inflammation, adhesions, bowel obstruction, transient CHF, and laparotomy
8. *Ovarian carcinoma antigen (CA 125).* 30 μ./ml.	8. Ovary, spinal cord, and germ cell tumors; pancreas	8. —
9. *Breast carcinoma antigen (CA 15-3).* 12.9–15.9 ml. in non-pregnant women	9. Breast	9. Addison's disease, adrenal hyperplasia
10. *Creatine kinase BB (CK-BB)*	10. Lung, colon, other antigen ACTH-producing tumors	10. Heart trauma and surgery, connective tissue disorders
11. *Neuron-specific enolase (NSE)*	11. Brain, endocrine, lung	11. —
12. *Lactic dehydrogenase (LDH)*	12. Seminoma, non-Hodgkin's lymphoma	12. Cellular injury and hemolyses
13. *Gross cystic disease fluid protein (GCDFP)*	13. Breast	
14. *Lipid-bound sialic acid (LSA)*	14. Lung, breast, prostate, melanoma, carcinoma, lymphoma	

   (b) Intermediate levels: found in persons with a predisposition to pulmonary emphysema
   (c) Low levels: found in patients with obstructive pulmonary disease and in children having cirrhosis of the liver
2. *Increased levels* indicate the following:
   (a) Acute and chronic inflammatory disorders
   (b) After infections of typhoid vaccine
   (c) Cancer
   (d) Thyroid infections
   (e) Use of oral contraceptives
   (f) Stress syndrome
   (g) Hematologic abnormalities
3. *Decreased levels* are associated with these progressive diseases:
   (a) Early-onset, chronic pulmonary emphysema in adults
   (b) Liver cirrhosis in children
   (c) Pulmonary disease
   (d) Severe hepatic damage
   (e) Nephrotic syndrome
   (f) Malnutrition

Interfering Factors
Serum levels may increase normally by 100% in pregnancy.

Patient Preparation
1. Instruct the patient about fasting if necessary.
2. Water is permitted.

Clinical Alert

Persons with deficient antitrypsin levels should be counseled to avoid smoking and occupations where significant levels of air pollutants such as fumes and dust can lead to respiratory inflammation. Because AAT deficiencies are inherited, genetic counseling may be indicated.

Tumor-Related Antigens as Cancer Markers

A number of tumor-associated antigens, enzymes and isoenzymes, and various hormones are valuable as biologic markers for cancer (Table 8-4). A problem in diagnosis of cancer by currently available tumor markers is that nonmalignant disease can also be associated with the same marker abnormalities. Useful tumor marker applications include detection, differentiating malignant from benign, monitoring, classification, staging, localization, and using cytotoxic agents directed to marker-containing cells. Pretreatment values have prognostic significance and a positive change in concentration during treatment should parallel the successful treatment of disease.

Clinical Alert

1. Persons especially prone to develop hepatocellular carcinoma are those with primary hemochromatosis and cirrhosis and those exposed to defoliation treatment used in the Vietnam War.
2. The carcioembryonic antigen (CEA) test is a nonspecific cancer test; it may be an aid in following inflammatory colon disease that places a patient at risk for developing malignant status.
   (a) CEA is also elevated in chronic cigarette smoking and at times without evident cause.
   (b) High levels indicate increased tumor volume and poorer prognosis, highest in metastatic colon neoplasia.
3. High levels of common acute lymphocytic leukemia antigen (CAL'LA or ALLA) signify a better prognosis than B or T cell antigen evidence.
4. In the presence of elevated calcitonin levels, a pentagastrin provocative test is done to confirm medullary thyroid cancer.

BIBLIOGRAPHY

American Association of Blood Banks: Blood Transfusion Therapy: A physician's Handbook, 1983

American Association of Blood Banks, Technical Manual of Blood Banking, 9th ed, 1985

Andruillu A, et al: Prospective evaluation of the diagnostic efficacy of CA19–9 asay as a marker for gastrointestinal cancers. Digestion 33:26–33, 1986

Bayer W, et al: Acquired cytomegalovirus infection in transfused premature neonates. Blood: 62 (Suppl. 1), 2329 (abs), 1983

Centers for Disease Control: Hepatitis Surveillance, Report Number 40, January, 1985

Curron JW, et al: Acquired immunodeficiency syndrome (AIDS) associated with transfusions. N Engl J Med 1984, 310:69–75

Honig CL, Bove JR: Transfusion-associated fatalities: Review of bureau of biological reports, 1976–78. Transfusion 20:653, 1980

Krebs B, et al: Role of CA125 as tumor marker in ovarian carcinomas. Obstet Gynecol 67:473, 1986

Leavelle DE (ed): Mayo Medical Laboratories Handbook. Rochester, MN, 1986

Mollison PL: Blood Transfusion in Clinical Medicine, 7th ed. Oxford, Blackwell
Scientific Publications, 1983

Ostchega Y, Culvane M: Tumor markers. Nurs '85:48–51, September 1985

Petz L, Swisher SN: Clinical Practice of Blood Transfusions. New York, Churchill–Livingstone, 1981

Wick MR, et al: Non-A, non-B hepatitis associated with blood transfusions.
Transfusion 25 (2):93, March–April 1985

NUCLEAR MEDICINE STUDIES

Introduction

Radionuclide studies are performed in a department of nuclear medicine. The success of a particular study depends on the existence of detectable differences in the concentrations of administered radioactive materials in normal and abnormal tissue in areas of the body under study.

Radionuclide imaging is used mainly to allow visualization of organs and regions within organs that cannot be seen on a simple radiograph. Space-occupying lesions, especially tumors, stand out particularly well. Generally, these lesions are represented by areas of reduced radioactivity; however, in some instances, such as in bone scanning, areas of increased activity represent pathology.

Radionuclide describes an unstable nucleus with its orbital or radioactive electrons. In an attempt to reach stability, the radionuclide emits one or more types of radiation, the most common examples being alpha particles, beta particles, and gamma electromagnetic radiation. In nuclear medicine, with the exception of therapy, gamma radiation is used in diagnostic procedures because of the absence of particulate radiation.

Principles of Nuclear Imaging

In general, gamma rays are those radioactive emissions used for imaging of organ systems or the specific functions of organs. Computerized radiation detection equipment, particularly *scintillation detectors*, show the presence of gamma rays by giving off a light flash, or scintillation. The imaging device outlines and photographs the organ under study and provides information on its size, shape, position, and functional activity. The nuclide scan should be thought of as a crude form of measurement or many organs. However, some measurements are specific, such as those obtained in nuclear cardiology, where very reliable and accurate information, such as ejection fractions, can be obtained.

The radioactive materials used in nuclear medicine in diagnostic imaging are called *radiopharmaceuticals*. These radiopharmaceuticals distribute throughout tissues, organs, and organ systems, depending on their biorouting and how they are administered. Radiopharmaceuticals exhibit different tissue specificities; that is, certain radiopharmaceuticals are more likely to concentrate in one organ or one organ system than another. Within these organs, the radioactive material shows distributions in normal tissue that differ from those in diseased tissue. The following are examples of tissue specificity in radiopharmaceuticals used in nuclear medicine imaging.

Radiopharmaceutical	*Tissue*
Technetium tagged to sulfur colloid	Liver
Technetium tagged to phosphate	Bone
DTPA (diethylenetriamine penta-acetic acid)	Brain or kidneys
^{131}I-Hippuran (iodohippurate sodium)	Kidneys
Thallium-201 (^{201}T1)	Heart
Krypton-81 m	Lung ventilation scan
Xenon-133	Lung
Technetium-99m pertechnetate and Iodine-123	Thyroid, Blood
^{99m}EHIDA or ^{99m}PIPIDA	Gallbladder

In the nuclear medicine *in vitro* laboratory, radionuclides are utilized in numerous ways. They may be tagged to proteins and used to measure emollients, or used in competitive protein binding studies. They also may be labeled to antibodies or antigens and used in radioimmunoassay (RIA) studies. These studies are in contrast to those in nuclear imaging described above.

Manufacture of Radionuclides

Manufacture of radionuclides can be explained in the following way:

1. A substance to be made radioactive is placed inside a reactor, where several processes may take place, one of which is the bombardment of the material by neutrons liberated by the fission process within the reactor. This bombardment raises the material to an unstable or excited state. This material in its excited state has a natural tendency to return to its stable or normal state. As it returns, or decays, it gives off energy in the form of particles of electromagnetic radiation. This form of production is called *neutron activation* and is one of the more common methods employed to produce materials used in nuclear medicine.

2. The only other method discussed in this text is the use of linear accelerators and cyclotrons. These devices are known as *particle accelerators*. They function by supplying sufficient energy to a charged particle so that it can overcome the repulsion effect of the nucleus, thereby penetrating the nucleus and causing an interaction. A source of particles is placed in the particle accelerator, is exposed to high energies, and is then directed to a target material to produce an altered nucleus, which is unstable. The cyclotron is generally used in preference to the linear accelerator because of the latter's space requirements and cost. The cyclotron can produce a variety of useful radionuclides with short half-lives that are free of contaminants, which is not the case with the nuclear reactor. It

might be added that the major disadvantage of the cyclotron is its high cost per unit compared to the nuclear reactor. The end product, however, is the same—an unstable nucleus attempting to return to a stable state.

Imaging Used in Nuclear Medicine

There are two major types of imaging. The first is known as *hotspot imaging,* in which an increased area of uptake of the radiopharmaceutical is compared to its normal distribution. The bone scan and brain scan are examples of hotspot imaging. The other type is *coldspot imaging,* in which an area of decreased uptake of the radiopharmaceutical is compared to the background. Examples of coldspot imaging are liver scanning and lung scanning.

Today there are several types of imaging devices used in the field of nuclear medicine; however, only two are in general use: the gamma camera and the rectilinear scanner. The gamma camera is placed over the target area, where it views the entire field at once. For routine imaging it does not move, nor does it require the patient to move. A picture is constructed similar to that used in time photography. The rectilinear scanner, on the other hand, is placed at the top or bottom of the target organ and is allowed to move from side to side, indexing either up or down with complete excursion.

Dual photo scanners are gaining acceptance in the evaluation of bone density of the lumbar spine, hip, and wrist. They are being used in the early diagnosis of osteoporosis. The device uses low-level radiation and is linked to a computer to determine mineral content of the bone. The resulting data can help determine the strength of the bones and risk of fracture. No radionuclides are administered to the patient, however. The test is mentioned here only because it is often done in the department of nuclear medicine.

The computed results of conventional imaging may be recorded in the following ways:

1. Black and white dot scan. The dot scan, whether it be recorded from impact paper or from an electronic stylus burning through conductive paper, does not give much quantitative information but, instead, allows the operator to visualize the image while it is being made, thereby adjusting his margins accordingly.
2. Gray scale photo images. These are recorded on special single-emulsion film; the varying count rate appears as lighter or darker shades of gray, thus using the complete spectrum of the gray scale. It gives a differential display of count and rate, whereas the black and white dot scan either records or does not record.
3. Color imaging. Color imaging involves a more complicated procedure than those described above and usually requires some sort of

computer processing. It gives a clear display of the differential count rate and is especially useful to those clinicians who are not used to gray scale imaging.

Variations in Nuclear Imaging

Emission Computer Tomography

There are two kinds of emission tomography used in nuclear medicine: single photon emission tomography (SPECT) and positron emission tomography (PET). Emission tomography involves the detection of photons emitted from radionuclides. Scintillation crystals or arrays of solid state detector material surround the patient in order to collect data from multiple angles. Emission tomography measures metabolism, hence, biological function; computerized tomography (CT) measures anatomy. Single-photon tomography (SPECT or ECT) involves the use of gamma-ray emitters such as iodine-123, thallium-201, or technitium-99m; while positron emission tomography (PET) involves the use of radionuclides that emit two gamma rays after the annihilation of a positron (positive electron) with a cyclotron. The cyclotron is needed to produce these labeled compounds (radioactive forms of natural elements) that can be detected externally. The positron is emitted from an isotope such as carbon-11, nitrogen 13, or rubidium 82. SPECT or ECT provides three-dimensional images (transaxial, sagittal, and coronal) of physiologic processes with greater image contrast and resolution than traditional imaging, and also has the capability for quantitation. By combining early lesion detection and quantitative SPECT imagery, greater therapeutic precision or oncology diagnosis and treatment can be offered to patients.

PET scanning is approximately 10 times more efficient than single-photon tomography for imaging the head and body. However, an advantage of single-photon tomography is the availability of radiopharmaceuticals without the need for a cyclotron. At this time, lesion detectability is in the 6 to 15 mm size range.

Uses of SPECT/ECT

1. Brain and cerebral blood flow with blood–brain barrier penetrating agent
2. Liver
3. Spleen
4. Cardiac infarct
5. Lungs
6. Indium, WBC for inflammation
7. Bone for special areas such as spine, knees, hips, temporomandibular joint (demonstrates a higher degree of lesion detection beyond other conventional approaches).

8. Heart thallium increases sensitivity and specificity for detecting coronary artery disease.

Normal procedures to be done more commonly in the future are monoclonal antibody imagery for the detection of breast, ovarian, lung, GI, and pancreatic malignancies.

There are some 157 positive-emitting radioelements available for radiopharmaceutical labeling. Only about 20 have been considered for such an application, excluding those that are natural constituents of organic molecules such as carbon, nitrogen, oxygen, and fluoride. The following are examples of tissue specificity in pharmaceuticals:

Principal Isotope	Radioisotopes in Pharmaceutical	Diagnostic Use
^{68}Ga	Proteins	Regional blood volume
	Microspheres	Regional blood flow
55Co	Bleomycin	Tumor tracer
	DTPA	CSF kinetics
^{82}Rb	-------	Myocardial blood flow
^{75,76}Bromine	Bromocriptine	Dopamine receptors
	Bromospiroperidal	Brain studies
^{73}Se	Methionine	Protein metabolism
^{51,52}Mn	Chloride	Myocardial imaging
	Chelate	Kidney function
^{122}I	-------	Cardiac angiography
^{19}Ne	-------	Local lung ventilation

General Procedure for Nuclear Medicine Scans

1. A radiopharmaceutical is administered orally or intravenously to the patient.

   Note: Before administration of the radioisotope, a blocking agent that is not radioactive may be administered to prevent tissues other than the organ under study from concentrating the radioactive substance. Examples of blocking agents include:

   (a) Lugol's solution, administered orally when iodine-tagged isotopes are used, except in thyroid studies.
   (b) Potassium perchlorate, administered orally to patients who are allergic to iodine. Blocks choroid plexus in brain.
   (c) Mercaptomerin, administered intravenously to block uptake of ^{197}Hg-chlormerodrin by the kidneys.

2. A sufficient time interval is allowed for the radioactive material to follow its specific metabolic pathway in the body and to concentrate in the specific tissue to be studied.

3. An imaging device outside the body reflects and records the concentration of the penetrating radiation that emerges from the radioisotope.

4. Total length of examining time depends upon:
   (a) Radioisotope used and time variable to allow for concentration in tissues
   (b) Type of imaging equipment used

Limitations of Procedure
1. Localizing tumors by scanning can be difficult when normal tissues surrounding the lesion absorb the radionuclide and produce fuzzy or ambiguous outlines.

Benefits and Risks
Benefits and risks should be explained prior to testing. Patients remain radioactive for relatively short periods of time. The radioactive energy does dissipate on its own, and some of the radiation will be eliminated in urine and feces.

Technetium, which is the most commonly used tracer, is significantly reduced in 6 hours and is virtually gone from the patient's body in 24 hours. Other tracers such as iodine and thallium take approximately 8 and 3 days, respectively, for half of the energy to dissipate.

Patients need to know that once the energy has been eliminated, they are no longer radioactive. A radiation hazard to the patient always exists. In all radionuclide procedures, the value and importance of the information gained must be weighed against the potential hazard of radiation to the patient. If a nuclide study will advance the solution of a difficult problem, or provide information that cannot be obtained in any other way, then it should be done. For example, some of the following factors may be considered:

(a) If a liver scan can be used to demonstrate hepatic metastases in a patient with lung carcinoma, thus sparing the patient from an unnecessary thoracotomy, the procedure is indicated.
(b) In almost all instances, radionuclide imaging exposes the patient to less radiation than would be received undergoing a similar procedure with diagnostic radiographs.
(c) With a radioisotope scan, metastatic disease to the bone can be found 6 months to a year before it can be detected with the usual bone radiograph. Also to be noted, the total body radiation from an injection of a bone agent tagged to ^{99m}Tc is about one-ninth as much as the unavoidable natural radiation that a person receives in 1 year from the ground and stars. In fact, this dosage is less than that received from a radiograph of the chest.

Clinical Considerations
The following information should be obtained prior to diagnostic testing:

1. Menstrual history of women of childbearing age: Pregnancy is a contraindication to radioisotope studies.
2. Whether a mother is breast-feeding her baby: This is very important because radioisotope studies are contraindicated in nursing mothers. The mother may be advised to stop nursing for a set period of time; for example, 3 to 4 days with ^{99m}Tc.
3. History of allergies: Certain patients may have adverse allergic reactions to some of the radioisotopes.
4. Knowledge of recent exposure to radionuclides: A history of any recent examination in which radionuclides were administered should be recorded and a body background taken in the nuclear medicine department. If for any reason it is suspected that a patient may have had an unreported examination in which a radionuclide was administered, again, a body background should be taken, because a previous study could seriously interfere with the clinician's interpretation of the current study.
5. Presence of any prostheses in the body: These must be recorded on the patient's history because certain devices can shield the gamma energy.
6. Current treatment or diagnostic measures: For example, telemetry, oxygen, and urine collection.
7. Age and current weight and height: This information is used to calculate the amount of the radioactive substance to be administered prior to imagery. If the patient is under 18, notify the examining department prior to testing.
8. Other special considerations regarding the patient's well-being should be communicated to the examining department.
   (a) Transportation, such as cart, wheelchair
   (b) If patient is on telemetry
   (c) Requires oxygen
   (d) Requires urine collection
   (e) Any allergies
   (f) An intravenous or nasogastric tube
   (g) If patient is a diabetic

Clinical Alert

Premenopausal women should be advised to practice effective birth control during the testing period. These tests may be harmful to a fetus. Nuclear medicine needs to be notified if the patient may be pregnant or is breast-feeding.

9. Thyroid scans need to be completed before radiographic examinations using contrast medicine (IVP, gallbladder, cardiac catheterization, and myelograms) are performed.

10. If possible, any medication containing iodine should not be given until thyroid scans are concluded. Notify the attending physician if thyroid studies have been ordered, together with interfering radiographs or medications.

Follow-Up Care
1. Advise the patient to empty his bladder when imaging is completed, to decrease radiation exposure time.
2. Documentation is important and should include assessment and education of the patient and significant others, how the patient tolerated the procedure, and the total examining time.

Part One
Nuclear Scans

Kidney Scan

Normal Values
Normal size, shape, position, and function of kidneys

Explanation of Test
This test is done to determine anatomical outlines and renal plasma flow in each kidney. It is also used to detect renal masses and to localize the kidney before needle biopsy. It can reveal positive evidence of renal disease when other tests are normal. The scan will also reveal lesions produced by vascular occlusion in the kidney. Parenchymal, tubular, and glomerular function can be ascertained with a number of renal imagery agents. Radioactive substances such as technetium-99m (^{99m}Tc), DMSA, GA, or DTPA are injected intravenously and a short time later will be concentrated and held in the kidneys. Scanning will demonstrate the size, shape, and position of the kidneys as well as the distribution of the radioisotope in the kidneys. Renal scans and renograms can be done simultaneously, giving both morphologic and functional data about the kidneys. The iodine-sensitive or azotemic patient who cannot tolerate an IVP can be evaluated in this way. In many instances, this study will be accompanied by a diagnostic ultrasound procedure.

Procedure
1. Scanning of the kidney area is done 30 minutes to 1 hour after the intravenous injection of the radioisotope. A renal blood flow and a 10-minute postinjection static film are taken in the sitting position.

2. Scans of the kidneys are then repeated at a later time or may be done at several different time intervals after the initial injection. This will depend on the patient's condition and the pharmaceutical used.
3. The patient must remain still during the delayed scans for 30 minutes or more, and usually, a prone position is used for this part of the procedure. Most often, both kidneys are scanned at the same time; however, they can be done separately.
4. In many nuclear medicine departments, this information is then processed by computer for further interpretation.

Clinical Implications
1. Abnormal results indicate
    (a) Space-occupying "cold" or nonfunctioning areas caused by tumors, cysts, or abscesses
    (b) Congenital abnormalities
    (c) Nonfunctioning kidneys
    (d) Infarction
    (e) Status of postrenal transplant
    (f) Severe renal insufficiency
2. In patients with uremia, the size, shape, and location of the kidneys can be demonstrated when no visualization occurs in the IVP.

Patient Preparation
1. Explain the purpose and procedure of the test.
2. Alleviate any fears the patient may have about radionuclide procedures.

Renogram (Renocystogram)

Normal Values
Right and left kidney blood flow is compared in healthy persons; flow is equal in both kidneys.
In 10 minutes, 50% of the isotope should be excreted.

Explanation of Test
This test is done to study the function of both kidneys and is used to detect renal parenchymal or vascular disease as well as defects in excretion. This is a dynamic study; blood flow is recorded as it is occurring. The test is indicated under the following conditions:

1. To detect the presence or absence of unilateral kidney disease
2. For long-term follow-up of patients with hydroureteronephrosis
3. To determine if recognized nephroureteral dilation represents significant obstruction

4. To study the hypertensive patient to determine a renal basis for the disease
5. To study the hypertensive obstetrical patient
6. To study the azotemic patient and the patient in whom urethral catheterization is contraindicated or impossible
7. To evaluate obstruction in the upper urinary tract
8. To study the kidney when an IVP cannot be done because of allergy to iodine

The radioactive drug ^{131}I-hippuran or Tc-99m DTPA is the nuclide administered intravenously and is selectively excreted by the kidney. The placement of the radiation detectors over the kidneys permits the monitoring of the uptake and the disappearance of the radioactivity. This information is usually displayed with a chart recording or put into a computer. The shape of this wave may be correlated with several measures of renal function such as tubular secretion and excretion.

Procedure
1. The patient is usually placed in an upright position in front of the recording device.
2. The radiopharmaceutical hippuran is injected intravenously. An IV diuretic may also be administered.
3. Imaging with the camera positioned midway through the test is started immediately upon injection.
4. A urine sample or a blood specimen may be obtained at the end of the procedure. Bladder catheterization is necessary in persons with suspected distal ureteral obstruction.
5. Total examination time is approximately 30 minutes.

Clinical Implications
Abnormal pattern results may be indicative of

1. Hypertension
2. Obstruction due to stones or tumors
3. Renal failure
4. Decreased renal function
5. Diminished blood supply

Patient Preparation
1. Have the patient's current weight available.
2. Explain the purpose and procedure of the test.
3. The patient should eat and be well hydrated with two to three glasses of water (unless contraindicated) before undergoing the scan. (10 ml. of water per kg. of body weight).
4. Alleviate any fears the patient may have concerning radioisotope procedures.

Clinical Considerations

A renogram may be performed in pregnant women when it is imperative that renal function be ascertained.

> **Clinical Alert**
>
> The test should not be done immediately after IVP because the patient needs to be at least normally hydrated.
> 1. Severe impairment of renal function or massive enlargement of the collecting system may impair drainage even without true obstruction.

Thyroid Scan

Normal Values

Normal or evenly distributed concentration of radioactive iodine; normal size, position, shape, site, weight, and function of thyroid

Explanation of Test

This test systematically measures the uptake of radioactive iodine (either ^{131}I or ^{123}I) by the thyroid. It is requested for the evaluation of thyroid size, position, and function. It is used in the differential diagnosis of masses in the neck, base of the tongue, or mediastinum. Thyroid tissue can be found in each of these three locations. In some instances, ^{99m}TC may be used in place of iodine for visualizing the thyroid.

Benign adenomas may appear as nodules of increased uptake of iodine ("hot" nodules), or they may appear as nodules of decreased intake ("cold" nodules). Malignant areas generally take the form of cold nodules. The most important use of thyroid scans is the functional assessment of these thyroid nodules.

Iodine (and, consequently, radioiodine) is actively transported by the thyroid gland, where it is incorporated into the production of thyroid hormone. The radioactivity of the gland is scanned by a scintillation imaging device, and this information is then transformed into a film or plotted on a CT scan, thus outlining the normal thyroid and demonstrating any areas of abnormality.

A thyroid scan performed with iodine is usually done in conjunction with a radioactive iodine uptake study, which is usually performed at 6 and 24 hours postdose when ^{131}I is used. The uptake and scan are performed the same day when ^{123}I is used. For a complete thyroid workup, thyroid hormone levels are usually measured by taking a blood specimen and performing radioimmunoassay tests as directed by the physician.

Procedure

1. The patient either swallows radioactive iodine in a tasteless capsule or a liquid or has the radionuclide injected intravenously.
2. Usually, the neck area is counted for uptake 6 or 24 hours later (or both). The area is scanned at 24 hours when ^{131}I is used and at 3 to 6 hours when ^{123}I is used.
3. The patient lies on his back on the examining table with his neck hyperextended.
4. Normal scan time is 20 minutes.

Clinical Implications

1. Cancer of the thyroid most often presents itself as a nonfunctioning cold nodule, which indicates an area of decreased uptake of radioiodine.
2. Abnormal results indicate
   (a) Hyperthyroidism represented by an area of increased uptake of radioiodine
   (b) Hypothyroidism represented by an area of decreased uptake of radioiodine
   (c) Graves' disease represented by an area of increased uptake of radioiodine
   (d) Autonomous nodules represented by an area of increased uptake of radioiodine
   (e) Hashimoto's disease represented by an area of decreased uptake of radioiodine

Interfering Factors

1. Ingested iodine and contrast diagnostic substances can interfere with a thyroid scan for up to 6 months. For this reason, thyroid scans should be completed before radiographic examinations using contrast media are performed.
2. Antithyroid medication
   Radioactive technetium is used when gallbladder radiograph or IVP has been done previously.

Limitations of Test

Measurements of total serum thyroxine (total T_4) and triiodothyronine by RIA are much more reliable tests for function of the thyroid.

Patient Preparation

1. Instruct the patient about the purpose, procedure, and special restrictions of the test.

2. Since the thyroid gland responds to small amounts of iodine, the patient must eliminate iodine intake for at least 1 week before the test. Restricted items include

(a) All thyroid drugs
(b) Weight control medicines
(c) Multiple vitamins
(d) Some oral contraceptives
(e) Gallbladder and other radiographic dyes containing iodine
(f) Cough medicine
(g) Iodine-containing foods, especially kelp, and "natural" foods

3. Alleviate any fears the patient may have about radioisotope procedures.

Clinical Alert

1. Thyroid scans are contraindicated in pregnancy. Thyroid testing in pregnancy is limited to blood testing.
2. This study should be completed before thyroid-blocking contrast agents for radiographs are administered and before thyroid or iodine drugs are given.
3. Occasionally, scans are done purposely with iodine or some thyroid drug in the body. In these cases, the doctor is testing the thyroid response to drugs. These stimulation and suppression scans are usually done to determine the nature of a particular nodule and to determine if the tissue is functioning or nonfunctioning.

Parotid or Salivary Gland Scan

Normal Values
No evidence of tumor type activity or blockage of ducts
Normal size, shape, position of glands

Explanation of Test
This study is helpful in the evaluation of swelling masses in the parotid region. This scan is done to detect blocked ducts of the parotid and submaxillary glands, tumors of parotid or salivary glands, and to diagnose Sjögren's syndrome in rheumatoid arthritis. The isotope injected intravenously is technetium-99m pertechnetate (^{99m}Tc). One of the limitations of the test is that it cannot furnish an exact preoperative diagnosis.

Procedure

1. A radioisotope (^{99m}Tc) is injected intravenously. Scanning is done immediately. There are three phases to imaging: blood flow; uptake or trapping mechanism; secreting capability.
2. The patient is examined in a sitting position.
3. Pictures of the gland are taken every few minutes for 30 minutes (two anteroposterior and one oblique).
4. If a secretory function test is being done to detect blockage of the salivary duct, three-fourths of the way through the test, the patient is asked to suck on a lemon slice. If the salivary gland is normal, it will cause the gland to empty. This is not done in tumor detection.
5. Total test time is 45 to 60 minutes.

Clinical Implications

1. The reporting of a hot nodule amidst normal tissue that accumulates the radioisotope is associated with tumors of the ducts as in
   (a) Warthin's tumor
   (b) Oncocytoma
   (c) Mucoepidermoid tumor
2. The reporting of a cold nodule amidst normal tissue that does not accumulate the radioisotope is associated with
   (a) Benign tumors or cysts, which are indicated by smooth, sharply defined outlines
   (b) Adenocarcinoma, which is indicated by ragged, irregular outlines

Patient Preparation

1. Explain the purpose and procedure of the test.
2. There is no pain or discomfort involved.
3. Alleviate any fears the patient may have concerning radioisotope procedures.

Liver Scan: Emission Computed Tomography (ECT); Single Photon Emission Computed Tomography (SPECT)

Normal Values

Normal size, shape, and position on the abdomen; normal size of cardiac impression on liver; normally functioning liver, gallbladder, patent common bile duct, and upper intestine.

Explanation of Test

This test is used to demonstrate the functions, anatomy, and size of the liver, gallbladder, and upper intestine. Alterations in function may indicate an obstruction, hepatitis, toxicity, gallbladder disease, and the cause of jaundice. It is helpful in determining the cause of right upper quadrant pain, in the detection of metastatic disease, cirrhoses, infarction due to trauma, and liver damage due to radiation therapy. The majority of liver scans still continue to be performed as part of a source for metastatic disease and in the differential diagnosis of jaundice.

A radioactive material, ^{99m}Tc-labelled IDA, is injected intravenously. Liver imaging is done using single photon emission computed tomography that gives a three-dimensional result of the radiopharmaceutical distributions.

Liver/Lung Combination Scan
There may be times when a liver/lung scan may be ordered in combination with a WBC or gallium scan to identify tumor masses or abscess formation in the subdiaphragmatic area. Procedure and patient preparation are the same as for a liver scan and lung scan.

Limitations of Test
1. Radionuclides have a short transit time through the liver with the advantage of a low radiation dose, but the scan must be done quickly, because the radioisotope, excreted by the hepatic parenchymal cells, is concentrated in the gallbladder and excreted into the gastrointestinal tract.

Procedure
1. The chosen pharmaceutical is injected intravenously.
2. After administration of the radioisotope, the patient lies on his back on an examining table for anterior pictures to determine liver uptake.
3. The entire study usually takes 80 minutes from injection to finish.
4. See also *Gallbladder Scan*.
5. Under certain conditions, the study can be performed without ECT at the bedside or in the emergency room.
6. Delayed images may need to be obtained at 2, 4, and 24 hours, postinjection.

Clinical Implications
1. Abnormal results will reveal abnormal patterns in
   (a) Cirrhosis
   (b) Hepatitis
   (c) Fatty metamorphosis
   (d) Diffuse cancer
   (e) Sarcoidosis
   (f) Tumor (primary or metastatic)
   (g) Cysts
   (h) Perihepatic abscess
   (i) Gumma
   (j) Tuberculoma
   (k) Common bile duct obstruction

   If the contrast is not seen in the intestines after a few hours, an obstructive process is present.

Interfering Factors
1. A recent meal induces gallbladder contractions with significantly decreased uptake in the normal gallbladder.

Patient Preparation
1. Explain the purpose and procedure of the test.
2. Alleviate fears about radiation.
3. If there is no history of cholecystectomy, fasting is necessary for two hours prior to testing to optimize visualization.
4. No discomfort is experienced during the examination.

Heart Scans

Normal Values
Normal heart: no areas of ischemia; blood flow equal throughout myocardium; normal ejection fractions and velocity
Normal stress test: ECG and blood pressure normal
Normal nitro test: blood pressure within expected limits
Normal shunt scan: pulmonary transit times and normal sequence or chamber filling

Explanation of Test
More than one type of myocardial scan may be performed. These scans are noninvasive and involve the intravenous injection of a radiopharmaceutical followed by imaging. These studies are indicated in the investigation of coronary artery disease, filling of the chambers of the heart, angina, aneurysm, infarct, cardiomyopathy, atypical chest pain, and pre- and postsurgical evaluation. New treatments have stimulated the use of radionuclide imagery in the early hours after infarction to determine myocardial tissue vitality.

1. *PYP heart scan* (Hotspot, myocardial infarct imaging)
   Technetium-99m stannous pyrophosphate is the radioactive imaging agent used to demonstrate the general location, size, and extent of myocardial infarction (MI) 24 to 96 hours after suspected MI and as an indication of myocardial neurosis, to differentiate between old and new infarcts. In some instances, the test is sensitive enough to detect an infarct 12 hours to 6 days after its occurrence. Acute infarction is associated with an area of increased radioactivity or hotspot on the myocardial image. This test is useful when ECG and enzyme studies are not definitive. PYP scans are commonly done the day before heart surgery and again postoperatively.
2. *Thallium stress heart scans*
   Thallium-201 (^{201}Tl) is the radioactive imaging agent used in conjunction with a bicycle ergometer or treadmill stress ECG test to

diagnose ischemic heart disease. It will reveal wall motor defects and heart pump performance during increased oxygen demands. These scans are also done before and after streptokinase treatment for coronary artery thrombosis. When thallium is injected at the time of maximum stress and is followed by imaging, areas of myocardial ischemia can be detected. Thallium-201 is a physiologic analog of potassium. The myocardial cells extract potassium, as do other muscle cells. Myocardial thallium activity is also dependent on blood flow. For this reason, when thallium-201 is injected during peak exercise, the normal myocardium will have much greater thallium activity than the abnormal myocardium, with maximum concentration normally occurring in about 10 minutes. A completely normal thallium stress study may eliminate the need for cardiac catheterization in the evaluation of chest pain and nonspecific abnormalities of the ECG.

3. *DPY-thallium and Persantine scans*
   Dipyridamole and Persantine imaging are indicated in persons unable to exercise to achieve desired cardiac stress and maximum cardiac vasodilation. These medications have been shown to have an effect similar to that of exercise on the heart. Persons who are candidates are those with lung disease, peripheral vascular disease with claudication, amputation, spinal cord injury, multiple sclerosis, and morbid phasing, and patients taking beta blockers. Persantine and DPY tests are also valuable as significant predictors of cardiovascular death, reinfarction, and of risk of postoperative ischemia events; these tests can also be used in reevaluation of unstable angina. The major disadvantage of DPY and Persantine imaging is the lack of information that would be provided by the ECG response to exercise.

4. *Gated equilibrium heart scan resting (multigated acquisition, MUGA); Ejection fractions*
   This method is similar to routine imaging except that scintillation events are distributed into not one, but multiple images during acquisition. Gated refers to the synchronizing of the imaging equipment and computer with the patient's ECG so that images are free of motion or blur. "First pass studies" refers to the image's mode when the bolus of radiopharmaceutical first passes through the right heart, lungs, and left heart. The distribution is regulated by synchronizing the recording of cardiac images with the ECG. This technique provides a means of obtaining information about cardiac output, end diastolic volume, ejection fraction, ejection velocity, and motion of the ventricles. This method of determining heart wall motion and ejection fraction (that portion of the ventricular volume ejected in systole) could only be measured by angiography

before use of this technique. This scan may also be performed with stress testing.

5. *Nitro Test*
   This procedure is an adjunct to MUGA studies to see the effect of drug intervention (using nitroglycerine) on heart performance.
6. *Heart Shunt*
   This angiographic study of the chambers of the heart using jugular vein injection of ^{99m}Tc is helpful in the study of heart chamber disorders, especially in the investigation of left-to-right and right-to-left shunts. Children are the usual candidates for this procedure.

Procedure for PYP Heart Scan
1. This myocardial scan involves a 30-minute to 3-hour waiting period for the patient after the intravenous injection of the radioisotope. During this waiting period, the radioactive material will accumulate in the heart muscle.
2. The imaging period takes 15 to 30 minutes, during which time the patient must lie quietly on an examining table.

Procedure for Thallium Stress Heart Scan
1. Before the stress test is begun, an IV is started, and ECG leads and blood pressure cuff are attached.
2. When the cardiologist has determined that the patient has reached maximum heart stress using the treadmill or bicycle ergometer (10 to 30 minutes), an injection of radioactive thallium is given. The patient then lies down on the scanning table.
3. After a waiting period of 10 to 15 minutes for the imaging substance to concentrate in the heart muscle, the scanning is begun and pictures are taken. The imaging period is about 1 hour. A repeat scan is done approximately four hours later at rest to check redistribution.

Procedure for MUGA
1. This is the same as the PYP scan except that two radionuclide injections may be necessary to obtain an assessment of wall motion in more than one position.
2. The scan may be performed with or without stress testing and is usually performed in conjunction with heart wall motion study.
3. The test could be performed at bedside if necessary.

Procedure for Nitro Test
1. A cardiologist should be present.
2. A resting MUGA is done for a baseline study.
3. Nitroglycerine is given, another scan is taken, nitroglycerine is given again, and scans are taken until the level of blood pressure desired by the cardiologist is reached.
4. Total study times is 1½ hours.

Procedure for Heart Shunt
1. A radioisotope is injected in the external jugular vein to ensure a compact bolus.
2. The patient lies on his back with his head slightly raised.
3. The total patient time is approximately 30 minutes; the actual scan time 5 minutes.
4. A resting MUGA is performed with *each* shunt study.

Procedure for Persantine Thallium
1. Persantine is infused intravenously over a 4-minute period prior to administration of thallium.
2. Blood pressure, heart rate, and ECG are monitored for any changes during Persantine infusion. Aminophylline will be given if vital signs change radically.

Procedure for DPY
1. After infusion and injection of DPY and thallium, precise positioning of the patient is done to ensure that the heart is visible in all of the 64 images acquired.
2. DPY may be given orally in some instances.
3. Under certain conditions the DPY procedures can be done at bedside. When tomographic views are obtained in the nuclear medicine department, results are more sensitive and specific.

Clinical Implications
1. Abnormal myocardial scans will reveal perfusion defects associated with
   (a) Ischemic heart disease
   (b) Location and extent of myocardial infarction
   (c) Progress of disease (estimated)
2. Larger perfusion defects have a much poorer prognosis than small defects.
3. When a scan is entirely normal in a person admitted with a diagnosis of "rule out myocardial infarction," this is an indication that an acute infarction is not present.
4. Specific and significant abnormalities in the stress ECG or myocardial scan are usually indications for cardiac catheterization or further studies.
5. Abnormal MUGA studies are associated with
   (a) Congestive cardiac failure
   (b) Change in ventricular function due to infarction
   (c) Persistent arrhythmias from poor ventricular function
6. Abnormal heart shunts reveal:
   (a) Left-to-right shunt   (c) Mean pulmonary transit
   (b) Right-to-left shunt   time

Patient Preparation
1. Explain the purpose and procedure of the test.
2. Fasting is necessary for at least 2 hours and no smoking is necessary for 2 hours and during the entire stress thallium test.
3. Advise the patient that the exercise stress period will be continued for 45 to 60 seconds after injection to allow the thallium to be cleared during a period of maximum blood flow.
4. Tests can be done at bedside in the acute phase of infarction if equipment is available.
5. A legal permit must be signed by the patient (parents or guardian of child) for a heart shunt scan.
6. No discomfort is experienced during the thallium series test (only feelings associated with stress testing).

Interfering Factors
1. False positive infarct avid (PYP) scans can occur in chest wall traumas, recent cardioversion, and unstable angina.
2. Neither PYP nor thallium studies are reliable in the evaluations of nontransmural infarction.
3. Long-acting nitrates affect coronary blood flow. For this reason, such medications should be discontinued 8 to 12 hours prior to testing.
4. Injection of DPY in the upright or standing positions or with isometric handgrip may increase myocardial uptake.
5. Gated and PYP studies will interfere with other nuclear tests such as liver, bone, or lung scan if they are done on the same day.

Clinical Alert

1. The stress study is contraindicated on patients who
   (a) Have right and left bundle branch block
   (b) Have left ventricular hypertrophy
   (c) Are using digitalis and quinidine
   (d) Are hypokalemic (because the results are difficult to evaluate)
2. Some defects seen immediately postexercise in a patient without infarction will disappear if imaging is repeated 2 to 3 hours later. Those defects that persist at the time of repeat imaging (4–24 hours later) are associated with the presence of a myocardial scar.
3. Contraindications to Persantine imaging are severe coronary artery disease and angina at rest.

4. Adverse short-term effects of DPY occur in 30% to 40% of patients and include nausea, headache, dizziness, facial flush, vomiting, angina, ST depression, and ventricular arrhythmia.

Lung Scans; Perfusion and Xenon Ventilation

Normal Values
Normal functioning lung
Normal pulmonary vascular supply
Normal gases exchanged

Explanation of Test
Lung scan is done for three major purposes: to detect the percentage of the lungs functioning normally; to diagnose and locate pulmonary emboli; and to assess the pulmonary vascular supply by providing an estimate of regional pulmonary blood flow. It is a simple method for following the course of embolic disease, since an area of ischemia will persist after apparent resolution on a radiograph of the chest. In the case of pulmonary emboli, the blood supply beyond an embolus is restricted. Imaging will reveal poor or no visualization of the affected area. Only three tests are positive immediately following pulmonary embolus: pulmonary arteriogram, measurement of physiological dead space, and lung scan. Assessment of the adequacy of pulmonary artery perfusion in areas of known disease can also be done reliably. As soon as a pulmonary embolism is suspected, a ventilated perfusion study should be considered and, if possible, should be performed within 2 days of the acute event.

Following the IV injection of a radioactive iodinated macroaggregated albumin (MAA) labeled with technetium, assessment of pulmonary vascular supply is done by scanning.

Krypton-81m, Xenon[133], or Technetium-99m is used in the ventilation lung scan. When inhaled, radioactive gas follows the same pathway as the air in normal breathing. In some pathological conditions affecting ventilation, there will be significant alteration in the normal ventilation process. The ventilation scan is performed with the lung perfusion scan and is significant in the diagnosis of pulmonary emboli. When the ventilation scan is performed in conjunction with the lung scan, it is helpful in diagnosing bronchitis, asthma, inflammatory fibrosis, pneumonia, chronic obstructive pulmonary disease, and lung cancer.

There are three types of lung scans: (1) the perfusion scan where the blood supply to the tissues in the lungs can be demonstrated; (2) the ventilation scan where the movement of air or lack of air in the lungs may be demonstrated; and (3) the inhalation scan where droplets of radioactive material can be administered by positive pressure ventilator. The aerosol is then breathed through a mouthpiece or facemask. A normal aerosol scan looks much like a perfusion scan except that the trachea and major airways are more visible.

Certain limitations exist with these tests. With a positive chest film and a positive scan, the differential possibilities are multiple: pneumonia, abscess, bullae, ateliosis, and carcinoma, among others. A pulmonary arteriogram is still necessary before an embolectomy can be attempted.

Procedure for Xenon Ventilation Scan

1. In addition to the above, the patient is asked to breathe radioaerosol for approximately 4 minutes through a closed, nonpressurized ventilation system. During this time, a small amount of radioactive gas will be administered into the system.
2. Breath-holding will be required for a brief period some time during the examination.
3. The examining time is 10 to 15 minutes. When performed with a lung perfusion scan, 30 to 45 minutes is the testing time (used in differential diagnosis of embolism).

Clinical Implications

1. Abnormal ventilation and perfusion patterns may indicate the possibility of
   (a) Tumors   (d) Atelectasis   (g) Inflammatory fibrosis
   (b) Emboli   (e) Bronchitis   (h) COPD
   (c) Pneumonia   (f) Asthma   (i) Lung cancer

Interfering Factors

1. False-positive scans occur in vasculitis, mitral stenosis, pulmonary hypertension, and when tumors obstruct a pulmonary artery with airway involvement.

Patient Preparation

1. Explain the purpose and procedure of the test.
2. Alleviate any fears the patient may have concerning radioisotope procedures.
3. It is important that a record of a recent radiograph of the chest be available.
4. The patient must be able to follow directions for breathing and holding his breath.

Brain Scan; Cerebral Blood Flow

Normal Values

Normal distribution and uptake in all regions of the brain
Normal extracranial and intracranial blood flow

Explanation of Test

A brain scan is a diagnostic procedure that follows a careful neurological history and examination. It is valuable in visualizing and localizing intradural lesions for *early* evaluation of patients with suspected intracranial pathology, such as subdural hematoma, cerebrovascular conditions, and for postoperative post-chemotherapy or postirradiation follow-up. This study is helpful in diagnosing superior sagittal sinus thrombosis, and in the evaluation of the intracranial cerebral arterial supply. In states where brain death is the legally accepted criterion of death, a radionuclide cerebral blood flow (also known as radionuclide cerebral angiography—RCA) is a valuable confirmatory test. The procedure is nonspecific, since neoplasms, vascular accidents, malformations, and extracerebral hematomas all present areas of increased activity on the scan. The brain scan is usually negative during the first week after a cerebrovascular accident (CVA). Most strokes will cause a positive scan in the third or fourth week. The brain scan is almost always performed in conjunction with cerebral flow study, which is a visualization of the intracranial and extracranial blood flow.

A radioactive isotope, usually ^{99m}TC or diethylenetriamine pentaacetic acid (DTPA), is injected intravenously. When it is introduced into the circulation, it will concentrate in or about a variety of intracerebral lesions, allowing visualization on scanning. The detection of a lesion rests on the differential between its uptake of radioactive materials and that in surrounding tissue.

Brain scanning is one of the testing systems in which lesions appear as an area of high radioactivity within the surrounding zone of low activity found in normal tissues. This relative increase in the concentration of radioactivity in brain lesions compared to the surrounding normal brain tissue occurs since most tracers fail to penetrate into normal brain tissue as a result of the blood-brain barrier. Tumors and other lesions of the brain interfere with the barrier, allowing a relatively high concentration of radioactive material to be localized. A change in the endothelium is one of the earliest changes in brain tumors. The blood-brain barrier is not a specific anatomical structure, but a complex system including capillary endothelium with closed intracellular clefts, a small or absent extravascular fluid space between endothelium and glial sheaths, and the membrane of the neurons themselves. To the extent that the blood-brain barrier is absent or has been rendered inoperative, the concentration of blood around a lesion increased, or the normal channels of flow altered, the existence and source of trouble is made apparent.

Procedure

1. An oral blocking agent taken in the form of stale-tasting liquid or a tasteless capsule may be given before testing. The blocking agent

reduces uptake of the isotope in the thyroid, choroid plexus, salivary glands, and mucosa of the mouth and sinuses.
2. Scanning will be done immediately following administration of the radioisotope for cerebral flow study and two hours later for an actual brain scan.
3. The actual scanning time for cerebral blood flow is 5 minutes. Waiting time is about 2 hours. The patient must be quiet during this time, with hands at the sides of the body.
4. Scanning can be done at bedside if the patient is suspected of being brain dead.

Clinical Implications
1. Abnormal results are indicative of
   (a) Brain tumors, such as astrocytomas, gliomas, and meningiomas
   (b) Aneurysms
   (c) CVAs
   (d) Hematomas
   (e) Malformations
   (f) Metastatic brain disease
   (g) Benign tumors
   (h) AV malformations
2. Lesions appear as areas of high radioactivity; normal surrounding tissue shows low radioactivity.
3. The scan does not reveal ventricular system, blood supply, or tumor type.
4. The cerebral blood flow in the presence of brain death will show a very distinct image of no tracer uptake in the anterior or middle cerebral arteries or the cerebral hemisphere along with the presence of uptake in the scalp.

Interfering Factors
1. If the patient coughs or changes position, the scan picture is altered.
2. Immediately after the injection of the radioisotope, the patient's saliva, tears, and urine become radioactive for a few hours. More ^{99m}Tc goes into saliva than the brain tissues. If the patient coughs into his hand and then scratches his head, he might contaminate his scalp. Although this is not harmful to the patient, the scan will record a false marking if this occurs.

Patient Preparation
1. Explain the purpose and procedure of the test.
2. Reassure the patient that the test is safe, nontoxic, and painless. The only discomfort is that he must remain very quiet and still.
3. In some instances, capsules of potassium iodide or Lugol's solution are given orally to block thyroid uptake of the radioiodine used in this procedure. If the patient is allergic to iodine, potassium perchlorate may be used. This substance causes gastric irritation in some persons.

4. If the patient will be unable to cooperate by lying perfectly still, obtain an order from the attending physician to give a sedative.

Gallbladder/Hepatobiliary Scan

Normal Values
Normal concentration pattern revealing normal size, shape, and function of gallbladder and ducts

Explanation of Test
This study, using ^{99m}Tc/D1SIDA or Disofenin tracers, is done to evaluate the gallbladder and biliary tract. It is indicated in the evaluation of acute cholecystitis and obstructive jaundice. Following the intravenous administration of the radionuclide, the substance will be excreted rapidly from the blood by the polygonal cells of the liver. The transit through the liver cells to the biliary tract is rapid, 10 to 30 minutes, and significant uptake occurs in the normal gallbladder.

Procedure
1. The radionuclide is injected intravenously.
2. Imaging starts immediately after injection and usually takes 1 hour.
3. Delayed views are usually done at 2, 4, and 24 hours, in the event of the discovery of severe parenchymal disease where bile duct obstruction is not noted. In these cases, bowel activity is generally detected somewhere between 24 and 48 hours postinjection. It is important to note that contributions from the right kidney may be mistaken for bowel activity. Also, 24 hours or longer may be indicated for a delayed view in cases of complete obstruction or other hepatobiliary disease.

Clinical Implications
1. Abnormal concentration patterns will reveal unusual bile communications.
2. Determine if the jaundiced patient is a surgical or nonsurgical candidate.
3. Gallbladder visualization excludes the diagnosis of acute cholecystitis with a high degree (close to 100%) of certainty.

Interfering Factors
1. Patients with high serum bilirubin (>10 mg/dl) may have less reliable test results.
2. Patients on total parenteral nutrition (TPN) or long-term fasting may not have GB visualization.

Patient Preparation
1. Explain the purpose and procedure of the test.
2. Fasting is required for 2 hours prior to testing.
3. If the patient has been without food for 48 hours or TPN, sincalide IV may be given one hour prior to testing to reduce cystic bile spasm and enhance gallbladder visualization.

Bone Scan

Normal Values
No areas of greater or lesser concentration of radioactive material in bones

Explanation of Test
This test is used primarily to evaluate and follow up persons with known or suspected metastatic disease and the majority of bone scans continue to be for this reason. Breast, prostate, lung tumors and lymphomas tend to metastasize to bone. Bone scans will demonstrate lesions 3 to 6 months before they appear in radiographs.

This scan is commonly used in the evaluation of patients with unexplained bone pain, and patients with primary bone tumors, arthritis, osteomyelitis, abnormal healing of fractures, fractures, shin splints, and compression fractures of the vertebral column. It is also used for patients with chronic renal failure in whom it is necessary to detect soft tissue calcification; and in pediatric patients with hip pain (Legg–Calvé-Perthes disease). It is also done to identify suitable bone biopsy sites, to evaluate those areas difficult to demonstrate radiographically, such as the sternum and the scapula, and to help determine the age and metabolic activity of traumatic injuries and infection.

Other indications are to evaluate candidates for knee and hip prostheses, to diagnose aseptic necroses, vascularity of the femoral head, and for presurgical assessment of viable bone tissue when amputation is necessary. Evaluation of prosthetic joints and internal fixation devices that are suspected of becoming loose or infected is also done.

TMJ Bone Scanning
This test is done to confirm the clinical impression of internal derangement of the temporomandibular joint (TMJ). The TMJ is the most actively used joint in the body. Single photon emission computed tomography (SPECT) has a sensitivity of 94% and a specificity of 70%.

A bone-seeking radiopharmaceutical is used to image the skeletal system. An example would be ^{99m}Tc-labeled phosphate injected intravenously. Imaging usually begins 2 to 3 hours after injection. The ex-

aminer will look for the distribution and concentration of the pharmaceutical in the bone. Abnormal pathology such as increased blood flow
to bone and increased metabolism will concentrate the radiopharmaceutical at a higher or lower rate than the normal bone. The radiopharmaceutical mimics the calcium physiology and, therefore, will concentrate more heavily in the areas of increased metabolic activity.

Procedure for Bone Scan
1. Radioactive ^{99m}Tc phosphate is injected intravenously.
2. A 2- to 3-hour waiting period is necessary for the radiopharmaceutical to concentrate in the bone. During this time, the patient may be
   asked to drink four to six glasses of water.
3. Before the scan begins, the patient is asked to urinate, since a full
   bladder will mask the pelvic bones.
4. The scan takes about 30 to 60 minutes to complete. The patient
   must be still during scanning. The table or the scanner will slowly
   move the patient under and over a sensitive radiation detector.

Procedure for TMJ Bone Scan
1. A radionuclide ^{99m}technetium MDP (methyline dyphosphate) is injected intravenously.
2. Scanning begins three hours after administration.
3. SPECT bone imaging as well as lateral plane views are done.
4. During SPECT, the patient must remain immobile for 21 minutes
   while the detector rotates around the person.

Interfering Factors
1. False-negative bone scans occur in multiple myeloma of bone.
   When this condition is known or suspected, the scan is an unreliable indicator of skeletal involvement.
2. Patients with follicular thyroid cancer may harbor metastatic bone
   marrow disease, but these lesions are often missed by scans.

Clinical Implications
Abnormal concentrations indicate

1. Very early bone disease and healing. This is detectable by radioiso-
   topic scan long before it is visible on radiographs. The latter are
   positive for bone lesions only after 30% to 50% decalcification (bone
   calcium decreased) has occurred.
2. Many disorders can be detected but not differentiated by this test
   (*e.g.*, cancer, arthritis, benign bone tumors, fractures, osteomyelitis,
   Paget's disease, and aseptic necroses). The findings must be interpreted in the light of the whole clinical picture, since any process
   inducing an increased calcium excretion rate will be reflected by an
   increased uptake in the bone.

3. Breast cancer-positive bone scan finding in the preoperative period depends on the staging of the disease and these scans are recommended prior to initial therapy. *Stages 1* and *2*: 4% will have positive bone scan. *Stage 3*: 19% will have positive bone scan. Yearly bone scans should be done for follow-up.
4. Multiple myeloma is the only tumor that shows better detectability with a plain radiograph than with a radionuclide scan.
5. Multiple focal areas of increased activity in the axial skeleton are commonly associated with metastatic bone disease. The reported percentage of solitary lesions due to metastasis varies on a site-by-site basis. With a single lesion in the spine or pelvis, the cause is more likely to be due to metastatic disease than one occurring in the extremities or ribs.

Clinical Implications of TMJ
Increased uptake with hot areas associated with increased osteoblastic activity about the margins of a displaced joint occur in

1. TMJ disk displacement
2. Bite abnormality
3. Congenital deformity of the mandible

Clinical Alert

1. The flare phenomenon occurs in patients with metastatic disease who are receiving a new therapy. In some persons, the bone scan may show increased activity or new lesions in persons with clinical improvement. It is due to a healing response in prostate and breast cancer within the first few months of a new treatment. These lesions should show marked improvement on scans 3 to 4 months later.
2. Radiographic correlation is necessary to rule out a benign process when solitary areas of increased or decreased uptake occur.
3. The TMJ examination should be deferred in women who are pregnant or who are breast-feeding infants.

Patient Preparation
1. Instruct the patient about the purpose and procedure of the test and his involvement. Alleviate any fears concerning the procedure. Advise the patient that frequent drinking and activity in the first 6 hours help to reduce excess radiation to the bladder and gonads.
2. The patient can be up and about during the waiting period.

3. If the patient is in pain or debilitated, assist him to void before the test. Otherwise, give a reminder about emptying the bladder before the test.
4. A sedative should be ordered and administered to any patient who will have difficulty lying quietly during the scanning period.

Deep Vein Thrombosis (DVT) Scan; ^{125}I-Fibrinogen Venogram; Fibrinogen Uptake Test

Normal Values
No areas of abnormal concentration in deep veins of lower legs

Explanation of Test
This scan is done to detect deep venous thrombosis in the lower extremities, from the ankle to the groin. These studies will demonstrate the early development of thrombi so that they can be managed with anticoagulant therapy before clots of significant size can form and, in some cases, embolize. The DVT scan is indicated in surgical patients and in high-risk medical and obstetrical patients where immobility and medical problems may be conducive to the formation of deep venous thrombosis. Patients with calf tenderness, positive Homan's sign, erythema, increased calf or thigh circumference, edema, or temperature differences are candidates for the procedure. The radioisotope injected intravenously is ^{125}I-fibrinogen.

Procedure
1. After administration of iodine or perchlorate intravenously (in surgical patients, it is usually injected in the recovery room), the lower extremities are marked from the ankle to the groin in approximately 2-inch segments along the course of the deep vein tract. The heart will also be marked at the same time for a body background count.
2. Daily readings are taken over these marked areas to determine whether the injected fibrinogen is being incorporated in the formation of clots.
3. The examination is done at the bedside with a portable scanner. The legs are elevated during the imaging procedure (7 to 10 minutes).
4. The scan is done daily, 7 days a week, for as long as 2 weeks.

Clinical Implications
1. Abnormal concentration will reveal
   (a) Deep venous thrombosis formation
   (b) Recurrence of thrombosis

2. Eighty-five percent of positive tests are evident within the first 24 hours after administration of ^{125}I-fibrinogen.

Patient Preparation

1. Explain the purpose and procedure of the test.
2. Reassure the patient that there is no discomfort and that the scan is safe and nontoxic.
3. Lugol's solution or potassium iodine should be given orally every day to block thyroid uptake of the radioiodine used in this procedure. If the patient is allergic to iodine, potassium perchlorate may be used instead.

Clinical Alert

Do not wash markings off thighs and legs when the patient is bathed.
Do not lower the patient's legs until you are certain that imaging has been completed at the bedside.

Gallium (^{67}Ga) Scans (Liver, Bone, Brain, Breast Scan)

Normal Values

No evidence of tumor-type activity

Explanation of Test

This test is used to detect the presence, location, and size of tumors, adhesions, abscesses, and inflammation in body cavities, primarily in the liver, bone, brain, and breast. It is most useful in differentiating malignant from benign lesions and determining the extent of invasion of known malignancies. The lymph nodes are also scanned for involvement. These studies are also used to stage bronchogenic cancer, Hodgkin's and nonHodgkin's lymphomas and to record tumor regression following radiation or chemotherapy, thereby noting the body response to therapy. The radioisotope injected intravenously is gallium citrate (^{67}Ga).

Areas of the body most often examined by this method are the lymph system, liver, bone, brain, and breast. Only 5% pathological activity is necessary for detection by this technique, while 45% activity is required for radiographic examination. The underlying mechanism for the uptake of ^{67}gallium citrate is not well understood. Uptake in some neoplasms may depend on the presence of transferrin receptors in tumor cells but this is only speculation.

Procedure
1. If imaging of the abdomen is to be performed, a laxative is usually given the evening before the scanning.
2. Laxatives, suppositories, or tap water enemas are often ordered before scanning. The patient may eat breakfast the day of imagery.
3. The radionuclide is injected 24 to 72 hours before imaging.
4. The patient must lie quietly without moving during the scanning procedure. Anterior and posterior views of the entire body are done.
5. Additional imaging may be done at 24 hours to differentiate normal bowel activity from pathologen concentrations.

Clinical Implications
1. An abnormal gallium concentration usually implies the existence of underlying pathology as in

   (a) Malignancy, especially lung, testes, and mesothelioma
   (b) Stages of lymphomas, melanoma, hepatoma, soft tissue sarcomas, primary tumors of bone and cartilage, neuroblastomas and leukemia
   (c) Abscesses
   (d) Tuberculosis
   (e) Thrombosis
   (f) Abscessed sarcoidosis

2. Further diagnostic studies are usually done to distinguish benign from malignant lesions.
3. Tumor uptake of ^{67}Ga varies with tumor type, among persons with tumors of some histologic types, and even with tumor sites in a given patient.
4. Tumor uptake of ^{67}Ga may be significantly reduced following effective treatment.

Interfering Factors
1. A negative study cannot be definitely interpreted as ruling out the presence of disease (40% false-negative results in gallium studies).
2. It is difficult to detect a single, solitary nodule such as in adenocarcinoma. Lesions smaller than 2 cm are detectable. Tumors near the liver are difficult to detect, as is interpretation of ileac nodes.
3. Because gallium does collect in the bowel, there may be an abnormal concentration in the lower abdomen. For this reason, enemas are ordered before testing.
4. Degeneration/necrosis of tumor and antineoplastic drugs immediately before scans cause false-negative results.

Patient Preparation
1. Explain the purpose and procedure of the test.
2. Reassure the patient that there is no pain involved.
3. Alleviate any fear the patient may have about radioisotope procedures.

4. Usually, no change need be made in eating habits before testing. However, some departments expect their patients to eat a low-residue lunch and clear liquid supper the day before examination.
5. The day before examination and after the procedure is completed, the patient is advised to drink large amounts of fluid to help excrete the gallium that is present in the gastrointestinal tract. The usual preparation includes oral laxatives beginning on the day of injection and continuing until imagery is completed and/or by enemas/suppositories prior to the examination. It is believed that these preparations clean normal gallium activity from the bowel.
6. Actual scanning time is 1 to 2 hours.

Clinical Alert

Breast-feeding should be discontinued for at least 4 weeks following testing.

^{131}I Total Body Scan

Normal Values
No functioning extrathyroid tissues outside of the thyroid gland

Explanation of Test
This study using ^{131}I or ^{123}I is done to search for any functioning thyroid tissue anywhere in the body. It is helpful in determining the presence of metastatic thyroid cancer and the amount and location of residual tissue following thyroidectomy.

Procedure
1. A radionuclide is administered orally in a capsule form.
2. Imaging will take place 24 to 72 hours after administration.
3. Imaging can take as long as 2 to 3 hours to perform.
4. Sometimes, thyroid-stimulating hormone (TSH) is administered intravenously before the radionuclide is given. This stimulates any residual thyroid tissue so it will take up enough ^{131}I or ^{123}I to be detected.

Clinical Implications
Abnormal uptake of iodine reveals
1. Areas of extrathyroid tissue such as
   (a) Stroma ovarii
   (b) Substernal thyroid
   (c) Sublingual thyroid

2. Residual tissue following thyroidectomy
3. Metastatic thyroid cancer

Clinical Alert

1. When possible, this test should be performed before any other radionuclide procedures and before using any iodine contrast medium, surgical preparation, or other form of iodine.
2. The test is most effective when endogenous TSH levels are high, in order to stimulate radioiodine uptake by metastatic neoplasm.

Patient Preparation
1. Explain the purpose and procedure of the test.
2. Advise the patient that the imaging process may take a long time.

Bone Marrow Scan

Normal Values
Normal reticuloendothelial and red blood cells and normal distribution of bone marrow

Explanation of Test
This study, using the radionuclide indium chloride, is used in determining the site of bone marrow biopsy sites, and is indicated in the differential diagnosis of myeloproliferative disorders, in detection of focal defects in bone marrow, and in differentiation of acute from chronic hemolysis, and of bone infarction from osteomyelitis in sickle cell disease. It is also helpful in staging lymphoma, Hodgkin's disease, and metastatic cancer in the bone marrow.

Procedure
1. A radionuclide is injected intravenously and imaging of the whole body follows 48 hours after injection of indium chlorine. If Tc sulfur colloid is used, scanning usually begins one hour after injection.
2. The patient must lie quietly on the scanning table during the entire examination. The body, from head to foot, is scanned.
3. Total imaging time is 1½ hours.

Clinical Implications
Abnormal filling patterns reveal

1. Bone marrow depression following radiation therapy
2. Bone marrow depression following chemotherapy

3. Extended marrow activity in polycythemia vera
4. Extended marrow activity in chronic hemolytic anemia
5. Nonvisualization in myelofibrosis

Patient Preparation
Explain the purpose and procedure of test. Reassure the patient that no discomfort will be experienced during the test. Instruct the patient to void before imaging occurs.

Cisternography; CSF Flow Scan

Normal Values
Unobstructed cerebrospinal fluid flow and normal reabsorption

Explanation of Test
This study, in which a radionuclide is injected by lumbar puncture, is a sensitive indicator of altered flow and reabsorption of cerebrospinal fluid. In the treatment of hydrocephalus, it aids in the selection of the type of shunt and pathway as well as in the prognosis of both shunting and hydrocephalus.

Procedure
1. A sterile lumbar puncture is performed after the patient has been positioned and prepared (see page 220 for procedure). At this time, a tracer dose of radionuclide is injected into the cerebrospinal circulation.
2. The patient must lie flat after the puncture; the length of time depends on the physician's order.
3. Imaging will be done at 2 to 6 hours postinjection, then again at 24 hours, 48 hours, and 72 hours in some cases.
4. Examining time is 1 hour for each scan.

Clinical Implications
Abnormal filling patterns reveal

1. Hydrocephalus
2. Subdural hematoma
3. Spinal mass lesions
4. Posterior fossa cysts

5. Third ventricle tumor
6. Parencephalic and subarachnoid cysts

Patient Preparation
1. Explain the procedures for both lumbar puncture and cisternography.
2. Advise the patient that it may take as long as 1 hour for each scan.
3. The patient must be taken by cart to the nuclear medicine department for the first scan, because of the preceding lumbar puncture.

Patient Aftercare
1. Follow instructions for lumbar puncture (see page 220).
2. Be alert to complications of lumbar puncture such as meningitis, allergic reaction to anesthetic, bleeding into spinal canal, and herniation of brain tissue.

Spleen Scan

Normal Values
Normal size of spleen, cell function, and blood flow to spleen
The amount of uptake in the spleen should always be less than the liver

Explanation of Test
This examination is performed to demonstrate anatomical changes in the spleen. Spleen imaging is accomplished by the use of a radioactive nuclide colloid such as ^{99m}Tc sulfur colloid. The amount of this pharmaceutical taken up by the spleen is dependent upon the blood flow to the spleen and its cell function. Resulting images allow the examiner to determine the size and condition of the spleen. This scan may also be used to demonstrate space-occupying lesions or accessory spleens, to visualize the infiltration of Hodgkin's or metastatic disease, and to evaluate trauma cases to rule out infarct. This procedure is performed in conjunction with a liver scan. Spleen imaging is performed using single photon emission computed tomography (SPECT).

Clinical Alert
1. It is essential that the nuclear medicine department know the purpose of the examination.
2. Additional views may be required for accurate diagnosis, as in trauma and suspected infarct.

Procedure
1. A patient history is obtained and recorded.
2. The radiopharmaceutical is injected intravenously.
3. A 10- to 20-minute wait is required to allow the injected radiopharmaceutical to be absorbed in the reticuloendothelial cells.
4. A minimum of three views is obtained. On some occasions, additional oblique views may be required.
5. Total examining time is approximately 80 minutes from injection to conclusion. The time involved will vary, due to the patient's ability to cooperate and the size and condition of the spleen. The

ability of the cells to accumulate the pharmaceutical will also affect the imaging time.

Clinical Implications
Abnormal concentrations reveal

1. Unusual splenic size
2. Infarction
3. Ruptured spleen
4. Accessory spleen
5. Tumors
6. Metastatic spread
7. Ivemark's syndrome
8. Kartagener's syndrome

Spleens greater than 14 cm. in size are abnormally enlarged; those less than 7 cm. are abnormally small. Areas of absent radioactivity or holes in the spleen scans are associated with abnormalities that displace or destroy normal splenic pulp.

Patient Preparation
1. Explain the purpose, procedure, benefits, and risks of the test. Radiation exposure is about 0.5 to 2.0 rads to the liver, slightly less to the spleen, and about 0.05 rads to the entire body. The whole body dose is about equal to 1 year of natural background radiation.
2. A thorough history must be obtained.
3. Whenever possible, schedule the scan before any test using barium as a contrast.
4. The test can be performed when a trauma case or when a ruptured spleen is suspected, at bedside, or in the emergency room. Electroconvulsive therapy (ECT) must be done in the department of nuclear medicine.

Interfering Factors
1. Possible artifacts may occur if the images are taken immediately after the administration of barium for radiologic colon examinations. Barium is a dense material and may attenuate some of the gamma radiation from technetium sulfur colloid, which is the pharmaceutical most often used.
2. About 30% of persons with Hodgkin's disease with spleen involvement will have a normal spleen scan.

Adrenergic Tumor Scan; ^{131}MIBG

Normal Values
No evidence of tumor sites
Normal salivary glands, urinary bladder, and vague shape of liver and spleen can be seen.

Explanation of Test
The purpose of this study is to obtain images that aid in identifying sites of certain tumors that produce excessive amounts of catechol-

amines: pheochromocytomas; paragangliomas; neuroblastomas; carcinoid tumors; or medullary carcinoma of the thyroid gland. This is accomplished by venous injection of a radionuclide [131]Iodine metaiodobenzylguanidine ([131]MIBG) followed by scans on the first, second, and third days or the second, third, and fourth days of the study.

This test is done to identify tumor sites when a reasonable probability exists (evidence of hormones and metabolites of norepinephrine and epinephrine) that pheochromocytomas are present. When laboratory tests do indicate a functional paraganglioma, it is sometimes difficult to locate the tumor anatomically. The recent development of radionuclides that are selectively taken up by paragangliomas, as in this study, has improved localization. Generally, three views are sufficient for a search: (1) anterior display of the pelvis and lower abdomen; (2) posterior display of abdomen and lower chest; and (3) upper chest and head. If metastasis is suspected, then the upper legs, the humeri, and all of the head are examined as well.

It is known that pheochromocytomas develop in cells that make up the adrenergic portion of the autonomic nervous system. A large number of these well-differentiated cells is found in adrenal medullas, paraspino-sympathetic ganglia, and periaortic organs of Zuckerkandl. In addition, a few cells are located elsewhere, as in the urinary bladder, heart, in an association with nerves, usually thought to be primarily parasympathetic, such as the vagus. Adrenergic tumors have been called paragangliomas when found outside the adrenal medulla, but many refer to all neoplasms that secrete norepinephrine and epinephrine as pheochromocytomas. Because the only definite and effective therapy is surgery to remove the tumor, identifying the site using this test, as well as CT scans and ultrasound, is an essential goal of treatment.

Procedure

1. The radionuclide, [131]MIGB, is injected intravenously.
2. Scans will be done on the second, third, and fourth days in most instances (Day 1 being the day of injection). Occasionally only one day of imaging will be necessary, while in a few patients, imagery will be required on the sixth and seventh days. Scanning will be done from the urinary bladder to the mastoid area when searching for a primary tumor.
3. Scanning time each day is approximately 30 minutes.

Clinical Implications

1. Abnormal results give substance to the "Rough Rule of Ten." This means that

   (a) Ten percent are in children.

   (b) Ten percent are familial.

   (c) Ten percent are bilateral in the adrenal glands.

   (d) Ten percent are malignant.

(e) Ten percent are multiple, in   (f) Ten percent are extrarenal.
   addition to bilateral, tumors.
2. Over 90% of primary pheochromocytomas occur in the abdomen.
3. Pheochromocytomas in children often represent a familial disorder.
4. Bilateral adrenal tumors often indicate a familial disease and vice versa.
5. Multiple extrarenal pheochromocytomas are often malignant.
6. The presence of two or more pheochromocytomas almost always indicates malignant disease.

Interfering Factors
Barium interferes.

Patient Preparation
1. Explain the purpose and procedure, benefits and risks. Radioactive exposure is comparable to computed tomography (CT scan) of the adrenal glands or conventional radiograph of the kidneys and adrenal glands.
2. To prevent uptake of radioactive iodine by the thyroid gland, Lugol's solution or potassium iodine will be given for a period of time before the test as well as after the test. For example, a common protocol is two days before injection of radionuclide and ten days after the injection.
3. Scans will usually be taken up to and including three successive days after injection. Occasionally patients will require imaging on four days. Even though most pheochromocytomas are readily defined on all three days, in some patients the tumor may not be seen on any day but will be best portrayed on Day 3; in others, the opposite will occur; the pheochromocytomas will be seen only on Day 1.

Patient Aftercare
1. Check the patient for discomfort or bruising at the site of injection.
2. Follow-up tests include:
   (a) Kidney and bone nuclear scans to give further orientation to abnormalities discovered in ^{131}I-MIBG tests.
   (b) CT scans if MIBG scans have failed to locate the tumor.
   (c) Ultrasound of pelvis if the tumor produces urinary symptoms.

Abscess Scan (WBC Inflammatory Imagery—Indium-111 Scan)

Normal Values
No signs of localization of leukocytes

Explanation of Test
This test, in which a sample of the patient's own leukocyta (white blood cells) has been isolated, labeled with indium oxine or chloride and reinjected, is used for the localization of abscess formation. The study is indicated in persons with signs and symptoms of a septic process, fever of unknown origin, and suspected intra-abdominal abscess. It is also helpful in determining the cause of complications of surgery, injury, or inflammation of gastrointestinal tract and pelvis. The test results are based on the fact that any collection of labeled white cells outside the liver, spleen, and functioning bone marrow indicates an abnormal area to which the WBCs are being attracted. This procedure is 90% sensitive and 90% specific for inflammatory disease and/or abscess formation.

Procedure
1. A venous blood sample of 40 ml is obtained for the purpose of isolating and labeling the white blood cells. This laboratory process takes about 3 hours to complete.
2. The WBCs are labeled with radioactive Indium-111 and injected intravenously.
3. After a waiting period, the patient returns for imagery at 24 and 48 hours.
4. Imaging time is about 1 hour each time.

Clinical Implications
Abnormal concentrations indicate

1. Abscess formation
2. Acute and chronic osteomyelitis and infection of orthopedic prostheses
3. Active inflammatory bowel disease

Interfering Factors
1. False-negative reactions are known to occur when the chematactic function of the WBC has been altered as in hemodialysis, hyperglycemia, hyperalimentation, steroid therapy, and long-term antibiotic therapy.
2. Gallium scans up to one month prior can interfere.
3. False-positive scans occur in the presence of GI bleeding and in upper respiratory infections and pneumonitis when patients swallow purulent sputum.

Clinical Considerations
1. If the patient does not have an adequate number of WBCs, then donor cells can be used. It is possible in some instances to do a successful study in persons who have less than 1000 WBC per cm.

Patient Preparation
1. Explain the purposes, procedure, benefits, and risks.
2. Assess for a history of recent Gallium scan.
3. If the patient is premenopausal, instructions are to be given to the patient to use effective birth control while being tested because the test may be harmful to the fetus.

Risks
Fetal radiation should be avoided whenever possible. The radiation dose to the fetus from this test is equal to the radiation from one abdominal radiograph.

Meckel's Diverticulum Scan

Normal Values
Normal blood flow in abdomen
Normal distribution of radiopharmaceutical
No evidence of ectopic tissue

Explanation of Test
This test is indicated in both children and adults with GI bleeding of unknown etiology, with undetermined abdominal pain and persistent guaiac positive stools with normal barium radiographs. Meckel's diverticulum can be difficult to detect by standard radiographic techniques. The radionuclide Tc^{99}m pertechnetate is taken up by the gastric mucosa following IV administration. This procedure detects the presence of abnormally situated gastric mucosa. Meckel's diverticulum frequently contains gastric mucosa that can be responsible for hyperacidity, causing bowel wall erosion and hemorrhage.

Procedure
1. Preferably, prior to the procedure, the patient should receive cimetidine orally every 6 hours for 24 hours. Cimetidine inhibits acid secretion and allows for a better scan. However, even without cimetidine secretion, the scan can be performed.
2. A radiopharmaceutical is injected intravenously.
3. There are two phases to imaging
   (a) Blood flow in the abdomen
   (b) Periodic imagery to determine uptake of radiopharmaceutical in duodenum
4. Total examining time is 60 minutes

Interfering Factors
Barium in the small or large bowel may mask radionuclide concentration.

Clinical Implications

Abnormal distributions indicate presence of Meckel's diverticulum, which is a remnant of the oomphalomesenteric duct. Only about 2% of the population will develop this disorder of the duodenum, and of this population, 25% will exhibit symptoms.

Clinical Considerations

A determination should be made that no recent barium studies have been done.

Patient Preparation

1. Explain the purpose and procedure of the test.
2. The patient should be NPO for at least 2 hours prior to the examination.

Parathyroid Scan

Normal Values

No areas of increased perfusion or uptake ratios in parathyroid and thyroid

Explanation of Test

This test is done primarily for presurgical localization of parathyroid adenomas in clinically proven cases of primary hyperparathyroidism. It is helpful in demonstrating intrinsic or extrinsic parathyroid adenoma. Two tracers, thallium and technetium, are used prior to imagery.

Procedure

1. The radionuclide thallium is injected and 20 minutes later imaging is done. This image is stored in the computer.
2. Without moving the patient, thallium (less than that used in a heart scan) is injected and a second image is obtained and computerized. Computer processing involves subtracting the technetium-visualized thyroid structures from the thallium accumulation in a parathyroid adenoma.
3. Total examination is 30 to 45 minutes.

Interfering Factors

1. Recent ingestion of iodine in food, medication, and recent tests with iodine content may reduce the effectiveness of the study.

Clinical Implications

Abnormal concentrations reveal parathyroid adenoma, both intrinsic and extrinsic, but cannot differentiate between benign and malignant parathyroid.

Clinical Considerations

Pregnancy is a relative contraindication. However, if primary hyperparathyroidism and surgical exploration is essential prior to delivery, the study may be performed.

Patient Preparation

1. Explain the purpose and procedure of the test.
2. Assess for the recent intake of iodine. However, this finding is not a specific contraindication to performing the study.
3. Inform the patient that the radiation exposure from this study is less than most fluoroscopic radiographs.
4. The thyroid should be carefully palpated because thallium may accumulate in thyroid adenomas.

Scrotal Scan Testicular Imaging

Normal Values

Normal blood flow to scrotal structures with even distribution and concentration of radiopharmaceutical

Explanation of Test

This test is performed on an emergency basis in the evaluation of acute, painful testicular swelling. It is used in the differential diagnoses of torsion of acute epididymitis and in the evaluation of injury, trauma, tumors, and masses. The radiopharmaceutical Tc^{99m} pertechnetate is used prior to imaging. The images obtained differentiate scrotal lesions associated with increased perfusion from those that are primarily ischemic.

Procedure

1. The patient lies on his back under the nuclear camera. The penis is gently taped back onto the lower abdominal wall.
2. A small tracer dose of radionuclide is injected intravenously.
3. Imagery is performed in two phases: first as a dynamic blood flow study of the scrotum and second, as an assessment of distribution of radiopharmaceutical in the scrotum.
4. Total examining time is 30 to 45 minutes.

Clinical Implications

Abnormal concentrations reveal:

1. Tumors
2. Hematomas
3. Infection
4. Torsions (with reduced blood flow)

The nuclear scan is most specific soon after the onset of pain, before abscess is a clinical consideration.

Patient Preparation
1. Explain the purpose, procedure, benefits, and risks of the test. There is no discomfort involved in testing.
2. If the patient is a child, a parent should accompany the boy. The examining department prefers the father.

Gastrointestinal (GI) Blood Loss Scan

Normal Values
No sites of active bleeding

Explanation of Test
This test has been documented as very sensitive in the detection and location of acute gastrointestinal bleeding that occurs distal to the ligament of Treitz. (Gastroscopy is the procedure of choice in diagnosing upper gastrointestinal bleeding). Prior to the refining of this diagnostic technique, barium enemas were used to identify lesions that reflect the site of bleeding, but these examinations are not specific and frequently miss small sites of bleeding such as that caused by diverticular disease and angiodysplasia. This scan is also indicated for detection and localization of recent hemorrhage, both peritoneal and retroperitoneal, as well as documentation and location of sites of pulmonary hemorrhage. In addition, this procedure is frequently done prior to angiography. For example, if a right lower quadrant bleed is detected, then the angiogram will begin by studying the superior mesenteric artery; if a left lower quadrant bleed is detected, then the inferior mesenteric artery will be the beginning point.

Procedure
1. Radiopharmaceutical ^{99m}technetium is injected.
2. Imaging is begun immediately and continued every few minutes, often with delayed images 2, 6 and sometimes 24 hours later, when necessary, to identify the location of active bleeding.
3. Images are obtained anteriorly over the abdomen at 5 minute intervals. If the study is negative at 1 hour, repeat images can be obtained throughout a 24-hour period without reinjection of radiopharmaceutical.
4. Total examining time varies.
5. Reexamination can be performed any time of the day or night, during a 24-hour period. Active bleeding must be occurring at the rate of .5 to 1 ml per minute to locate the bleeding site.

Clinical Considerations
1. This test is contraindicated in those who are hemodynamically unstable. In these instances, angiography or surgery should be the procedures of choice.

2. Assess patients for signs of active bleeding during the examining period. The procedure will be performed by the department of nuclear medicine any time during a 24-hour period.

Clinical Implications
Abnormal concentration of RBCs with areas of radioactivity greater than the background activity are associated with

1. Approximate geographic location of active GI bleeding, both peritoneal as well as retroperitoneal.
2. Non-GI sites of hemorrhage, such as in the lungs, can also be identified, up to 24 hours postinjection.

Interfering Factors
Presence of barium in GI tract may obscure the site of bleeding. This is because of the high density of barium and the inability of the technetium to penetrate the barium.

Patient Preparation
1. Explain the purpose and procedure, benefits and risks of the test.
2. Determine whether or not the patient has received barium as a diagnostic agent in the last 24 hours. If the presence of barium in the GI tract is questionable, an abdominal radiograph may be ordered.
3. Advise the patient that delayed repeat images may be necessary if barium is present. Also, if active bleeding is not seen on initial scans, additional images must be obtained for as long as 24 hours postinjection, whenever the patient has clinical signs of active bleeding.

Part Two
Radionuclide Laboratory Procedures
(Other Than Radioimmunoassay
[RIA] Studies)

Introduction
Minute quantities of radioactive materials may be detected in blood, feces, urine, other body fluids, and glands. Therefore, very small amounts of radioactive substances may be administered to patients, and then their body fluids and glands may be assayed for concentrations of radioactivity.

The majority of nuclide procedures check the ability of the body to absorb the administered radioactive compound. An example of this type of study is the Schilling test. Other procedures, such as radioactive iodine uptake or blood volume determination, test the ability of the body to localize or dilute the administered radioactive substance.

The use of radionuclides in analysis depends on the fact that the radioactive atoms of a substance such as iodine react chemically just as nonradioactive iodine does, but the radionuclide can be readily detected because of its radioactivity.

Part II of this chapter includes a sampling of tests that employ the use of radionuclides in the study of disease. Imaging may or may not be part of these procedures.

Schilling Test

Normal Values
Excretion of 8% or more of test dose of cobalt-tagged vitamin B_{12} in urine

Explanation of Test
This 24-hour urine test is used to diagnose macrocytic anemia, pernicious anemia, and malabsorption syndromes. It is an indirect test of intrinsic factor deficiency, evaluates ability to absorb vitamin B_{12} from the gastrointestinal tract, and is based on the anticipated urinary excretion of radioactive vitamin B_{12}. In this test, the fasting patient is given an oral dose of vitamin B_{12} tagged with radioactive cobalt (^{57}Co). One hour later, an intramuscular injection of vitamin B_{12} is given to saturate the liver and serum protein-binding sites and to allow radioactive B_{12} to be absorbed in the GI tract and to be excreted in the urine. A 24-hour urine specimen is then collected. The amount of the excreted radioactive B_{12} is determined and expressed as a percentage of the given dose. Normal persons will absorb (and therefore excrete) a large proportion of the radioactive vitamin B_{12}, for they can absorb vitamin B_{12} from the GI tract. Patients with pernicious anemia absorb little of the oral dose and thus have little radioactive material to excrete in the urine.

Procedure
1. The patient must fast for 12 hours before the test. (Breakfast is delayed 2 hours or until the intramuscular injection of vitamin B_{12} is administered.)
2. Tasteless capsules of radioactive B_{12} labeled with cobalt-57 and -58 are administered orally by a medical technologist.

3. One hour later, nonradioactive B_{12} is given by intramuscular injection by an RN or nuclear medical technologist.
4. Total urine is collected for 24 to 48 hours from the time the patient receives the injection of vitamin B_{12}
    (a) Obtain a special 24-hour urine container from the laboratory. No preservative is needed.
    (b) Take care that there is no contamination of the urine with stool.
    (c) Follow the procedure for 24-hour urine collection (see Chapter 3).
    (d) In presence of renal disease, a 48-hour collection may be necessary.

Clinical Implications
1. An abnormally low value (*e.g.*, <8%), borderline, 8%–10%, allows two interpretations:
    (a) Absence of intrinsic factor
    (b) Defective absorption in the ileum
2. When the absorption of radioactive vitamin B_{12} is low, the test must be repeated with intrinsic factor to rule out intestinal malabsorption (confirmatory Schilling test).
    (a) If the urinary excretion then rises to normal levels, it indicates a lack of intrinsic factor, suggesting the diagnosis of pernicious anemia.
    (b) If the urinary excretion does not rise, malabsorption is considered the cause of the patient's anemia.

Interfering Factors
1. Renal insufficiency may cause reduced excretions of radioactive vitamin B_{12}. If renal insufficiency is suspected, a 48- to 72-hour urine collection is advised since eventually nearly all the absorbed material will be excreted and urine specific gravity and volume are checked.
2. The single most common source of error in performing the test is *incomplete collection of urine*. Some laboratories may require a 48-hour collection to allow for a small margin of error.
3. Urinary excretion of B_{12} is depressed in elderly patients, diabetics, patients with hypothyroidism, and those with enteritis.

Patient Preparation
1. Explain the purpose and procedure of the test.
2. Give a written reminder to the patient about fasting and collection of urine specimen. Water is permitted during the fasting period.
3. Food and drink is permitted after the intramuscular dose of vitamin B_{12} is given. The patient is encouraged to drink as much as can be tolerated during the entire test.

4. Be certain the patient receives the nonradioactive B_{12}. If the intramuscular dose of vitamin B_{12} is not given, the radioactive vitamin B_{12} will be found in the liver.

Clinical Alert
1. No laxatives are to be used during the test.
2. Bone marrow aspiration should be done before the Schilling test, since the vitamin B_{12} administered in the test will destroy the diagnostic characteristics of the bone marrow.

Total Blood Volume Determination; Plasma Volume; Red Cell Volume

Normal Values
Total blood volume: 55–80 ml./kg.
Chromium-51 red cell volume: 20–35 ml./kg. (greater in men than in women)
Plasma volume: 30–45 ml./kg.
Note: Since adipose tissue has a sparser blood supply than lean tissue, the patient's body type can affect the proportion of blood volume to body weight, which is why test findings should always be reported. in ml./kg.

Explanation of Test
The purpose of this test is to determine circulating blood volume, to help evaluate the bleeding or debilitated patient, and to determine the origin of hypotension in the presence of anuria or oliguria when dehydration may be the cause. This determination is one way to monitor blood loss during surgery; it is used as a guide in replacement therapy following blood or body fluid loss and in the determination of whole body hematocrit. The results are useful in determining the most appropriate blood component for replacement therapy (*e.g.,* whole blood, plasma, or packed red cells).

Total blood volume determinations are of value in the following situations:

1. To evaluate gastrointestinal and uterine bleeding
2. To aid in the diagnosis of hypovolemic shock
3. To aid in the diagnosis of polycythemia vera
4. To determine the required blood component for replacement therapy as in persons undergoing open heart surgery

These tests will reveal a decreased blood or plasma volume and decreased total red cell mass. A sample of the patient's blood is mixed with a radioactive substance, incubated at room temperature, and reinjected. Another blood sample is obtained 15 minutes later. The most commonly used tracers in blood volume determination are serum albumin tagged with ^{131}I or ^{125}I and patient or donor RBCs tagged with ^{51}Cr. The combination of procedures or total blood volume is the only true blood volume. Other volume studies are plasma volume and ^{51}Cr red cell volume.

Plasma volume may be done separately and is the most commonly requested and performed blood volume. It is used to establish a vascular baseline, to determine changes in plasma volume pre- and post-surgically, and to evaluate fluid and blood replacement in gastrointestinal bleeding, burn, and trauma cases.

Chromium-51 red cell volume study is done to see what percentage of the circulating blood is composed of red cells. This procedure is performed only in connection with red cell survival, gastrointestinal blood loss, or ferrokinetic studies.

Procedure
1. Record the patient's height and current weight.
2. Venous blood samples are obtained and one sample is mixed with a radionuclide.
3. Fifteen to 30 minutes later, the blood is reinjected.
4. About 15 minutes later, another venous blood sample is obtained.

Clinical Implications
1. A normal total blood volume with a decreased red cell content indicates the need for a transfusion of packed red cells.
2. Polycythemia vera may be differentiated from secondary polycythemia.
   (a) Increased total blood volume, plasma volume, and red cell mass suggest polycythemia vera.
   (b) Normal or decreased total blood volume and plasma volume suggest secondary polycythemia.

Clinical Alert

If intravenous therapy is ordered for the same day, the blood volume determination should be done before the IV is started.

Patient Preparation
1. Explain the purpose and procedure of the test.
2. The patient should be weighed just before the test if possible.

Red Blood Cell (RBC) Survival Time Test

Normal Values
Normal half-time ^{51}Cr red blood cell survival is approximately 28 days. However, a normal value is determined by the nuclear medicine physician/radiologist. In the body, RBCs live about 100–120 days. Radioactivity: Half the radioactivity of plasma disappears in 1 to 2 hours.
Chromium-51 in stool: <3 ml./24 hr.

Explanation of Test
This blood test has its greatest use in the evaluation of known or suspected hemolytic anemia and is also indicated when there seems to be an obscure cause for anemia, to identify accessory spleens, and to determine abnormal red cell production and destruction. A sample of the patient's RBCs is mixed with a radioactive substance (^{51}Cr), incubated at room temperature, and reinjected. Blood specimens are drawn at the end of a 24-hour period and at regular intervals for at least 3 weeks. After counting, the results are plotted and the red cell survival time calculated. Results are based on the fact that disappearance of radioactivity from the circulation corresponds to the disappearance of the RBCs, thereby determining overall erythrocyte survival.

Scanning of the spleen is often done as part of this test. RBC survival is usually ordered in conjunction with blood volume determination and radionuclide iron uptake and clearance tests. When stool specimens are collected for three days, the test is often referred to as the GI blood loss test, which is different from the study on page 562.

Procedure
1. A venous blood sample of 20 ml. is obtained.
2. Ten to 30 minutes later, the blood is reinjected after being tagged with a radioisotope, ^{51}Cr.
3. Blood samples are usually obtained the first day, again at 24, 48, 72 and 96 hours, then at weekly intervals for 3 weeks. Time may be shortened depending on the outcome of the test. As part of this procedure, a radioactive detector may be used over the spleen, sternum, and liver to assess the relative concentration of radioactivity in these areas. This external counting helps to determine if the spleen is taking part in excessive sequestration of red blood cells as a causative factor in anemia.
4. In some instances, a 72-hour stool collection may be ordered to detect gastrointestinal blood loss. At the end of each 24-hour collection period, the total stool is to be collected by the department of nuclear medicine. This test can be completed in 3 days.

Clinical Implications
1. Shortened red cell survival may be the result of blood loss, hemolysis, and removal of RBCs by the spleen, as in
   (a) Chronic lymphatic leukemia
   (b) Congenital nonspherocytic hemolytic anemia
   (c) Hemoglobin C disease ·
   (d) Hereditary spherocytosis
   (e) Idiopathic acquired hemolytic anemia
   (f) Paroxysmal nocturnal hemoglobinuria
   (g) Elliptocytosis
   (h) Pernicious anemia
   (i) Megaloblastic anemia of pregnancy
   (j) Sickle cell anemia
   (k) Sickle cell hemoglobin C disease
   (l) Uremia
2. Prolonged red cell survival time may be the result of abnormality of red cell production as in thalassemia minor.
3. If hemolytic anemia is diagnosed, further studies are needed to establish whether RBCs have intrinsic abnormalities or whether anemia results from immunologic effects of the patient's plasma.
4. Results will be normal in
   (a) Hemoglobin C trait
   (b) Sickle cell trait
   (c) Elliptocytosis without hemolysis or anemia
5. Half of the radioactivity of plasma may not disappear for 7 to 8 hours.

Patient Preparation
1. Explain the purpose and procedure of the test. Emphasize that this test requires a minimum of 2 weeks of the patient's time with trips to the diagnostic facility for venipunctures.
2. If stool collection is required, advise the patient of the importance of saving all stool and that stool be free of urine contamination.

Clinical Alert
1. The test is usually contraindicated in an actively bleeding patient.
2. Record and report signs of active bleeding.
3. Transfusions should not be given when the test is in progress. If it is necessary to do so, notify the nuclear medicine department to terminate the test.

Radioactive Iodine (RAI); ¹³¹I Uptake Test

Normal Values

1%–13% absorbed by thyroid gland after 2 hr. ⎫
2%–25% absorbed by thyroid gland after 6 hr. ⎬ laboratory-
15%–45% absorbed by thyroid gland after 24 hr. ⎭ dependent

Explanation of Test

This direct test of the function of the thyroid gland measures ability of the gland to concentrate and retain iodine. When radioactive iodine is administered, it is rapidly absorbed into the bloodstream. This procedure measures the rate of accumulation, incorporation, and release of iodine by the thyroid. The rate of absorption of the radioactive iodine (which is determined by an increase in radioactivity of the thyroid gland) is a measure of the ability of the thyroid gland to concentrate iodide from the blood plasma.

This procedure is indicated in the evaluation of hypothyroidism, hyperthyroidism, thyroiditis, goiter, pituitary failure, and post-treatment evaluation. The patient who is a candidate for this test may have a lumpy or swollen neck or complain of pain in the neck, be jittery and ultrasensitive to heat, or may be sluggish and ultrasensitive to cold. The test is more useful in the diagnosis of hyperthyroidism than in hypothyroidism.

Procedure

Note: The test is usually done in conjunction with a thyroid scan.
1. A fasting state is preferred. A good history and listing of all medications is a must for this test.
2. A tasteless capsule of radioiodine or a lipid is administered orally. However, it can be administered intravenously if a quick test is desired. The patient is usually instructed not to eat for 1 hour after isotope administration.
3. Two, 6 and 24 hours later, the amount of radioactivity is measured by a scan of the radioactivity in the thyroid gland. There is no pain or discomfort involved.
4. The patient will have to return to the laboratory at the designated time, for the exact time of measurement is crucial in determining uptake.

Clinical Alert

1. This test is contraindicated in pregnant or lactating women, in children, and in infants.

2. Whenever possible, this test should be performed before any other radionuclide procedures are done, before any iodine medications are given, and before any radiographs using iodine contrast medium are done.

Clinical Implications

1. Increased uptake (*e.g.*, 20% in 1 hr., 25% in 6 hr., 50% in 24 hr.) suggests hyperthyroidism.
2. Decreased uptake (*e.g.*, 0% in 2 hr., 7% in 6 hr., 15% in 24 hr.) may be caused by hypothyroidism, but it is not diagnostic for it.
   (a) If the administered iodine is not absorbed, as in severe diarrhea or intestinal malabsorption syndromes, the uptake may be low even though the gland is functioning normally.
   (b) Rapid diuresis during the test period may deplete the supply of iodine, causing an apparently low percentage of iodine uptake.
   (c) In renal failure the uptake may be high, even though the gland is functioning normally.

Interfering Factors

1. The chemicals, drugs, and foods that interfere with the test by *lowering uptake* are
   (a) Iodized foods and iodine-containing drugs such as Lugol's solution, expectorants (SSKI), saturated solutions of potassium iodide, and vitamin preparations that contain minerals (1–3 weeks' duration time for the effect of these substances in the body)
   (b) Radiographic contrast media such as Diodrast (iodopyracet), Hypaque (sodium diatrizoate), Renografin, Lipiodal, Ethiodol, Pantopaque (isophendylate), Telepaque (iopanoic acid). One week to a year or more duration. Consult with nuclear medicine laboratory for specific times.
   (c) Antithyroid drugs such as propylthiouracil and related compounds (2–10 days' duration)
   (d) Thyroid medications such as desiccated thyroid, thyroxine (1–2 weeks' duration)
   (e) Miscellaneous drugs—thiocyanate, perchlorate, nitrates, sulfonamides, orinase, corticosteroids, PAS, isoniazid, Butazolidin (phenylbutazone), Pentothal (thiopental), antihistamines, ACTH, aminosalicylic acid, amphenone, cobalt, coumarin anticoagulants. Consult the diagnostic department for duration times, which may vary.

2. The compounds and conditions that interfere by *enhancing uptake* are

(a) TSH
(b) Estrogens
(c) Cirrhosis
(d) Barbiturates
(e) Lithium carbonate
(f) Phenothiazines (1 week)

Patient Preparation

1. Explain the purpose and procedures of the test, which takes 24 hours to complete.
2. Advise that iodine intake is restricted for at least 1 week before testing.

^{131}I Thyroid Stimulation Test; Thyroid-Stimulating Hormone (TSH) Test

Normal Values

TSH: less than 5 μU./ml.
In normal persons, TSH, T_4 and RAI uptake is increased within 8 to 10 hours after TSH is given.

Explanation of Test

This test measures the response of the thyroid gland to an injection of thyrotropin-releasing hormone, which should activate the release of TSH. This examination is used in conjunction with the RAI uptake test. It is done to differentiate primary from secondary hypothyroidism, to determine the level of thyroid gland activity, especially borderline thyroid function, and to evaluate thyroid hormone therapy. It is indicated in the evaluation of hypopituitarism and to demonstrate the presence of normal suppressed thyroid tissue in persons with autonomous hyperfunctioning nodules. The thyroid gland may have impaired RAI uptake because of intrinsic disease (primary hypothyroidism) or insufficient stimulation by the pituitary gland (secondary hypothyroidism). Patients who have a decreased amount of functioning thyroid gland, as in subtotal thyroidectomy radiation therapy or thyroiditis, may have a normal RAI uptake and still fail to respond to TSH stimulation. Such persons have a low thyroid reserve and need continued observation to prevent myxedema.

Procedure

1. *Day 1*: patient receives 10 units TSH intramuscularly.
2. *Day 2*: background counts over thyroid are taken and 10 more units TSH administered (IM). Radioactive iodine^{123} is also given at this time.
3. Patient returns in 2–6 hours for uptake.
4. *Day 3*: 24-hour thyroid uptake and thyroid scan performed.

> **Clinical Alert**
>
> TSH should be administered by a physician because the patient may have a reaction to this hormone.

Clinical Implications
1. No response to TSH is seen in the following conditions:
   (a) Primary untreated hypothyroidism (increase ranges from three times normal to 100 times normal in severe myxedema)
   (b) Hashimoto's thyroiditis
2. TSH positive response is seen in the following conditions (secondary hypothyroidism):
   (a) Hypothalamic hypothyroidism
   (b) Pituitary hypothyroidism

Interfering Factors
Iodine intake will invalidate ^{131}I uptake results.

Patient Preparation
1. Explain the purpose and procedure of the test, which takes several days to complete. Check with the appropriate department for the protocols to be used.
2. Advise that iodine intake is restricted for at least 1 week before testing.
3. Inform the patient that TSH is given intramuscularly.

^{131}I Perchlorate Suppression Study/Iodide Washout Test

Normal Values
In normal persons, the uptake of radioactive iodine will not change appreciably following the administration of perchlorate.

Explanation of Test
The perchlorate test is used to evaluate patients with suspected Hashimoto's disease or to demonstrate an enzyme deficiency within the thyroid gland. The procedure is used to identify defects in the iodide organifaction process within the thyroid. This study is based on the fact that potassium perchlorate competes with and displaces the iodide ions that are not organified. Perchlorate also stops the further trapping of iodide at the time of administration. Iodine is concentrated within the thyroid gland, is quickly bound to the protein thyroglobulin, and

normally becomes organified. The administration of perchlorate will stop any further trapping of iodide as well as the release of any unbound iodide within the thyroid gland, thus stopping the normal process. When iodine is trapped within the gland, it becomes bound to thyroxine, and the perchlorate will not remove the iodine from the gland. In the case of a patient with enzyme deficiency, the perchlorate will remove any unbound iodide from the gland as well as prevent further trapping. Patients with an enzyme deficiency will show a drop in their uptake greater than 15% after the administration of perchlorate.

Procedure
1. A complete patient history is taken.
2. Body background is measured for residual radiation by imaging.
3. A small tracer dose of radioactive iodine is administered orally.
4. An uptake is performed at 1 and 2 hours after administration.
5. After the 2-hour uptake is performed, the patient is given 400 mg. to 1 g. of potassium perchlorate orally.
6. Uptakes are performed every 15 minutes for the first hour post-dose perchlorate and then 30 minutes thereafter for the next 2 to 3 hours.
7. Uptakes performed after the administration of perchlorate are compared to the 2-hour uptake before perchlorate.
8. The results are recorded on linear graph paper as counts over the thyroid versus time in minutes of the uptake.

Clinical Implications
Abnormal results reveal
1. Enzyme deficiency within a thyroid gland
2. Hashimoto's disease

Note: Both disease processes will interfere with the organification process.

Patient Preparation
1. Explain the purpose and procedure of the test.
2. The patient should be fasting for this procedure.
3. Advise that no form of iodine should be ingested for at least 1 week before testing; this includes medications, foods, and contrasts used in radiographs.

^{131}I Thyroid Cytomel Suppression Test

Normal Values
Euthyroid patients with normal thyroid uptakes can expect a depression of the second uptake of at least 50% following Cytomel.

Explanation of Test
This test measures the response of the thyroid metabolic system to the administration of oral triiodothyronine. The uptake of iodine by a normal thyroid gland will decrease following the administration of oral triiodothyronine.

A patient who has a high initial uptake due to iodine deficiency or a dyshormonogenesis condition, or who is recovering from a subacute thyroiditis, will have a sharp decline, usually about one-half the baseline value, after the administration of Cytomel. Some patients will not be suppressed by the administration of Cytomel. In most instances, those patients will be hyperthyroid due to a toxic goiter (Graves' disease), a toxic multinodular goiter, or a toxic autonomously functioning thyroid adenoma. In some instances, a nonhypothyroid patient will not suppress after administration of Cytomel. An example would be a person with euthyroid Graves' disease.

Procedure
1. A careful patient history must be taken before the administration of Cytomel.
2. If the physician agrees that the Cytomel will not have an adverse effect, the patient is started on 75 g. to 100 g. per day for a period of 5 to 10 days (25 μg. every 8 hours for 5 days).
3. The patient must return to the nuclear medicine department 1 day before the last dose of Cytomel is taken.
4. On that day, a body background is taken for residual radioactive iodine from the previous uptake and recorded.
5. A new tracer dose of radioactive iodine is given and amount, date, and time are recorded.
6. The patient returns after the last dose of Cytomel is taken, and an uptake is performed (2- and 6-hour uptakes are usual after I^{123} is used).

Clinical Implications
1. The euthyroid patient who is iodine deficient will normally have a high uptake initially and a decreased second uptake following the administration of Cytomel.
2. A patient with a hyperthyroid condition demonstrating a high initial uptake will show no appreciable change on the second uptake following the administration of Cytomel.
3. Other abnormal findings
   (a) TSH-dependent tissue will be suppressed.
   (b) Autonomous nodules will not be suppressed.
   (c) Patients with thyroid cancer may or may not be suppressed.
   (d) Destroyed thyroid tissue due to therapy or disease will remain unchanged.

(e) A scan of the thyroid performed before and after the administration of Cytomel will demonstrate an autonomous nodule or tissue since it is unaffected by TSH.

Patient Preparation
1. Explain the purpose and procedure of the test, including the time involved and the proper administration of Cytomel.
2. Advise the patient not to consume any products containing iodine or take any medication that would affect this study.

Iron-59 Ferrokinetic Studies (Iron Utilization)

Normal Values
Red cell volume: based on patient's height and weight
Plasma iron disappearance rate: Normal patients with adequate iron reserves will show a clearance rate of 1 to 2 hours.
Red cell iron uptake: 85% of dose in circulating RBCs within 10 days
Red cell sequestration: Liver–spleen precordium ratio is 1 : 1.

Explanation of Test
These studies are performed using radioactive iron-59 and chromium-51 to provide information about the hematological system such as red cell volume, sequestration of RBCs, iron uptake by RBCs, and disappearance rate from plasma. Indications for this procedure include investigation of anemia, suspected abnormalities in iron metabolism, suspected sequestration, and other disorders of the hematologic system.

Procedure
1. An intravenous line is established and remains for approximately 3 hours while many blood samples are obtained.
2. The radionuclide is injected intravenously. Blood samples are drawn at various times during a 2–2½ hour period and measured for radioactivity. Blood samples will also be obtained three times a week for the next 3 weeks.
3. Many areas of the patient's body will be identified with a permanent mark. Sequestration readings will be done by imaging over those areas.
4. These markings must not be removed until the entire procedure is completed.

Clinical Implications
1. The uptake of radioactive iron by RBCs is markedly decreased in
   (a) Hypoplastic anemia
   (b) Pernicious anemia
   (c) Myeloid metaplasia

2. The uptake of iron by the RBCs is increased in
   (a) Iron deficiency anemia   (c) Polycythemia vera
   (b) Hemolytic anemia   (d) Blood loss
3. Plasma clearance of radioactive iron is markedly decreased in
   (a) Hemolytic anemia
   (b) Iron deficiency anemia
   (c) Polycythemia vera
4. Plasma clearance of radioactive iron is increased in
   (a) Aplastic anemia
   (b) Hemachromatosis
   (c) Myelofibrosis

Patient Preparation
Explain the purpose and procedure of the test. Advise the patient that the test will require a minimum of 2 weeks to complete and that he must return to the testing facility several times to have blood examined and to have counts made of liver, spleen, and heart.

Part Three
Positron Emission Tomography (PET)

Normal Values
Normal patterns of tissue metabolism based on oxygen, glucose, and fatty acid utilization, protein synthesis, and blood volume and flow

Explanation of Test
Positron emission tomography (PET) is the combined use of positron emitting isotopes and emission-computerized axial tomography to measure regional tissue function (see page 523 for SPECT and PET). Like a CT scan, the PET scanner, which is shaped like a giant tire, does transverse imagery. The injected or inhaled radionuclide will emit radioactivity in the form of positrons that are identified and transformed into a visual display by a computer. The most commonly used positron-emitting radiolabels are oxygen 15 and fluorene 18-fluorodeoxyglucose.

PET studies are noninvasive tests used most commonly to determine physiological function of the brain and heart. However, the technique is applicable to the examination of all parts of the body for the diagnosis and staging of disease and monitoring therapy. Unlike MR and CT scans, PET can provide physiologic, anatomic, as well as biochemical data. At this time, PET's use is mainly in large medical centers with a large number of experimental studies being done.

Uses of PET
1. Blood flow
2. Tissue metabolism
3. Blood volume
4. Tissue density

Procedure for Brain Studies
1. An intravenous line will be inserted into both hands or arms—one is for injecting the radionuclide, the other is for drawing blood samples.
2. The patient will sit in a reclining couch next to the scanner. A radionuclide is injected intravenously into an arm vein. Scanning will begin 45 minutes later if the brain is to be examined. This is the period of time needed for the radioactive substances to concentrate the brain tissue.
3. If a mental activity such as speech or reading is to be checked, the patient will be asked to do letter recognition activities or read. Some reasoning or remembering functions will be determined by asking the patient to recite the Pledge of Allegiance to himself, to think of words beginning with a specific letter.
4. The patient will be blindfolded and ears plugged with cotton to remove stimuli.
5. The test takes 45 to 60 minutes to complete. At the present time, it takes 3 to 5 persons to operate the scanner and cyclotron for just one test.

Clinical Implications
Abnormal results are associated with several disorders

1. In epilepsy focal areas with increased metabolism have been seen during the actual stage of epilepsy, and decreased oxygen utilization and blood flow during the interictal stage. It is proving to be the best test for locating damaged brain tissues in persons with severe forms of epilepsy. In these cases it is possible to remove this tissue surgically with greater precision.
2. Profound striatal hypometabolism in Huntington's disease
3. In stroke, an extremely complex pathophysiological picture is being revealed: anaerobic glycolysis, depressed oxygen utilization, and decreased blood flow. In a CVA, if the patient cannot speak, the test can determine if part of the brain that controls speech is still viable.
4. In dementia the hypothesis of chronic cerebral anoxia has been refuted and instead is beginning to reveal focal disturbances of protein synthesis in this disease. PET is used to differentiate Alz-

heimer's disease and other types of dementia from depression in older persons.

5. In schizophrenia, some studies using labelled glucose indicate reduced metabolic activity in the frontal region. PET scans can also distinguish the developmental stages of cranial tumors and give information about operability of such tumors.

6. Heart: In coronary artery disease, during exercise-induced ischemia, focal disturbances of cation extraction occur in the myocardium. These changes persist beyond the time the ECG changes have reverted to normal and angina pain has ceased. PET can be used to monitor heartbeat and is one of the best ways to determine how much of the heart has been damaged.
   (a) Future use as a screening tool for coronary artery disease.
   (b) Study of the metabolic state of the heart to determine the rate at which fatty acids are used for energy (a crucial factor in the development of myopathies).
   (c) PET may provide more information than other modalities concerning the state and extent of myocardial infarctions.

7. Presence of chronic pulmonary edema. In pneumonia, it has been possible to measure uptake of C-labeled erythromycin. The concentration of antibiotic at the site of infection is related to minimum inhibitory concentration of the microorganisms.

8. In brain tumors, data have been collected concerning oxygen use and blood flow relationships for these tumors. Gliomas have relatively good perfusion in comparison to their decreased O_2 utilization. The high uptake of ^{18}FDG in gliomas is reported to correlate with the tumor's histological grade.

9. Breast tumors show a relatively high rate of vascularity.

Interfering Factors
1. Excessive anxiety can ruin test results when brain function is being tested.

Clinical Considerations
1. Diabetics should take final pretest dose of long-acting insulin prior to eating a meal 3–4 hours before testing. After that time, no insulin or any other drug that alters glucose metabolism should be taken.
2. Tranquilizers cannot be given before the test because they alter glucose metabolism.
3. Thorough preparation for the testing experience will make the difference between a successful or unsuccessful outcome and production of usable results.

Patient Preparation
1. Advise the patient to abstain from alcohol, caffeine, and tobacco for 24 hours.

2. Explain the purpose, procedure, benefits, and risks of the test. The level of radiation is short-lived and approximate to that from 5 to 6 radiographs of the chest and less than a quarter of the radiation absorbed during a CT scan of the brain. Repeat or sequential studies can be carried out over short periods of minutes to hours.
3. Advise the patient that lying as still as possible during the scan is necessary. However, the patient is not to fall asleep or count to pass the time.
4. Use measures to reduce anxiety and help the patient manage stress, such as progressive relaxation and breathing techniques.

Patient After Care

1. The patient is cautioned not to stand up too quickly after the test is completed to prevent postural hypertension.
2. Advise that urination should occur soon after the scan to clear the radiopharmaceutical from the bladder.

BIBLIOGRAPHY

Bauer JD: Clinical Laboratory Methods, 9th ed. St. Louis, CV Mosby, 1982

Baum S, et al. (eds.): Atlas of Nuclear Medicine Imaging. New York, Appleton-Century-Crofts, 1981

Berkow R (ed.): Merck Manual of Diagnosis and Therapy, 14th ed. Rahway, NJ, Merck Sharp & Dohme, 1982

Early PJ, Sodee DB: Principles and Practice of Nuclear Medicine. St. Louis, CV Mosby, 1985

Ell PJ, Holman BL: Computed Emission Tomography. Oxford, Oxford University Press, 1982

Fordham EW, et al. (eds): Atlas of Total Body Radionucleotide Imaging. Philadelphia, Harper & Row, 1982

French RM: Guide to Diagnostic Procedures, 5th ed. New York, McGraw-Hill, 1980

Honigman RE: Thyroid function tests. Nursing 12(4):68–71, 1982

Pantaleo N et al.: Thallium myocardial scintography and its use in the assessment of coronary artery disease. Heart and Lung 10(1):61–71, 1981

Ravel R: Clinical Laboratory Medicine, 4th ed. Chicago, Year Book Medical Pub, 1984

Rocha AR, Harbert JC: Textbook of Nuclear Medicine and Clinical Applications. Philadelphia, Lea & Febiger, 1979

Thorell JI, Larson SM: Radioimmunoassay and Related Techniques: Methodology and Clinical Applications. St. Louis, CV Mosby, 1978

Wallach J: Interpretation of Diagnostic Tests: A Handbook Synopsis of Laboratory Medicine, 4th ed. Boston, Little, Brown & Co., 1986

Vinocur B: PET asserts itself in heart, brain imaging. Diagn Imaging, p 68–72, October, 1984

COMMON X-RAY STUDIES

10

Introduction

General Principles

X-ray studies (also known as *radiographs* or *roentgenograms*) are used to examine the soft and bony tissues of the body. X-rays (roentgen rays) are electromagnetic vibrations of very short wavelength produced when fast-moving electrons hit various substances. They are similar to light rays except that their wavelength is only 1/10,000 the length of visible light rays. Because of their short wavelength, x-rays have the ability to penetrate very dense substances and to produce an image or shadow that can be recorded on photographic film. The entire principle of radiography depends on differences in density between various body structures, which produce shadows of varying intensity on the x-ray film.

In x-ray examinations, a high-voltage electric current is passed through a "target" made of tungsten in a vacuum tube. Less than 1% of the high-speed electrons (cathode rays) are transformed into x-rays; the rest of the energy is transformed into heat.

X-rays travel in straight lines at the speed of light. When a beam of rays passes through matter, its intensity is reduced by absorption. The greater the density of matter, the greater the degree of absorption. A photographic film is affected by x-rays, just as it is affected by light. The sensitive silver emulsion of the film undergoes a chemical change when it has been exposed to radiation. The film is subsequently processed by development and fixation, resulting in an image that is black, white, and various tones of gray. This image will be an accurate representation of the variable densities of the tissue through which the beam has passed. Third generation x-ray equipment uses high resolution techniques, TV screens, digital magnetic records, and laser driven printers that produce much sharper pictures of bones and organs.

Use of Contrast Media

Many radiographic techniques can use the natural contrasts that exist in body tissue—air, water (in soft tissue), fat, and bone. The lungs and gastrointestinal tract normally contain gases; certain body structures are encased in a fatty envelope, and bone has naturally occurring mineral salts. However, diagnosis of certain pathologic conditions at times requires the visualization of details not revealed through plain film radiography. These details can be highlighted through administration of *contrast media*, which can be inserted orally, rectally, or through injection.

The ideal contrast medium should be harmless, inert, and should not interfere with any physiologic function. It may be either radiopaque (not permitting the transmission of x-rays) or radiolucent (permitting the transmission of x-rays but still offering some resistance). However, there is really no safe contrast media; any foreign material put into the body can cause reactions.

Certain contrast media are used routinely in radiographic studies.

1. Barium sulfate (radiopaque)
   (a) Used in gastrointestinal studies
   (b) Prepared in a colloidal suspension
   (c) Effectively demonstrates small filling defects
2. Organic iodides (radiopaque)
   (a) Examples: sodium diatrizoate, meglumine diatrizoate, metrizamide and the new, "nonionic" agents
   (b) Used for studies of the kidney, liver, blood vessels, urinary bladder, and urethra
   (c) Water-soluble iodide used in myelography (study of the spinal cord after contrast media have been injected)
3. Iodized oils (radiopaque)
   Used in myelography, bronchography (study of the lung after contrast media have been injected), and lymphangiograms
4. Oxygen, helium, air, carbon dioxide, nitrous oxide, and nitrogen (radiolucent substances)
   Used for visualization of the brain, joints, subarachnoid space, pleural space, peritoneal cavity, and pericardial space

Adverse Reactions to Contrast Media
The administration of contrast media can sometimes cause allergic reactions in certain persons. The degree of reaction may range from mild (causing such symptoms as nausea and vomiting) to severe (causing cardiovascular collapse, CNS depression, and death, if untreated).

Table 10-1 indicates the range of possible adverse reactions to iodine contrast media.

Clinical Considerations When Iodine Contrast Media Is Used
1. The highest incidence of side-effects occurs in patients 20 to 49 years of age; the lowest incidence, after 70 years of age.
2. The patient who has had an allergic reaction to iodine contrast media should have this fact noted on his medical records. Such a patient possibly can have subsequent adverse reactions; the risk rises 3 to 4 times, although the second reaction is not necessarily more severe. The patient should also be told that he has had an allergic response to a specific substance.
3. Check to see when the patient last had a full meal before sending him to the x-ray department. Except in an extreme emergency, iodine contrast media should never be administered intravenously sooner than 90 minutes after eating. In most instances, the patient

Table 10-1

Signs and Symptoms of Reactions to Iodinated Contrast Media

Type	Cardiovascular	Respiratory	Cutaneous	Gastrointestinal	Nervous	Urinary
Mild	Pallor Diaphoresis Tachycardia	Sneezing Coughing Rhinorrhea	Erythema Feeling of warmth	Nausea Vomiting Metallic taste	Anxiety Headache Dizziness	
Intermediate	Bradycardia Palpitations Hypotension	Wheezing Acute asthma attack	Urticaria Pruritus	Abdominal cramps Diarrhea	Agitation Vertigo Slurred speech	Oliguria
Severe	Acute-pulmonary edema Shock Congestive heart failure Cardiac arrest	Laryngospasm Cyanosis Laryngeal edema Apnea	Angioneurotic edema	Paralytic ileus	Disorientation Stupor Coma Convulsions	Acute renal failure

(Daffner RH: Introduction to Clinical Radiology: A Correlative Approach to Diagnostic Imaging. St. Louis, CV Mosby, 1978)

should be NPO the night before any radiographic testing employing iodine contrast media.

4. Be aware that death from an allergic reaction can occur if severe symptoms go untreated. Staff in attendance must be able to give cardiopulmonary resuscitation.

5. Promptly administer oral antihistamines per the physician's order if mild to moderate reactions to iodine contrast substances occur.

6. When coordinating x-ray testing that uses contrast media, keep in mind that iodine and barium do not mix.

7. Some physiologic change can be expected whenever an iodine contrast substance is injected, as in an intravenous pyelogram (IVP). The types of changes that can be seen are hypotension, hypertension, tachycardia, or arrhythmias. For this reason, always check the blood pressure, pulse, and respiration before and following these tests.

8. Instruct patients that large amounts of fluids should be taken to promote frequent urination to flush the iodine from the body.

9. Assess for these additional contraindications to iodinated contrast
   (a) Patients with sickle cell anemia—use may increase sickling effect
   (b) Patients with syphilis—use may lead to nephrotic syndrome
   (c) Patients in long-term steroid therapy—some of drug may be rendered inactive by contrast
   (d) Patients with pheochromocytoma—use may produce a sudden, perhaps fatal, rise in blood pressure
   (e) Patients with hyperthyroidism

Clinical Alert

1. Prevent the need for repeat examination through careful preparation. Because any diagnostic radiogram has some risk, there is a great responsibility to monitor and guide patients carefully. This responsibility is amplified when examinations using contrast media are employed.

2. Risks are involved in repeated x-ray testing and use of contrast media. There is really no safe contrast medium; any foreign material put into the body can cause reactions. For example, in cancer diagnosis, the benefit of early detection outweighs the dangers of cumulative radiation. In a person undergoing a work-up for cancer, the risks of x-ray testing should be deemphasized to help reduce anxiety that can be overwhelming in these persons. However, the facts about risk must be given because the patient has a legal right to this information.

Clinical Considerations When Barium Contrast Is Used

There is always a danger when introducing barium sulfate or similar contrast media into the gastrointestinal tract.

1. Barium radiography may interfere with many other abdominal examinations. There are a number of studies including other x-rays; tests using iodine, ultrasound procedures, radioisotope studies, tomograms, computerized scanning, and proctoscopy which must be scheduled prior to barium studies. Consult with the x-ray department for the best sequencing of barium studies with other ordered examinations.
2. Emphasize that a laxative should be taken after a procedure is completed if barium sulfate is used during the examination.
3. Elderly, inactive persons should be checked for impaction. The first sign of impaction in the elderly may be fainting.
4. Observe and record stools for color and consistency to determine that the barium has been evacuated. Stools should be checked for at least 2 days. Stools will be light in color until all barium has been expelled. Outpatients should be given a written reminder to inspect stools for two days.
5. Avoid giving narcotics, especially codeine, when barium x-rays are ordered because there is a tendency for these drugs to interfere with the elimination of barium from the gastrointestinal tract.
6. Be prepared for complications. Barium may aggravate acute ulcerative colitis or cause an obstruction in the bowel, ranging from partial to complete obstruction.
7. Barium should *not* be used as a contrast for intestinal study when a bowel perforation is suspected. Leakage of barium through a perforation may cause peritonitis. Iodinated contrasts should be used when perforations are suspected.

There are special clinical considerations for ostomy patients undergoing bowel preparation for contrast x-ray testing of the GI tract (barium enema, colon x-ray, upper GI series, and gallbladder study/oral cholecystogram).

1. A successful outcome depends upon communications of specific, objective information that differs from the standardized information usually given by a radiology department.
2. In most cases the standard dietary restrictions and medications will apply, but modifications are made in procedures involving mechanical bowel cleansing with enemas, and physiologic cleansing with laxatives.

Clinical Alerts for Patients with Ostomies

1. An enema and laxatives should never be given to a person with an ileostomy in preparation for x-ray filming or endoscopy. Administering an enema would put the person with an ileostomy at risk for dehydration and electrolyte imbalance. However, a person with a sigmoid colostomy needs an enema for x-ray or endoscopy. For this reason, it is very important to identify the type of stoma the patient has because not all colostomies need irrigation. For example, a person with an ascending right-sided colostomy will normally pass a liquid, pasty stool, high in H_2O content, and digestive enzymes; such a patient may have laxatives, and no enema.
2. Notify the radiology staff that the person has an ostomy, so that department can be prepared.
3. Advise patients, both hospitalized and outpatient, to have extra pouches with them during tests, especially if the pouch needs to be removed for the procedure.

See page 607 for specifics of barium enema preparation for ostomies, ileostomies, and colostomies.

Xeroradiography: Overview

Xeroradiography differs from traditional x-ray examinations in that the image is created on a photoconductive surface of selenium rather than on a silver halide film. The selenium plate is housed in a cassette to protect it from rough handling and from light.

Xeroradiography is a photoelectric process; traditional film radiography is primarily a photochemical process. This relatively new technique uses the technology of the office copier to process x-ray images on paper.

Several distinct advantages exist in the use of this method: it offers a very high degree of resolution; small point densities can be easily distinguished because of greater contrast, and the xeroradiographs are easily interpreted.

Xeroradiography has been found useful in radiography of the extremities and especially in soft-tissue studies. Radiographic study of the breast is the prime use of this technique. Patient exposure during a xeromammogram is less than 1 radiation absorbed dose (rad).

Computed Tomography (CT): Overview

Computed tomography (CT), also called CT scanning and computerized axial tomography (CAT), uses x-rays similar to those used in conventional radiography but with a special machine having a scanner system. The x-rays in conventional radiography pass through the body, and an image of bone, soft tissues, and air is projected onto film. In CT scans, a computer provides rapid complex calculations determining the degree of multiple x-ray beams that are not absorbed by all the tissue in its path. The single most valuable function of CT scanning is to provide the geography and characteristics of tissue structures within solid organs. Because it is basically an anatomical technique, which measures the attenuation coefficient of tissue, it is not useful for measurement of tissue perfusion, metabolism, or vessel blood flow. For this reason, it is not the best technique to evaluate small atrioventricular (AV) malformation, early ischemic disease of the brain, or subdural hematomas.

Digital Radiography and Fluorography: Overview

Digital radiography is very similar to CT in that it is a computer-based imaging modality with exceptionally high spatial resolution. An ordinary x-ray beam contains far more information about body structure and physiology than it is possible to record in x-ray film, and some information is lost. The lost information includes the compression of three dimensional data to two dimensions, some decrease in spatial resolution, a reduction in ability to visualize soft tissue, organs, and vascular structures, and the inability to obtain accurate information about blood flow, volume, and ejection fractions. This information is regained to a great extent by digital radiography. At the present time, there are several variations in commercial systems for digital video-angiography, which accounts for the variety of terms used to describe the technique. This system incorporates image-processing technology originally intended for high-altitude military systems. The main use for this technique is to obtain images of the carotid arteries leading to the brain. To obtain this information, a standard x-ray picture of an area is taken, with all the bone and tissue obscuring the view. About 40 to 60 ml. of iodine dye is then injected intravenously into the femoral or antecubital area, and another picture is taken. A computer then processes the two pictures, superimposing a reversed image over the other. Specially designed electronics convert the x-ray image into digital form. These images can be acquired at rates up to 30 frames per second. The images can then be displayed or enhanced. The result is a view of the arteries highlighted by dye, with almost everything else blocked out. In addition, the electronics of this technology allow the instant recall of radiological images for review.

Digital subtraction images (DSA) are produced in this way: basically, a fluoroscopic image is converted from analog to digital form; the image is stored digitally as a matrix, with a varying number of picture elements (pixels); after each image is converted to digital form, the first image or mask is subtracted from the object image, pixel by pixel. As in computed tomography, the number of pixels into which the image is divided influences the quality of the image, the complexity of the computer needed, and the speed at which images can be processed.

Limitations
1. The patient risk is about the same as that of a conventional intravenous urography (IVU) examination.
2. For examination of the abdomen and lower extremities, inadequate field size necessitates multiple iodine injections.
3. This procedure is not for everyone. It is well suited for many persons in the 40 to 65 age group. It is not appropriate for the extremely sick or for those with preinfarction angina.

Advantages
1. 120 ml. required by standard angiography is reduced to 30 ml. This reduces the risks of contrast toxicity and injury to the blood vessels.
2. Contrast can be infused through a smaller catheter, a No. 5 French rather than a No. 8. The likelihood of complications following the procedure is less and enables the procedure to be done on an outpatient basis in many cases.
3. Improved recording—digital system records on disks for less than one minute.
4. Computer measurements of percentage of blocking can be made.
5. High-quality, computer-enhanced images filtered in real time can be instantly replayed on a TV monitor. This information can be taped and stored on standard video cassettes.
6. Can enhance standard arteriograms. For example, using this technique, the small blood vessels are hard to visualize with a standard arteriogram. In addition, selective studies can be performed with a much smaller amount of contrast.

Magnetic Resonance Imaging, MR, NMR: Overview
Magnetic resonance (MR), formerly called nuclear magnetic resonance (NMR), is a new noninvasive, nonionic technique that produces cross-sectional images of the human anatomy obtained by exposure to magnetic energy sources, but without using radiation. A description is given in this chapter because, although it is not an x-ray method, it is a diagnostic service offered by many x-ray departments in larger medical centers. This versatile device is used primarily in three diagnostic areas: to study blood flow and determine the condition of blood vessels; for *in vivo* spectroscopy to infer tissue *p*H and energy state; and in whole body imaging to detect tumors, sites of infection, and differentiation of diseased tissues from healthy tissues. MR machines are essentially large magnets fitted with a group of field control coils. Atomic nuclei, when placed in a magnetic field and stimulated by a particular radio frequency, emit measurable radio signals that are influenced by

the type and condition of tissue composed of these nuclei. These radio signals are detected and are converted to a visual display on a computer monitor or etched on magnetic tape for later playback on a video screen.

Angiography: Overview

Angiography is a method of using x-ray examinations to study the vascular structures of the body. This method involves the injection of an organic cc. trast solution (such as iodine) by a catheter inserted into the femoral artery (the usual site, but the brachial artery is also used). The catheter is placed selectively into the artery under fluoroscope control by the radiologist performing the examination. After satisfactory x-ray films have been obtained, the catheter is removed and direct pressure is held on the puncture site until bleeding is controlled. The patient is usually instructed to remain at complete bedrest for approximately 6 hours.

The terms given to the variety of studies performed are based on the vascular structure to be studied and the method of injection. *Arteriography* refers to contrast studies of arterial vessels. Venous structures can also be seen in later stages of these examinations. *Venography* is a contrast study of peripheral or central veins. *Lymphography* is a contrast study of lymph vessels and nodes. *Angiocardiography* is an investigation of the interior of the heart using a contrast solution. During this examination the great vessels such as the pulmonary arteries can be seen. *Aortography* refers to a contrast study of either the thoracic aorta (*thoracic aortography*) or the abdominal aorta (*abdominal aortography*) and *lumbar aortography*.

Angiographic examinations may also be named by the route of injection. For example, *renal arteriography* is performed by inserting a catheter into the abdominal aorta and then into the renal artery. In *peripheral arteriography*, an injection may be made directly into the vessel under study, such as the femoral artery. The injection may also be done by the venous method. For example, in venous aortography, a large bolus of contrast medium is injected into a peripheral vein. As the contrast flows through the right side of the heart, lung, and left side of the heart, x-ray films are taken.

Indications for Angiography
1. Examination of cervical carotid arteries
2. Examination of intracranial arteries
3. Before transphenoidal hypophysectomy
4. Postoperative evaluation
5. Detection of superior sagittal sinus thrombosis
6. Identification of renal and iliac arteries in relation to an abdominal aortic aneurysm
7. Accurate screening examination for renovascular hypertension. In

this instance, the study can be performed before a routine IVP using the same dose of contrast material.

8. Periodic reevaluation of arterial angioplasty
9. Vascular integrity can be confirmed in traumatic lesions
10. Vascular grafts can be followed for patency

Interfering Factors

Very small lesions or abnormalities may be missed using this technique.

Orthopedic Radiography: Overview

Orthopedic x-ray testing is a general radiographic examination of a particular bone, group of bones, or a joint of the body. The bony or osseous system has five functions of radiologic significance. They are support of the body, locomotion, housing of red marrow, calcium storage, and protection of underlying vessical structures.

Most of the orthopedic x-ray examinations require the person to be sitting or recumbent and to remain motionless. Various devices may be used to immobilize the patient. In order to produce a thorough study of the body part, at least two projections are required, usually 90° to one another. For examination of more complex structures such as the spine and skull, multiple projections are required, thus increasing the length of time of the examination. Medical hardware used to stabilize the traumatized area can obscure the area of interest and may have to be removed. This is done only with the consent of the attending physician and possibly requires nursing staff assistance.

Abnormal results are indicated by the following pathology:

1. Fractures
2. Dislocations
3. Arthritis
4. Osteoporosis
5. Osteomyelitis
6. Degenerative joint disease
7. Hydrocephalus
8. Sarcoma
9. Aseptic necrosis
10. Paget's disease
11. Gout
12. Acromegaly
13. Metastases
14. Myeloma
15. *Osteochondrosis, i.e.,* Legg–Calvé–Perthes, Osgood–Schlatter
16. Bone infarcts
17. Histeocytosis X
18. Bone tumors (benign and malignant)

Clinical Alert

Orthopedic radiography generally does not provide information about associated soft tissue structures such as cartilage, tendons, or ligaments.

Risks of Radiation

Exposure of the human body to x-rays carries certain risks. These risks are of two types: genetic and somatic. If the genital organs are exposed to radiation, the reproductive cells (specifically, the DNA within the chromosomes) may undergo mutations. These mutations can cause changes in the offspring of the patient. Somatic changes (those occurring in body tissue other than the reproductive cells) may occur in parts of the patient's body receiving excessive doses of radiation or receiving repeated exposure.

The dangers of exposure to radiation arise not only from the absorption of relatively large amounts of radiation received over a short period of time but also from the cumulative effects of very small amounts received over months or years. Moreover, the cumulative effects of radiation may not become evident for several years. Radiation can increase the risk of cancer after a latent period of many years.

Table 10-2
Estimated Mean Dose to Uterus/Embryo From Common X-Rays and Scans

Beam Radiation*	Dose Equivalent (rem)
Skull	<0.01
Chest	<0.01
Upper GI series	0.048
Barium enema	0.822
Cholecystogram	<0.02
Intravenous pyelogram	0.814
Abdomen, KUB	0.263
Lumbosacral spine	0.639
Pelvis	0.194
Hip	0.128
Radionuclide Scans†	**Dose Equivalent (rem)**
Liver (4mCi Tc–99m)	0.028
Bone (20mCi Tc–99m)	0.500
Gallium (5mCi Ga–67)	1.250
Thyroid (5mCi Tc–99m)	0.135

* For the type of radiation used in hospitals, rads and rems are interchangeable. Radiation dose absorbed by the body is measured in rems or rads (mrem or nrad).

† After Kereiakes JG, Rosenstein M: Handbook of Radiation Doses in Nuclear Medicine and Diagnostic X-Ray, p 211. Boca Raton, FL, CRC Press, 1980, and Husak V, Wiedermann M: Radiation absorbed dose estimates to the embryo from some nuclear medicine procedures. Eur J Nucl Med 5(3):205–207, 1980

A woman in the first trimester of pregnancy especially is at risk. A developing embryo or fetus that is exposed to high levels of ionizing radiation is very likely to be born with abnormalities. See Tables 10-2, 10-3, and 10-4.

Safety Measures
Certain precautions must be taken to protect medical/nursing personnel, patients, and any technical staff assisting in the x-ray examination from unnecessary exposure to radiation.

General Precautions
1. Patients, radiologists, and other staff in the radiology laboratory should wear lead aprons and gloves.
2. The x-ray tube housing should be checked periodically to prevent leakage.
3. The patient's medical records should be carefully checked to determine the frequency of diagnostic radiologic examinations and the dosage received with each study.
4. X-ray tubes should have additional layers of aluminum to act as filtering devices that will reduce the exposure to radiation without sacrificing detail.
5. Fast film as well as a screen enhancing the action of x-rays should be used.
6. Adjustable or fixed cones as well as diaphragms can be used to reduce exposure to the lowest possible level. These devices will restrict the area being radiated, avoiding excessive peripheral exposure.
7. The gonads should be shielded on all patients capable of producing children unless the examination is of the abdomen or the gonad area.

Table 10-3
Estimated Genetic Effects of Radiation
per Million Liveborn Offspring*

Genetic Disorder	Incidence	Additional Effects of Exposure of 1 rem per 30-Year Generation	
		First Generation	Later Generations
Autosomal dominant and X-linked	10,000	5–65	40–200
Irregularly inherited	90,000	Very few	20–900
Recessive	1,000	Very few	Very slow increase
Chromosomal aberrations	6,000	<10	Slight increase

* After National Research Council Committee on the Biological Effects of Ionizing Radiation: The Effects on Populations of Exposure to Low Levels of Ionizing Radiation, p 85 (BEIRIII). Washington, DC, National Academy Press, 1980

Table 10-4
Understanding Radiation Risks; Gonad and Bone
Marrow Doses of Common X-Ray Procedures (Continued)

Gonad dose is estimated amount of radiation absorbed by the ovaries and testes. Exceeding this dose may have genetic effects. Bone marrow dose is estimated amount of radiation absorbed by bone marrow.

Relatively High Gonad Dose—Adult (over 100 mrad)	Moderate Gonad Dose—Adult (10–100 mrad)	Low Gonad Dose—Adult (less than 10 mrad)
Lumbar spine, lumbo-sacral vertebrae	Stomach and upper gastrointestinal tract	Head (including cervical spine)
Pelvis	Cholecystography, cholangiography	Dental (full mouth)
Hip and femur (upper third)	Femur (lower two-thirds)	Arm (including forearm and hand)
Urography		Bony thorax (ribs, sternum, clavicle, shoulder)
Retrograde pyelography		Dorsal spine
Urethrocystography		Lower leg, foot
Lower gastrointestinal tract		Chest (heart, lung) including mass miniature radiography)
Abdomen		
Obstetric abdomen		
Pelvimetry		
Hysterosalpingography		
Lumbar spine, lumbo-sacral vertebrae	Dorsal spine	Head (including cervical spine)
	Stomach and upper gastrointestinal tract	
Pelvis		Dental (full mouth)
Hip and femur (upper third)	Cholecystography, cholangiography	Arm (including forearm and hand)
Urography	Femur (lower two-thirds)	Bony thorax
Retrograde pyelography	Abdomen	Lower leg, foot
Urethrocystography		Chest (heart, lung) including mass miniature radiography
Lower gastrointestinal tract		

(Continued)

Table 10-4
Understanding Radiation Risks; Gonad and Bone
Marrow Doses of Common X-Ray Procedures (Continued)

Relatively High Bone-Marrow Dose— Adult (400–2000 mrad)	Moderate Bone-Marrow Dose— Adult (50–400 mrad)	Low Bone-Marrow Dose—Adult (less than 50 mrad)
Pelvimetry	Retrograde pyelography	Femur, hip
Lower gastrointestinal tract	Urethrocystography	Head, chest, heart, lung
Urography	Hysterosalpingography	Dental (full mouth)
	Stomach and upper gastrointestinal tract	Extremities (hand, foot)
	Lumbar or dorsal spine, lumbosacral	
	Pelvis, abdomen	
	Cholecystography, cholangiography	
	Bony thorax (ribs, sternum, clavicle, shoulder)	

Precautions to be Used With Pregnant Patients

1. Women of childbearing age who possibly could be in the first trimester of pregnancy should *not* have x-ray examinations. A brief menstrual history should be taken to determine if the woman is or could be pregnant. If any doubt exists about whether the woman is pregnant, she should *not* risk having the examination until a pregnancy test is done.
2. Pregnant patients (at any time during the pregnancy) should avoid radiographic studies of the pelvic region, lumbar spine, and abdomen, or procedures involving serial film or fluoroscopy.
3. If films are made for obstetric reasons, *repeat films* should be avoided.
4. If x-ray studies are made of body parts other than the pelvic area (*e.g.*, of the teeth), the woman should wear a lead apron to cover the abdominal and pelvic regions.

Responsibilities in Ordering and Scheduling X-Ray Examinations

All radiology requisitions should include the correct spelling of the patient's name, age, and diagnosis. The purpose and procedure of the x-ray examination should be carefully explained to the patient. Written instruction sheets with directions for the x-ray examination are most beneficial.

When a complete GI series is scheduled for the same day, the order of x-ray examination is: 1. Gallbladder x-ray; 2. Barium enema; 3. Upper GI x-ray.

Barium studies should be scheduled *after* gallbladder studies because the barium will interfere with the results of the gallbladder x-rays. Thyroid scans and ^{131}I uptake tests must be performed prior to the gallbladder x-ray because the oral iodine contrast will adversely alter nuclear test results.

X-ray examinations that do not require preparation and that can be ordered when the radiology department and the patient agree on a mutual time are chest x-ray, extremity x-rays, KUB (kidney, ureter, bladder) x-rays, and mammograms.

Chest Radiography

Normal Values
Normal chest

Normal bony thorax (all bones present and in position, symmetry, and shape)
Normal soft tissues
Normal mediastinum
Normal lungs (proper number of lobes, position, and alteration)
Normal pleura
Normal heart (aortic arch and abdominal arteries)

Explanation of Test
The chest x-ray is the radiograph requested most frequently. This examination is very important in the diagnosis of cancer, tuberculosis, and other lung diseases, pulmonary disease, and diseases of the mediastinum and bony thorax. The chest x-ray is also a record of the presence or absence of disease on the date it was taken, and any x-ray studies that follow this date determine progress or development of the disease. This study can also give valuable information on the condition of the heart, lungs, gastrointestinal tract, and thyroid gland. It is also important that a chest x-ray be done after the insertion of chest tubes and subclavian catheters to determine the position of these devices and possible pneumothorax. In addition, positions of other devices such as nasogastric tubes and enteric feeding tubes are easily determined. Without x-ray or fluoroscopy it cannot be ascertained that enteral feeding tubes are positioned beyond the pylorus.

Procedure
1. Routine radiography consists of an anterior, posterior, and lateral, A and P (front. back, and side) view of the chest. It is usually per-

formed with the patient in a standing position. Upright films of the chest are of utmost importance, since films taken with the patient supine will not demonstrate fluid levels. This is especially important to observe when testing persons confined to bed.
2. Clothing is removed to the waist.
3. The patient is asked to take a deep breath and exhale; then he is required to take a deep breath and hold it while the picture is taken.
4. The procedure takes only a few minutes.

Clinical Implications
1. Abnormal results will indicate these conditions of the lungs:
   (a) Aplasia
   (b) Hypoplasia
   (c) Cysts
   (d) Lobar pneumonia
   (e) Bronchopneumonia
   (f) Aspiration pneumonia
   (g) Pulmonary brucellosis
   (h) Viral pneumonia
   (i) Lung abscess
   (j) Middle lobe syndrome
   (k) Pneumothorax
   (l) Pleural effusion
   (m) Atelectasis
   (n) Pneumonitis
   (o) Congenital pulmonary cysts
   (p) Pulmonary tuberculosis
   (q) Sarcoidosis
   (r) Pneumoconiosis (*e.g.*, asbestosis)
   (s) Westermark's sign indicates decreased pulmonary vascularity, sometimes thought to suggest pulmonary embolus
2. Abnormal results will indicate these conditions of the bony thorax:
   (a) Scoliosis
   (b) Hemivertebrae
   (c) Kyphosis
   (d) Trauma
   (e) Sarcoma
   (f) Bone destruction

Interfering Factors
An important consideration in interpreting chest radiographs is whether the film is in "full inspiration." Certain conditions do not allow the patient to inspire fully. The following conditions should be considered when radiographs are evaluated:

1. Obesity
2. Severe pain
3. Congestive heart failure
4. Scarring of lung tissue

Chest Tomography

Normal Values
Same as for chest x-ray

Explanation of Test

Chest tomograms are particularly useful in the study of patients with pulmonary tuberculosis, the compressed lung beneath a thoracoplasty, and study of lung abscess. They are also used to outline detailed anatomy of the lung, mediastinum, and thoracic structures in which an abnormality is observed in the chest film and to outline the vascular pattern in emphysema, pulmonary hypertension, and pulmonary vascular abnormalities.

Clinical Implications

Abnormal results will reveal

1. Cavities and nodular infiltration in tuberculosis that is not visible on routine x-ray films
2. Bronchiectasis associated with tuberculosis
3. Outline of tumor in patients with bronchogenic carcinoma
4. Calcium in small parenchymal nodules
5. Site of a bronchial occlusion

Radiography and Tomography of the Paranasal Sinuses

Normal Values

Normal sinuses are radiolucent because of their air content. The paranasal sinuses are paired cavities lined by mucous membranes that arise as outpouchings from the nasal fossa and extend into the maxillary, ethmoid, sphenoid, and frontal bones. They are named according to the bones in which they develop.

Explanation of Test

Radiographs of the sinuses are to detect the unilateral or bilateral diseases that may affect them and that may cause detectable alterations. Tomograms of the sinuses are usually done to outline foreign bodies, to determine the presence or extent of bony tumor involvement, and to determine the extent and location of fractures of the bony walls of the sinuses and nasal bones.

Procedure

1. If possible, the patient should be in an upright sitting position during the examination of the sinuses. This will allow demonstration of fluid levels when they are present.
2. The patient is usually required to have his head placed in a padded vice headbrace that restricts movement but is comfortable.
3. The examination may take 10 to 15 minutes to complete.

Clinical Implications
Abnormal results will reveal

1. Acute sinusitis
2. Chronic sinusitis
3. Cysts (retention and nonse-
   creting)
4. Mucocele
5. Polyps

6. Tumors of the bone and soft
   tissue
7. Allergic reactions
8. Trauma
9. Foreign bodies

Patient Preparation
Explain the purpose and procedure of the test.

Cardiac Radiography

Normal Values
Normal size and shape of heart, aorta, pulmonary arteries, and pulmonary vascularity

Explanation of Test
Diagnosis of cardiovascular disorders may involve a wide range of diagnostic procedures. There are, however, three routine radiographic imaging techniques that are used for the evaluation of the heart.

1. Plain film radiography
2. Fluoroscopy
3. Cardiac series

The heart may also be evaluated by more sophisticated radiographic studies (*e.g.*, cardiac catheterization) or by procedures that are discussed in more detail in other chapters (*e.g.*, ultrasound studies, radioisotope scans).

Use of Routine Procedures
Plain film radiography

1. Routine screening technique with all suspected cardiac patients
2. Useful for determining cardiac size

Fluoroscopic examination

1. For assessing heart motion and dynamics
2. For determining whether calcification exists in heart
3. For investigating suspected pericardial effusion
4. For verifying position of pacemaker electrodes
5. For guiding movement of catheter in cardiac catheterization

Cardiac series
This radiographic procedure is a four-view exam. Generally, the patient will be asked to swallow barium during the following views:

1. Posteroanterior view
2. Lateral view
3. Right anterior oblique view
4. Left anterior oblique view

Cardioangiography (angiography of the heart)
This procedure is technically quite difficult and places the patient at risk. A large quantity of contrast material must be introduced rapidly into the blood vessels, and films must be exposed rapidly so that the blood vessels can be visualized. A radiopaque contrast material containing iodine is injected directly into one of the heart chambers, the greater vessels, or the coronary arteries by a catheter. See *Cardiac Catheterization* in Chapter 15 for more information.

Note: Cardioangiography is the most invasive and thus the most potentially dangerous of all the diagnostic procedures. In many medical facilities, the technique is being replaced by CT scanning, echocardiography, or digital subtraction.

Abdominal Plain Film or KUB (Kidney, Ureters, Bladder)

Normal Values
Normal abdominal structures

Explanation of Test
This radiographic study, which does *not* use contrast media, is done to diagnose intra-abdominal diseases such as nephrolithiasis, intestinal obstruction, soft tissue masses, or a ruptured viscus. It is also the preliminary step in the examination of the gastrointestinal tract, the gallbladder, or the urinary tract. The study is done before an IVP or before any renal study. It is also useful in the study of abnormal accumulations of gas and of ascites within the GI tract and of the size, shape, and position of the liver, spleen, and kidneys. This type of study is also called a "scout film" and was formerly called the "flat plate."

Procedure
1. The patient is not required to fast.
2. During the test the patient lies on his back on an x-ray table. He may also have a second film taken when he is standing or sitting.
3. If the patient cannot sit or stand, he is asked to lie on his left side with his right side up.

4. There is no discomfort involved, and the test takes only a few minutes.

Clinical Implications
Abnormal results reveal

1. Calcium in blood vessels, lymph nodes, cysts, tumors, or stones
2. Ureters cannot be defined, but calculi may be detected along the course of the ureters.
3. The shadow cast by the urinary bladder can often be identified, especially when it contains urine of a high specific gravity along with fusion anomalies and horseshoe kidneys.
4. Abnormal size, shape, and position of kidney
5. Presence of appendicolithiasis
6. Presence of foreign bodies
7. Abnormal fluid; ascites

Interfering Factors
Because of the interference of barium, this examination should be done before any barium studies.

Patient Preparation
Explain the purpose and procedure of the test.

Clinical Alert
Abdominal plain films are not useful with conditions such as esophageal varices and bleeding peptic ulcer.

Gastric Radiography (Including Upper GI Examination)

Normal Values
Normal size, contour, motility, and peristalsis of the stomach.

Explanation of Test
This x-ray and fluoroscopic examination is done to visualize the form and position, mucosal folds, peristaltic activity, and motility of the stomach.

Preliminary film without contrast media is useful in detecting perforation, presence of metallic foreign substances, thickening of the gastric wall, and displacement of the gastric air bubble, indicating a mass outside of the stomach wall.

The use of an oral contrast substance such as barium sulfate or

Gastrografin (diatrizoate meglumine) will demonstrate a hiatal hernia, pyloric stenosis, gastric diverticulitis, undigested food, gastritis, congenital anomalies (*e.g.,* dextroposition and duplication), and diseases of the stomach (*e.g.,* gastric ulcer, cancer, and stomach polyps).

If this examination includes the esophagus, duodenum, and upper part of the jejunum, it is called the *upper GI examination.*

Procedure

1. The patient lies on the examining table in the x-ray department while a preliminary film is made.
2. The patient swallows the chalky contrast substance while standing in front of the fluoroscopy machine. All the chalky substance must be swallowed.
3. The contrast agent swallow is followed by x-ray filming; 24-hour films may also be taken.
4. Examining time is 45 minutes.

Clinical Implications

Abnormal results reveal

1. Congenital anomalies
2. Gastric ulcer
3. Carcinoma of stomach
4. Gastric polyps
5. Gastritis
6. Foreign bodies
7. Gastric diverticula
8. Pyloric stenosis
9. Hiatal hernia
10. Volvulus of the stomach

Note: The normal contour may be deformed by intrinsic tumor or consistent filling defects as well as stenosis accompanied by dilatation.

Interfering Factors

1. Because of poor physical condition of the patient, examination is sometimes difficult, and it may be impossible to visualize adequately all parts of the stomach.
2. Retention of food and fluid residues may cause difficulty and lead to errors.

Patient Preparation

1. Explain the purpose and procedure of the test. Give a written reminder.
2. No food or liquid is permitted from midnight until the examination is completed.

Patient Aftercare

1. Provide fluids, food, and rest after the test.
2. Administer laxatives if ordered. If barium sulfate or diatrizoate meglumine is used during the exam, a laxative should be taken after the procedure.

3. Observe and record stools for color and consistency to determine that all of the barium has been evacuated.

Radiography and Fluoroscopy of the Small Intestine

Normal Values
Normal contour, position, and motility of the small intestine.

Explanation of Test
This radiographic and fluoroscopic study is done to diagnose diseases of the small bowel (*e.g.*, ulcerative colitis, tumors, active bleeding, or obstruction). The patient swallows a contrast material such as barium sulfate or meglumine diatrizoate to aid in the diagnosis of Meckel's diverticulum, congenital atresia, obstruction, filling defects, regional enteritis, lymphoid hyperplasia, tuberculosis of small intestine (malabsorption syndrome), sprue, Whipple's disease, intussusception, and edema. This test is usually scheduled in conjunction with an upper GI examination.

The mesenteric small intestine begins at the duodenojejunal junction and ends at the ileocecal valve. The mesenteric small intestine is not included routinely as part of the upper GI study.

Procedure
1. A preliminary plain film study is made while the patient lies on the examining table.
2. While in a standing position in front of the fluoroscopy machine, the patient swallows a chalky contrast material. (All of the chalky substance must be swallowed.)
3. The contrast agent swallow is followed by x-ray filming. Timed films are taken, usually every 30 minutes
4. Examining time is variable. The examination is not completed until the ileocecal valve has filled with contrast. This may take several minutes (for those patients having a bypass) or several hours.

Clinical Implications
Abnormal results indicate

1. Anomalies of the small intestine
2. Errors of rotation
3. Meckel's diverticulum
4. Atresia
5. Neoplasms
6. Regional enteritis
7. Tuberculosis
8. Malabsorption syndrome
9. Intussusception

10. Round worms (ascariasis)
11. Intra-abdominal hernias

Interfering Factors
1. Delays in motility in the small intestine can be due to
   (a) Use of morphine
   (b) Severe or poorly controlled diabetes
2. Increases in motility in the small intestine can be due to
   (a) Fear
   (b) Excitement
   (c) Nausea

Patient Preparation
1. Explain the purpose and procedure of the test. Give a written reminder.
2. Advise the patient that no food or liquids are permitted from midnight until the examination is completed.

Patient Aftercare
1. Provide fluids, food, and rest after the examination.
2. Administer laxatives if ordered. If a barium sulfate swallow is used during the examination, a laxative should be taken after the examination is finished. No laxatives for an ileostomy patient.
3. Check stools for color and consistency to determine that all the barium has been evacuated.

Barium Enema Radiography of the Colon; "Air-Contrast" Study

Normal Values
Normal position, contour, filling, rate of passage of barium, movement, and patency of colon.

Explanation of Test
This examination of the large intestine, or colon, uses x-ray films and fluoroscopy to visualize the position, filling, and movement of the divisions of the colon. It is an aid in determining the presence or absence of disease such as diverticulitis, cancer, polyps, colitis, any form of obstruction, and active bleeding. Barium or Hypaque is used as a contrast medium and instilled through a rectal tube. The radiologist observes the barium through a fluoroscope as it flows into the large intestine. X-ray films are taken.

For a satisfactory examination, the colon must be cleansed thoroughly of fecal matter. This is most important if a search is being made for a source of bleeding. The accurate identification of small polyps is possible only when there are no confusing shadows caused by retained lumps of stool.

If polyp formation is suspected, an air-contrast colon examination may be ordered. The procedure for this test is basically the same as for the barium enema. However, it does require that more complex radiographs be taken in several positions. A "double contrast" of air and barium is instilled into the colon under fluoroscopy.

Procedure
1. In the x-ray department, the patient is asked to lie on his back while a preliminary film is made.
2. The patient lies on his side, and the barium is introduced by enema. When barium is given by rectal enema in the x-ray department, it goes through the rectum, up through the sigmoid, descending, transverse, and ascending colon, up to the ileocecal valve. Barium contrast opacifies the bowel mucosa and outlines the haustra folds of the large intestine.
3. The patient is instructed to retain barium until x-ray films are taken. Following fluoroscopic examination, which includes several "spot films," conventional x-ray films are taken. After completion of the films, the patient is asked to go into the bathroom to expel the barium. After evacuation, another film is made.
4. Total examining time may be up to 1¼ hours.

Clinical Implications
1. Abnormal results indicate
   (a) Lesions
   (b) Obstructions
   (c) Megacolons
   (d) Fistulae
   (e) Inflammatory changes
   (f) Diverticulae
   (g) Chronic ulcerative colitis
   (h) Stenosis
   (i) Right-sided colitis
   (j) Hernias
   (k) Polyps
   (l) Intussusception
   (m) Carcinoma
2. Size, position, and motility of the appendix can be determined by this examination; however, a diagnosis of chronic appendicitis *cannot* be made from x-ray findings. A diagnosis of appendicitis is made from the presence of typical signs and symptoms.

Interfering Factors
A poorly cleansed bowel is the most common interfering factor. Unless fecal matter is satisfactorily cleansed from the colon, small polyps or a source of blockage will not show up well on the x-ray film.

Patient Preparation
Preparation requires a three-step process over a one-to-two day period:
1) diet restrictions; 2) physiologic cleansing of large bowel with oral

laxatives; 3) mechanical cleansing with enema. Twelve and eighteen hour protocols are common. Check with the examining department for specifics.

1. Explain the purpose and procedure of the test.
2. Give a written reminder of the following intructions:
   (a) A clear liquid diet before testing
   (b) Stool softeners, laxatives, and enemas will be given in order to obtain the clearest possible x-ray films. Giving agents such as X-Prep, citrate of magnesia, and bisacodyl will result in emptying of the ascending and right-to-mid-transverse colon (proximal large bowel). Administering enemas cleanses the left transverse descending and sigmoid colon and rectum of stool. Suppositories may also be used to empty the rectum.
   (c) No food is to be eaten after the evening meal, and no liquids are to be taken from midnight until the examination is completed. Oral medications are not permitted. Unless otherwise contraindicated, drinking eight glasses of water each day until ordered restrictions before testing.

Patient Aftercare

1. Provide food, fluids, and rest after the examination is completed. This examination is the most fatigue-producing of all x-ray studies. Patients may be weak, thirsty, or tired after the test is finished.
2. A laxative should be given for at least 2 days following the x-ray studies or until stools are normal in consistency and color.
3. Stools must be checked and recorded for color and consistency for at least 2 days in order to determine whether all the barium has been evacuated. Stools will be light in color until all barium has been expelled. Outpatients should be given a written reminder to inspect stools for 2 days.

Clinical Alert

1. See page 586 for clinical considerations for barium.
2. The use of multiple enemas prior to diagnostic procedure as an enema until clear, especially on a person at risk for electrolyte imbalances, could induce a rather rapid hypokalemia. Enema fluid, if not expelled from the body, can be absorbed through the bowel wall, thereby diluting it in the interstitial space and ultimately in all extracellular space.
3. A judgment should be made about the administration of cathartics or enemas in the presence of acute abdominal pain,

ulcerative colitis, or obstruction. Consult the physician or radiology department and consider the following points:

(a) When giving enemas, remember that introducing large quantities of water into the bowel should be avoided in patients with megacolon because of the danger of water intoxication. In general, patients with toxic megacolon should *not* be given enemas.

(b) If any obstruction is suspected in the colon, the water from large enemas may be reabsorbed and impaction can occur.

(c) If there is an obstruction in the rectum, it will be difficult or impossible to give the cleansing enemas, for the fluid will not flow into the colon. Consult the physician or radiology department in these matters.

4. Strong cathartics in the presence of obstructive lesions and acute ulcerative colitis can be hazardous or lifethreatening.

5. The danger of introducing barium into the colon and the preparation for the procedure should always be considered. Be prepared for complications when barium sulfate or a similar contrast medium is introduced into the GI tract.

6. Barium may aggravate acute ulcerative colitis or cause a partial to complete obstruction.

7. NPO also includes oral medications.

8. Preparations for the test will vary from one x-ray department to another.

9. Barium should not be used as a contrast for intestinal studies when a bowel perforation is suspected. Leakage of barium through a perforation may cause peritonitis. Iodinated contrasts should be used when perforation is suspected.

Special Considerations for Barium Enema with Colostomy

1. See page 586 for assessment criteria.
2. Laxatives can be taken.
3. Suppositories are useless.
4. Usually a suggested diet can be followed.
5. If irrigation is needed, use a preassembled colostomy irrigation kit or use a soft 28 Foley catheter attached to a disposable enema bag.
6. In those persons with a double-barreled colostomy, the irrigation solution may be expelled through the rectum as well as the stoma.
7. Advise the patient that a Foley catheter is used to introduce the barium into the stoma.

Aftercare of Patients with Stomas

Persons with descending or sigmoid colostomies may need a normal saline or tap water irrigation to wash out the barium.

Advise those who normally irrigate the colostomy to wear a disposable pouch for several days until all the barium has passed.

Cholecystography (Gallbladder Radiography)

Normal Values

Normal functioning gallbladder and ducts without stones

Explanation of Test

This x-ray study involving the use of an oral iodine contrast substance such as Telepaque (iopanoic acid), Oragrafin (sodium spodate), and Priodax (iodoalphionic acid) is done to evaluate the functioning of the gallbladder (filling, concentration, contraction, and emptying) and to determine the presence of disease or gallstones. Since gallstones are not usually radiopaque, it is necessary to fill the gallbladder with a radiopaque substance that permits stones to show up as shadows. After administration of the iodinated substance, it takes about 13 hours for it to reach the liver and to be excreted into the bile, where it is stored in the gallbladder. This test is effective only if the liver cells are functioning normally and are capable of excreting the radiopaque dye into the bile.

Procedure

Ultrasound studies of the gallbladder are commonly used alone or in conjunction with oral cholecystography, because of a high degree of accuracy and ease of performance. Calculi or diseases that are suggested but not positively identified by one type of imaging procedure are often verified by the other type of study.

1. A series of up to three x-ray examinations is made with the patient assuming the following positions: lying on his abdomen, lying with the right side of his body elevated away from the table, sitting, or standing. Total examining time is 1 hour.
2. In some instances, a high-fat drink may be given to make the gallbladder contract, and after 20 to 60 minutes another x-ray examination is conducted. Sincalide, when injected intravenously, also causes contraction of the gallbladder in 5 to 15 minutes and subsequent evacuation of bile.

Clinical Implications

Abnormal results reveal

1. Cholelithiasis (gallstones)
2. No evidence of gallbladder

Note: If the gallbladder is chronically inflamed or contains stones, it may not show up at all. This will provide presumptive evidence of disease if on two different occasions the gallbladder cannot be demonstrated.

3. Presence of gas within the gallbladder or ducts, which is always abnormal
4. Papillomatous or adenomatous tumors of the gallbladder
5. Congenital anomalies
6. Obstruction of cystic duct

Scheduling of Test
1. Thyroid scans, ^{131}I uptake, and protein-bound iodine (PBI) must be performed before a gallbladder examination.
2. Barium studies should be performed after gallbladder studies are completed, since barium may interfere with the results.
3. When a series of GI x-ray studies is made in a single day, the usual order of examination is (1) gallbladder, (2) barium enema, and (3) upper GI x-ray film.

Patient Preparation
1. Explain the purpose and procedure of the test.
2. Tell the patient that this test often has to be repeated, so if it is requested again, there is no need to be alarmed.
3. Emphasize the importance of drinking a large amount of water with the contrast capsules. Give a written reminder.
4. Be familiar with the procedures of your medical facility. Prepare the patient with the following information:
   (a) A low-fat meal is eaten the evening before the x-ray examination.
   (b) An oral laxative or stool softener is given after the meal.
   (c) The iodine contrast is given orally, usually in the form of tasteless capsules. Some departments prefer two doses of oral contrast given on consecutive days before x-ray filming, others prefer a single dose followed by a second dose only if the first is unsuccessful.
   (d) Some x-ray departments require the patient to have an enema.
   (e) No food is permitted from the time the contrast is given until the examination is completed. Usually, water and coffee or tea without cream and sugar are permitted if the examination is not done in conjunction with intestinal studies.

Patient Aftercare
1. Provide fluids, food, and rest after the examination is completed.
2. Observe the patient for allergic reaction to the iodine contrast substance.

Clinical Alert

These tablets may act as a laxative in some patients with right-sided colostomies or ileostomies. If this happens, the patient needs extra oral fluids at once.

1. This examination is contraindicated in
   (a) Jaundiced patients who will be unable to metabolize and concentrate the iodine in the gallbladder because of liver disease
   (b) Patients sensitive to iodine
   (c) Vomiting patients
   (d) Patients with diarrhea
2. Observe for reactions to iodine. See page 583 for additional assessment criteria.

T-Tube Cholangiography; Intravenous Cholangiography

Normal Values
Patent common duct

Explanation of Test
The intravenous cholangiogram is an examination done to study the biliary ducts. It is usually performed after nonvisualization of the gallbladder following an oral choledochogram. A contrast is injected intravenously and followed by radiographic and tomographic evaluation. With intravenous injection of contrast there can be visualization of the gallbladder in persons unable to take oral contrast media or unable to absorb them from the GI tract.

The T-tube cholangiogram is done after gallbladder surgery to evaluate the patency of the common bile duct before removal of the T-tube (a T-tube is a self-retaining drainage tube that is attached to the common bile duct during surgery). An iodine contrast dye is injected into the T-tube; then a fluoroscopic examination is made. This test is usually done about 10 days after the operation.

Procedure
For T-tube cholangiogram

1. The patient lies on the x-ray table while a contrast medium such as Hypaque is injected into the T-tube.
2. Normally no pain or discomfort is experienced. Some persons may feel pressure upon injection.

3. The procedure takes at least 15 minutes. On leaving the x-ray department, the T-tube should be unclamped and draining freely unless otherwise ordered. This avoids prolonged, often irritating, contact of the residual dye with the bile duct.

For intravenous cholangiogram

1. A "scout film" of the right upper quadrant is made.
2. The patient lies on the x-ray table while a contrast agent, usually Cholografin, is injected. This process takes about 15 minutes.
3. Films are taken every 15 to 30 minutes until the common bile duct visualizes.
4. Following visualization of the biliary ducts, tomographic studies are performed.
5. If the patient's gallbladder has not been removed, the examination may include fluoroscopy of the gallbladder with the patient standing.

Clinical Implications
Results will reveal whether the lower end of the duct is clear.

Patient Preparation
1. Explain the purpose and procedure of the test.
2. The meal before the x-ray study is omitted. If the examination is in the morning, hold breakfast; if the exam is in the afternoon, hold lunch. Decrease the patient's fluid intake as well. A laxative may be administered the afternoon before the examination, and after midnight nothing can be eaten. Fluids are usually allowed upon completion of infusion.
3. The intravenous cholangiogram is a lengthy procedure requiring 2 to 4 hours and, in some instances, longer.

Patient Aftercare
1. After the test, nausea, vomiting, and transient elevated temperature may occur as a reaction to the iodine contrast.
2. Record observations and notify the physician.

Clinical Alert

1. Persistent fever, especially with chills, may signify inflammation of the bile duct.
2. Follow-up care to monitor for hemorrhage, pneumothorax, and/or peritonitis is essential after percutaneous transhepatic cholangiography.

Other Tests Used in the Examination of the Biliary System

Intravenous cholangiography—Radiographic visualization of the large hepatic ducts and the common ducts after intravenous injection of a contrast medium

Operative cholangiography—Performed by cannulation of the exposed cystic duct or common bile duct at laparotomy and subsequent injection of a contrast agent.

Percutaneous transhepatic cholangiography—A needle or catheter is introduced percutaneously into the liver and bile duct. The contrast agent is then injected, and opacification of the hepatic and common ducts occurs. The dilated biliary tree is opacified up to the point of obstruction, usually in the common duct. It is done on the jaundiced patient whose liver cells are unable to transport contrast when administered by oral or intravenous routes.

T-tube (or postoperative) cholangiography—The hepatic and common ducts can be opacified by injecting a contrast agent through the external opening of a drainage T-tube that has been placed in the common duct during surgery.

Intravenous cholecystography—Radiographic visualization of the gallbladder after intravenous injection of a contrast agent

Oral cholangiography—Radiographic visualization of the biliary ducts after oral administration of a contrast agent

Oral cholecystography—Radiographic visualization of the gallbladder after ingestion of an opaque medium

---

Esophageal Radiography

Normal Values

Normal size, contour, swallowing, movement of material through the esophagus; peristalsis of esophagus

Explanation of Test

Usually, the esophagus is examined together with the stomach, duodenum, and upper part of the jejunum. By common usage, this examination is referred to as an upper GI series (UGI series). In addition, the esophagus may be examined separately because of specific complaints pertaining to this region of the GI tract.

This x-ray and fluoroscopic examination is done to visualize the position, patency, and contour of the esophagus. The technique of examination will vary, depending on such factors as the presence or absence of a lesion and the amount of obstruction. Preliminary films without contrast media are made to identify opaque foreign bodies in the neck and thorax, displacement of trachea, or air or fluid in mediastinal tissues or pleural cavities.

The use of an oral contrast medium, barium sulfate or diatrizoate meglumine, will permit visualization of the lumen of the esophagus. Swallowing small pledgets of cotton soaked in barium is useful when the esophagus is being examined for the presence of small or sharp foreign bodies such as fish bones. Congenital abnormalities of the esophagus can be detected by this method as well as esophageal involvement in scleroderma, diverticulae, cancer, stricture with inflammation, and spasms. It is difficult to identify esophageal varices, but if present, they are an indication of cirrhosis of the liver.

Procedure
1. The patient lies on the examining table in the x-ray department while a preliminary plain film study is made.
2. Barium sulfate or diatrizoate meglumine is swallowed while the patient is in a standing position in front of the fluoroscope. All of the chalky substance must be swallowed.
3. The barium swallow is followed by x-ray studies. Twenty-four hour films may also be done.
4. Examining time is 45 minutes.

Clinical Implications
1. Abnormal results indicate
   (a) Congenital abnormalities
   (b) Esophageal involvement in scleroderma
   (c) Diverticulae
   (d) Cancer
   (e) Stricture with inflammation and spasm
   (f) Acute ulcerative esophagitis
   (g) Chronic fibrosing esophagitis
   (h) Peptic ulcer of the esophagus
   (i) Achalasia (cardiospasm)
   (j) Chalasia (cardioesophageal relaxation)
   (k) Polyps
   (l) Foreign bodies
   (m) Rupture
   (n) Paralysis
2. Esophageal varices may be difficult to identify but, if present, they are an indication of cirrhosis of the liver.

Patient Preparation
1. Explain the purpose and procedure of the test. Give a written reminder. Since barium has a chalky taste, it is often flavored.
2. No food or liquids are permitted from midnight until the examination is completed.

Patient Aftercare
1. Provide food and fluids after the test is completed.
2. If barium is used during the examination, a laxative should be given after the examination is completed.
3. Check stool for barium (color and consistency) to determine that all the barium has been evacuated.

Intravenous Urography (IVU) (Excretory Urography or IV Pyelography)

Normal Values
1. Normal size, shape, and position of the kidneys, ureters, and bladder. Normal kidneys are approximately as long as three and one-half vertebral bodies. Size of kidneys is estimated in relation to the shadows cast against the vertebra on the x-ray film.
2. Normal renal function
   (a) Two to five minutes after the injection of the contrast material the kidney outline will appear. Threadlike strands of the contrast material will be seen in the calyces.
   (b) When the second film is taken 5 to 7 minutes after the injection, the renal pelvis can be noted.
   (c) In the last stages of film-taking, the ureters and bladder can be visualized as the contrast material makes its way down the lower urinary tract.
3. No signs of residual urine should be found on the postvoid film.

Explanation of Test
An IVU is one of the most frequently ordered tests in instances of suspected renal disease or urinary tract dysfunction. A radiopaque iodine contrast substance, such as sodium diatrizoate (Hypaque) or n-methylglucamine iothalamate (Conray) is injected intravenously, concentrating the contrast substance in the urine. Then a series of x-ray films is made at set intervals over a 20- to 30-minute period. A final postvoid film is taken after the patient has been asked to empty his bladder.

The result allows for visualization of the size, shape, and structure of the kidneys, ureters, and bladder, and the ability of the bladder to empty sufficiently. Renal function is reflected by the length of time it takes the contrast material to appear and be excreted in each kidney. Kidney disease, ureteral or bladder stones, and tumors can be detected with this test.

An IVU is indicated in the initial investigation of any suspected urologic problem, especially in the diagnosis of lesions of the kidney and ureters and in the determination of renal function. The term *intra-*

venous urogram is preferred to IVP because urogram implies visualization of the entire urinary tract, whereas pyelogram refers specifically to the kidneys.

Tomography of the kidney may also be done at this time to obtain better visualization of renal pathology and tumors. This will increase the examination time, for more films will be taken. If kidney tomography or nephrotomogram is ordered separately, the procedure and preparation are the same as for IVU.

Procedure
1. A preliminary x-ray film is taken with the patient in a supine position in order to assure that the bowel has been properly emptied and that kidney placement can be visualized.
2. The contrast material is injected intravenously, usually by the antecubital vein.
3. During and following the IV injection, the patient should be forewarned that he may experience the following sensations: warmth, flushing of the face, salty taste, and nausea.
   (a) Should these sensations occur, the patient should be instructed to take slow deep breaths.
   (b) As a precaution, an emesis basin should be handy.
   (c) Other untoward signs should be watched for, such as respiratory difficulty, heavy sweating, numbness, and palpitations.
4. Following injection of the contrast material, at least three x-ray films are taken at set intervals.
5. The patient is then asked to go to the bathroom to void, after which another film is taken to determine bladder emptying.
6. Total examination time is about 45 minutes.

Clinical Implications
1. Abnormal IVU findings reveal
   (a) Altered size, form, and position of the kidneys, ureters, and bladder
   (b) Duplication of the pelvis or ureter
   (c) The presence of only one kidney
   (d) Hydronephrosis
   (e) A supernumerary kidney
   (f) Renal or ureteral calculi (stones)
   (g) Tuberculosis of the urinary tract
   (h) Cystic disease
   (i) Tumors
   (j) The extent of renal injury following trauma
   (k) Prostate enlargement (male)
   (l) Very large kidneys suggesting obstruction or polycystic disease
   (m)Evidence of renal failure with kidneys of normal size, suggesting an acute rather than a chronic process

(n) Irregular scarring of the renal outlines, suggesting chronic pyelonephritis
2. A delay in the appearance time of the radiopaque contrast indicates renal dysfunction. No contrast may indicate very poor function or no function at all.

Interfering Factors
1. Feces or gas not cleared from the intestinal tract will obscure the view of the urinary tract.
2. Retained barium and the resulting gaseous distention from a previous barium examination can obscure the kidneys. (For this reason, barium tests should be scheduled to follow an IVU when possible.)

Patient Preparation
1. Explain the purpose and procedure of the test. Give a written reminder.
2. Since dehydration is necessary for the contrast material to be concentrated in the urinary tract, instruct the patient that no food, liquid, or medication is to be taken 12 hours before the examination. This usually means NPO after the evening meal.

   Note: Elderly or debilitated patients with poor renal reserves may not tolerate dehydration procedures (NPO, laxatives, enemas). In such instances, consult with the radiologist or the patient's physician to see if these procedures are contraindicated and if the patient should be given fluids during the normal NPO period.

   For infants and small children, the NPO time will usually vary from 6 to 8 hours preceding the test. However, be sure to obtain specific orders since each child will require different limits.

3. Usually, a laxative is prescribed for the evening before the examination and an enema the day of the examination.
   (a) Patients with intestinal disorders such as ulcerated colitis probably should not be given a cathartic. Special orders should be obtained in such instances.
   (b) Elderly patients need special attention for possible assistance to the bathroom.
4. Children under 7 years should not be given cathartics or enemas before the examination. Should the preliminary x-ray film show gas obscuring the kidneys, a few ounces of formula or carbonated drink may help push the gas aside.
5. Check stool and abdomen for distention to assure that barium from a previous enema has been eliminated and that the bowel evacuation efforts have been successful.
6. See page 586 for assessment criteria.

Patient Aftercare
1. Provide fluid and food immediately after the examination.
2. Inform the patient about the importance of drinking fluids to overcome dehydration and feelings of weakness.
3. Encourage bedrest following the examination, up to 8 hours for elderly and debilitated patients.
4. Observe and record any of the following mild reactions to the iodine material: hives, skin rashes, nausea, swelling of the parotid glands (iodinism).
   (a) Consult with the physician if the signs and symptoms persist.
   (b) Administration of oral antihistamines may relieve the more severe symptoms.

Clinical Alert

1. Contraindication to an IVU include
   (a) Hypersensitivity to iodine preparation
   (b) The presence of combined renal and hepatic disease
   (c) Oliguria
   (d) A BUN of more than 40 mg. per 100 ml. (40 mg. per dl.)
   (e) Multiple myeloma, unless the patient can be kept well hydrated during and after the study
   (f) Advanced pulmonary tuberculosis
   (g) Patients receiving drug therapy for chronic bronchitis, emphysema or asthma
2. Whenever a radiopaque iodine substance is injected, some physiologic changes can be expected. Hypertension, hypotension, tachycardia, arrhythmia or other ECG changes are the types of conditions expected to occur.
3. Radiopaque contrast media containing iodine are given with caution to patients with hyperthyroidism or a history of asthma, hay fever, or other allergies.
4. Patients should be observed for any anaphylactic or severe reaction to iodine as evidenced by signs of shock, respiratory distress, a precipitous drop in blood pressure, fainting, or convulsions.
5. In all cases except emergencies, the contrast media should not be injected sooner than 90 minutes after eating.
6. Intravenously injected iodine can be highly irritating to the intima of the veins and may cause a painful vascular spasm.
   (a) Intravenous injection of 1% procaine solution may help relieve vascular spasm and pain.
   (b) Sometimes local vascular irritation is severe enough to

induce thrombophlebitis. The area may be treated with warm compresses to relieve pain. The attending physician should be notified. In some cases, anticoagulant therapy is prescribed.

7. Patients should be observed for local reaction to iodine as evidenced by extensive redness, swelling, and pain at the injection site. A leakage of even a small amount of iodine contrast into the subcutaneous tissues can ultimately cause sloughing of the area, which may require skin grafting.
   (a) When extravasation is recognized, the local injection of hyaluronidase may hasten reabsorption of the iodine and resolution of the reaction.
   (b) The use of local applications of warm saline packs may alleviate discomfort, but it does not prevent sloughing.

Retrograde Pyelography

Normal Values
Normal contour and size of ureters and kidneys

Explanation of Test
This test is generally used to confirm findings suspected on the IVU. This test is also indicated when the IVU yields insufficient results because of nonvisualization of kidney (congenital absence of the kidney), decreased renal blood flow that restricts renal function and obstruction, when the IVU shows that one kidney is not working properly or provides evidence of a stone, or when the patient is allergic to intravenous contrast material. This x-ray examination of the upper urinary tract uses cystoscopy to introduce catheters into the ureters to the level of the renal pelvis. An iodine contrast dye is injected into the catheter and films are taken. The chief advantage of retrograde pyelography is that a dense contrast substance can be injected directly under controlled pressure so that visualization is good. The extent of impairment of renal function that may be present does not influence the degree of visualization.

Procedure
1. The examination is usually done in the surgical department in conjunction with cystoscopy.
2. The examination is preceded by sedation and analgesia and insertion of a local anesthetic into the urethra (see *Cystoscopy*). General anesthesia may be used.
3. Total examination time is less than 1½ hours.

Clinical Implications
Abnormal results reveal
1. Intrinsic disease of ureters and pelvis of the kidney
2. Extrinsic disease of the ureters such as obstructive tumor or stones

Interfering Factors
Because of the tendency of barium to interfere with the test results, these studies must be done before barium x-rays.

Patient Preparation
1. Explain the purpose and procedure of the test.
2. A legal consent form must be signed before examination.
3. The patient is allowed no foods or liquids after midnight before the test.
4. Cathartics, suppositories, or enemas are usually ordered before the examination.

Patient Aftercare
1. Observe for allergic reaction to iodine contrast dye.
2. Following the examination, check vital signs for at least 24 hours (every 15 minutes times 4, then every hour times 4, then every 4 hours times 4). If general anesthetic was used, care is the same.
3. Record accurate urine output and appearance for 24 hours. Hematuria and dysuria are common for several days after the examination.
4. Administer analgesics if necessary. Pain is common the first few days following the examination and may require something stronger than aspirin (*e.g.*, codeine).

Clinical Alert
If ordered, renal function tests of blood and urine must be completed before this examination is done.

Other Tests Used in Examination of the Urinary System
Excretion urography or intravenous pyelography (IVP)—After intravenous injection of a contrast agent, the collecting system (calyces, pelvis, and ureter) of each kidney is progressively opacified. Radiographs are made at intervals of 5 to 15 minutes until the urinary bladder is opacified.

Drip infusion pyelography—A modification of conventional pyelography. Increased volume of a contrast agent is administered by continuous intravenous infusion.

Cystography—The urinary bladder is opacified by introduction of a contrast agent through a urethral catheter. After the patient has voided, air may be introduced to obtain a double contrast study.

Retrograde cystourethrography—After catheterization, the bladder is filled to capacity with a contrast agent; radiographic techniques then visualize the bladder and urethra. ⁻

Voiding cystourethrography—After contrast material has been instilled into the urinary bladder, films are made of the bladder and urethra during the act of voiding.

Lymphangiography

Normal Values
Normal lymphatic vessels and nodes

Explanation of Test
This x-ray examination of the lymphatic channels and lymph nodes uses a radiopaque iodine contrast oil, such as Ethiodol, injected into the small lymphatics of the foot. The test is commonly ordered for patients with Hodgkin's disease and cancer of the prostate to check for nodal involvement. Lymphography is also indicated in diagnosing edema of an extremity with an unknown cause, in evaluating the extent of adenopathy and the staging of lymphomas, and in localizing affected nodes for treatment planning, either surgery or radiotherapy.

Procedure
1. The patient is asked to lie on the examining table in the x-ray department.
2. A blue dye is injected intradermally between each of the first three toes of each foot in order to stain the lymphatic vessels.
3. Under local anesthesia, a 1 to 2 inch incision is made in the dorsum of each foot about 15 to 30 minutes later.
4. The lymphatic vessel is identified and a cannula attached for an extremely *low* pressure injection of the iodine contrast medium.
5. When the contrast medium reaches the level of the third and fourth lumbar vertebra (as seen in fluoroscopy), the injection is discontinued.
6. Films taken of the abdomen, pelvis, and upper body demonstrate the filling of the lymphatic vessels.
7. A second set of films is obtained in 12–24 hours to demonstrate filling of the lymph nodes.
8. The nodes in the equinal, external iliac, common iliac, and para-aortic areas, as well as the thoracic duct and supraclavicular nodes can be visualized.

9. When the injection is made in a lymphatic of the hand, the axillary and supraclavicular nodes are demonstrated.
10. Because the dye persists in the nodes for 6 months to a year, repeat studies can be used to confirm disease activity and follow the results of treatment without injection of dye.
11. The total examination time may take up to 3 hours, which can be very tiring.
12. The patient returns to the x-ray department for additional films in 24 hours.

Clinical Implications
Abnormal results indicate

1. Retroperitoneal lymphomas in patients with Hodgkin's disease
2. Metastasis to lymph nodes
3. Abnormal lymphatic vessels

Patient Preparation
1. Explain the purpose and procedure of the test. A legal permit must be signed.
2. No fasting is necessary; the patient can eat and drink during the procedure if he desires.
3. There may be some discomfort when the local anesthetic is injected into the feet.
4. An oral antihistamine is administered to any patient the physician suspects may be allergic to the iodized oil used as a contrast medium.

Patient Aftercare
1. Check the patient's temperature every 4 hours for 48 hours after the examination.
2. Allow the patient to rest after the test.
3. If ordered, elevate the legs to prevent swelling.
4. Be aware of complications such as delayed wound healing or infection at site of incision, edema of legs, allergic dermatitis, headache, sore mouth and throat, skin rashes, transient fever, lymphangitis, and oil embolism.

Clinical Alert
1. The test is usually contraindicated in
   (a) Known iodine hypersensitivity
   (b) Severe pulmonary insufficiency
   (c) Cardiac disease
   (d) Advanced renal or hepatic disease

2. The major complication of the procedure is related to emboli-
   zation of the contrast media into the lungs. This will diminish
   pulmonary function temporarily and, in some patients, may
   produce lipid pneumonia.

Mammography

Normal Values
Essentially normal breasts. If calcification is present, it is evenly distributed—normal duct contrast with gradual narrowing of branches of
the ductal system.

Explanation of Test
Soft tissue mammography is the securing of an x-ray image of the
breast on photographic film or on paper using the technology of the
Xerox office copier. Its primary use is to discover cancers that escape
detection by all other means. Cancers of less than 1 cm. in size cannot
be regularly detected by routine clinical examination. Since the average cancer has probably been present in a woman's breast for 10 to 12
years before it reaches the clinically palpable size of 1 cm., the prognosis for cure is excellent if breast cancer is detected in this preclinical or
presymptomatic phase. Breast cancer can be detected as early as 2 to 3
years before clinical appearance.

Mammography (x-ray diagnosis of breast disease) is based on gross
characteristics. A low-energy x-ray beam is required to delineate the
breast structures on mammograms. This radiation dose is quite acceptable for use in frequent reexamination, particularly when one con-
siders that only a relatively small volume of tissue is in the low-energy
x-ray beam and that the radiation to the eyes and gonads of the patient
is too small for measurement.

Benign lesions push breast tissue aside as they expand while malignant lesions may invade the surrounding breast tissues. The x-ray criteria for diagnosing lesions of the breast are 85% accurate in identifying carcinomas and give less than 10% false-positive diagnoses.

Background
1. Most breast lumps are not malignant. Eight out of ten are benign.
2. For women over age 40, the benefits of using low-dose mammography to find early, curable cancers outweigh a possible risk from
   radiation.

Indications for Mammography
1. To detect clinically nonpalpable cancers in women over age 40
2. When signs and symptoms of breast cancer are present

    (a) Skin changes

    (b) Nipple or skin retraction

    (c) Nipple discharge or erosion

3. Breast pain
4. "Lumpy" breast; multiple masses or nodules
5. Pendulous breasts that are difficult to examine
6. Survey of opposite breast after mastectomy
7. Patients at risk for having breast cancer (*e.g.*, having family history of breast cancer)
8. Adenocarcinoma of undetermined site
9. Previous breast biopsy
10. Examination of tissue biopsied from breast

Note: The American Cancer Society recommends a baseline mammogram for all women between 35 and 40 years of age, an annual or biannual mammogram for ages 40 to 49, and a yearly mammogram after 50 years of age.

Procedure

1. The patient is asked to identify the area of lumps or thickening, if any.
2. The breasts are exposed and held in position on the film holder to reduce air pockets, skin folds, and wrinkles in order to get the clearest films.
3. Two views are usually taken of each breast.
4. Following x-ray examination, the radiologist or technologist will often palpate the breasts.
5. Total examining time is about one half hour.

Clinical Implications

1. Abnormal findings reveal
   (a) Benign breast mass. On mammogram it appears as a round, smooth mass with definable edges. If there are calcifications in the mass, they are usually coarse.
   (b) Cancerous mass. On mammogram it appears as an irregular shape with extensions into the adjacent tissue. An increased number of blood vessels are present. Primary and secondary signs of breast cancer are apparent.
2. Speculated mass, on occasion, may be smooth and regular.
3. Calcification in malignant mass (duct carcinoma) or in adjacent tissue (lobular carcinoma) is described as innumerable punctate calcifications resembling fine grains of salt or rodlike calcifications when thin, branching, and curvilinear.
4. The likelihood of malignancy increases with the number of calcifications in a cluster. However, a cluster with as few as three calcifications, particularly if they are irregular, can occur in cancer.
5. Typical parenchymal patterns:

N_1: Normal
P_1: Mild duct prominence or less than one quarter of the breast
P_2: Marked duct prominence
DY:Dysplasia. Some diagnosticians believe that the dysplasia group is 22 times more likely to develop breast cancer than those with normal results

6. Findings of breast cancer when contrast is injected is associated with extravasation of contrast, filling defects, obstruction, an irregular narrowing of ducts.
   (a) Intraductal papilloma. Contrast mammography (ductograms, galactograms) is a most valuable aid in diagnosing intraductal papillomas. Mammary duct injection is used when cytologic examination of breast fluid is abnormal and in cases of breast discharge. In contrast mammography, about 1 ml of a radiopaque substance such as 50% sodium diatrizoate is injected after careful cannulation of a discharging duct in the breast with a blunt 25-gauge needle.

7. Difficult diagnoses
   (a) Colloid (gelatinous or mucinous) and medullary (circumscribed) carcinomas are difficult to diagnose by mammography.
   (b) Soft-tissue mammography is notoriously poor in the localizing of nonpalpable intraductal papillomas. Sometimes the calcifications of cancer and sclerosing adenosis may be indistinguishable, particularly if the adenosis is not bilateral.

Patient Preparation

1. Explain the purpose, procedure, benefits, and risks of the test. Mammography is the single best method for detecting breast cancer in a curable stage. Some discomfort is experienced when the breast is compressed.
2. Instruct the patient not to use any deodorant, perfume, powders, or ointment in the underarm area of the breasts on the day of the examination. Residue on the skin from these preparations can obscure the mammograms.
3. Advise the patient to wear a blouse with a skirt or slacks rather than a dress, since it is necessary to remove the clothing from the upper half of the body.
4. Suggest that patients who have painful breasts refrain from coffee, tea, cola, and chocolate 5 to 7 days before testing.

Transillumination Light Scan of Breast; Diaphanography

Normal Values
Normal tissue light absorption patterns

Explanation of the Test

This study projects red and infrared light through the breasts to differentiate benign and malignant tumors. It is known that light in the red and near-infrared spectrum varies in its absorbency and scattering characteristics as it passes through tissue. The basic premise of light scanning is that a soft tissue organ such as the breast acts as a light filter. The manner in which the breast filters light differs from a very dense glandular breast to a fatty breast. The process is similar to shining a flashlight beam through a person's hand and it does not include x-ray filming. A computerized television camera, focused on the breast, converts the light into images. The test is most useful in young women, women with dense breasts, and women with fibrocytic breasts in which benign tumors occur with the breast connective tissue. The technique is also valuable in the evaluation of women with nipple discharge, for those who are afraid of the radiation risk of mammography and refuse x-rays, silicone-injected and silicone-augmented breasts, and patients requiring frequent follow-up. It is particularly helpful in the evaluation of patients with mammary dysplasia, a disease difficult to assess by mammography. The scar tissue of mastectomy patients can also be examined for recurrence of carcinoma.

Procedure

1. The test is performed in a darkened room with the patient leaning far forward so that lesions near the chest wall are not missed.
2. The examiner moves a hand-held emitter similar to a flashlight over each breast.
3. Total examining time is 15 to 20 minutes.

Clinical Implications

1. Tissue variations are shown in computer-enhanced hues of blue and red. Malignancies often show as deep purple.
2. Areas of malignancy will absorb more light than benign tissues and appear to transilluminate to a lesser degree.

Interfering Factors

False positives are associated with hematoma, mastitis, sclerosing adenosis, fibroadenoma, and papillomatosis.

Patient Preparation

Explain the purpose and procedure of the test, its benefits and its no known risk factors. There is no discomfort involved.

Clinical Alert

This test is not a substitute for mammography.

Computed Tomography (CT) of the Brain/Head
(Computerized Axial Tomography [CAT])

Normal Values
No evidence of tumor or pathologic activity
Typically low electron and tissue density areas appear black, and high electron and tissue density areas appear as shades of gray. The whiter the shading, the higher the density.

Explanation of Test
Computed tomography of the head is a simple, routine x-ray examination that uses a special machine with a scanner system to evaluate suspected intracranial pathology. A narrow beam of attenuated x-rays, that allows little internal scatter of radiation, is transmitted through the body part being evaluated and measured by special detectors. A computer provides rapid, complex calculations and determines the degree of multiple x-ray beams that are not absorbed by all the tissue in their path. The result is a three-dimensional picture of the anatomical structure of the head that includes the internal structure of the cranium, brain tissue, and surrounding CSF. This transverse image of the head is similar to a view of the head looking down from the top.

The basic parameter measured by CT method is the attenuation coefficient of tissue. This reflects the electron density as well as the elemental composition of tissue. When there is more phosphorous in gray matter than in white matter (a change in elemental composition) the result is a difference in attenuation coefficient for low-energy x-rays, even though the densities of these tissues are the same. Because clotted blood, cystic fluid, bone, CSF, and air have somewhat different coefficients, it is possible to demonstrate the anatomical distribution in these tissues.

By rotation of the x-ray source around the head, several attenuation readings are obtained and computer-processed. These detailed cross-sectional, three-dimensional pictures of the head are free of blurred images, are displayed on a screen, photographed, and are stored in an x-ray film. In the procedure, the patient's head is placed in the scanner and is then scanned in successive "slices." Destructive, atrophic, space-occupancy intracranial pathology and such congenital abnormalities as hydrocephalus may be diagnosed. A CT scan can demonstrate minor differences in density and composition of different structures. For this reason, it is helpful in differentiating tumors from soft tissues, air spaces from CSF, and normal blood from clotted blood. If there is a disruption in permeability, such as a break in the blood–brain barrier, the accumulation of contrast after IV administrations can also be demonstrated by the basal increase in attenuation coefficients.

CT scanning is a noninvasive diagnostic technique that has virtually eliminated the use of pneumoencephalography and sometimes eliminated angiography. The scope of the information afforded by CT scanning is such that a large number of patients requiring investigation for neurological complaints need be subjected only to plain skull x-ray, a radioisotope brain scan, or a computerized head scan. In neurologic practice, the common lesions that require identification are cerebral neoplasms, inflammation, hematomas, infarctions, infections, and cerebral edema that often accompanies these lesions. The CT scan is the best screening test for this purpose.

In interpreting the scan, the radiologist identifies structures by appearance: their shape, size, symmetry, and position. On a typical CT brain scan, CSF appears black, bones appear white, and the brain appears to be various shades of gray. The radiologist then looks for changes in the tissue density. Usually, a space-occupying lesion will produce a characteristic displacement or deformity of some part of the ventricular system, and the extent of tissue change is defined. Scans for specific indications can be done in different planes, using thinner slices when the examination is one for the evaluation of small, intracranial structures such as the pituitary gland, optic nerves, and ossicles in the middle ear. These studies require a good deal of cooperation from the patient.

Procedure
1. Each examination takes 20 to 40 minutes to complete (10 scans per examination). During this time the patient must lie perfectly still, but there is no other discomfort involved.
2. The patient lies on a motorized couch with his head resting in a head holder set in a movable frame (gantry) that revolves around the head. The face is not covered. No movement is experienced by the patient. A monotonous sound is heard that some people compare to a dulled sound of a broken washing machine. The head is enclosed and braced as if the patient were sitting under a hair dryer in a beauty salon.
3. If tissue density enhancement is desired (a questionable area that needs further clarification), an iodinated radiopaque substance may be injected intravenously. This contrast material can induce vomiting in some patients.
4. More pictures are taken after a short waiting period.
5. During and following the IV injection, the patient may experience the following sensations: warmth, flushing of the face, salty taste, and nausea.
   (a) If these sensations occur, instruct the patient to take slow, deep breaths.
   (b) Have an emesis basin ready as a precaution.

(c) Watch for other untoward signs, such as respiratory difficulty, heavy sweating, numbness, and palpitations.

Clinical Implications

Tissues with Increased Density

Tissue abnormalities can be identified by the tissue density alterations they exhibit in the scan pictures. Calcium is an important factor contributing to the increased density of a lesion. Meningiomas and low-grade astrocytomas are neoplasms that may show up as white areas because of their high tissue density. Calcium also collects in angiomas, aneurysms, and degenerative and infected tissue. Any hematoma can be distinguished easily. In intracranial hemorrhage, once clotting has occurred, serum is absorbed and tissue density is much higher than in the normal brain. Hemoglobin and calcium ions play an important part in this increase of average density. From a surgical point of view, the demonstration of a hematoma, its size, relationship to ventricles, or the extent of surrounding edema may be valuable. In subarachnoid hemorrhage, scans may be used to locate a small hematoma. Where aneurysms are multiple, this may be a valuable means of identifying or confirming which aneurysm has, in fact, ruptured. In craniocerebral trauma, computerized scanning provides an easy method of distinguishing between extradural, subdural, or intracerebral hematoma and cerebral edema resulting from brain damage.

Tissues With Decreased Density

Diminished tissue density on scanning is caused by many pathological conditions. The breakdown of cell structure in infarctions, infections, necrosis in malignant tumors, cyst formation, degenerative processes, benign cysts, and edema are the main changes that will reduce tissue density and are observed as darker areas on the scan pictures.

Tissues Requiring Contrast Media

Lesions having tissue densities that are the same as those of the surrounding normal brain are difficult to identify in the routine scan. The basis for use of this contrast enhancement is that the breakdown of the brain blood–brain barrier permits small amounts of administered contrast substances to pass into the abnormal brain. Contrast enhancement is indicated when there is evidence of a tumor, multiple sclerosis, aneurysm, or vascular abnormality. Contrast enhancement is used in 80% to 85% of patients with a history of headache and seizures. A quantity of 300 ml. of a radiopaque sodium-iodine solution is given by an IV infusion, and scans must be repeated. By administering venous contrast, abnormal areas can be enhanced, thus helping to detect underlying processes.

Interfering Factors

1. A false-negative CT result may occur in identifying areas of hemorrhage. One of the limitations of the test is that, as hematomas age, their appearance on CT scans changes from a high intensity to a low intensity level. This is partly due to the fact that older hematomas become more transparent to x-rays.
2. Movement will result in inaccurate pictures.
3. Because it is basically an anatomical technique, it is not useful for measurement of tissue perfusion, metabolism or vessel blood flow. For this reason it is not the best technique for evaluating small A-V malformations, early ischemic disease of the brain, or subdural hematomas.

Patient Preparation

1. Explain the purpose and procedure of the test. Provide written explanation and reminders. The patient should be aware of risks that include possible adverse effects such as radiation exposure and possible allergic reactions to iodine contrast media. The x-ray dose per examination is essentially the same as in a routine skull x-ray.
2. Generally, the patient should not eat or drink 2 to 3 hours prior to the test if contrast study is planned. Prescribed medications can be taken prior to CT studies. Diabetics should take their insulin and be allowed to eat. CT scanning time can be adjusted so that the examination does not interfere with the patient's medications.
3. Reassure the patient that scanning results in no more radiation than in conventional x-ray studies.
4. Check for allergy in food or drugs that contain iodine. If a contrast iodine intravenous substance is administered during the test (indications may not be present before testing), nausea and vomiting, warmth, and flushing of the face may occur. See page 583 for additional assessment criteria.
5. Reassure the patient that claustrophobic fears of being in the machine are common. Show a picture of the scanner.
6. Administer analgesics and sedatives to patients with painful neck stiffness or injuries to the back of the head, and to those who are unable to cooperate by lying still. Any movement by the patient will give poor results.

Patient Aftercare

1. Determine whether or not an iodine contrast substance was used during the test. If the contrast material was used, observe and record any of the following mild reactions to the iodine material: hives, skin rashes, nausea, swelling of parotid glands (iodism).
2. Consult with the physician if the signs and symptoms persist.

3. Administer oral antihistamines to possibly relieve the more severe symptoms.
4. Documentation should include assessment of need for information, patient instruction given, time examination was completed, how the patient tolerated the procedure, and any signs or symptoms of reaction to contrast.

Computed Tomography (CT) of the Body (Computerized Axial Tomography [CAT] Body Scan; Computerized Transaxial Tomography [CTT] Body Scan)

Normal Values
No tumor or pathological activity is evident. Air appears black on CT scans, bone appears white, soft tissue appears in shades of gray. The pattern of shades and their correlation to different densities in the body, with the added dimensions of depth, assist in identifying normal body structures and organs.

Explanation of Test
The body scanner is used primarily to give a clear, computerized image of the chest, abdomen, and pelvis and as an important diagnostic aid in the identification of neoplastic and inflammatory diseases. CT scanning of the neck, spine, and extremities can also be done. CT examination of the lumbar spine is also a reliable test for the evaluation of disc herniation or stenosis. Rapid scanning at a certain level can be done to determine changes in blood flow as in instances of aortic dissection and in determining vascularity of a mass (simple level dynamic scan technique).

The body scanner is 100 times more sensitive than the traditional x-ray machine in critical areas. Ordinary machines take a flat picture, with organs in the front of the body appearing to be superimposed over organs in the back of the body. The result is a two-dimensional picture of a three-dimensional object. The scanner also produces a two-dimensional picture, but by taking many cross-sectional views of organs of the body and displaying the pictures in turn on an x-ray film, a three-dimensional appearance is created. Typical x-rays show only major contrasts between body densities such as bones, soft tissue, and air. Fine density differences, as between structures within the liver, do not usually register on an x-ray film but will appear on a body scan. CT scanning of the abdomen, chest or pelvis will, in most cases, require administration of iodinated contrast material before and during the examination.

Procedure

1. The patient lies on his back in a comfortable position in the scanner. His head remains outside of the scanning unit.
2. The patient should be still and follow breathing instructions.
3. No movement is felt by the patient as the x-ray beam makes a 180° scan of the body, one degree at a time, in three or four different planes.
4. A television picture of the inside of the living body is seen almost immediately.
5. If there is a questionable area that needs further clarification, such as unusual tissue densities, a contrast iodine substance is injected intravenously and more pictures are taken after a short waiting period. In addition, all patients having CT scans of the pelvis will be given a barium contrast enema. Furthermore, all female patients undergoing pelvic testing will require the insertion of a vaginal tampon.
6. During and following the IV infusion or injection, the patient may experience warmth, flushing of the face, salty taste, and nausea.
   (a) If these sensations occur, instruct the patient to take slow, deep breaths.
   (b) Have an emesis basin available as a precaution.
   (c) Watch for other untoward signs, such as respiratory difficulty, heavy sweating, numbness, and palpitations.
7. The total examination time is 40 to 60 minutes.

Clinical Implications

Abnormal CT scan findings reveal

(a) Tumors, nodules, and cysts of the whole body
(b) Ascites
(c) Abscessed or fatty liver
(d) Aneurysm of abdominal aorta
(e) Lymphoma
(f) Enlarged lymph nodes
(g) Pleural effusion
(h) Radioactive iodine used in previous testing
(i) Cancer of pancreas
(j) Liver metastasis
(k) Retroperitoneal lymphadenopathy
(l) Collection of blood, fluid, or abnormal fat
(m) Skeletal metastasis
(n) Cirrhosis of liver

Interfering Factors

1. Retained barium can obscure organs in the upper and lower abdomen. (Barium tests should be scheduled to *follow* a CT scan when possible.)
2. Inability of the patient to lie quietly. Movement will result in inaccurate pictures.

Patient Preparation
1. Explain the purpose and procedure of the test. Provide written explanation and reminders. The patient should be aware of the benefits and risks, which are the same as for CT scanning of head.
2. Prescribed medications can be taken prior to CT studies. Diabetics should take their insulin and be allowed to eat. CT scanning time can be adjusted so that the examination does not interfere with a patient's medication.
3. Inform the patient that an iodine contrast substance may be administered before and during the examination. Elicit any history of allergy to iodine. See page 583 for additional assessment criteria. Pelvic CT examinations usually require both intravenous and rectal contrast administration.
4. Abdominal cramping and diarrhea may occur in some patients. For this reason, drugs such as glucagon, Lipomul, or Donnatal will be ordered to decrease side-effects.
5. Caution the patient not to eat solid foods on the day of the examination. Clear liquids are usually permitted up to 2 hours before examination. Check with the diagnostic department for specific protocols, because instructions concerning eating will vary. For CT of the abdomen, the patient is usually NPO.
6. Warn the patient that if a contrast iodine intravenous substance is administered during the test (indications are usually not present before testing), he may experience warmth, flushing of the face, salty, metallic taste, and nausea or vomiting.
7. Reassure the patient that claustrophobic fears of being in the machine are common. Show a picture of the scanner.
8. Sedation and analgesics may be ordered if it is difficult for the patient to lie quietly for a long period of time.

Patient Aftercare
If an iodine contrast material was used, observe the patient and record any of the following mild reactions to the iodine material: hives, skin rashes, nausea, swelling of parotid glands (iodism).
1. Consult with the physician if the signs and symptoms persist.
2. Administer oral antihistamines to relieve the more severe symptoms.
3. Document the preparation and instruction of the patient or significant others, the time the procedure was completed, and how the patient tolerated the procedure. Record the use of a control substance and the presence or absence of reaction to iodine contrast material.

Digital Subtraction Angiography (DSA) (Transvenous Digital Subtraction)

Normal Values
Normal carotid and vertebral arteries, normal abdominal aorta and branches, normal renal arteries, normal peripheral vessels.

Explanation of Test
Digital angiography is a computer-based imaging method of vascular study that uses venous or arterial catheterization to examine the arteries of the body, especially the carotids. However, the intracranial vessels, aortic arch, and abdominal and renal arteries are also examined for patency and flow using this method. Digital subtraction angiography was first used as an intravenous technique, but because of its limitations, other methods of iodine contrast administration have been investigated. For this reason, intra-arterial injection may be needed for evaluation of viscera and detailed vascular anatomy. The presence of the contrast blocks the path of x-rays and makes the blood vessels visible on x-ray film. Basically, what happens is that an image taken just before contrast injection is subtracted from that taken when the contrast material is in the vascular system. The resulting image shows only the distribution of the contrast substance. Digital subtraction is used to isolate a clinically relevant subset of information; this technique is particularly useful in preoperative and postoperative evaluations for vascular and tumor surgery.

In addition to reducing the risk associated with arterial puncture, the procedure precludes the potential trauma and emboli complications associated with arterial catheterization techniques. Because arterial punctures are not always necessary, this test may be routinely performed on an outpatient basis with considerably less risk and at lower cost than conventional angiography.

Visualization of the extra- and intracranial carotid and vertebral vasculature is possible in patients with a history of stroke, transient ischemic attacks, bruit, or subarachnoid hemorrhage. In the latter indication, the procedure may be used as an adjunct to CT scanning and may be performed just before the CT scan in cases where there is evidence of an aneurysm, vascular malformation, or hypervascular tumor.

Procedure
1. A local anesthetic is administered following careful cleansing of the antecubital area in the right arm. The basilic vein is easier to cannulate than the cephalic. For some studies the femoral vein is used.
2. The catheter is usually advanced over a guide wire into the superior vena cava. The catheter is connected to a 250-ml. bottle of normal

saline that is administered slowly. Also connected to the catheter is a power injector that administers an iodine substance very rapidly after a variable delay to allow the contrast substance to clear the pulmonary circulation (depending on vessels being studied). Pictures are taken and stored on magnetic tapes or videodiscs.

3. As soon as the vessels being studied have been defined, the procedure is terminated and the catheter is removed.
4. A bandage is placed over the venous insertion site. Pressure is applied to the puncture site for about 5 minutes.
5. Total examining time is 30 to 45 minutes.

Clinical Implications
Abnormal results reveal:

1. Stenosis of arteries
2. Large aneurysms
3. Large jugular tumors and masses
4. Total occlusion of arteries
5. Thoracic outlet syndrome
6. Large or central pulmonary emboli
7. Vascular parathyroid adenoma
8. Pheochromocytoma
9. Ulcerative plaque
10. Tumor circulation
11. Abnormalities that can be identified with 65% accuracy:
    (a) Total occlusion of internal carotid arteries
    (b) Ulcers without web stenosis of thrombosis
    (c) Aortic arch occlusion
    (d) Subclavian steal
    (e) Meningiomas

Interfering Factors
1. All examinations, especially intracranial, are very sensitive to minimal amounts of patient motion such as respiration. Motion artifacts result in poor images. For this reason, uncooperative or agitated patients cannot be studied. Swallowing in the cooperative person also results in unsatisfactory images. Measures to reduce swallowing, such as having the patient hold his breath, bite on a block, or exhale through a straw, do not yield consistent results.
2. Vessel overlap of external and internal carotid arteries makes it almost impossible to obtain a select view of an individual artery. This is because contrast fills both arteries almost simultaneously. Incidence of uninterpretable studies ranges from 6% to 16%.
3. The examination is not totally reliable in ruling out small aneurysms, severe stenoses of intracranial arteries, and arteriovenous malformations.

Clinical Alert

Tests should be used cautiously in renal insufficiency and unstable cardiac disease. Assess for contraindications to the iodinated contrasts listed on page 583.

Patient Preparation

1. Explain the purpose and procedure of the test and document any instructions given. Explain the benefits and risks (see number 5, below). The patient must be able to hold his breath when so instructed and to be very still during the test. A legal permit must be signed.
2. Determine whether or not allergy exists to iodine or contrast medium. See page 583 for additional assessment criteria.
3. In many instances, glucagon is administered intravenously just before any abdominal examinations. This will reduce motion artifacts by stopping peristalsis.
4. No food or fluids should be taken within 2 hours of the study in order to prevent possible vomiting if there is a reaction to the iodine contrast.
5. The patient needs to be aware of the risk and benefits. This method of testing is decidedly less risky than conventional arteriography: less radiation than conventional x-ray; no known fatalities, and no known strokes. However, risks will vary from one testing center to the next. Risks include these rare complications: thrombosis of a vein; infection; overall, the risks are less than in routine angiography, especially when the lower pressure venous circulation is catheterized. By the venous route, the arteries, which are already under high pressure, are able to free through normal circulation and at their own rate. For this reason, there is less risk of loosening plaque. Another benefit to the patient is that all of the arteries in a specific area are visualized in one series of exposures. This overview gives the radiologist the advantage of being able to evaluate the entire blood supply to an area of interest at one time. In routine angiography, one specific artery at a time is visualized.

Patient Aftercare

1. Check vital signs for stability.
2. Observe the site of venous insertion for signs of infection, hemorrhage, or hematoma and use infection control measures for site care.
3. Observe for signs of allergic reaction to iodine. Mild side-effects of iodine that may occur are nausea, vomiting, dizziness, or urticaria. Watch for complications that can include abdominal pain, hyper-

tension, congestive heart failure, angina, and MIs. The possibility of renal failure in susceptible persons exists because there is a higher contrast level given than in conventional arteriograms.

4. Instruct the patient to increase fluid intake up to 2000 ml. over the next 24 hours to facilitate excretion of the iodine contrast.

Arthrography

Normal Values
Normal filling of structures of encapsulated joint: joint space, bursae, menisci, ligaments, and articular cartilage.

Explanation of Test
Multiple x-ray examinations in specific positions of the soft tissue structures of encapsulated joints are made following the injection of a contrast agent or agents into the capsular space. The knee is the most frequent site of study for the evaluation of menisci and ligaments. This test is indicated in the investigation of persistent unexplained joint discomfort and is done using sterile technique. However, the shoulder, hip, elbow, wrist, and temporomandibular joints may also be examined using this method. These examinations are performed using local anesthetics and under careful aseptic conditions.

Procedure
1. The patient is asked to lie on his back on the examining table.
2. Skin over the joint is cleansed using sterile technique.
3. A local anesthetic is injected around the puncture site. It is usually not necessary to anesthetize the joint space itself.
4. Any effusion in the joint is aspirated by the examining physician. Then a contrast agent or agents (gas, water, or soluble iodine) is injected. After the needle is removed, the joint is manipulated to ensure distribution of the contrast material. In some cases, the patient may be asked to walk around the room and exercise the joint for a few minutes.
5. During the examination, other positions will be assumed by the patient to obtain multiple x-ray views of the joint.
6. A special frame may be attached to widen the joint space under investigation. Cotton pillows and sandbags are also used for this purpose.
7. Actual examining time is 30 to 40 minutes.

Clinical Implications
Abnormal results reveal

1. Arthritis
2. Dislocation
3. Tears of ligaments
4. Rupture of rotor cuff
5. Synovial abnormalities

Patient Preparation
1. Explain the purpose and procedure of the test.
2. Determine whether or not the patient has any known allergies to iodine or contrast substance.

Patient Aftercare
1. The joint should be at rest for 12 hours.
2. An elastic bandage is applied to the knee joint for several days.
3. Ice can be applied for swelling if it occurs. Some persons will experience pain requiring a mild analgesic.
4. Cracking or clicking noises may be heard in the joint for 1 or 2 days following the test. This is normal. Notify the physician if crepitant noises persist.

Myelography

Normal Values
Normal lumbar or cervical myelogram

Explanation of Test
Myelography is a radiographic study in which iodine contrast material is introduced into the spinal subarachnoid space so that the spinal cord and nerve roots may be outlined and any distortion of the dura mater may be detected.

The test is done to detect neoplasms, ruptured intravertebral disks, or extraspinal pathology such as arthritic lumbar stenosis and cervical ankylosing spondyloses. This examination is indicated when compression of spinal or posterior fossa neural structure or nerve roots is suspected. The test is usually requested when surgical treatment for a ruptured vertebral disk or release of stenosis is considered. Persons who are candidates for testing are those with unrelieved back pain, pain radiating down the leg, those with absent ankle and knee reflexes, claudication of neurospinal origin, and persons with past history of cancer who lose leg and bladder control.

Three types of myelograms are done: positive contrasts using water-soluble iodine, iodized oil, and negative air contrast. The water-soluble contrast is the commonly used substance for myelograms. Both water and air contrast are followed by CT scanning that improves visualization. In low dose myelograms, a very small amount of water contrast is injected, followed immediately by scanning. An air myelogram is often a last resort examination and is also the test of choice for persons who are too large for the conventional CT myelogram and for those in traction, because of unstable spinal fractures.

Procedure
1. The test is usually done in the x-ray department.
2. The puncture area is shaved if necessary.
3. The patient is positioned lying on his abdomen during the procedure.
4. The procedure is the same as for lumbar puncture (see Chapter 5, page 220), except for the added procedure of injection of the contrast substance and fluoroscopic x-ray films; with water-soluble contrast, a narrow-bone needle (22 gauge) may be used. A lumbar puncture is done when lumbar pathology is suspected and a cervical puncture for cervical pathology so that there will be a higher concentration of contrast in the area of interest. In children, the lumbar puncture level is much lower than in adults to avoid the risk of puncturing the spinal cord. Depending on the specific contrast used, the substance may be removed (oil) or left to be absorbed by the body (water or air).
5. The table is tilted during the procedure. A shoulder and foot brace help to maintain correct position.
6. Total examining time is 30 to 90 minutes.

Clinical Implications
Abnormal results will reveal distortion of the outline of the subarachnoid space indicating

1. Ruptured intervertebral disk
2. Compression and stenosis of spinal cord
3. Exact level of intravertebral tumors
4. Obstruction of spinal canal
5. Avulsion of nerve roots

Patient Preparation
1. Explain the purpose, procedure, benefits, and risks of the test. Disadvantages of water and air contrast include poor visualization, and, in air contrast, painful headache because of difficulty in controlling gas as it is introduced. Disadvantages of oil contrast studies are irritation of tissues and poor absorption of the oil on subarachnoid space. This oily substance is still visible in x-ray examination up to one year following the original examination. About 1 in 20 examinations uses oil; air is rarely used.
2. A legal consent form must be signed by the patient before the test may be administered.

3. Explain that the examination table may be tilted during the test, but that the patient is securely fastened and will not fall off the table.
4. Advise the patient that clear liquid intake is encouraged to lower any incidence of headache post-test. If the test is scheduled close to a meal time, there may be a food restriction.
5. There is usually minimal discomfort associated with the myelogram itself. However, if the patient has trouble moving, a pain reliever may be ordered to make it easier for positioning and movement during the test.

Patient Aftercare
1. Bedrest is necessary for several hours after the test. If water-soluble contrast is used, the head of the bed is kept elevated at 45° for 8 to 24 hours and the patient is advised to lie quietly. This position will reduce the rate of upward dispersion of the medium and keep contrast out of the head where it can cause headache. If oil contrast is used, the patient will usually be prone for 2 to 4 hours, then on his back for 2 to 4 hours. If all the oil contrast has not been withdrawn, the head will be elevated to prevent the substance from flowing into the brain.
2. Fluid intake is encouraged to hasten absorption of any retained contrast media, to replace cerebrospinal fluid (CSF), and to reduce chance of headache.
3. Check for bladder distention and the ability to void adequately, especially if metrizamide has been used.
4. Check vital signs every 4 hours for at least 24 hours after the examination.

Clinical Alert

1. Observe the patient for possible complications including nausea, headache, fever, seizure, paralysis, arachnoiditis (inflammation of the coverings of the spinal cord), drowsiness, stupor, stiffness of the neck, sterile meningitis reaction (severe headache and symptoms of arachnoiditis, slow wave patterns on EEGs).
2. Manipulation of CSF pressure may cause an acute exacerbation of symptoms, which may require immediate surgical intervention. No lumbar punctures should be done unless really needed.
3. This test is to be avoided unless there is strong and sufficient reason to suspect a lesion. Multiple sclerosis, for example, may be worsened by the procedure.

4. Be certain to determine whether water-soluble oil or air contrast is used in the procedure, because aftercare interventions will differ.
5. If nausea or vomiting occurs after a water-soluble contrast has been used, do not administer phenothiazine antinauseants such as Compazine.

Magnetic Resonance Imaging (MR, MRI, NMR)

Normal Values
Normal relaxation times, spin densities, and flow velocities, pulse and spin echo frequencies. Rapid blood flow annihilates signals. Relaxation times are age dependent and probably reflect tissue dehydration of aging. These parameters are different for every type of tissue.

Explanation of Test
This noninvasive method of fluid-filled soft tissue study, as well as the study of structural dynamics of molecules, produces cross-sectional images of the anatomy by placing patients in strong magnetic fields and bombarding them with radio waves. This causes the hydrogen atoms to emit their own signals, which are converted to computerized images. These images are based on body water content. The hydrogen atom is most commonly measured in these studies because it is the most abundant atom on the human body and has the highest sensitivity to nuclear resonance. We know of course that water is composed of hydrogen and oxygen and that human tissue is about 70% H_2O (see Table 10-5).

This technique is used primarily to study the condition of blood vessels and determine blood flow, body imagery to differentiate diseased tissue from healthy tissue, and proton basic spectroscopy to eval-

Table 10-5
Major Measurement Parameters of Magnetic Resonance Imaging*

	Related to
Proton relaxation time	Water and iron concentrations
Nuclear density	Intracellular sodium concentrations
Chemical shifts	Currents of specific molecular constituents
Flow and perfusion	Physiological movements with a specific manner of signals

* Local coils are in use that improve the resolution to very restricted areas of the body, such as the knee and spine.

uate pyruvate, phosphate, water, fat, and lactic acid metabolism. These studies are helpful in detecting ischemia and infarctions, location of thrombi, follow-up of antineoplastic agents, viability of transplants, and to differentiate benign from malignant masses and degenerative brain diseases from psychiatric disorders. It has superior value in imaging the central nervous system, especially the brain.

Procedure
There are two procedures in common use: blood flow and body imaging.

Blood Flow in Extremities
1. The patient will be lying down or sitting during the test and will be as motionless as possible.
2. The limb to be examined is extended and rests in a cradlelike support. Prior to testing, a finger plethysnograph is applied. Reference sites are marked: the ankle or knee for a leg; the wrist or elbow for the arm.
3. The examination table rotates to accommodate upper and lower extremities. The patient's limb is moved into and out of the flow cylinder during each extremity study.
4. If both leg and arm studies are to be performed, the leg study will be done first.
5. Flow data are computed and projected in a graphics monitor and can be stored for evaluation at another time. Completed data reveal critical flow rates and waveform information for selected arteries of an extremity at a given cross-section.
6. Total examining time is 15 minutes for upper and 15 minutes for lower limbs.

Procedure for Body Imagery
1. The patient lies down on a narrow pallet that slides in and out of the cylindrical magnetic core. The super conducting magnet circles around the body, causing the hydrogen nuclei in the body to align themselves to the magnetic field.
2. If a head scan is done, a clear plastic cylinder containing antenna is placed around the head.
3. A monotonous clanging noise produced by the machine can be heard by the patient.
4. It is necessary for the patient to be completely still during imaging.
5. Total examining time is 60 to 90 minutes.

Interfering Factors
Respiratory motion causes severe artifacts in abdominal and thoracic imaging.

Clinical Implications

Changes in the waveforms, signal intensity and spectral peaks are associated with

1. Coronary occlusion
2. Myocardial infarction
3. Ischemia of cardiac and skeletal muscle and bone
4. Significant atherosclerosis
5. Brain iron deposits in neurodegenerative disease
6. Tumors
7. Anaerobic metabolism
8. Infection sites
9. Changes in blood fats

Clinical Alert

1. Contraindications to examination are pacemakers, surgical clips, metallic implants, neuro- or musculoskeletal stimulators, and patients on life support equipment and infusion pumps.
2. Patients who are critically ill or medically unstable are not candidates for upper body or whole body scanning because it is impossible to monitor cardiac rhythm and other signs inside the scanner.
3. Pregnancy is a contraindication because the long-term effects of magnetization are not known at this time.

Patient Preparation

1. Explain the purpose, procedure, and risks. Major potential risks are tissue heating and heating of metallic prosthetic implants from absorption of energy. No adverse effects have been reported and the standard examination does not require contrast and there is no radiation risk. No discomfort is felt during the test. A tingling sensation may be felt in metal fillings.
2. Assess for contraindications to testing and obtain a relevant history regarding implanted heart valves, surgical and aneurysm clips, and internal orthopedic screws and rods.
3. Help the patient to remove anything metal, such as dental bridges and appliances, credit cards, keys, hairclips, shoes, belts, jewelry, or clothing with metal fasteners.
4. Those who are to have body imagery may experience a closed-in feeling that can be avoided if the patient keeps his eyes closed during the entire test. Explain to these persons that it is better not to eat a large meal at least one hour before testing to reduce physiological demands in the body and possible emesis that could occur in claustrophobic persons.

5. Patients who are having blood flow testing should abstain from alcohol, caffeine, and iron prescription drugs to avoid unexpected vasoconstriction or dilatation. No smoking should be permitted before the test.
6. The patient should be helped to relax and remain as motionless as possible during testing.

After Care

No special after care is needed.

BIBLIOGRAPHY

Alteresm KB: What about special procedures. Am J Nurs 1363–1367, December 1985

Ballinger PW: Merrill's Atlas of Roentgenographic Positions and Standard Radiologic Procedures, 6th ed. St. Louis, CV Mosby, 1985

Boteler J: Digital radiography. Diagn Imagery 51(5):18–20, 1982

Douglas E et al: Digital Subtraction Angiography of the Heart and Lungs. Orlando, Grune & Stratten, 1981

Federle M: Computed Tomography in the Evaluation of Trauma, 2nd ed. Baltimore, Williams & Wilkins, 1981

Felson B: The chest roentgenologic workup: What and why? Respir Care 25(9):955–959, 1980

Greenfield GB: Radiology of Bone Diseases, 4th ed. Philadelphia, JB Lippincott, 1986

Griffiths HS, Sarno RC: Contemporary Radiology: An Introduction to Imaging. Philadelphia, WB Saunders, 1979

Grossman ZD et al: The Clinician's Guide to Diagnostic Imaging. New York, Raven Press, 1983

Gyll C, Black NS: Pediatric Diagnostic Imaging. New York, John Wiley & Sons, 1986

Heiken JP: Manual of Clinical Magnetic Resonance. New York, Raven Press, 1986

Hoffman DA et al: Effects of Imaging Radiation on the Developing Embryo and Fetus: A Review. HHS Publication No. (FDA 81-8170), Washington, DC, U.S. Government Printing Office, 1981

Kereiackes JB, Rosenstein M: Handbook of Radiation Doses in Nuclear Medicine and Diagnostic X-Ray. Boca Raton, FL, CRC Press, 1980

Kreel L, Paris A (eds): Clark's Positioning in Radiography, Vol 2. Chicago, Year Book Medical Pub, 1981

Levy JM et al: Digital subtraction angiography. Diagn Imaging (3):423–28, 1982

Marshall V et al: Diaphanography as a means of detecting breast cancer. Radiology 150(2):339–343, 1984

McIntosh DMF: Breast light scanning. J Can Assoc Radiol 34:258–289, December, 1983

Meschan I: Synopsis of Radiologic Anatomy with Computed Tomography. Philadelphia, WB Saunders, 1980

Milbrath JR et al: Mammography. Tumor Imaging 115–129, 1982

Seeram E: Computed Tomography Technology. Philadelphia, WB Saunders, 1982

Van Breda A, Katzen B: Digital Subtraction Angiography: Practical Aspects. Thorofare, NJ, Charles B. Slack, 1986

Whitehouse WM (ed): Diagnostic Radiology. Chicago, Year Book Medical Pub, 1982

CYTOLOGY AND GENETIC STUDIES

11

CYTOLOGY STUDIES

Introduction

Cytologic Study

Exfoliated cells in body tissues and fluid are studied to (1) count the cells, (2) determine the type of cells present, and (3) detect and diagnose malignant and premalignant conditions. The staining technique developed by Dr. George N. Papanicolaou has been especially useful in diagnosis of malignancy and is now routinely used in the cytologic study of the female genital tract, as well as in many types of nongynecologic specimens.

Some cytologic specimens (*e.g.*, smears of the mouth, genital tract, and nipple discharge) are relatively easy to obtain for study. Other samples are from less accessible sources (*e.g.*, amniotic fluid, pleural effusions, and cerebrospinal fluid), and special techniques such as fine needle aspiration (see page 647), are required for collection. Tissue samples obtained in surgery are also examined, and skin biopsies for fibroblast culture are done. In all studies, the source of the sample and its method of collection must be noted so that the evaluation can be based on complete information.

Specimens for cytologic study are usually composed of many different cells. Some are normally present, while others indicate pathologic conditions. Under certain conditions, cells normally observed in one sample may be indicative of an abnormal state when observed elsewhere. All specimens are examined for the number of cells, cell distribution, surface modification, size, shape, appearance and staining properties, functional adaptations, and inclusions. The cell nucleus is also examined. Any increases or decreases from normal values are noted.

Gynecologic specimens are smeared and fixed in 95% alcohol. (Some types of spray fixative are also available.) Nongynecologic specimens are generally collected without preservative, and they must be handled carefully to prevent drying or degeneration. Check with your individual laboratory for collection requirements. It is important for all cytology specimens to be sent to the laboratory as soon as they are obtained to prevent disintegration of cells or any other process that could cause alteration of the material for study.

Clinical Alert

1. The test is only as good as the specimen received.
2. Specimens collected from patients in isolation should be clearly labelled on the specimen container and requisition

form with appropriate warning stickers. The specimen container should then be placed in two protective bags before transporting it to the laboratory.

In practice, cytologic studies will be commonly reported as

1. Inflammatory
2. Benign
3. Atypical

4. Suspicious for malignancy
5. Positive for malignancy (*in situ* versus invasive)

Histology
Material submitted for tissue examination may be classified according to the histologic or cellular characteristics. A basic method for classifying cancer according to the histologic or cellular characteristics of the tumor is Broder's classification of malignancy.

Grade I   Tumors showing a marked tendency to differentiate; 75% or more of cells differentiated
Grade II   75%–50% of cells differentiated, slight to moderate dysplasia and metaplasia
Grade III   50%–25% of cells differentiated, marked dysplasia, marked atypical, and cancer *in situ*
Grade IV   25%–0% of cells differentiated

The TNM system is a method of identifying tumor stages according to spread of the disease. This system evolved from the work of the International Union Against Cancer and the American Joint Committee on Cancer. In addition, the TNM system further defines each specific type of cancer, such as breast, head, or neck. This staging system (on pages 648 and 649) is employed for previously untreated and treated cancers and classifies the primary site of cancer and its extent and involvement, such as lymphatic and venous invasion.

Cytologic Study of Fine Needle Aspiration

Normal Values
Negative. No abnormal cells present.

Explanation of Test
Fine needle aspiration is a method of cytologic study that is gaining recognition as a method for obtaining diagnostic material with a minimal amount of trauma to the patient. Bacteriologic studies may also be done on material obtained during fine needle aspiration. Unfixed material, either left in the syringe or on a needle rinsed in sterile saline, may be taken to the microbiology department for study.

TNM System

Three capital letters are used to describe the extent of the cancer:

T   Primary tumor
N   Regional lymph nodes
M   Distant metastasis

Chronology of Classification

c   Clinical-diagnostic
p   Postsurgical treatment—pathologic
s   Surgical-evaluative
r   Retreatment
a   Autopsy

This classification is extended by the following designations:

T Subclasses (Extent of Primary Tumor)

TX	Tumor cannot be adequately assessed
T0	No evidence of primary tumor
Tis	Carcinoma *in situ*
T1, T2, T3, T4	Progressive increase in tumor size and involvement

N Subclasses (Involvement of Regional Lymph Nodes)

NX	Regional lymph nodes cannot be assessed clinically
N0	Regional lymph nodes demonstrably abnormal
N1, N2, N3, N4	Increasing degrees of demonstrable abnormality of regional lymph nodes

Histopathology

GX   Grade cannot be assessed
G1   Well-differentiated grade
G2   Moderately well differentiated grade
G3, G4   Poorly to very poorly differentiated grade

Metastasis

MX   The minimum requirements to assess the presence of distant metastasis cannot be met
M0   No evidence of distant metastasis
M1   Distant metastasis present
     Specify sites of metastasis_____

(Continued)

TNM System (Continued)

The category M1 may be subdivided according to the following notations:

Pulmonary	PUL	Bone marrow	MAR
Osseous	OSS	Pleura	PLE
Hepatic	HEP	Skin	SKI
Brain	BRA	Eye	EYE
Lymph nodes	LYM	Other	OTH

In certain sites further information regarding the primary tumor may be recorded under the following headings:

Lymphatic Invasion (L)

LX   Lymphatic invasion cannot be assessed
L0   No evidence of lymphatic invasion
L1   Evidence of invasion of superficial lymphatics
L2   Evidence of invasion of deep lymphatics

Venous Invasion (V)

VX   Venous invasion cannot be assessed
V0   Veins do not contain tumor
V1   Efferent veins contain tumor
V2   Distant veins contain tumor

Residual Tumor (R)

This information does not enter into establishing the stage of the tumor but should be recorded for use in considering additive therapy. When the cancer is treated by definitive surgical procedures, residual cancer, if any, is recorded.

Residual Tumor Following Surgical Treatment

R0   No residual tumor
R1   Microscopic residual tumor
R2   Macroscopic residual tumor
       Specify _____

(Adapted from Beahrs OH, Myers MH [eds]: Manual for Staging of Cancer, 2nd ed. Philadelphia, JB Lippincott, 1983)

Procedure

1. Superficial or palpable lesions may be aspirated without radiologic aid, but nonpalpable lesions are aspirated with radiographic aid in placement of the needle.
2. After the needle is properly positioned, the plunger of the syringe is retracted to create negative pressure. The needle is moved up and down, and sometimes at several different angles. The plunger of the syringe is released and the needle is removed.
3. The material obtained is expressed onto slides that are then smeared together and fixed immediately. The needle may be rinsed in sterile saline or 50% alcohol for further studies.

Clinical Implications

Abnormal results are helpful in identifying

1. Infectious processes. The infectious agent may be seen or characteristic cellular changes may indicate the infectious agent that is present.
2. Benign conditions. Some characteristic cellular changes may be present, indicating the presence of a benign process.
3. Malignant conditions, either primary or metastatic. If the disease is metastatic, the findings may be reported out as consistent with the primary malignancy.

Patient Preparation

Explain the purpose and procedure, benefits, and risks.

Patient Aftercare

Assess the patient for signs of inflammation and use site care infection control measures. Pain may be common in sensitive areas such as the breast, nipple, and scrotum.

Clinical Alert

1. Traumatic complications are rare. Fine needle aspiration of the lung infrequently results in pneumothorax. Local extension of the malignancy is a consideration, but studies have shown this to be an extremely rare occurrence.
2. A negative finding on a fine needle aspirate does not rule out the possibility that a malignancy is present. The cells aspirated may have been from a necrotic area of the tumor, or a benign area adjacent to the tumor.

Cytologic Study of the Respiratory Tract

(See also Chapter 7, under "Respiratory Tract Cultures.")

Normal Values
Negative

Background
The lungs and the passages that conduct air to and from the lungs form the respiratory tract, which is divided into the upper and lower respiratory tracts. The upper respiratory tract consists of the nasal cavities, the nasopharynx, and the larynx; the lower respiratory tract consists of the trachea and the lungs. Cytologic studies of sputum and bronchial specimens are quite important as diagnostic aids because of the frequency of cancer of the lung and the relative inaccessibility of this organ. Also detectable are cell changes that may be related to the future development of malignant conditions and to inflammatory conditions.

Sputum is composed of mucus and cells. It is the secretion of the bronchi, lungs, and trachea and is therefore obtained from the lower respiratory tract (bronchi and lungs). Sputum is ejected through the mouth but originates in the lower respiratory tract. Saliva produced by the salivary glands in the mouth is *not* sputum. A specimen can be correctly identified as sputum in microscopic examination by the presence of dust cells (carbon dust-laden macrophages). Although the glands and secretory cells in the mucous lining of the lower respiratory tract produce up to 100 ml. of fluid daily, the healthy person does not cough up sputum.

Procedure

For Obtaining Sputum
1. The preferred material is an early-morning specimen. Three specimens are usually collected on three separate days.
2. The patient must inhale air to the full capacity of the lungs and then exhale the air with an expulsive deep cough.
3. The specimen should be coughed directly into a wide-mouthed clean container containing 50% alcohol. (Some cytology laboratories prefer the specimen to be fresh if it will be delivered to the laboratory immediately.)
4. The specimen should be covered with a tight-fitting sterile lid.
5. The specimen should be labeled with the patient's name, age, date, diagnosis, and number of specimens (1, 2, or 3) and sent immediately to the laboratory.

For Obtaining Bronchial Secretions
1. Bronchial secretions are obtained during bronchoscopy (see Chapter 12). Bronchoscopy involves removal of bronchial secretions and tissue for cytologic and microbiologic studies.

For Obtaining Bronchial Brushings
Bronchial brushings are obtained during bronchoscopy. The material collected can be smeared directly on all-frosted slides and immediately fixed, or the actual brush may be placed in a container of 50% ethyl alcohol or saline (check with the laboratory for their preference) and delivered to the cytology laboratory.

Bronchopulmonary Lavage
Bronchopulmonary lavage may be used to evaluate patients with interstitial lung disease. Saline is injected into the distal portions of the lung and aspirated back through the bronchoscope into a specimen container. This essentially "washes out" the alveoli. The fresh specimen should be brought directly to the laboratory. A total cell count and a differential cell count are performed to determine the relative numbers of macrophages, neutrophils, and lymphocytes.

Patient Preparation
1. Explain the purpose and procedure of the test.
2. Emphasize that sputum is not saliva.
3. Advise the patient to brush his teeth and rinse his mouth well before obtaining the specimen to avoid introduction of saliva into the specimen.

Clinical Implications
Abnormalities in sputum and bronchial specimens may sometimes be helpful in detecting

1. Benign atypical changes in sputum as in
   (a) Inflammatory diseases
   (b) Asthma (Creola bodies, Curschmann's spirals and eosinophils may be found, but they are not diagnostic of the disease.)
   (c) Lipid pneumonia (Lipophages may be found, but they are not diagnostic of the disease.)
   (d) Asbestosis (ferruginous or asbestos bodies)
   (e) Viral diseases
   (f) Benign diseases of lung such as bronchiectasis, atelectasis, emphysema, and pulmonary infarcts
2. Metaplasia, which is the substitution of one adult cell type for another. Severe metaplastic changes are found in patients with
   (a) History of chronic cigarette smoking

(b) Pneumonitis
(c) Pulmonary infarcts
(d) Bronchiectasis
(e) Healing abscess
(f) Tuberculosis
(g) Emphysema
(Metaplasia often adjoins a carcinoma or a carcinoma *in situ.*)
3. Viral changes and the presence of virocytes (viral inclusions may be seen), as in
   (a) Viral pneumonia
   (b) Acute respiratory disease caused by adenovirus
   (c) Herpes simplex
   (d) Measles
   (e) Cytomegalic inclusion disease
   (f) Varicella
4. Degenerative changes, as seen in viral diseases of the lung
5. Fungal and parasitic diseases (in parasitic diseases, ova or parasite may be seen)
6. Tumor (benign and malignant)

Interfering Factors
False negatives may be due to

1. Delays in preparation of the specimen, causing a deterioration of tumor cells
2. Sampling error (Diagnostic cells may not have exfoliated into the material examined.)

Note: Incidence of false negatives is about 15%, in contrast to about 1% in studies for cervical cancer. This high incidence occurs even with careful examination of multiple deep cough specimens.

Cytologic Study of the Gastrointestinal Tract

Normal Values
Negative. Squamous epithelial cells of the esophagus may be present.

Explanation of Test
Exfoliative cytology of the gastrointestinal tract is useful in diagnosis of benign and malignant diseases. However, it is not a specific test for these diseases. Many benign diseases, such as leukoplakia of the esophagus, esophagitis, gastritis, pernicious anemia, and granulomatous diseases, may be recognized because of their characteristic cellular changes. Response to radiation may also be noted from cytologic studies.

Procedure

1. For esophageal studies, a nasogastric Levin tube is passed approximately 40 cm. (to the cardioesophageal junction) with the patient in a sitting position.
2. For stomach studies, a Levin tube is passed into the stomach (approximately 60 cm.) with the patient in a sitting position.
3. For pancreatic and gallbladder drainage, a special double lumen gastric tube is passed orally to 45 cm., with the patient in a sitting position. Then the patient is placed on his right side and the tube is passed slowly to 85 cm. It takes about 20 minutes for the tube to reach this distance. Tube location is confirmed by biopsy. Lavage with physiologic salt solution is done during all upper GI cytology procedures.
4. Specimens can also be obtained during endoscopy procedures.
5. During endoscopy, cytologic brushings may be taken of suspicious areas. The material obtained may be smeared on a slide and immediately fixed, or the brush may be placed in a specimen cup containing 50% alcohol or saline (check with the cytology laboratory for their preference) and taken to the laboratory for processing.

Patient Preparation

1. The patient should be told the purpose of the test, the nature of the procedure, and to anticipate some discomfort from the procedure.
2. A liquid diet is usually ordered 24 hours before testing. The patient is encouraged to take fluids throughout the night and in the morning before the test.
3. No oral barium should be administered for the preceding 24 hours.
4. Laxatives and enemas are ordered for colon cytology studies.
5. Since insertion of the nasogastric tube can cause considerable discomfort, the patient and clinician should devise a system (e.g., raising a hand) to indicate discomfort.
6. The patient should be informed that panting, mouth-breathing, or swallowing can help to ease the insertion of the tube.
7. Sucking on ice chips or sipping through a straw also makes insertion of the tube easier.

Clinical Alert

Immediately remove the tube if the patient shows signs of distress: coughing, gasping, or cyanosis.

Patient Aftercare
1. The patient should be given food, fluids, and rest after the tests are completed.
2. Provide rest. Patients having colon studies will be feeling quite tired.

Clinical Implications
1. The characteristics of benign and malignant cells of the gastrointestinal tract are the same as for cells of the rest of the body.
2. Abnormal results in cytologic studies of the esophagus may be a nonspecific aid in the diagnosis of
   (a) Acute esophagitis, characterized by increased exfoliation of basal cells with inflammatory cells and polymorphonuclear leukocytes in the cytoplasm of the benign squamous cells
   (b) Vitamin B_{12} and folic acid deficiencies, characterized by giant epithelial cells
   (c) Malignant diseases characterized by typical cells of esophageal malignancy
3. Abnormal results in studies of the stomach may be a nonspecific aid in the diagnosis of
   (a) Pernicious anemia characterized by giant epithelial cells. An injection of vitamin B_{12} will cause these cells to disappear within 24 hours.
   (b) Granulomatous inflammations seen in chronic gastritis and sarcoid of the stomach, which are characterized by granulomatous cells
   (c) Gastritis, characterized by degenerative changes and an increase in the exfoliation of clusters of surface epithelial cells
   (d) Malignant diseases, most of which are gastric adenocarcinomas. Lymphoma cells can be differentiated from adenocarcinoma. The Reed–Sternberg cell, a multinucleated giant cell, is the characteristic cell found along with abnormal lymphocytes in Hodgkin's disease.
4. Abnormal results in studies of the pancreas, gallbladder, and duodenum may reveal
   Malignant cells (usually adenocarcinoma), but it is sometimes difficult to determine the exact site of the tumor
5. Abnormal results in examination of the colon may reveal
   (a) Ileitis, characterized by large multinucleated histocytes (bovine tuberculosis commonly manifests itself in this area)
   (b) Ulcerative colitis, characterized by a hyperchromatic nuclei surrounded by a thin cytoplasmic rim
   (c) Malignant cells (usually adenocarcinoma)

Interfering Factors
The barium and lubricant used in Levin tubes will interfere with good results, because their presence will distort the cells and prevent accurate evaluation.

Cytologic Study of the Female Genital Tract
(Papanicolaou Smear)

Normal Values
Normal: no abnormal cells
Maturation Index (MI): The MI is a ratio of parabasal to intermediate to superficial cells. The following are representative ratios:

Normal child	80/20/0
Preovulatory adult	0/40/60
Premenstrual adult	0/70/30
Pregnant adult (2nd mo.)	0/90/10
Postmenopausal adult (age 60)	65/30/5

Explanation of Test
The Papanicolaou (Pap) smear is used principally for diagnosis of precancerous and cancerous conditions of the genital tract, which includes the vagina, cervix, and endometrium. This test is also used for hormonal assessment and for diagnosis of inflammatory diseases. Because the Pap smear is of great importance in the early detection of cervical cancer, it is recommended that all women over the age of 20 have the test at least once a year.

The value of the Pap smear depends on the fact that cells readily exfoliate (or can be easily stripped) from genital cancers. Cytologic study can also be used for assessing response to the effect of administered sex hormones. It should be noted that the microbiologic examination on cytology samples is not as accurate as bacterial culture, but it can provide valuable information.

Specimens for cytologic examination of the genital tract are usually obtained by vaginal speculum examination or by colposcopy with biopsy. Material from the cervix, endocervix, and posterior fornix is obtained for most smears. Smears for hormonal evaluation are obtained from the vagina.

All Pap smears are usually reported on a five-point scale. The meaning of the classes varies, however, and is not universally agreed upon. The following is the scale:

1. Absence of atypical or abnormal cells, negative
2. Atypical cytology, dysplastic, borderline but not neoplastic
3. Cytology suggestive of but not inclusive of malignancy (*suspect* is term often used)

4. Cytology strongly suggestive of malignancy or strongly suspect
5. Cytology conclusive of malignancy, cancer cells present

Clinical Alert

It is important to remember that cytologic findings alone do not form the basis of a diagnosis of cancer or other diseases. Often they are used to justify further procedures, such as biopsy.

Cells are also examined for hormonal effect and organisms. Cells examined for hormonal effect may be reported on a six-point scale.

1. Marked estrogen effect
2. Moderate estrogen effect
3. Slight estrogen effect
4. Atrophic
5. Compatible with pregnancy
6. No evaluation—specimen too bloody or inflamed or scanty

Cells can also be examined for microorganisms using routine staining techniques. These cells may be reported on a five-point scale.

1. Normal flora
2. Scanty or absent
3. *Trichomonas*
4. *Monilia*
5. Other (cocci, coccobacilli, mixed bacteria)

Background
Characteristic physiologic cellular changes occur in the genital tract from birth through the postmenopausal years. Hormonal evaluation by cytologic examination should be performed only on vaginal smears taken from the lateral vaginal wall or from the vaginal fornix. Smears from the ectocervix or endocervix cannot be used for hormonal evaluation because certain conditions, such as metaplasia and cervicitis, interfere with a correct assessment. There are three major cell types occurring in a characteristic pattern in vaginal smears.

1. Superficial squamous cells (mature squamous, usually polygonal, containing a pyknotic nucleus)
2. Intermediate squamous cells (mature squamous, usually polygonal, containing a clearly structured vesicular nucleus, which may be either well preserved or peptolytically changed as a result of bacterial cytolysis)
3. Parabasal cells (immature squamous, usually round or oval, containing one or, rarely, more than one relatively large nucleus. These

cells occur either well preserved or in proteolytic clusters as a result of degeneration or necrosis).

Note: Deviation from physiologic cell patterns may be indicative of pathologic conditions.

Hormonal cytology is valuable in the assessment of many endocrine-related conditions, especially ovarian function.

Procedure

1. The patient is usually asked to remove clothing from the waist down.
2. The patient is placed in a lithotomy position on an examining table.
3. A speculum lubricated only with water is inserted into the vagina to expose the cervix.
4. The posterior fornix and external os of the cervix are scraped with a wooden spatula and obtained material is spread on slides and placed in preservative or fixative.
5. Label the specimen with name, date, woman's age, reason for examination, last menstrual period, and area from which specimen is obtained.
6. Examination takes only about 5 minutes.

Note: The best time to take a Pap smear is 5 to 6 days after the end of the menstrual period.

Procedure for Hormonal Smears, "Maturation Index"
Obtain a specimen by scraping the proximal portion of the lateral wall of the vagina, avoiding the cervical area. Otherwise the same as above.

Clinical Implications

1. Abnormal cytology responses can be classified as protective, destructive, reparative (regenerative), or neoplastic.
2. Inflammatory reactions and microbes can be identified to help in the diagnosis of vaginal diseases.
3. Precancerous and cancerous lesions of the cervix can be identified. The stages of neoplastic disease can be arbitrarily classified as dysplasia (mild, moderate, and severe), carcinoma *in situ* (preinvasive carcinoma), microinvasive carcinoma, and invasive carcinoma.
4. Hormonal cytology reports will include several factors.
   (a) Hormonal cell pattern: The report will state that the pattern is, or is not, compatible with the age and menstrual history of the patient. The reason for noncompatibility is given.
   (b) Maturation Index (MI): MI is a proportion of the major cell types (parabasal, intermediate, and superficial) in each 100 cells counted. The MI will be expressed as a ratio (*e.g.*, MI = 100/0/0). See "Normal Values" for representative MI's.
5. The following facts should be kept in mind when hormonal cytology reports are reviewed (see Table 11-1).

degrees of estrogenic effects or estrogen deficiencies, since more than one hormonal stimulus is involved (estrogen, progesterone, and adrenal hormones).

(b) Surgical removal of the ovaries does not necessarily result in epithelial atrophy.

(c) Only two cell types can be identified with accuracy if the age and menstrual history of the patient are not known.

Table 11-1
Vaginal Cytologic Smear Findings in Gynecologic and Related Endocrinopathies

Condition	Usual Smear Types
Adrenal hyperplasia, congenital	Atrophic to atypical intermediate proliferation
Adrenogenital syndrome (hyperplasia)	Atrophic to atypical intermediate proliferation
Adrenal tumor (masculinizing)	Usually atrophic; sometimes "multihormonal" with cells from all layers
Chiari–Frommel syndrome	Markedly atrophic
Cushing's syndrome	Intermediate proliferation or atypical regressive types
Eunuchoidism, ovarian	Atrophic
Feminizing testicular syndrome	Proliferative; nuclear sex chromatin negative
Follicular cytosis	Persistently high estrogen index (EI) and karyopyknotic index (KI)
Gonadal dysgenesis	Atrophic; nuclear sex chromatin negative in 80%
Hirsutism, genetic	Normal cycling
Hypothalamic (psychogenic) amenorrhea	Most often atrophic to slight proliferation but great variation from atrophic to highly proliferative
Menopausal syndrome	At first highly proliferative, some with cycling; later, intermediate proliferation or atrophic
Ovarian tumors, feminizing	Proliferative, some with high EI and KI, occasionally regressive
Ovarian tumors, masculinizing	Variation, many atrophic, some with atypical proliferation or "multihormonal"
Precocious puberty, constitutional	Proliferative, some with high EI and KI, some with cycling
Pituitary hypogonadism	Atrophic to slight proliferation
Pseudocyesis	"Progestational" types with varying regression
Stein–Leventhal syndrome	Variation; most with intermediate proliferation, occasionally highly proliferative
Uterine defect (congenital absence or irresponsiveness)	Normal cycling

(Alter Rakoff AI: Hormonal cytology in gynecology. Clin Obstet Gynecol 4:1045–1061, 1961) In Keebler CM, Reagan JW (eds): Manual of Cytotechnology, 6th ed. Chicago, American Society of Clinical Pathologists, 1983

        (1) Abundant superficial squamous cells, indicative of unequiv-
        ocal estrogenic effect
        (2) Parabasal cells, indicative of lack of cell maturation due to
        lack of hormone stimulation
    (d) From a single specimen it is impossible to predict whether ovu-
    lation will occur, whether it has recently occurred, or what
    stage of menstrual cycle the patient is in. Serial specimens must
    be examined to obtain the above results.
    (e) An intermediate cell type is always intermediate, regardless of
    its size.
    (f) No hormonal assessment should be made without knowing the
    age of the patient, her menstrual history, and her history of
    hormone administrations.

Interfering Factors
1. Medications such as tetracycline and digitalis, which affect the
   squamous epithelium, will alter test results.
2. The use of lubricating jelly in the vagina and recent douching will
   interfere with test results by distorting the cells and preventing
   accurate evaluation.
3. The presence of infection will interfere with hormonal cytology.
4. Heavy menstrual flow may make the interpretation of the results
   difficult and may obscure atypical cells.

Patient Preparation
1. Explain the test purpose and procedure.
2. Instruct the patient not to douche for 2 to 3 days before the test
   because this may remove the exfoliated cells.
3. Have the patient empty her bladder and rectum prior to examination.
4. Ask the patient to give the following information:
   (a) First day of last menstrual period
   (b) Use of hormone therapy or birth control pills
   (c) All medications taken
   (d) Any radiation therapy
   This information must be sent to the laboratory along with specimens for cytology.

Cytologic Study of Aspirated Breast Cysts and Nipple Discharge

Normal Values
Negative for neoplasia

Background
Nipple discharge is normal only during the lactation period. Any other nipple discharge is abnormal and when it occurs, breasts should be examined for mastitis, duct papilloma, or intraductal cancer. Certain situations increase the possibility of finding a normal nipple discharge, such as pregnancy, perimenopause, and use of birth control pills. About 3% of breast cancers and 10% of benign lesions of the breast are associated with abnormal nipple discharge.

The contents of all breast cysts obtained by needle biopsy are examined to detect malignant cells.

Procedure
1. Breast cyst
   The contents of the identified breast cyst are obtained by percutaneous aspiration.
2. Nipple discharge

   Note: This procedure should be confined to patients who have no palpable masses in the breast or other evidence of breast cancer.

   (a) The nipple should be washed with a cotton pledget and patted dry.
   (b) The nipple is gently stripped, or milked, to obtain a discharge.
   (c) Fluid should be expressed until a pea-sized drop appears.
   (d) The patient may assist by holding a bottle of fixative beneath the breast so that the slide may be dropped in immediately.
   (e) The discharge is spread immediately on a slide and then dropped into the fixative bottle containing 95% alcohol.
   (f) The specimen is identified with pertinent data, including from which breast it was obtained.
   (g) The specimen is sent without delay to the laboratory.

Clinical Implications
Abnormal results are helpful in identifying
1. Benign breast conditions, such as mastitis and intraductal papilloma.
2. Malignant breast conditions, such as papilloma intraductal cancer or intracystic infiltrating cancer

Clinical Alert

Any discharge, regardless of color, should be examined. A bloody or blood-tinged discharge is especially significant.

Interfering Factors
Use of drugs that alter hormone balance, such as phenothiazines, digitalis, diuretics, and steroids, often results in a clear nipple discharge.

Cytologic Study of Urine

(See also Chapter 3, especially "Microscopic Examination of Sediment.")

Normal Values
Negative. Epithelial and squamous cells are normally present in urine.

Explanation of Test
Cells from the epithelial lining of the urinary tract exfoliate readily into the urine. Urine cytology is most useful in the diagnosis of cancer and inflammatory diseases of the bladder, the renal pelvis, the ureters, and the urethra. This study is also valuable in detecting cytomegalic inclusion disease and other viral diseases and in detecting bladder cancer in high-risk populations, such as workers exposed to aniline dyes, smokers, and patients previously treated for bladder cancer. A Papanicolaou stain of smears prepared from the urinary sediment, filter preparations, or cytocentrifuged smears are useful to identify abnormalities.

Procedure
1. Obtain a clean voided urine specimen of at least 180 ml. (adults) and 10 ml. (children).
2. Obtain a catheterized specimen, if possible, if cancer is suspected.
3. Deliver the specimen immediately to the cytology laboratory. Urine should be as fresh as possible when it is examined.

Clinical Implications
1. Findings possibly indicative of *inflammatory conditions* of the *lower urinary tract*
   (a) Epithelial hyperplasia
   (b) Atypical cells
   (c) Abundance of red blood cells
   (d) Leukocytes

   Note: Inflammatory conditions could be due to any of the following:

   (a) Benign prostatic hyperplasia
   (b) Adenocarcinoma of the prostate
   (c) Kidney stones
   (d) Diverticula of bladder
   (e) Strictures
   (f) Malformations

2. Findings indicative of viral diseases
   (a) Cytomegalic inclusion disease: large intranuclear inclusions

   Note: Cytomegalic inclusion disease is a viral infection that usually occurs in childhood but is also seen in cancer patients
   treated with chemotherapy and in transplant patients
   treated with immunosuppressives. The renal tubular epithelium is usually involved

   (1) Cytomegaloviruses or salivary gland viruses are related to
       the herpes varicella agents.
   (2) Infected people may excrete virus in the urine or saliva for
       months.
   (3) About 60% to 90% of adults have experienced infection.
   (4) In closed populations such as the mentally retarded or
       households, high infection rates may occur at an early age.
   (b) Measles: characteristic cytoplasmic inclusion bodies may be
       found in the urine preceding the appearance of Koplik's spots.
3. Findings possibly indicative of malacoplakia and granulomatous
   disease of the bladder or upper urinary tract
   (a) Histiocytes with multiple granules in an abundant, foamy cyto-
       plasm
   (b) Michaelis-Gutmann bodies in malacoplakia
4. Cytologic findings possibly indicative of malignancy
   If the specimen shows evidence of any of the changes associated
   with malignancy, cancer of the bladder, renal pelvis, ureters, kidney, and urethra may be suspected. Metastatic tumor should be
   ruled out as well.

Cytologic Study of Cerebrospinal Fluid (CSF)

Normal Values
1. Total cell count
   Adult: 0–10/cu. mm. (all mononuclear cells)
   Infant: 0–20/cu. mm.
2. Negative for neoplasia
3. A variety of normal cells may be seen. Large lymphocytes are most
   common; small lymphocytes are also seen, as are elements of the
   monocyte–macrophage series.
4. The CSF of a healthy person should be free of all pathogens.

Explanation of Test
Spinal fluid obtained by lumbar puncture is examined for the presence
of abnormal cells and for an increase or decrease in the normally
present cell population. Most of the usual laboratory procedures for

study of CSF involve an examination of the white cells and a white blood cell count; chemical and microbiological studies are also done. In recent years, cell studies of the CSF have been used to identify neoplastic cells. These studies have been especially helpful in the diagnosis and treatment of the different phases of leukemia disorders. The nature of neoplasia is such that for tumor cells to exfoliate, they must actually invade the CSF circulation and enter such areas as the ventricle wall, the choroid plexus, or the subarachnoid space.

Procedure
1. Usually, three specimens of at least 1 to 3 ml. are obtained by lumbar puncture (see Chapter 5, page 220).
2. Generally, only one specimen of 1 to 3 ml. goes to the cytology laboratory. Other tubes are sent to different laboratories for examination.
3. The specimen is labeled with the patient's name, date, and type of specimen.
4. The sample is sent immediately to the cytology laboratory for processing.

Clinical Alert

The laboratory should be given adequate warning that a CSF specimen will be delivered. Time is a critical factor; cells begin to disintegrate if the sample is kept at room temperature for more than 1 hour.

Clinical Implications
1. Cerebrospinal fluid abnormalities may be helpful in the detection of
   (a) Malignant gliomas that have invaded the ventricles or cortex of the brain. WBC $\leq$ 150/cu. mm. (The sample may be normal in 75% of patients.)
   (b) Ependymoma (neoplasm of differentiated ependymal cells) and medulloblastoma (a cerebellar tumor) in children
   (c) Seminoma and pineoblastoma (tumors of the pineal gland)
   (d) Secondary carcinomas
       (1) Secondary carcinomas metastasizing to the CNS have multiple avenues to the subarachnoid space through the bloodstream.
       (2) The breast and lung are common sources of metastatic cells exfoliated in the CSF. Infiltration of acute leukemia is also quite common.

(e) Central nervous system leukemia
(f) Fungal forms
    (1) Congenital toxoplasmosis
        WBC 50–500/cu. mm. (mostly monocytes present)
    (2) Coccidioidomycosis
        WBC 200/cu. mm.
(g) Various forms of meningitis
    (1) Cryptococcal meningitis
        WBC 800/cu. mm. (Lymphocytes are more abundant than polynuclear neutrophilic leukocytes.)
    (2) Tuberculous meningitis
        WBC 25–1000/cu. mm. (mostly lymphocytes present)
    (3) Acute pyogenic meningitis
        WBC 25–10,000/cu. mm. (mostly polynuclear neutrophilic leukocytes present)
(h) Meningoencephalitis (primary amebic meningoencephalitis)
    (1) WBC 400–21,000/cu. mm.
    (2) Red blood cells are also found.
    (3) Wright's stain may reveal amebas.
(i) Hemosiderin-laden macrophages, as in subarachnoid hemorrhage
(j) Kipophages from CNS destructive processes
2. Characteristics of neoplastic cells
    (a) Sometimes marked increase in size, most likely sarcoma and carcinomas
    (b) Exfoliated cells tend to be more polymorphic as the neoplasm becomes increasingly malignant.

Interfering Factors
The lumbar puncture can occasionally cause contamination of the specimen with squamous epithelial cells or spindly fibroblasts.

Cytologic Studies of Effusions

Normal Values
Negative for abnormal cells

Background
Effusions are accumulations of fluids. They may be exudates, which generally accumulate as a result of inflammation, or transudates, which are fluids not associated with inflammation. Below is a comparison of these two effusions.

Exudate
1. Accumulates in body cavities and tissues because of malignancy or inflammation
2. Associated with an inflammatory process
3. Viscous
4. High content of protein, cells, and solid materials derived from cells
5. May have high WBC content
6. Clots spontaneously (because of high concentration of fibrinogen)
7. Malignant cells as well as bacteria may be detected
8. Specific gravity >1.015

Transudate
1. Accumulates in body cavities from impaired circulation
2. Not associated with an inflammatory process
3. Highly fluid
4. Low content of protein, cells, or solid materials derived from cells
5. Has low WBC content
6. Will not clot
7. Malignant cells may be present
8. Specific gravity <1.015

Fluid contained in the pleural, pericardial, and peritoneal or abdominal cavities is a serous fluid. Accumulation of fluid in the peritoneal cavity is called *ascites*.

Explanation of Test
Cytologic studies of effusions—either exudates or transudates—are sometimes helpful in determining the cause of these abnormal collections of fluids. The effusions are found in the pericardial sac, the pleural cavities, and the abdominal cavities. *The chief problem in diagnosis is in differentiating malignant cells from reactive mesothelial cells.*

Procedure
Material for cytologic examination of effusions is obtained by either thoracentesis or paracentesis. Both of these procedures involve surgical puncture of a cavity for aspiration of a fluid.

Thoracentesis
1. Chest roentgenograms should be available at the patient's bedside so that the location of fluid may be determined.
2. The patient may be administered a sedative.
3. The chest is exposed. The physician inserts a long thoracentesis needle with a syringe attached.
4. At least 40 ml. of fluid is withdrawn. It is preferable to withdraw 300 ml. to 1000 ml of fluid.
5. The specimen is collected in a clean container and heparin may be added, particularly if the specimen is very bloody (5–10 units heparin per 1 ml. fluid). Alcohol should *not* be added.
6. The specimen should be labeled with the patient's name, date, source of the fluid, and diagnosis.

7. The covered specimen should be sent immediately to the laboratory. (If the specimen cannot be sent at once, it may be refrigerated.)

Paracentesis (Abdominal)
1. The patient should be asked to void.
2. The patient is placed in the Fowler's position.
3. A local anesthetic is given.
4. A #20 needle is introduced into the patient's abdomen and the fluid
is withdrawn, 50 ml. at a time, until 300 ml. to 1000 ml. is withdrawn.
5. Follow the same procedure as in #5, 6, and 7 of *Thoracentesis*,
above.

Clinical Alert

Paracentesis may precipitate hepatic coma in a patient with
chronic liver disease. The patient must be watched constantly for
indications of shock: pallor, cyanosis, or dizziness. Emergency
stimulants should be ready.

Clinical Implications
1. All effusions contain some mesothelial cells. (Mesothelial cells comprise the squamous layer of the epithelium covering the surface of
all serous membranes.) The more chronic and irritating the condition, the more numerous and atypical are the mesothelial cells.
Histiocytes and lymphocytes are common.
2. Evidence of abnormalities in serous fluids is characterized by
(a) Degenerating RBCs, granular red cell fragments, and histiocytes containing blood. Presence of these structures means that
injury to a vessel or vessels is part of the condition causing fluid
to accumulate.
(b) Mucin, which is suggestive of adenocarcinoma
(c) Large numbers of polymorphonuclear leukocytes, which is indicative of an acute inflammatory process such as peritonitis
(d) Prevalence of plasma cells, which suggests the possibility of
antibody formation
(e) Numerous eosinophils, which suggest parasitic infestation,
Hodgkin's disease, or a hypersensitive state
(f) Presence of many reactive mesothelial cells together with hemo-
siderin histiocytes, which may indicate
(1) Leaking aneurysm
(2) Rheumatoid arthritis
(3) Lupus erythematosus
(g) Malignant cells

3. Abnormal cells may be indicative of
   (a) Malignancy. The most important criterion of cancer is the arrangement of chromatin within the nuclei.
   (b) Inflammatory conditions

Interfering Factors
Vigorous shaking and stirring of specimens will cause altered results.

Patient Preparation
Explain the purpose of the test and procedure.

Cutaneous Immunofluorescence Biopsy

Normal Values
A descriptive interpretative report is made.

Explanation of Test
Biopsy of the skin for direct epidermal fluorescent studies is indicated in the investigation of certain disorders such as lupus erythematosus, blistering disease, and vasculitis. Skin biopsies are also used to confirm the histopathology of skin lesions to rule out other diagnoses and to follow the results of treatment.

Procedure
A 4-mm. punch biopsy specimen of involved or uninvolved skin is obtained.

Clinical Implications
Biopsy of skin will show

1. The lesions of discoid lupus erythematosus as a bandlike immunofluorescence of immunoglobulins and complement components. Similar findings in a biopsy of the normal skin are consistent with systemic lupus erythematosus and may be used to follow the results of treatment.
2. In blistering diseases such as pemphigus and pemphigoid, where circulating antibodies may not be present, a lesion may show intercellular epidermal antibody of pemphigus or basement membrane antibody of pemphigoid.

Estradiol Receptor and Progesterone Receptor in Breast Cancer (ERA, PRA)

Normal Values
Estradiol: Negative; ≤3 femtomoles/mg. of protein
Progesterone: Negative; ≤5 femtomoles/mg. of protein

Explanation of Test

Estrogen and progesterone receptors in the cells of breast cancer tissues are measured to determine whether or not a tumor is likely to respond to endocrine therapy or to the removal of the ovaries.

Procedure

A 1-g. specimen of quickly frozen tumor is examined for saturation and expressed in a Scatchard Plot.

Clinical Implications

1. Positive test for estrogen occurs at levels greater than 3 femtomoles and for progesterone binding at levels of 5 femtomoles and above.
2. Approximately 55% of estrogen receptor–*positive* tumors will respond to endocrine therapy.
3. Estrogen receptor–*negative* tumors rarely respond to endocrine therapy.
4. The finding of positive progesterone increases the predictive value of selecting patients for hormonal therapy. There is some incidence to suggest that progesterone receptor synthesis is estrogen dependent.

STUDIES OF INHERITED OR INBORN DISEASES

The diagnosis of inherited and inborn diseases includes chromosomal diseases such as Down syndrome and disorders such as inherited metabolic diseases, hemolytic disease, and neural tube effects.

Indications for Testing

1. Prenatal (See Chapter 16) to identify genetic and biochemical defects so that prenatal treatment can be initiated.
2. Test results are used as bases for genetic counseling. A determination about the nature of the birth defect must be precisely established. This is because environmentally produced defects may mimic genetic defects. An accurate family history (2 or more generations back) is obtained.

The usual body tissues used in genetic study are blood, amniotic fluid, bone marrow, skin, or buccal smears.

This chapter gives a very brief overview of chromosomal tests and tests for lysosomal storage disorders. Other disorders are discussed in hematology and prenatal studies.

Introduction

Chromosomes are the cellular constituents of heredity. Each chromosome possesses a large amount of deoxyribonucleic acid (DNA) and there are thousands of genes within each chromosome.

Among this vast number, a few are likely to be abnormal; thus, each of us carries some faulty genes. Most genetic diseases occur only if both parents transmit the same faulty gene; although some genetic diseases are caused by a single faulty gene. When a disease is caused by a faulty gene, there is always some risk that it will recur in a family, though the chance may be less than feared. On the other hand, genetic disease may be caused by a chromosome defect affecting a specific pregnancy. There usually is little risk that this type of genetic error will be transmitted to other children in the family or to succeeding generations, due to the nature of most chromosome errors.

Genetic defects may be transmitted in varying degrees of severity from generation to generation in one of four ways.

1. *Dominant Inheritance*
   An affected child usually has a parent with the same disorder. This affected parent has a single faulty gene (D) that dominates its normal counterpart (N). Each child's chances of inheriting either the D or the N from the affected parent are 50%. Almost 2000 autosomal dominant disorders have been catalogued. Examples are hypercholesterolemia and polydactyly (extra fingers or toes).
2. *Recessive Inheritance*
   Both parents, usually unaffected, carry a normal gene (N) that takes over its faulty recessive counterpart (r). The odds for each child are:
   (a) 25% risk of inheriting a double dose of *r* genes, that may cause a severe birth defect
   (b) 25% chance of inheriting 2 *N*s, thus being unaffected
   (c) 50% chance of being a carrier, as are both parents
   Examples are sickle cell disease and phenylketonuria.
3. *X-linked (sex-linked) Inheritance*
   In the most common form, the female sex chromosomes of an unaffected mother carry one faulty gene (X) and one normal gene (Y). The father has the normal male X and Y chromosome complement.
   (a) The odds for each *male* child are 50/50—50% chance of inheriting disorders and 50% of inheriting normal chromosomes.
   (b) The odds for each *female* child are 50% risk of inheriting one faulty X and being a carrier, and 50% chance of inheriting *no* faulty gene.
   Examples are color blindness and muscular dystrophy.
4. *Multifactorial Inheritance*
   Many genetic defects are the result of the interaction of many genes with other genes or with environmental factors. The transmission pattern is not well defined. The chances of having the same defect with one affected child in the family are 5% or less. Examples are cleft palate and diabetes mellitus.

Chromosome Analysis

Normal Values
Females: 44 autosomes + 2X chromosomes; karyotype: 46,XX
Males: 44 autosomes + 1X and 1Y chromosome; karyotype; 46,XY

Background
The 46 chromosomes present in every normal human somatic cell carry the genes that determine inherited characteristics. Errors in chromosome number or structure can occur before or after fertilization and lead to duplication or deletions of these genes. Chromosome analysis is the study of the chromosomes, which are the cellular structures.

Two major factors are studied: number of chromosomes and structure of chromosomes. Alteration in the total number of chromosomes or in their structure can result in a genetic disorder and may be the cause of many other less well-defined entities.

Most chromosome analyses are used as an aid in genetic counseling and diagnostic evaluation. This includes the study of chromosomes of fetal cells obtained by amniocentesis.

Studies are indicated in the following conditions:

1. Multiple malformation
2. Failure to thrive
3. Mental retardation
4. Ambiguous genital organs and hypogonadism
5. Frequent miscarriages
6. Infertility (Klinefelter syndrome)
7. Primary amenorrhea or oligomenorrhea
8. When parents have children with known genetic disorders
9. When prospective mothers are over 35 years of age
10. When either parent has produced a child with a chromosome abnormality
11. When either parent is a mosaic or carrier of a balanced chromosome anomaly such as a translocation
12. Delayed puberty (Turner syndrome)
13. Sex determination
14. Relatives of persons with chromosomal abnormalities

Clinical Alert
Genetic counseling often depends on precise chromosome analysis.

Source of Specimen
Specimens used for chromosome analysis are generally taken from

1. Leukocytes from peripheral blood
2. Bone marrow
3. Buccal or vaginal smears
4. Fibroblasts from skin or other tissues
5. Amniotic fluid
6. Products of conception
7. Autopsy

Of the sources, leukocytes are used most often because blood is the most easily obtained specimen.

Bone marrow cytogenetics may be helpful in many hematologic disorders. For example, a Ph[1] or t (9:22) abnormality is indicative of chronic granulocytic leukemia and a t (8:21) defines a subset of patients with acute nonlymphocytic leukemia. Cytogenetics may also identify the onset of a blast crisis and has been used to monitor patients in remission as an indicator of prognosis and as a basis for evaluating the extent of therapy.

Chromosome studies on products of conception may provide useful information concerning the cause of the miscarriage and its inheritance potential. For this reason, chromosome studies on the parents may be indicated. However, in approximately one-half of all miscarriages there are no viable cells, and in others there is contamination. Therefore, fibroblast cultures for chromosome analysis can be established in only about half of spontaneously aborted products of conception.

Skin tissue may be used for chromosome analysis in special cases when the results of blood are inconclusive as in suspected mosaicism, confirmation of a new chromosome disorder, or dermatologic disorders.

Postmortem chromosome analysis may be desirable in severely malformed abortions and neonates, particularly if there is a family listing of frequent miscarriages. Chromosome analysis may also be indicated if the body has malformations that correspond to the classic chromosome syndromes, and when the diagnosis is doubtful.

Karyotyping
To evaluate chromosomes for anomalies in number or structure, a *karyotype* is prepared. A karyotype is an arrangement of pairs of chromosomes according to their size and structure, with the largest chromosomes placed first and the smallest placed last. The 23 pairs of chromosomes are arranged in seven groups—A through G. The sex chromosomes (two Xs in normal females and an X plus a Y in a normal male) are usually placed apart from the autosomes but belong to the C

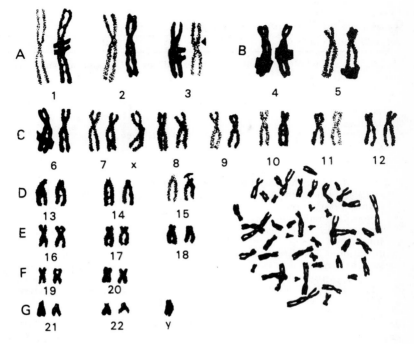

Figure 11-1
A human karyotype. Pairs of homologous chromosomes are arranged in seven groups (A–G) according to total length. This figure shows a normal human male chromosome complement. (Koss LG: Diagnostic Cytology and Its Histopathologic Bases, 3rd ed. Philadelphia, JB Lippincott, 1979)

group (X) and the E group (Y). (See Figure 11-1 for a karyotype of a male.)

Individual chromosomes are distinguished by several characteristics.

1. Length
2. Location of the centromere position or the primary constriction
3. Arm ratios
4. Presence of secondary constrictions
5. Presence of satellites
6. Staining patterns

Explanation of Test

Chromosome analysis can be the single most important test for screening for or definitely establishing certain common genetic disorders, for identifying numerical chromosomal abnormalities, and for making

Table 11-2
Guidelines for Chromosome Analysis

Purpose and Conditions	Test

Identification of whole chromosomal abnormalities
  Down syndrome
  Klinefelter syndrome
  Turner's syndrome
  Trisomy 18
  Trisomy 13–15
  XYY syndrome
  XXX syndrome
	Chromosome analysis, routine

Identification of 2 or more populations of cells from mosaics in any of the above conditions and identification of deletions, duplications, translocations and isochromosomes
  Mental retardation
  Congenital malformations
  Spontaneous abortions
  Infertility
	Chromosome analysis, extended study

Identification of Ph[1] chromosome in chronic granulocytic leukemia	Chromosome analysis, Philadelphia chromosome
Identification of fetal chromosomal abnormalities *in utero* and determination of fetal sex (helpful in instances of X-linked recessive defective genes)	Chromosome analysis, amniotic
Identification of fetal chromosomal abnormalities involved in repeated spontaneous abortions, or chromosome abnormalities in any other tissue	Chromosome analysis, tissue (fetal or other)

(After Bio-Science Handbook, 12th ed., p 213. Van Nuys, CA, Bio-Science Laboratories, 1979)

definite sex determinations in cases of ambiguous genitalia (see Table 11-2).

Nomenclature of the Karyotype

Placement of the letters and numbers of the karyotype has been agreed on at international symposia. These conventions are followed:

1. The first number is the total number of chromosomes.
2. The complement of sex chromosomes follows.
3. Then the chromosomes that are missing, extra, or abnormally formed are so indicated.

These principles are illustrated in the following examples:

Normal female	46,XX
Normal male	46,XY
Male with an additional No. 21 chromosome	47,XY,+21

Female with the short arm of No. 5 chromosome
shorter than normal   46,XX,5p−

Procedure
1. Cells are cultured in the laboratory.
2. Time is allowed for the cells to undergo mitosis and to enter metaphase.
3. Further mitotic division is halted through chemical treatment of the cell culture.
4. Chromosomes are released when cell membrane is ruptured.
5. Chromosomes are placed on a glass slide, stained, and observed through a microscope.
6. Photomicrographs are taken of the chromosomes.
7. Individual chromosomes in the photo are cut apart and assembled to form the karyotype.
8. The patient's abnormalities are evaluated with respect to the karyotype.

Prenatal Chromosome Analysis
Certain genetic disorders, such as Down syndrome, can be detected in the early stages of a pregnancy through chromosome analysis of fetal cells. A small amount of amniotic fluid is withdrawn through a needle inserted into the pregnant woman's abdominal wall. The fetal cells are analyzed as described above under "Procedure." Results are available within 2 to 3 weeks.

Clinical Implications
A. Chromosomal abnormalities involve whole chromosomes or parts of them. There may be too few or too many chromosomes, parts of a chromosome may be missing, or parts may be broken off and reattached to another chromosome. Common chromosomal disorders include
   1. Down's syndrome (formerly called *mongolism*). Three types of cytogenetic abnormalities have been identified.
      (a) *Trisomy 21*. This is the most common form of Down syndrome and is caused by an additional complete No. 21 chromosome. (There are three No. 21 chromosomes rather than a pair, giving a total chromosome count of 47.) This condition results in multiple defects with mental retardation, limb and facial anomalies, heart defects, and infertility in males. The disorder is due to failure of the two chromosomes of pair 21 to separate during sperm or egg development, resulting in an abnormal zygote with 47 chromosomes and a child with trisomy 21. Older women are much more likely than younger women to give birth to a child with Down syndrome—for example, at 34 the risk is higher than at 27.

(b) *Translocation 21 trisomy.* This is rare and caused by extra chromosome 21 material attaching to chromosome 15. The same symptoms are produced as in standard trisomy 21. The actual chromosome count is the normal 46; however, persons with this form of Down syndrome have a longer No. 15 chromosome because the No. 21 chromosome is attached to it. This may be familial. When a parent, especially the mother, carries a chromosome 21 translocation, there is a substantial risk that her child will have Down syndrome.

(c) *Mosaicism.* This is rare in Down syndrome. It is due to a mistake in the embryonic cell division and not a fault in the ovum or sperm formation. The affected individual has cells of different No. 21 chromosome counts dispersed throughout the body. The same symptoms as listed above are found, but the abnormalities are often less severe. This type of trisomy is not familial. Studies have shown that approximately 20% of pregnancies will end in spontaneous abortion if mosaicism is present.

B. Sex chromosome abnormalities include
1. *Intersexuality.* In persons with ambiguous genitalia, chromosome studies are helpful to establish their cellular sex. This information is important in guiding medical and surgical management.
2. *Turner syndrome.* The person with only one X chromosome, missing either an X or a Y chromosome, has Turner syndrome. This condition is associated with shortness of stature, infertility, heart disease, and other manifestations.
3. *Klinefelter syndrome.* This is a major type of male hypogonadism and is caused by an extra X chromosome (karyotype is 47,XXY). Klinefelter syndrome can be detected by sex chromatin smears, since the second X chromosome forms a Barr body as in normal females, but it should be confirmed by chromosome analysis.

C. Chromosome analysis and cancer
1. *Solid tumors.* Cells from many solid tumors can be characterized as having a broader range of chromosome count than found in normal tissue. However, there is little correlation between the type of chromosomal makeup and tumor histology.
2. *Leukemia.* A particular chromosomal aberration, the Philadelphia chromosome (Ph[1]), can be found in about 80% of patients with chronic granulocytic leukemia. The Philadelphia chromosome is a deleted chromosome No. 22. It may be found in bone marrow cells even during remissions. Blast crisis is associated with trisomy 8, isochromosome 17, q-arm and multiple Ph[1] chromosomes.

3. The Philadelphia chromosome is also associated with Burkitt lymphoma.

Fibroblast Culture

Normal Values
Dependent on lysosomal enzyme being determined.

Explanation of Test
Cultures of skin fibroblasts are helpful in diagnosing many of the lyso-somal storage disorders, such as sphingolipidosis or mucopolysac-charidosis. Persons with lysosomal disorders generally show delayed or regressing psychomotor performance, abnormal bone development, and eye abnormalities.

Clinical Alert

Fibroblasts offer the advantage of an unlimited supply of sample, and they normally contain very high levels of the enzyme in ques-tion. However, because the skin biopsy procedure is considered more invasive than venipuncture and because a 4-week culturing period is required, appropriate blood samples are often per-formed.

Procedure
A skin biopsy using a 4-mm. punch is obtained. Keep the culture sterile and do not freeze it. Only one fibroblast culture is required for each enzyme or all enzymes requiring this technique.

Clinical Implications
Fibroblast culture will reveal the enzymes that are responsible for ge-netic storage disorders (see Table 11-3) as in

1. Sphingolipidosis
2. Mucopolysaccharidosis
3. Disorders involving glycoprotein or multiple storage products

³⁵S Mucopolysaccharide Turnover

Normal Values
Normal versus abnormal turnover

Table 11-3

Tests for Lysosomal Storage Disorders

Genetic Storage Disorders	Enzyme	Sample (In order of preference)
I. Sphingolipidoses		
Niemann–Pick	Sphingomyelinase	Fibroblasts; WBCs
Gaucher's	Beta-glucosidase	Fibroblasts; WBCs
Globoid cell leukodystrophy (Krabbe's)	Galactosylceramide-beta-galactosidase	Fibroblasts; WBCS
Metachromatic leukodystrophy	Arylsulfatase-A	Serum; Urine; Fibroblasts; WBCs
Fabry's	Alpha Galactosidase	Plasma; Fibroblasts; WBCs
Tay–Sachs (G_{M2})	Hexosaminidase A and Total (Beta-N-acetyl-glucosaminidase A)	Serum; Fibroblasts; WBCs
Sandhoff's	Beta-N-acetylglucosaminidase A and B	Serum; Fibroblasts; WBCs
Generalized gangliosidoses, G_{M1}	Beta-galactosidase	Fibroblasts; WBCs
II. Mucopolysaccharidoses		
Mucopolysaccharidoses Types I, II, III, VI, VII	^{35}S labeled mucopolysaccharide turnover	Fibroblasts: Normal/abnormal turnover
Hurler's (MPS I)	Alpha-L-iduronidase	Fibroblasts
Sanfilippo's Type A	Heparan sulfamidase	Fibroblasts
Sanfilippo's Type B (MPS IIIb)	Alpha-N-acetylglucosaminidase (Alpha-hexosaminidase)	Serum; Fibroblasts
Maroteaux–Lamy (MPS VI)	Arylsulfatase-B	Fibroblasts
Glucuronidase deficiency (MPS VII)	Beta-glucuronidase	Fibroblasts
III. Disorders Involving Glycoprotein or Multiple Storage Products		
Fucosidosis	Alpha-fucosidase	Fibroblasts; WBCs
Mannosidosis	Alpha-mannosidase	Fibroblasts; WBCs
Xylosidosis	Beta-xylosidase	Fibroblasts
Mucolipidosis I	Neuraminidase	Fibroblasts
Mucolipidoses II, III	^{35}S labeled mucopolysaccharide turnover	Fibroblasts

(After Bakken CL [ed]: Mayo Medical Laboratories Handbook. Rochester, Mayo Clinic Laboratories, 1981)

Explanation of Test

In addition to specific enzyme tests for lysosomal storage disorders, the evaluation of the rate of turnover of ^{35}S labeled mucopolysaccharides in cultures of skin fibroblasts can be used as a general approach to determine if a person has any of the mucopolysaccharidoses, with the exception of Morquio syndrome. Cultured fibroblasts that are deficient in an enzyme required for the breakdown of mucopolysaccharides will accumulate polysaccharides.

Procedure
A specimen obtained by skin biopsy using a 4-mm. punch is required.

Clinical Implications
Abnormal turnover is associated with mucopolysaccharidoses I, II, III, VI, and VII.

Sphingomyelinase

Normal Values
1.53–7.18 U./g.

Explanation of Test
This test using cultured skin fibroblasts is done to diagnose Niemann–Pick disease. This disorder is caused by a deficiency of sphingomyelinase resulting in extensive storage of sphingomyelin and cholesterol in the liver, spleen, lungs, and to a lesser degree, in the brain.

Procedure
A skin biopsy using a 4-mm. punch is done.

Clinical Implications
Decreased levels are associated with Niemann–Pick disease.

1. Large lipid-laden foam cells are characteristic of the disease.
2. Deficiency of sphingomyelinase can be demonstrated in leukocytes or cultured skin fibroblasts from patients with the most severe types of A and B.

Beta-Glucosidase

Normal Values
0.28–4.71 U./g.
Fibroblast: 3.76–8.7 U./g.
WBC:
Adults: 8.8–39.4 U./10^{10} cells
Children: 11.9–67 I.U./10^{10} cells

Background
Beta-glucosidase is a lysosomal enzyme that is required for the hydrolysis of glucocerebroside. This enzyme is normally present in many body tissues, including the fibroblasts and white blood cells.

Explanation of Test

This test based on a skin biopsy is done to detect Gaucher's disease, an autosomal recessive disease that is due to a deficiency of beta-glucosidase.

Procedure

A skin biopsy using a 4-mm. punch is obtained.

Clinical Implications

1. A decreased level of beta-glucosidase is associated with Gaucher's disease. This deficiency results in increased storage of glucosylceramide.
2. Gaucher's cells are characteristic of this disease along with large histiocytes derived from endothelial cells.

BIBLIOGRAPHY

Bauer JD: Clinical Laboratory Methods, 9th ed. St. Louis, CV Mosby, 1982
Beahrs OH, Myers MH (eds): Manual for Staging of Cancer, 2nd ed. Philadelphia, JB Lippincott, 1983
Dallenbach–Hellweg G: Histiopathology of the Endometrium. New York, Springer–Verlag, 1981
Fine BA, Paul NW (eds): Strategies in Genetic Counseling: Clinical Investigations Studies. White Plains, NY, March of Dimes Birth Defects Foundation, 1984
Genetic Counseling Booklet. White Plains, NY, March of Dimes Birth Defects Foundation, 1984
Halsted CH, Halsted JA (eds): The Laboratory in Clinical Medicine, 2nd ed. Philadelphia, WB Saunders, 1981
Harper PS: Practical Genetics Counseling, Baltimore, University Park Press, 1981
Isselbacher KJ et al (eds): Harrison's Principles of Internal Medicine, 11th ed. New York, McGraw-Hill, 1987
Jackson LG, Schimke RN (eds): Clinical Genetics. New York, John Wiley & Sons, 1979
Koss LG: Diagnostic Cytology and Its Histological Bases, 3rd ed. Philadelphia, JB Lippincott, 1979
Koss LG et al: Aspiration Biopsy: Cytological Interpretation and Histological Basis. Tokyo, New York, Igaku–Shoin, 1984
Leavelle DE: Mayo Medical Laboratories Handbook. Rochester, Mayo Clinic, 1986
Livolsi VA: Practical Clinical Cytology. Springfield, IL, Charles C. Thomas, 1980
Milbeck R: Cytogenetic examination: Specimen acquisition and handling. Lab Med 13(7):416–419, 1982
Muench KH: The Genetic Basis for Human Disease. New York, Elsevier–Dutton, 1979
Wisniewski LP, Hirschbaum K: A Guide to Human Chromosome Defects. White Plains, NY, March of Dimes Birth Defects Foundation, 1980

COMMON ENDOSCOPIC STUDIES

Introduction

A group of diagnostic devices, known generically as *fiberoptic instruments*, is used for direct visual examination of various internal body structures. Each of these instruments has a lighted mirror–lens system attached to a rigid or flexible tube. Flexible scopes are the state of the art. In fiberoptics, light travels through an optic fiber by multiple reflections. Fiberoptic instruments, comprised of a fiber bundle system, are designed to redirect and transmit light around any number of twists and bends in the cavities and hollow organs of the body. An image fiber and a light fiber allow for visualization at the distal tip of the scope. A suction port allows for instilling anesthetic and lavaging of fluids, insertion of brushes and forceps, and for suctioning. The tube can be inserted into orifices and tracts of the body not easily accessible or directly visualized by other means. The insertion can be for both diagnosis of pathologic conditions and for therapy, such as in the removal of foreign objects. These examinations are done using local or general anesthetics. Biopsies are submitted for histologic examination. This chapter will include discussions of the following procedures:

1. Mediastinoscopy: for examination and biopsy of lymph nodes in the mediastinum
2. Bronchoscopy: for visualization of the trachea and bronchi
3. Esophagogastroduodenoscopy (EGD): for gastroscopy—for visual examination of the upper gastrointestinal tract (UGI)
4. Esophageal manometry: not an endoscopic examination, but included here because it is often done for patients who need EGD. These pressure readings are done to evaluate esophageal muscle contraction
5. Endoscopic retrograde cholangiopancreatography (ERCP): for visualization of pancreatic and bile ducts
6. Colposcopy: for direct visualization of the vagina and cervix
7. Cervicography: not an endoscopic examination, but included here because this photography of the cervix is often done in conjunction with colposcopy
8. Proctoscopy, sigmoidoscopy, proctosigmoidoscopy: for visualization of the rectum and sigmoid colon
9. Colonoscopy: for examination of the large intestine
10. Peritonoscopy or laparoscopy: for visualization of liver or uterus, fallopian tubes, and ovaries
11. Cytoscopy: for inspection of the bladder, urethra, orifices of the ureters, and prostate (in males). Ureteroscopy can also be done to examine both ureters.
12. Urodynamic studies: not an endoscopic examination, but included because those procedures are often done in conjunction with cytos-

copy. These tests are performed to study voiding patterns and identify possible causes of incontinence.
13. Arthroscopy: for examination of knee or shoulder joint

Mediastinoscopy

Normal Values
No evidence of disease; normal lymph glands

Explanation of Test
This examination, which is performed under general anesthesia, involves the insertion of a lighted mirror lens instrument, similar to a
bronchoscope, through an incision at the base of the neck. This procedure is done to biopsy the lymph nodes in the mediastinum. These
nodes receive lymphatic drainage from the lungs, and biopsies may
identify such diseases as carcinoma, granulomatous infection, and sarcoidosis. Mediastinoscopy has virtually replaced biopsy of the scalene
fat pad for suspected nodes on the right side of the mediastinum. Mediastinoscopy is the routine method for establishing a tissue diagnosis of
the stage of lung cancer and to demonstrate the spread of a lung tumor.
Nodes on the left side of the chest are usually biopsied through a limited left anterior thoracotomy (mediastinotomy) or, occasionally, by
scalene fat pad biopsy.

Procedure
1. The procedure is performed under general anesthesia in the surgical department.
2. The biopsy is done through a suprasternal incision.
3. The total procedure time is 1½ hours.

Clinical Implications
1. Abnormal results in the examination aid in diagnosing
   (a) Sarcoidosis
   (b) Tuberculosis
   (c) Histoplasmosis
   (d) Hodgkin's disease (This condition commonly involves the
   lymph nodes.)
   (e) Granulomatous infections
   (f) Lung cancer
2. The procedure helps to demonstrate the spread of lung tumors.

Patient Preparation
1. Explain the purpose and procedure of the test.
2. A legal permit must be signed before the examination.

3. Preoperative care is the same as for any patient having general anesthesia and surgery.
4. The patient must be NPO for 12 hours before the test.

Patient Aftercare

Following the examination, care is the same as for any patient who has had surgery and a general anesthetic.

Clinical Alert

1. Previous mediastinoscopy is a contraindication to another examination because adhesions make an adequate dissection of nodes extremely difficult and sometimes impossible.
2. The main complication of the procedure results from the general anesthesia.

Bronchoscopy

Normal Values

Normal trachea, bronchi, and alveoli

Explanation of Test

This test permits visualization of the trachea and bronchi with a flexible or rigid bronchoscope. The procedure is used to diagnose tumors, coin lesions, or granulomatous lesions, to find the site of hemorrhage, to biopsy, to take brushings for cytologic examinations, to improve drainage, to identify inflammatory infiltrates, and to lavage and to remove foreign bodies. In addition, bronchoscopy is used to determine resectability of a lesion as well as to obtain a definite diagnosis of bronchogenic cancer.

The examination is usually done under local anesthetic in an outpatient department, diagnostic center, or in the small operating room of a surgical suite. It can also be done in an intensive care unit when patients are unresponsive or for ventilator-assisted patients.

Procedure

1. A local anesthetic is administered. The back of the nose, tongue, pharynx, and epiglottis are sprayed and swabbed with a local anesthetic. In some cases a nebulizing atomizer will be used. If the patient has a history of bronchospasms, steroid and aminophylline will be administered before the procedure is started.
2. The flexible bronchoscope is inserted carefully through the mouth or nose into the pharynx and trachea.

3. Because of sedation with Valium or Demerol, the patient is not uncomfortable. When the bronchoscope is passed, the patient may feel that he cannot breathe or that he is suffocating.
4. Total examining time is 30 to 45 minutes, depending on technique: nasal approach, one half hour; endotracheal intubation with local anesthetic takes longer.
5. A 4-hour postbronchoscopy arterial blood gas is desirable. Arterial blood oxygen may remain below normal 1 to 4 hours after the procedure. In addition, a 12-hour postbronchoscopy sputum specimen is often ordered for cytology or culture and sensitivity.

Clinical Implications
Abnormalities that will be revealed include

1. Abscesses
2. Bronchitis
3. Carcinoma (right lung more than left)
4. Tumors (usually appear more often in larger bronchii)
5. Tuberculosis
6. Alveolitis
7. Signs of nonresectability by surgery (*e.g.*, involvement of tracheal wall by tumor growth, immobility of a main stem bronchus, widening and fixation of the carina)

Clinical Considerations
Prior to the procedure, this data base must be available: chest x-ray, recent ABG's, and ECG if the patient is over age 40 or has heart disease.

Patient Preparation
1. Explain the purpose, procedure, benefits and risks of the test. Tell the patient that anesthetic has a bitter taste. Anesthesia occurs in 5 to 10 minutes. It is followed by feelings of a thickened tongue and a sensation that there is something in the back of the throat that cannot be coughed out or swallowed. These sensations will pass.
2. An informed consent must be signed.
3. The patient must be NPO for 4 to 6 hours before the procedure to reduce the risk of aspiration before reflexes are blocked.
4. Dentures and contact lenses must be removed before the examination.
5. Analgesics or tranquilizers/sedatives and atropine are ordered and administered one-half to one hour before bronchoscopy. The patient must be as relaxed as possible before and during the procedure. The patient needs to know that it is normal to feel anxious.
6. Use relaxation techniques to help the patient relax and continue to breath normally during the entire procedure. The more relaxed the patient, the easier it will be to complete procedure.

Patient Aftercare
1. Usually the patient is NPO for 2 hours. Be certain that swallowing and coughing are present before allowing food or liquids.
2. Provide gargles to relieve mild pharyngitis that may persist for 4 to 48 hours after the examination.
3. For 4 hours postprocedure, monitor TPR and color q1h.
4. Oxygen per mask or nasal cannula may be ordered for 4 hours postprocedure.

Clinical Alert

Observe for possible complications including

1. Cardiac arrhythmias
2. Hypoxemia
3. Laryngospasm
4. Bronchospasm (pallor and increasing dyspnea are signs)
5. Infection with gram-negative bacteria
6. Pneumothorax
7. Respiratory failure
8. Bleeding following biopsy (rare, but can occur if excessive friability of airway or massive lesions)
9. Anaphylactic drug reactions

Esophagogastroduodenoscopy (EGD) (Endoscopy, Gastroscopy)

Normal Values
Essentially normal upper GI tract

Explanation of Test
This test allows the physician to visualize the lumen of the upper gastrointestinal tract (UGI) with a fiberoptic instrument. This instrument is a tube that incorporates a lighted mirror–lens system. This examination is indicated for all patients with dysphagia and weight loss, especially those patients with moderate to heavy alcohol and tobacco consumption. This method is valuable in determining the cause of UGI bleeding, to confirm suspicious findings on x-rays, to establish a diagnosis in a symptomatic patient with a negative x-ray report, to biopsy UGI lesions, and to diagnose hiatal hernia and esophagitis. It is also valuable in helping to determine if a gastric ulcer is benign or malignant and postgastrectomy follow-up.

Note: *Endoscopy* is a general term denoting visual inspection of any body cavity with an endoscope. Endoscopic examination of the upper GI tract, therefore, may be called any of the following when ordered: panendoscopy, esophagoscopy, gastroscopy, duodenoscopy, esophagogastroscopy or esophagogastroduodenoscopy.

Procedure

1. This examination is usually done in a gastrointestinal (GI) laboratory setting or in a surgical suite.
2. A topical anesthetic is applied to the throat in the form of gargle or spray.
3. An intravenous tranquilizer is often given by the physician before the procedure. The medication is injected slowly into a vein until the patient becomes relaxed and somewhat sleepy.
4. The endoscope is gently inserted into the esophagus and advanced slowly into the stomach and duodenum. Air is insufflated through the scope to distend the area being examined and to permit good visualization of the mucosa. Biopsies and brushings for cytology may be obtained during the examination. Photos may also be taken.
5. Feelings of pressure or bloating are normal, but there is no pain involved.
6. Immediately after completion of the examination, the patient will be asked to sit up and deep-breathe, cough, and expectorate.
7. Examining time is about 10 to 20 minutes.

Clinical Implications

Abnormal results indicate

1. The site of hemorrhage
2. Hiatal hernia
3. Esophagitis
4. Neoplastic tissue
5. Gastric ulcers, benign or malignant

Patient Preparation

1. Explain the purpose, procedure, benefits and risks of the test. Tell the patient that the flexible tube is thinner than most food that is swallowed. Tell the patient that many persons fall asleep during EGD.
2. Instruct the patient that no food or water is to be ingested 8 hours before the examination. In the hospital, this restriction is usually begun at midnight, before the examination. Give the patient a written reminder of the fasting. A legal permit must be signed.
3. With outpatients, oral hygiene is to be done before coming to the laboratory. With hospital patients, give assistance with oral care if needed.
4. The patient is encouraged to urinate and defecate before the examination.
5. A tranquilizing medication may be given by injection 30 minutes before an examination if ordered.

Patient Aftercare

1. Be certain the patient is able to swallow before offering liquids.
2. After the test is completed, no food or liquids are permitted for 2 hours or longer if the patient cannot swallow.
3. Blood pressure, pulse, and respirations are checked every 30 minutes times four.
4. A side-lying position in bed with the side rails up is to be maintained until the sedative has worn off, usually 2 hours. This position is used to prevent the patient from aspirating.
5. Encourage the patient to belch to expel the air that was inserted into the stomach during the examination.
6. The patient should experience no discomfort or side-effects once the sedative has worn off.

Clinical Alert

1. Complications are rare but can occur.

   (a) Perforation
   (b) Bleeding
   (c) Local irritation of vein
   (d) Drug reactions
   (e) Complications from unrelated diseases such as MI and CVA
   (f) Death is extremely rare, but is a remote possibility

Esophageal Manometry

Normal Values
Normal esophageal and stomach pressure readings
Normal contraction, no acid reflux

Explanation of Test
This explanation is a way of testing to see if the esophagus, a tubelike muscle, is contracting properly. Pressure measurements of the esophagus and stomach are obtained. These results are helpful in determining whether or not the esophageal musculature is contracting normally.

Indications for Testing

1. Abnormal esophageal muscle function
2. Difficulty in swallowing
3. Heartburn
4. Chest pain of unknown cause
5. Regurgitation
6. Vomiting

Other tests often done in conjunction with manometry are the acid reflux tests and Bernstein test. These measurements are useful in evaluating heartburn, esophagitis and chest pain of uncertain cause.

Procedure
1. A local anesthetic is applied to the nasal passage with a cotton swab.
2. A small tube is passed through the nose while the patient is sitting. Tiny holes in the sides of the tube allow for the measurement of pressure within the esophagus and stomach.
3. After the tube is passed, the patient lies on his back for the remainder of the test.
4. Small amounts of water or jello are placed in the mouth and the patient is asked to swallow.
5. Examining time for this part of the test is 40 minutes.
6. *Acid reflux testing*
   A second small tube is passed alongside the one already in place. This tube is actually a probe that is sensitive to acid. When the valve at the bottom of the esophagus is not functioning, acid from the stomach comes back up the esophagus. When this occurs, the acid is sensed by the probe sitting in the esophagus.

Clinical Implications
Abnormal results reveal

1. Achalasia
2. Esphageal spasm
3. Acid reflux

Patient Preparation
1. Explain the purpose, procedure and benefits of the test. No serious complications have been known to occur.
2. No food or drink for 6 hours prior to testing.
3. If the patient is diabetic, the testing department should be notified.

Patient Aftercare
1. Advise the patient that a sore throat is common within the first 24 hours.
2. The nose may be slightly irritated from passage of the tube.

Endoscopic Retrograde Cholangiopancreatography (ERCP)

Normal Values
Patent pancreatic ducts, common bile ducts, duodenal papilla, and normal gallbladder (if present)

Explanation of Test
This examination of the gallbladder and pancreas is done using an endoscope followed by instillation of contrast medium into the duodenal papilla or ampulla of Vater. It is used to evaluate obstructive jaundice and as a follow-up study in confirmed or suspected pancreatic disease. ERCP manometry can also be done to obtain pressure readings in the bile duct, pancreatic duct, and sphincter of Oddi at the papilla. Measurement is obtained by a catheter that is inserted into the endoscope and placed within the sphincter zone.

Procedure
1. Before the procedure is begun, a flat plate of the abdomen (KUB) is done to be certain that no barium is present, which could obscure the view.
2. The patient is asked to gargle with a topical anesthetic.
3. An IV is started, and drugs such as Valium and Demerol are administered before and during the procedure as needed for appropriate sedation. Surprisingly, the very ill patient often needs only a small amount of sedation.
4. A left lateral position is assumed by the patient while the endoscope is inserted through the esophagus to the duodenum. At this point, a prone position is assumed.
5. Glucagon may be given during the procedure to relax the duodenum so that the papilla can be cannulated. Anticholinergics are often administered during the study.
6. A catheter is passed into the ampulla of Vater and a contrast substance such as Renografin is instilled to outline the pancreatic and common bile ducts.
7. Several x-rays are taken at this time.
8. Biopsies or cytology brushings may also be done before the endoscope is removed.

Clinical Implications
Abnormal results will reveal the presence of stones, stenosis, and other abnormalities that are indicative of

1. Biliary cirrhosis
2. Primary sclerosing cholangitis
3. Cancer of bile ducts
4. Pancreatic cysts
5. Pseudocysts
6. Pancreatic tumor
7. Cancer of head of pancreas
8. Chronic pancreatitis
9. Pancreatic fibrosis
10. Cancer of duodenal papilla
11. Papillary stenosis

Patient Preparation
1. Explain the purpose, procedure, benefits, and risks of the test.
2. A legal permit must be signed.
3. No food or fluids are permitted for 12 hours before the procedure.

Patient Aftercare
1. Check vital signs for 4 hours after the test.
2. No food or fluids are permitted for at least 2 hours or until the gag reflex has returned. Determine that the patient can swallow before offering liquids or food.
3. Urinary retention may be a complication.
4. Observe the patient for signs of complications such as
   (a) Cholangitis
   (b) Pancreatitis
5. Check for elevation in temperature, which may be the first sign of inflammation.

Colposcopy

Normal Values
Essentially normal vagina and cervix

Explanation of Test
Colposcopy is the examination of the vagina and cervix with a colposcope, which is an instrument with a magnifying lens that is inserted into the vagina for visualization of the vagina and cervix. This examination is an aid in the diagnosis of benign and preclinical cancerous lesions of the cervix. It is now common to examine by colposcope all patients who have abnormal Papanicolaou (Pap) smears. With colposcopy, it is possible to do biopsies and take scrapings of cells under direct visualization. Colposcopy is also valuable in assessing persons with a history of exposure to diethylstilbestrol.

The most common criteria for biopsy are whitish areas of epithelium (leukoplakia), areas of mosaic staining pattern, and irregular blood vessels. Leukoplakia vulvae is a precancerous condition characterized by white to grayish infiltrated patches on the vulvar mucosa. The colposcope has a definite advantage in detecting atypical epithelium, which is designated in the literature as *basal cell activity*. Atypical epithelium may be considered epithelium that cannot be called benign and yet does not fulfill all the criteria for a diagnosis of carcinoma *in situ*. Its detection is of value in cancer prophylaxis.

Patients receiving colposcopy may often be spared a conization (the removal of a cone of tissue from the cervix), which is a surgical procedure requiring hospitalization.

Procedure
1. The vagina and cervix are exposed with a speculum, as is usual in a gynecologic examination. No part of the colposcope is inserted into the vagina (see Figure 12-1). There is no discomfort when the speculum is inserted, just feelings of slight pressure.

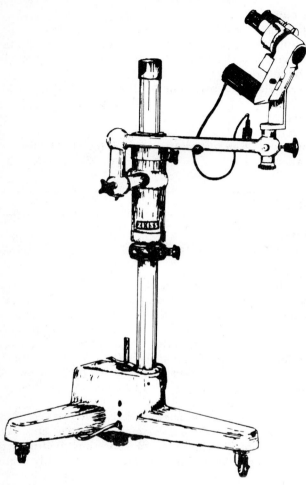

Figure 12-1
The colposcope. (Courtesy of Carl Zeiss, Inc., New York)

2. Long cotton applicator sticks are used to wash and remove any cervical secretions.
3. The cervix and vagina are usually swabbed with acetic acid to improve contrast of the epithelial tissues. A mosaic pattern is usually consistent with dysplasia of some degree.
4. Suspicious lesions are drawn on a diagram for the patient's record and photographs are made.

5. Biopsies of the lesions are done with a fine biopsy forceps. Some patients note discomfort at this time and others do not.
6. Total examining time is 10 to 15 minutes.
7. A small amount of vaginal bleeding for a few hours is not abnormal. A vaginal tampon may be inserted to absorb the flow.

Clinical Implications

A description is given of any abnormal lesions or unusual epithelial patterns.

1. Leukoplakia
2. Abnormal blood vessels
3. Slight-to-moderate-to-marked dysplasia

Patient Preparation

1. Explain the purpose of the examination and procedure.
2. Inform the patient that there will be a slight sensation of pressure when the speculum is inserted and that there may be a few hours of bleeding from the biopsy.

Patient Aftercare

Insert a vaginal tampon to absorb any bleeding.

Cervicography

Cervicography is now being done in conjunction with colposcopy. It is a photographic method used to record a colposcopic image of the entire cervix. After application of 5% acetic acid, photographs of the whole cervix are taken with a specially designed optical instrument with a 35 mm lens; the photographs are then processed into slides (cervigrams). The procedure allows the entire cervix to be visible on one slide. Cervicography also provides evidence for colposcopic consultations. In addition, the cervigram can be done in conjunction with a routine gynecological examination. It has been shown to be more sensitive than the PAP smear in the early detection of cervical intraepithelial neoplasia (CIN) and invasive cervical cancer.

Proctoscopy; Sigmoidoscopy; Proctosigmoidoscopy

Normal Values

Essentially normal rectum and sigmoid

Explanation of Test

These tests involve the examination of a 31-cm. (or 12-inch) area of the rectum and sigmoid with a proctoscope or sigmoidoscope. In some departments, flexible proctoscopes are being used. These instruments are 30 to 60 cm. long. Both devices are essentially tubes incorporating a lighted mirror–lens system for illuminating the rectum and sigmoid. The main use of these studies is the detection and diagnosis of cancers. In cancer screening of persons over 40, these examinations should be routine.

Note: Men over 45 are the high-risk group for this form of malignancy.

These tests are also indicated in the evaluation of hemorrhoids, when blood is present in the stool, when bowel symptoms are present, and in unexplained anemia.

Procedure
1. The patient is placed in a knee-chest position for the examination, and the proctoscope or sigmoidoscope is carefully inserted. When the flexible proctoscope is used, the patient must be in the left lateral position.
2. The examination can be done with the patient in bed or on a special tilt table.
3. Usually, the procedure takes 3 to 5 minutes; when the longer, flexible instrument is used, examining time is 5 to 30 minutes.
4. The patient may feel a very strong urge to defecate, which is a natural reaction.

Clinical Implications
Findings (edematous, red, or denuded mucosa, granularity, friability, ulcers, gray, yellow, pseudomembranes, spontaneous bleeding on examination and normal rectal mucosa) may help to confirm or rule out any of the following conditions:

1. Ulcerative, amebic, pseudo-membranous, or granulomatous colitis
2. Inflammation of rectosigmoid area
3. Tumors of rectosigmoid area
4. Irritable bowel syndrome
5. Crohn's disease

Patient Preparation
1. Explain the purpose and procedure of the test.
2. The patient does not need to fast, but he may be placed on a light diet the evening before the test.
3. Laxatives and an enema may be given the night before the examination, or one or two enemas or a suppository may be administered an hour before the procedure. (In young, active patients, a small enema 1 hour before the scheduled examination is ample preparation.)

Clinical Alert

1. Patients having acute renal symptoms, particularly those with suspected ulcerative or granulomatous colitis, should be given the examination *without* any preparation—that is, without enemas, laxatives, or suppositories.
2. Perforation of the intestinal wall is an infrequent complication of these tests.
3. Do not give laxatives or enemas to pregnant women.

Colonoscopy

Normal Values
Normal mucosa of large intestine

Explanation of Test
Colonoscopy is the examination of the large intestine with a fiberoptic instrument. This examination permits visualization of the colon by the use of a colonoscope, which is inserted through the anus to the ileocecal valve. The technique is valuable in differentiating inflammatory disease from neoplastic disease or in evaluating polypoid lesions beyond the reach of the sigmoidoscope. It is also helpful in evaluating suture lines after resection and anastomosis for colon cancer and for surveillance of groups at high risk for colon cancer. Polyps, foreign bodies, and specimens can be removed with the colonoscope, and photographs can be taken. Before colonoscopy was available, major abdominal surgery was the only way to remove colon polyps to determine if they were benign or malignant. Periodic colonoscopy is a valuable test for the follow-up of persons with previous polyp, colon cancer, or a family history of colon cancer. Air, which passes through an accessory channel of the colonoscope, is used to distend the intestinal walls.

Clinical Implications
Abnormal results indicate

1. Polyps
2. Tumor
3. Areas of ulcerative colitis

Procedure
1. A clear liquid diet is usually ordered 48 to 72 hours before the examination, and the patient must fast for 8 hours before the procedure. Laxatives may be ordered for 1 to 3 days before the test, and enemas are often ordered for the night before. To be effective, a

purgative must be taken to produce fluid diarrhea, which shows that unaltered small intestinal contents are emerging and the colonic residue has been cleared. Enemas must be repeated until no solid matter remains.

2. Another common form of preparing the patient involves the administration of an oral saline iso-osmotic and isotonic (with respect to bowel contents) laxative. This washout solution may contain a number of salts such as potassium, chloride, sodium, bicarbonate, and sulfate, an additive such as polyethylene glycol, and distilled or deionized water. The glycol acts as an osmotic agent so there is no net ion absorption or loss. Water and electrolyte balances should not change significantly. The patient is asked to drink 3 to 6 liters over a 2 to 3½ hour period. The typical dosage per patient is one gallon. It can be administered by nasogastric tube if necessary. This laxative acts quickly and first results can be expected in ½ to 1 hour. Ingestion is continued until defecation is clear liquid. No special diet, laxative, or enemas are required with this solution.

3. The examination is done under analgesia using combinations of medications such as Demerol (meperidine hydrochloride) and Valium (diazepam). The patient should be alert enough to inform the doctor of any gross complication during the examination.

4. Intravenous anticholinergics and glucagon are used when needed to relax local bowel spasms.

5. The patient is placed on his left side or in Sims's position, and the rectum is dilated. Feelings of pressure are felt, but pain is usually not experienced.

6. The examination may take from ½ to 2 hours and is done by an endoscopist, who maneuvers the colonoscope through the twists and turns of the colon. Better views are obtained during withdrawal than during insertion, so a more careful examination is performed during withdrawal.

Clinical Considerations

1. Keep colon electrolyte lavage preparations refrigerated. Use within 48 hours and discard any unused portion.

2. Prior to testing, CBC, current ProTime, platelet count and PTT results should be available.

3. Preparation for colostomy and paralyzed patients will be the same and they will usually receive at least 4 liters of oral prep solution.

4. Persons with known heart disease will receive ordered antibiotics before testing.

5. Patients should not mix or drink anything with the liquid preparation. Do not add ice.

Patient Preparation

1. Explain the purpose, procedure, benefits, and risks of the test. One large glass of liquid prep is to be taken every 10 minutes (one

glass = 12 oz.). Each gallon has nine glasses. The entire gallon should be taken in 2 hours, if possible. Time is important. Slow drinking does not clean the colon.

2. Some patients will be on a clear liquid diet 72 hours before the test and are usually NPO except for medications after a clear liquid supper the evening before the test.
3. Administer purgatives and cleansing enemas as ordered. Preparation is complete when fecal discharge is clear. If returns are not clear after 4 liters of solution have been ingested, continue until returns are clear (up to *6 liters total*).
4. Some protocols call for Reglon liquid to be given in the first 2 doses of oral preparation.
5. A legal consent form must be signed by the patient.
6. Iron preparations should be discontinued 3 or 4 days before the examination. This is because iron residues produce an inky black stool that interferes with inspection and can make the stool viscous and difficult to clear. Aspirin/aspirin-containing products should also be discontinued one week before the examination.
7. Some protocols call for a capped IV in the forearm or hand.
8. Persons with heart valve disease usually receive antibiotics before the test.

Patient Aftercare
1. The patient should be NPO for 2 hours after the examination.
2. The stools should be observed for gross bleeding. The patient should be alert to abdominal pain because perforation and hemorrhage are possible complications.
3. Vital signs should be checked for 2 hours.
4. Most frequent adverse reactions to oral purgatives are nausea, vomiting, bloating, and rectal irritation.

Clinical Alert

1. Solid food should never be given <2 hours prior to the oral cleansing regime.
2. Orally administered colon lavage is contraindicated in
   (a) Actual or suspected ulcers
   (b) Gastric outlet obstruction
   (c) Weight <20 kg
   (d) Toxic colitis
   (e) Megacolon
3. Relative contraindications for colonoscopy include
   (a) Perforating disease of the colon
   (b) Peritonitis
   (c) Acute conditions of the anus and rectum

    (d) Recent abdominal surgery
    (e) Recent myocardial infarction

4. Observe for possible complications including
    (a) Perforations
    (b) Hypotensive episodes
    (c) Cardiac or respiratory arrest, which can be provoked by the combination of oversedation and intense vagal stimulus from instrumentation
    (d) Hemorrhage, especially if polypectomy has been performed
    (e) Death is extremely rare but remains a remote possibility

5. If oral colon lavage preparations are administered to the unconscious or to those with impaired gag reflexes, observe for aspiration or regurgitation, especially if a nasogastric tube is in place.

6. No barium studies are to be done during the preparation period.

Peritoneoscopy, Laparoscopy

Normal Values

GYN examination: normal size and shape of uterus, fallopian tubes, and ovaries

Medical examination: normal liver, gallbladder, spleen, and greater curvature of the stomach

Explanation of Test

This examination of the peritoneal cavity is done using a laparoscope inserted through the anterior abdominal wall. The pelvic organs as well as all of the abdominal organs such as the greater curvature of the stomach and liver can be viewed. Two separate types of examinations are done: peritoneoscopy (medical laparoscopy) and gynecologic (GYN) laparoscopy.

The most common use of the peritoneoscopy is evaluation of liver disease and to obtain a biopsy. This procedure is done when the liver is too small, when previous liver biopsy proves inadequate, when contraindications to percutaneous liver biopsy exist (ascites), when there is unexplained portal hypertension, unexplained liver function abnormalities and when the liver cannot be palpated before obtaining a conventional liver biopsy. It also does away with the need to do a blind liver biopsy. Other indications for peritoneoscopy are unexplained ascites, staging of lymphoma, staging and follow-up of ovarian cancer and abdominal masses. It is also recommended that patients with advanced primary chest, gastric, pancreatitis, advanced endometrial and rectal tumors should be evaluated by peritoneoscopy before attempted surgical cure. Peritoneoscopy/laparoscopy is usually done using a local anesthetic.

GYN laparoscopy is used to diagnose cysts, adhesions, fibroids, and the presence of infection in persons with pelvic and abdominal pain. Evaluation of the fallopian tubes can also be done in infertile patients. It is also commonly done to remove adhesions, obtain biopsies, treat endometrial implants in fulguration, and do tubal ligations for sterilization purposes. GYN laparoscopy is commonly performed using a general anesthetic.

Use of these techniques has replaced laparotomy because it is less stressful to the patient, uses a small incision, can be performed in a shorter period of time, may be performed using local or general anesthetics, reduces potential for formation of adhesions, and hastens healing time.

Procedure Using Local Anesthetic

1. The patient lies on his back during the procedure.
2. The skin is cleansed and a local anesthetic is injected.
3. An IV is started and analgesics and anticholinergic drugs are given intravenously before or during the procedure.
4. A sterile field is maintained.
5. A small incision is made near the umbilicus through which a trocar is introduced, followed by passage of the laparoscope. Double puncture peritoneoscopy is also done. Nitrous oxide is introduced into the peritoneal cavity, so that the organs can be visualized by causing the omentum to rise from the organs. The organs are viewed and biopsy specimens may be obtained.
6. Two stitches are usually needed to close the site of examination. Band–Aid bandages are applied as dressings.
7. Total examining time is about 1 hour for medical examination and about 30 minutes for GYN procedure.

Clinical Implications

Abnormal results reveal the presence of

1. Endometriosis
2. Ovarian cysts
3. Pelvic inflammatory disease
4. Spread and stage of cancer
5. Uterine fibroids
6. Abscesses
7. Enlarged fallopian tubes (hydrosalpinx)
8. Ectopic pregnancy
9. Infection
10. Adhesions
11. Ascites
12. Cirrhosis
13. Nodules on liver, which are often an indication of cancer
14. Engorged vessels in the peritoneum that correlate with portal hypertension

Clinical Alert

This procedure is contraindicated in persons known to have

1. Advanced abdominal wall cancer
2. Severe respiratory or cardiovascular disease with impaired reserve
3. Intestinal obstruction
4. Palpable abdominal mass
5. Large abdominal hernia
6. Chronic tuberculosis
7. History of peritonitis

Patient Preparation

1. Explain the purpose and procedure of the test; advise the patient about the type of anesthesia to be used (general or local).
2. A legal permit must be signed.
3. No food or fluids are permitted for 12 hours before the procedure.

Patient Aftercare

1. Check blood pressure hourly for 4 hours.
2. Observe for signs of complications such as infection, hemorrhage, and bowel and bladder perforation.
3. Advise the patient that shoulder discomfort may be present for 1 to 2 days because of nitrous oxide gas that may remain in the abdominal cavity.
4. If the patient has a general anesthetic, follow the usual cautions that are involved in the care of any person having a general anesthetic.

Cystoscopy

Normal Values

Normal structure and function of the bladder, urethra, orifices of the ureters, and prostate (in males)

Explanation of Test

This examination is indicated in the evaluation of hematuria, urinary incontinence, and urinary trace infection and provides a view of the interior of the bladder, urethra, and prostatic urethra by means of the cystoscope, which is a tubular, lighted, telescopic lens. The procedure is done to observe bladder function and to detect deformation of the bladder, ureters, and prostate. The function of each kidney may be studied separately by means of catheterization of the ureters and collection of urine from each kidney.

The cystoscope is used not only for diagnostic but also for therapeutic purposes. Small stones and other foreign bodies may be removed from the urethra, ureter, and bladder. Biopsy specimens can be obtained, bladder stones can be crushed, bladder tumors can be fulgurated, and strictures can be relieved by dilatation. Ureteroscopy is also done to determine the cause of hematuria, detect tumors and stones, and for stone manipulation.

Procedure
1. The examination is performed in a cystoscopy room, which is part of the operating room suite of the hospital. It is also performed safely in the urologist's office.
2. The external genitalia are scrubbed and sprayed with an antiseptic solution such as Betadine (povidone-iodine).
3. The patient is placed in the lithotomy position with legs in stirrups.
4. A local anesthetic in the form of jelly is instilled into the urethra. In the male patient, the anesthetic is held in the urethra by a clamp applied near the end of the penis. For best results the local anesthetic is applied 5 to 10 minutes before passage of the cystoscope.
5. The cystoscope is connected to an irrigation system.
6. The actual examination takes 15 minutes; however, the patient's time in the examining room may be about 1 hour.

Clinical Implications
1. Cystoscopy is the most important and precise of all urologic diagnostic methods. This procedure may be indicated with the following conditions:
   (a) Unexplained hematuria
   (b) Recurrent urinary tract infection
   (c) Infection resistant to medical treatment
   (d) Unexplained urinary symptoms (e.g., dysuria, frequency, urgency, hesitancy, intermittency, and straining)

   Note: In an intravenous pyelogram (IVP) it is almost impossible to see the area from the neck of the bladder to the end of the urethra. Cystoscopy makes it possible to diagnose abnormalities in this area of the body.

2. Abnormal conditions that are revealed by this method include
   (a) Prostatic hyperplasia
   (b) Cancer of the bladder
   (c) Bladder stone
   (d) Urethral stricture
   (e) Prostatitis

(f) Vesical neck contracture

(g) Urinary blood fistulas

Patient Preparation

1. Explain the purpose and procedure of the test. Advise the patient that there is little pain or discomfort from cystoscopy. (Most persons will complain of more discomfort from a catheterization procedure.)
2. If cystoscopy is performed in the hospital, have the patient sign a legal consent form.
3. The patient is permitted a full liquid breakfast the morning of the examination, and liquids are permitted until the time of the examination.
4. Intravenous medications such as Valium and Versed are administered during the examination to relax the patient. Amnesia is a side-effect. Men up to 60 years of age experience more pain and discomfort than do older men. Women require less sedation because the urethra is shorter.

Patient Aftercare

1. For 24 hours following cystoscopy, the patient's capacity to void should be determined, as well as whether his bladder emptying is complete.
2. When the patient is able to void, fluids should be encouraged.
3. Any bleeding that occurs should stop because clots will form. Report heavy bleeding to the urologist.
4. Inability to void or to empty the bladder completely may signify large clot formation.
5. Frequency of urination and some dysuria or urethral burning is anticipated following cystoscopy.
6. Antibiotics are usually given 1 day before and 3 days after examination to prevent infection.
7. The urethra is such a vascular organ that any break in the tissues allows bacteria to enter directly into the bloodstream. Observe and report chills and fever (urethral chill) and back pain to the urologist.

Clinical Alert

1. If urethral dilatation has been part of the procedure, the patient is advised to rest and increase fluid intake.
2. Edema may induce sufficient reaction to cause urinary retention, hesitancy, small urinary stream, or urinary dribbling. These symptoms can occur within hours or up to 7 days after

cystoscopy. Warm sitz baths and urinary analgesics may be helpful until the edema subsides. However, an indwelling catheter will be necessary to relieve retention.

Urodynamic Studies, Cystometrogram (CMG), Urethra Pressure Profile, and Rectal Electromyography

Normal Values
Normal sensation of fullness, heat, and cold
Low voiding pressure without dyssynergia and with detrusor reflex contraction that can be suppressed on command. Normal rectal electromyographic (EMG) readings. Urethra pressure profile (UPP) reveals normal closing mechanism of urethra.

Explanation of Test
These techniques are used to identify abnormal voiding patterns in incontinent persons. The primary purpose of these studies is to determine if a detrusor reflex exists. The response in the cystometrogenic part of the test reflects intactness of the neuroanatomic connections via the spinal cord from the brain to the bladder. These studies are indicated when there is evidence of neurologic disease: spina bifida, myelomeningocele, cord injury, extensive pelvic dissection, cordotomy, neurectomy, or a specific neuropathy such as multiple sclerosis, cord tumor, diabetes, and tabes dorsalis. This examination is also useful in evaluating patients with known neurologic disease but with symptoms of dysuria, small or weak urinary stream, frequency, enuresis, overflow or stress incontinence, residual urine, or recurrent infection. This examination is often done in conjunction with cystoscopy.

Procedure
Cystometrogram Procedure
1. A catheter is inserted and is then connected to the cystometer. (A cystometer is a device for studying the neuromuscular mechanism of the bladder by measuring capacity and pressure.) The bladder is then filled with water or a gas.
2. During the cystometric examination observations are recorded about these sensations: heat and cold, bladder fullness, urge to void, and ability to inhibit voiding when contractions occur.
3. The patient is asked to void, and the urine flow rate and voiding pressure are recorded.
4. The patient is asked to report sensations that are related to the neurologic stimulation of the bladder and sphincter muscles.

(a) Flushing   (d) Nausea
(b) Sweating   (e) Bladder fullness
(c) Pain   (f) Strong urge to void

5. During the examination, cholinergic and anticholinergic drugs (*e.g.*, Banthine [methantheline bromide], atropine, and Urecholine [bethanechol chloride]) may be administered to determine their effects on bladder function.
   (a) Is an atonic bladder capable of being stimulated by cholinergic parasympathomimetic drugs such as Urecholine, or are detrusor muscle fibers so decompensated that no response can be elicited?
   (b) Can overactive motor stimuli be altered sufficiently with cholinergic blocking parasympatholytic drugs such as atropine to allow a near-normal bladder volume that will produce an acceptable voiding pattern?
   To determine the effect of these drugs, a cystometric study is performed as a control (see procedure for cystometry), followed by another tracing 20 to 30 minutes after injection of the drugs.
6. A change in posture from supine to standing or walking may be required during the examination.
7. *Sleep examination* may be used in conjunction with electroencephalogram to evaluate persons with nocturnal incontinence.

Rectal EMG Procedure
1. Electrodes are applied close to the anus and a ground is attached to the thigh.
2. These electrodes record EMG activity during voiding and give a simultaneous recording of urine flow rate.
3. A needle electrode may be introduced into the periurethral striated muscle.

Urethral Pressure Profile, UPP Procedure
A special catheter, connected to a transducer, is slowly withdrawn and the pressures along the urethra are recorded.

Clinical Implications
Abnormal results reveal motor and sensory defects, abnormal patterns that point to inappropriate or absent contractions of the pelvic floor muscle and internal sphincter during voiding.

1. The most common cause of incontinence is a vesical-sphincter dyssynergia that is a disturbance of muscular coordination between the external urethral sphincter/pelvic floor musculature and the detrusor muscle. The dyssynergia is thought to be responsible for incomplete emptying of the bladder, inappropriate voiding, perineal dampness, and predisposition to urinary tract infections.
2. Detrusor hyperreflexia is a detrusor reflex that the patient cannot suppress on command due to Loop I lesions or spinal portion of

Loop II as in

(a) CVA

(b) Parkinson's

(c) Multiple sclerosis

(d) Cervical spondylosis

(e) Spinal cord injury above
conus medullarus

Urethrovesical causes of hyperreflexia are benign prostatic hypertrophy and stress urge incontinence.

3. Detrusor areflexia in which the detrusor reflex cannot be evoked because the peripheral innervation of the detrusor muscle has been interrupted. Persons with detrusor areflexia have difficulty in initiating voiding without residual volume. If it is due to interrupted peripheral innervation of the detrusor muscle, the cause may be associated with these disease processes: trauma to cauda equina or conus medullarus, spinal arachnoiditis, spinal cord birth defects, diabetic neuropathy, anticholinergic effects of phenothiazides. In postmenopausal women, the UPP may be altered because the mucosal sphincter is estrogen deprived.

Patient Preparation

1. Explain the purpose and procedure of the test.
2. There may be embarrassment and slight discomfort associated with the procedure.

Arthroscopy of the Knee

Normal Values

Normal knee joint: normal vasculature and color of the synovium, patellofemoral compartment, suprapatellar pouch, menisci, intercondylar notch, lateral compartment, ligaments, and articular cartilage

Explanation of Test

This visual examination of the knee joints using an arthroscope and conducted under sterile conditions is used most commonly in the diagnosis of athletic injuries and in the differential diagnosis of acute and chronic disorders of the knee. For example, degenerative processes can be accurately differentiated from a disorder resulting from injury. Torn ligaments can be identified and the extent of arthritis determined. Irrigation and corrective surgery can also be performed at the time of examination. With the information provided by arthroscopy, effective rehabilitation programs can be initiated that will shorten recovery time from trauma. Arthroscopy can also be done to assess response to treatment and to help identify those persons in whom arthrotomy or other corrective procedures are indicated.

Although the knee joint is the site most frequently examined, in some instances the shoulder, ankle, hip, elbow, wrist, and metacarpophalangeal joints can be explored. Calcium deposits, bone spurs, meniscus or cartilage, and scar tissue can be removed when examination is done.

Clinical Implications
Abnormal results reveal
1. Torn and displaced meniscus or cartilage in persons who complain of clicking, locking, and swelling
2. Trapped synovium
3. Loose fragments of osteochondral and chondral fractures
4. Torn ligaments
5. Osteochondritis dissecans
6. Chronic inflammatory arthritis
7. Secondary osteoarthritis
8. Chondromalacia of femoral condyle or wearing down of back of kneecap in persons who complain of grinding

Procedure
The examination is usually conducted under general anesthesia for several reasons

The knee is already painful.
If a lesion is found, definitive treatment can be done at once.
There is no discomfort if a tourniquet is inflated.
Complete muscle relaxation permits a thorough examination including assessment of ligament stability and eliminates any risk of inadvertent patient movement while the instrument is in the joint.

1. A tourniquet is applied to the upper thigh. Some surgeons will choose not to inflate the tourniquet unless bleeding occurs that cannot be cleared by irrigation.
2. Skin is cleansed and sterile drapes (some are waterproof) are applied. A double layer of stockinette is applied to lower leg and foot.
3. The contents of the knee joint are aspirated with a 15- or 16-gauge needle inserted in the suprapatellar pouch. A specimen is sent to the laboratory for analysis. The joint is then injected with 75 to 100 ml. of normal saline to distend the joint before inserting the arthroscope.
4. The arthroscope is inserted as close to the patellar tendon and upper surface of the tibia as possible without penetrating or passing beneath the meniscus or damaging the patellar tendon.
5. Joint washings are collected and examined for loose bodies or cartilage fragments.
6. All parts of the knee are carefully examined, and photographs may be taken.
7. As the arthroscope and irrigating needles are slowly withdrawn, the suprapatellar pouch is compressed to squeeze out excess fluid.

8. The wound is closed with a single deep stitch or closed with Steri Strips.
9. A small, sterile dressing is applied and an elasticized bandage is wrapped around the knee or a long leg cast is used if more extensive surgery is performed.
10. Total examining time varies (45 minutes to 1½ hours) Longer if more than a diagnostic procedure is done (*i.e.*, if meniscus is removed).

Patient Preparation

1. Explain the purpose and procedure of the test. The patient should be NPO from midnight before the examination.
2. A legal permit must be signed by the patient.
3. A cream preparation is used to remove obvious hairs 6 inches above and below the joint.
4. The same preparations are carried out as for any person who is to have a general anesthetic. Usually, no analgesia is ordered before the procedure.
5. Crutch walking should be taught before the examination.

Patient Aftercare

1. Vital signs are checked carefully along with neurologic and circulatory status.
2. The dressing is examined for bleeding. Ice is applied immediately to minimize swelling and pain. Twenty-four hours later, the bandage can be removed and Band–Aid bandages applied over puncture sites and sutures.
3. Advise the patient that sutures will be removed in approximately 7 days.
4. The patient can be up and about when recovered from the anesthetic. Crutches are to be used for the first 2 days. The patient is advised that as soon as he can walk without a limp, the crutches are no longer needed.
5. Instructions are given to do straight leg raises every hour after surgery. Gradually, weights are to be added over the next 7 days so that by the seventh day, at least 5 pounds and up to 12 pounds can be raised. These exercises increase the strength of the joint and reduce swelling.

Clinical Alert

1. Arthroscopy is usually contraindicated if ankylosis is present. It is almost impossible to maneuver the examining instrument in a joint that is stiffened by severe adhesions.

2. If there is any risk of sepsis, the procedure should be postponed.

3. Arthroscopy is usually not done less than 7 to 10 days after arthrography because chemical synovitis caused by a contrast medium can adversely affect the visual examination. However, it may be necessary to perform arthroscopy if the patient is experiencing severe pain. In this case, the knee joint will be thoroughly irrigated to remove all contrast medium.

BIBLIOGRAPHY

Beck ML: Guiding your patient a step at a time through a colonoscopy. Nursing 11(6):28–31, 1981

Beck ML: Preparing your patient psychologically for an esophagogastroduodenoscopy. Part I, Nursing 11(1):28–31, 1981; Part II, 11(2):88–91, 1981

Brunner, LS, Suddarth DS: The Lippincott Manual of Nursing Practice, 3rd ed. Philadelphia, JB Lippincott, 1982

Cotton PB, Williams CB: Practical Gastrointestinal Endoscopy. Boston, Blackwell Scientific Publications, 1982

Cunningham JT: Peritoneoscopy: Indications, technique, and diagnostic yield. Hosp Med, 128–144, August, 1985

Farrell J: Arthroscopy. Nursing 12(5):73–75, 1982

Friedman, EA (ed): Atlas Of Colposcopy. Philadelphia, WB Saunders, 1981

Hollen EM, Toomley IV, Given S: Bronchoscopy. Nursing 12(6):120–122, 1982

Isselbacher KJ et al. (eds): Harrison's Principles of Medicine, 9th ed. New York, McGraw-Hill, 1980

Kasugal T (ed): Endoscopic Diagnosis in Gastroenterology. Tokyo, Igaku–Shoin, 1982

Sugarbaker PH: Endoscopy in cancer diagnosis and management. Hosp Pract 111–112, November, 1984

ULTRASOUND STUDIES

Introduction

Overview

Ultrasonography is a noninvasive procedure for visualizing soft tissue structures of the body by recording the reflection of ultrasonic waves directed into the tissues. This diagnostic procedure, which requires very little patient preparation, is now being used in many branches of medicine for accurate diagnosis of certain pathologic conditions. It may be used diagnostically with the obstetric and gynecologic patient, the cardiac patient, and in patients with abnormal conditions of the kidney, pancreas, gallbladder, lymph nodes, liver, spleen, thyroid, and peripheral blood vessels. Frequently, it is used in conjunction with radiography or nuclear medicine scans. The procedure is relatively quick (often requiring only a few minutes to an hour) and causes little discomfort. At this time, no harmful effects have been established at the low intensities that are used (under 100 mW./cm.²). However, the ultrasound technique is a relatively new procedure, and long-term effects have not been documented. As with any diagnostic procedure, ultrasound must be weighed by its benefit and risk and should not be used frivolously.

Principles of the Technique

Ultrasound employs high frequency sound waves to examine the position, form, and function of anatomical structures (*e.g.*, the heart) and beautifully demonstrates fetal movements. Using principles first employed in sonar, ultrasound involves transmission of a sound frequency higher than that detectable by the human ear. Sonar stands for *sound visualization and ranging* and is akin to radar. Ultrasonograms are really echo reflection maps. The visualization of even a very early fetus *in utero* is simply a scaled down version of submarine detection and copies the miniaturization technique of metal flaw detection in modern engineering practice.

The two basic parameters measured by ultrasound are tissue acoustic impedance differences and sound frequency shifts due to motion. The ways in which these basic parameters are obtained are

1. An ultrasound beam is directed into the patient's body.
2. By vibration, the beam is propagated through body tissue.
3. The body tissue, being composed of structures of different acoustic impedances, reflects the sound waves in various ways. Flow through the carotid arteries is manifested by a frequency shift in the echoes reflected from moving blood cells.
4. Reflected sound waves are electronically processed and shown on imaging displays.
5. Recordings of the reflected sound waves may be made on Polaroid

film, x-ray film, chart paper, slides, or videotape. The record may be called a scan.

Evidences of pathology are detectable because lesions are of a different density and elasticity than the surrounding normal tissue. However, ultrasound cannot be used diagnostically with the air-filled lung or the gas-filled intestine because the ultrasound beam is almost totally reflected by air-containing organs. For this reason, the ultrasound beam cannot be employed where air-filled lung, gas-filled intestine or bone will come between the beam and the part of the body being studied.

Display Techniques

The complexities of the ultrasonic equipment used in ultrasound studies as well as the physical principles involved are beyond the scope of this text. However, it is helpful to have a general understanding of the types of equipment used and the techniques for displaying the image.

A cathode ray tube (CRT) displays the amplitude of the echoes and the time required for the reflection of the sound waves. Several different types of imaging displays are available.

1. A-mode display (amplitude modulated)—the earliest type of display used. All other displays are derived from it. Time and amplitude are given. It was commonly used in echoencephalography and is now used in echocardiography, and as an adjunct to B-mode displays for more accurate measurement.
2. B-mode (brightness modulated)—a two-dimensional display that provides a cross-sectional image. B-mode or scan displays echo information in various levels of gray according to the returning amplitude of the echo. An image (B scan) of the object scanned can be built up in the face of the tube as the transducer is moved through many locations and orientations.
3. Real-time display—a high-speed scanner that allows for visualization of moving structures such as the living fetus, heart, blood vessels, gallbladder, and pelvic organs. Real time uses transducer arrays that have more than one transducer element. If images are generated rapidly and repetitively to present many per second of the same section through tissue, motion of interfaces can be observed. We know this technique as *real-time scanning.*

Recording Display Images

Images are displayed on a cathode ray tube. However, a permanent record of the pattern is needed so that the images can be carefully studied and kept for legal reasons. The following are some of the methods used now:

1. Photographs may be taken of A-mode or B-mode scans that are displayed on nonstorage oscilloscopes.
2. Real-time imaging systems are recorded on hard copy such as Polaroid, x-ray film, or videotape.
3. M-mode uses sensitized paper to provide a permanent record of scannery in echocardiography.
4. Scan converter memories are devices used to store the echo signals electronically before sending them respectively to a television CRT display to give a constant echo presentation.

Doppler Method
Doppler effect is also used in a continuous ultrasound method. The Doppler effect relates to the alteration in the frequency of sound waves reflected from a moving target, such as a pulsating structure or moving cells within a blood vessel. The difference in reflected transmitted sound is converted to audible signals.

Methods of recording the echoes of ultrasound include

1. A-mode (amplitude)
2. B-mode (brightness)
3. M-mode (motion)
4. Real-time (like a movie in which you see several frames to examine)
5. Doppler method, continuous ultrasound

Note: Variations between internal textures of various organs are displayed on a television screen in varying shades of gray (gray scale).

Uses of Ultrasound
1. Obstetrical use of ultrasound is the most common application of this diagnostic modality. This is because the fluid-filled uterus is an ideal environment from which to gain information with diagnostic ultrasound. It is used in the perinatal as well as the prenatal and neonatal periods.
2. Ultrasound has been used frequently in diagnosis of brain disorders to determine shifts in the intracranial midline structures; however, this technique is used less often since the advent of computed tomography (CT) of the head. Ultrasound studies are still useful when CT and radionuclide studies are not available. Real-time study may also be used in following young children with hydrocephalus and in the evaluation of intracranial hemorrhage.
3. Other uses of ultrasound include studies of the genitourinary system, with promising results identified in the examination of the urinary bladder, scrotum, prostate, and in the diagnosis of renal masses.
4. A 98.8% accuracy rate has been reported in use of ultrasound to detect aortic aneurysms.

5. Diagnostic ultrasound also permits direct visualization of the pancreas. As with the procedures already mentioned, it has both advantages and disadvantages. Major advantages are that the pancreas can be seen in its normal state and that ultrasound gives information different from x-rays, since it is dealing with acoustic properties. Tissue echogenicity is an important aid in scanning; thinner patients yield the highest quality scans. The major disadvantage of ultrasound is related to its high reflectivity at bone and air interfaces. Adequate visualization of the pancreas is often obscured by ribs, stomach, and colon. Even with its inherent drawbacks, diagnostic ultrasound has found an important role in the work-up of a patient with suspected pancreatic pathology. Its noninvasive aspect makes serial examination possible, and this allows us to follow the progress of pathological states. Tissue character information can also narrow the diagnostic possibilities.

6. Echograms of the neck include thyroid, parathyroid, lymph nodes, and carotids. Echograms of the thyroid have their greatest value when used in conjunction with palpation of the gland by an experienced clinician. It is useful in differentiating cysts from tumors. Real time Doppler ultrasound is commonly used in the evaluation of carotid vascular disease.

7. Echograms of the eye aid ophthalmologists in removal of foreign bodies and allow the ophthalmologist to study the posterior parts of the eye, especially when the lens is opaque (as in cataracts or in vitreous hemorrhage). It is also helpful in evaluating retinal detachment.

8. Ultrasound studies of the gallbladder will detect disease as well as gallstones. The overall accuracy of gallbladder ultrasound is approximately 90%. Diseases of the gallbladder often are not detected when conventional x-ray techniques are used because the organ cannot concentrate the contrast used in testing. Ultrasonography does not depend on organ function and, thus, can be used even in the presence of significant jaundice, which would interfere with radiologic techniques dependent on organ function. Liver and spleen ultrasound studies are also done.

9. Well-circumscribed, solitary breast masses greater than 1 cm. in diameter can be evaluated. Under certain circumstances, it is possible to make a determination of the nature of mass as either cystic or solid.

10. Gallium scanning combined with ultrasound is a very useful method of evaluating suspected abscesses, and aspiration of pus collections can also be aided by ultrasound.

11. Ultrasound can also be used in evaluating persons with increasing abdominal girth and suspected ascites.

Procedure (General)

1. A gel or lubricant such as mineral oil or glycerin is applied to the skin over the area to be examined. The oil or gel acts as a conductor of the sound waves.
2. In certain cases, water is used as the conductor. The patient is then either immersed in a water bath or a water bath is hung over the area to be scanned.
3. A transducer is held by an examiner, who watches a screen while moving this device over a specific area of the body. Often a sweeping or brushing motion is used.
4. The examination is performed by a technician called an ultrasonographer.
5. Scan pictures of the recorded images are made.
6. The examination causes no physical discomfort. However, if the examining time is long, the patient could become very tired.
7. Tests usually take at least 35 to 45 minutes. This test time refers to the actual time the patient is in the examining department.
8. Some examinations require fasting and enemas.
9. Certain tests are best performed with a full urinary bladder.
10. Each individual examining department will determine its own guidelines.

Contact Technique vs. Water Bath Technique

Since air provides a poor medium for transmission of ultrasound beams, another medium must be used to couple the ultrasonic energy from the probe into the patient. Two major kinds of coupling agents have been used: water and various kinds of oils and gels.

1. *Water bath*—Early scanning devices relied heavily on the immersion of the patient in a water bath. This method provided good detail of internal structure and good sound beam control, but it was cumbersome, and the condition of the patient often made immersion inadvisable. Several newer ultrasound devices have returned to the water bath as a coupling agent. This is especially true when visualizing small organs such as the eye, the thyroid, and breast.
2. *Contact method*—This technique uses oils, glycerin, and water-soluble gels that are applied directly to the patient's skin. The transducer is swept across the skin with a brushing motion, with the probe always moving along a layer of the coupling material. Advantages of this technique are that it is easy to use and the device is portable.

Rectal and vaginal transducers have recently been introduced for the evaluation of prostate, uterine, and adnexal regions. The advantage is that these devices can often supply information in organs that were otherwise difficult to visualize sonographically because of overlying intestinal gas.

Benefits and Risks of Ultrasound Studies

1. Noninvasive procedure (with no radiation risk)
2. Requires little, if any, patient preparation
3. Procedure is safe for both patient and examiner. (To date, the procedure has been shown to be safe even for the developing fetus.)
4. As far as we know, examination can be repeated as many times as necessary without being injurious to patient. There is no harmful cumulative effect proven to date.
5. Studies can obviate the need for extended hospitalization.
6. Since ultrasound studies demonstrate structure rather than function, they may be useful with patients whose organ function is impaired.
7. Useful in detection and examination of moving parts, such as the heart
8. Does not require the injection of contrast materials, isotopes, or ingestion of opaque materials
9. Fasting is not required in many instances.

Disadvantages of Ultrasound Studies

1. An extremely skilled technician is required to operate the transducer. The scans must be read immediately and interpreted for adequacy. If the scans are not satisfactory, the examination must be repeated.
2. Air-filled structures (e.g., lungs) cannot be studied by ultrasonography.
3. Certain patients (e.g., restless children, extremely obese patients) cannot be studied adequately unless they are specially prepared.

Patients Difficult to Study

The following general categories of patients may provide some difficulties in ultrasound studies:

1. Postoperative patients—If possible, dressings should be removed and a sterile coupling agent and probe should be applied gently to the skin.
2. Patients with abdominal scars—The scar tissue causes attenuation of the ultrasound.
3. Children—Since the procedure requires the patient to remain very still, some children may need to be sedated so that their movements do not cause artifacts. However, the technologist remains with the child during the entire procedure so in most cases, there is little apprehension and little need for sedation.

4. Obese patients—Certain patients cannot be studied adequately in any case. For example, it may be very difficult to obtain an accurate scan on a very obese patient due to the alteration of the sound beam. There is no prep that would help in this case.

Interfering Factors
1. Barium has an adverse effect on the quality of abdominal studies, so echograms should be scheduled before barium studies are done.
2. If a patient has a large amount of gas in the bowel, the examination will be rescheduled because air (bowel gas) is a very strong reflector of sound and will not permit visualization.
3. Because gel or lubricant on the skin is used as a conductor, the examination cannot be performed over an area of open wounds or dressings.

Inadequate contact between the skin and the probe may be one of the causes of unsatisfactory scans. Sufficient quantities of the coupling agent, such as oil, must be applied to the skin and frequently reapplied.

Obstetric Sonogram

Normal Values
Normal pattern image reported in B-mode and real-time of fetal and placental position and of normal size, motion, cardiac, and breathing activity. Beta-scan fetal biparietal diameter at 36 weeks—approximately 8.9 cm. Fetal maturity and term pregnancy—biparietal diameter: >9.5 cm. Gestational age is estimated within 2 to 3 weeks by measuring crown to rump length, biparietal diameter, thoracic circumference, or a combination of measurements.

Explanation of Test
Ultrasound studies of the obstetric patient are valuable in (1) confirming pregnancy; (2) facilitating amniocentesis by locating a suitable pool of amniotic fluid; (3) determining fetal age; (4) confirming multiple pregnancy; (5) ascertaining whether fetal development is normal, through sequential studies; (6) determining fetal viability; (7) localizing the placenta; (8) confirming masses associated with pregnancy, and (9) postmature pregnancy (evaluation of amount of amniotic fluid and degree of placental calcification). A pregnancy can be dated with considerable accuracy if one sonogram is done at 20 weeks and a follow-up is done at 32 weeks. There is a good reliability between those two points in fetal growth. This validation is most important when early delivery is anticipated and prematurity is to be avoided. Conditions in which determination of pregnancy duration are useful are maternal diabetes, Rh immunization, preterm labor, and any medical condition that is worsening with the progress of labor. See Table 13-1.

Table 13-1

Major Uses of Obstetric Sonography

First Trimester	Second Trimester	Third Trimester
Confirm pregnancy	Establish or confirm dates†	If no fetal heart tones
Confirm viability	If no fetal heart tones	Clarify dates/size discrepancy
Rule out ectopic pregnancy	Clarify dates/size discrepancy	Large for dates—rule out
Confirm gestational age*	Large for dates—rule out	Macrosomia (diabetes mellitus)
Birth control pill use	Poor estimate of dates	Multiple gestation
Irregular menses	Molar pregnancy	Polyhydramnios
No dates	Multiple gestation	Congenital anomalies
Postpartum pregnancy	Leiomyomata	Poor estimate of dates‡
Previous complicated pregnancy	Polyhydramnios	Small for dates—rule out
Caesarean delivery	Congenital anomalies	Fetal growth retardation
Rh incompatibility	Small for dates—rule out	Oligohydramnios
Diabetes mellitus	Poor estimate of dates	Congenital anomalies
Fetal growth retardation	Fetal growth retardation	Poor estimate of dates‡
Clarify dates/size discrepancy	Congenital anomalies	Determine fetal position—rule out
Large for dates—rule out	Oligohydramnios	Breech
Leiomyomata	If history of bleeding—rule out total placenta	Transverse lie
Bicornuate uterus	previa	If history of bleeding—rule out
Adnexal mass	If Rh incompatibility—rule out fetal hydrops	Placenta previa
Multipel gestation		Abruptio placentae
Poor dates		Determine fetal lung maturity
Molar pregnancy		Amniocentesis for lecithin/sphingomyelin ratio
Small for dates—rule out		Placental maturity (grade 0–3)
Poor dates		If Rh incompatibility—rule out fetal hydrops
Missed abortion		
Blighted ovum		

* Accuracy ±3 days
† Accuracy ±1 to 1½ weeks
‡ Accuracy only ±3 weeks
(After Jensen MD, Bobak I: Maternity and Gynecologic Care, the Nurse and the Family, 3rd ed. St. Louis, CV Mosby, 1985)

The pregnant uterus is ideal for echographic evaluation because the amniotic fluid-filled uterus provides strong transmitting interfaces between the fluid, placenta, and fetus. Ultrasonography has become the method of choice in evaluating the fetus, thus eliminating the need for potentially injurious x-ray studies previously used. Since ultrasonography as used in obstetrics is about 98% accurate in detecting placental site, radionuclide studies of the pregnant patient have been abandoned. Static scans are complemented by real-time scanning which can be performed in any plane. Real-time scanning gives valuable information about cardiac activity and fetal motion.

Procedure

1. The pregnant woman lies on her back with her abdomen exposed during the test. This may cause some shortness of breath and supine hypotensive syndrome and can be relieved by elevating the upper body.
2. The patient is usually scanned with a full bladder, except when ultrasound is used to locate the placenta prior to amniocentesis, the last weeks of pregnancy, and in labor and delivery. A full bladder allows the examiner to assess other structures, especially the vagina and cervix in relation to the bladder. This is especially important when vaginal bleeding is noted and placenta previa is the suspected cause. Since the full bladder repositions the uterus and cervix for better visibility, it serves as a reference point. It also acts as a sonic window to the pelvic organs.
3. A coupling agent (*e.g.*, special transmission gel, mineral oil, olive oil) is applied liberally to the skin to prevent air from absorbing sound waves. The sonographer slowly moves the transducer over the entire abdomen to obtain a picture of the uterine contents.
4. The examining time is about 30 minutes.

Clinical Implications

1. *In the first trimester* the following information can be obtained:
   (a) Number, size, and location of gestational sacs
   (b) Presence or absence of fetal cardiac and body movement
   (c) Presence or absence of uterine abnormalities (*e.g.*, bicornuate uterus, fibroids) or adnexal masses (*e.g.*, ovarian cysts, ectopic pregnancy)
   (d) Pregnancy dating (*e.g.*, biparietal diameter, crown–rump length)
   (e) Coexistence and location of an intrauterine device (IUD)
2. *In the second and third trimesters*, ultrasound can be performed to obtain the following information:

(a) Fetal viability, number, position, gestational age, growth pattern, and structural abnormalities

(b) Amniotic fluid volume

(c) Placental location and maturity, abnormalities

(d) Uterine fibroids and anomalies

(e) Adnexal masses.

Early diagnosis of fetal structural abnormalities makes the following choices possible: (1) intrauterine surgery or other therapy to fetus if possible; (2) discontinuation of pregnancy and (3) preparation of family for care of child with a disorder or plan or other options.

3. *Fetal viability:* Fetal heart activity can be demonstrated as early as 6 to 7 weeks by real-time scanners, 10 to 12 weeks by Doppler ultrasound. This information can be utilized in management of a woman who has vaginal bleeding. Incomplete, complete and missed abortions can be differentiated. A molar pregnancy can be diagnosed but may be misdiagnosed by 9 to 10 weeks.

4. *Gestational age:* Indications for G.A. include uncertain dates for the last menstrual period or last normal menstrual period; recent discontinuation of oral hormonal suppression of ovulation; bleeding episode during the first trimester; amenorrhea of at least 3 months' duration; uterine size that does not agree with dates; previous cesarean birth, and other high-risk conditions. Four methods of gestational age estimation are: (1) determination of gestational sac dimensions (about 8 weeks): (2) measurement of crown–rump length (between 7 and 14 weeks); (3) measurement of femur length (after 12 weeks); and (4) measurement of the biparietal diameter (BPD) (starting at about 12 weeks). Fetal age determinations are not accurate in the second trimester.

5. *Fetal growth:* Some of the conditions that serve as indicators for ultrasound assessment of fetal growth include the following: poor maternal weight gain or pattern of weight gain; previous intrauterine growth retardation (IUGR); chronic infections; ingestion of drugs such as anticonvulsants or heroin; maternal diabetes; pregnancy-induced or other hypertension; multiple pregnancy, and other medical and/or surgical complications. Serial evaluations of BPD and limb length can differentiate between wrong dates and true IUGR. IUGR can be symmetrical (the fetus is small in all diameters) or asymmetrical (head and body growth vary). Symmetrical IUGR may be due to low genetic growth potential, intrauterine infection, maternal undernutrition and/or heavy smoking, or chromosomal aberration. Asymmetrical IUGR may reflect placental insufficiency secondary to hypertension, cardiovascular disease, or renal disease. Depending on the probable cause, the therapy varies.

6. *Fetal anatomy:* Depending on the gestational age, the following structures may be identified: head (including blood vessels and ven-

tricles), neck, spine, heart, stomach, small bowel, liver, kidneys, bladder, extremities. Structural defects may be identified prior to delivery. The following are examples of structural defects that may be diagnosed by ultrasound. Hydrocephaly, anencephaly, and mye-lomeningocele are often associated with polyhydramnios. Potter's syndrome (renal agenesis) is associated with oligohydramniosis. These can be diagnosed prior to 20 weeks, also skeletal defects (dwarfism, achondroplasia, osteogenesis imperfecta) and fat disorders. Other structural anomalies that can be diagnosed by ultrasound are pleural effusion (after 20 weeks), intestinal atresias or obstructions (early to second trimester), hydronephrosis and bladder outlet obstruction (second trimester to term and fetal surgery available). Two dimensional studies of the heart, together with echocardiogram, allow diagnosis of congenital cardiac lesions and prenatal treatment of cardiac arrhythmias.

7. *Detection of fetal death:* Inability to visualize the fetal heart beating and the separation of bones in the fetal head are signs of death. With real-time scanning, the absence of cardiac motion for three minutes is diagnostic of fetal demise.

8. *Placental position and function:* The site of implantation such as anterior, posterior, under, or in lower segment can be described, as well as the location of the placenta on the other side of midline. The pattern of uterine and placental growth and the bladder fullness influence the apparent location of the placenta. For example, in approximately 15% to 20% of all pregnancies when ultrasound scanning is done in the second trimester, the placenta seems to be overlying the os; at term, the evidence of placenta previa is only 0.5%; therefore, the diagnosis of placenta previa can seldom be confirmed until the third trimester. Placenta abruptia (premature separation of placenta) can also be identified.

9. *Fetal well-being:* The following physiologic measurements can be accomplished with ultrasound: heart motion; beat-to-beat variability; fetal breathing movements (FBM); urine production (following serial measurements of bladder volume); fetal limb and head movements, and analysis of vascular wave forms from fetal circulation. FBM are decreased with maternal smoking and alcohol use, and increased with hyperglycemia. Fetal limb and head movements serve as an index of neurologic development. Identification of amniotic fluid pockets is also used to evaluate fetal status. A pocket of amniotic fluid measuring at least 1 cm. is associated with normal fetal status. The presence of one pocket measuring less than 1 cm. or the absence of a pocket is abnormal. It is associated with increased risk of perinatal death.

10. *Assessment of multiple pregnancy:* It may be seen after 6 to 7 weeks—two or more gestational sacs each containing an embryo. Of those

diagnosed in the first trimester, only approximately 30% will deliver secondary to loss or absorption of one. Of value is the assessment of the relative fetal growth of twins, where IUGR or twin-to-twin transfusion is suspected. One cannot unequivocally diagnose whether they are monozygotes or heterozygotes, with ultrasound alone. Routine ultrasound cannot be totally relied upon to exclude the possibility of triplets or quadruplets, instead of only twins.

11. Male sex can be determined if fetal position is favorable; the genitalia of the male fetus may be identifiable. However, this is not the purpose of ultrasound. There is a low incidence of sex determination from the examination.

Interfering Factors
1. Artifacts can be produced when the transducer is moved out of contact with the skin. This can be resolved by adding more coupling agent to the skin and repeating the scan.
2. Artifacts (reverberation) may be produced by echoes emanating from the same surface several times. This can be avoided by careful positioning of the transducer.
3. A posterior placental site may be difficult to identify because of the angulation of the reflecting surface or insufficient penetration of the sound beam due to the patient's size.
4. Schedule uterine examination before barium x-ray examination whenever possible because barium will deflect the ultrasound beam.

Patient Preparation
1. A brief explanation of procedure to be performed is given, emphasizing that it is not uncomfortable or painful, or that it does not involve ionizing radiation that may be harmful to the mother and fetus. The studies can be repeated without harm, but the procedure is being studied carefully to determine whether there are any adverse side-effects. Benefits of the procedure should be explained.
2. The patient is asked to drink five to six glasses of fluid (coffee, tea, water, juice, soda) approximately 1 to 2 hours before the examination. If she is unable to do so, intravenous fluids may be administered. She is asked to refrain from voiding until the examination is completed. Tell the patient the examination will be done when she has a strong urge to void. Discomfort due to pressure applied over a full bladder may be experienced. If the bladder is not sufficiently filled, three to four eight-ounce glasses of water should be ingested, and rescanning is done 30 to 45 minutes later. The examination will not be conducted if the bladder is empty.
3. Explain that a liberal coating of coupling agent must be applied to the skin so that there is no air between the skin and the transducer, and so that the transducer will pass easily across the skin. A sensa-

tion of warmth may be felt. The woman should be advised not to wear good wearing apparel.

4. The woman may face the screen, and the sonographer can explain and interpret the picture. The father of the baby is encouraged to observe the testing. Some institutions provide a Polaroid photograph for the family to keep.

Clinical Alert

1. A full bladder may not be needed or desired in patients in the late stages of pregnancy or active labor. However, if a full bladder is required, and the woman has not been instructed to report with a full bladder, at least another hour of waiting time may be required before the examination can begin.
2. Fetal age determinations are most accurate in the second trimester.
3. Ultrasound cephalometry (head-size measurement) at term has a plus or minus 2-week margin of error.

Gynecologic Sonogram; Pelvic and Uterine Mass Diagnosis

Normal Values
Normal pattern image of bladder, uterus, ovaries, fallopian tubes, and vagina, and the prostate in men.

Explanation of Test
Pelvic ultrasound examines the area from the umbilicus to the pubic bone in both men and women. Ultrasound studies may be used in the evaluation of pelvic masses, postmenopausal bleeding, and to aid in the diagnosis of cysts and tumors. Information can be provided on the size, location, and structure of the masses. These examinations cannot give definitive diagnoses of pathology, but they can be used as an adjunct procedure when the diagnosis is not readily apparent. These studied are also used in treatment planning and follow-up radiation therapy of gynecologic cancer

With this test, a full bladder is necessary. The distended bladder serves four purposes: (1) it acts as a "window" for transmission of the ultrasound beam; (2) it pushes the uterus away from the pubic symphysis, thus providing a less obstructed view; (3) it pushes the bowel out of the pelvis, and (4) it may be used as a comparison in evaluating the internal characteristics of a mass under study.

Procedure
1. The patient lies on the back on the examining table during the test.
2. A coupling agent is applied to the area under study.
3. The active face of the transducer is placed in contact with patient's skin and swept across the area being studied.
4. A contact B-scanner or real-time scanner is used. A 3.5 MHz transducer is most commonly used with a 5.0 or 2.25 MHz transducer used in specific situations.
5. Examination time is about 30 minutes.

Interfering Factors
1. Results may be only fair, may vary with the patient's habits and preparation (see *Clinical Implications*), and can only be used in conjunction with other studies. However, masses as small as 1 cm. can be seen with new high resolution equipment.
2. Sonograms are difficult to do in the pelvic area unless the bladder is fully distended. This is because of the superimposition of the gas-filled intestine and interference of the symphysis pubis.
3. Whenever possible, schedule the pelvic examination before a barium x-ray.

Clinical Implications
1. Ultrasound studies may raise the suspicion that a uterine fibroid exists; such studies, however, cannot confirm this diagnosis. It may be difficult to differentiate a uterine fibroid from a solid adnexal tumor.
2. Adnexal masses smaller than 3 cm. in diameter may not be demonstrated by ultrasound studies. Large masses studied with this technique can provide information on size and consistency.
3. *Cysts:*
    (a) Ovarian cysts (the most common ovarian mass detected by ultrasound) will appear as smoothly outlined, well-defined masses. Cysts cannot be confirmed as either malignant or benign, but ultrasound studies can increase the suspicion that a particular mass is malignant.
    (b) A corpus luteum cyst is a single simple cyst commonly visualized in early pregnancy.
    (c) Theca-lutein cysts are associated with hydatidiform mole, choriocarcinoma, or multiple pregnancy.
    (d) Parovarian cysts are thin-walled cystic masses that can become quite large. When the urinary bladder is not distended, these large cysts are often situated low in the pelvis and confused with the urinary bladder.
    (e) Since normal ovaries often have numerous visible small cysts, the diagnosis of polycystic ovaries is difficult on the basis of ultrasound alone.

(f) Dermoid cysts or benign ovarian teratomas are found in the young adult female and have an extremely variable appearance. Because of their echogenicity, they are often missed on ultrasound. The only initial clue may be an indentation of the urinary bladder. When a dermoid is suspected on ultrasound, a pelvic x-ray should be obtained.

4. Solid ovarian tumors such as fibromas, fibrosarcomas, Brenner tumors, dysgerminomas, and malignant teratomas are not distinguishable by diagnostic ultrasound. Ultrasound will document the presence of a solid lesion, but can go no further in narrowing the diagnosis.

5. Metastatic tumors of the ovary are common and may be solid or cystic in ultrasonic appearance. They are quite variable in size and may be bilateral. Since ascites is often present, the pelvis and remainder of the abdomen should be scanned for fluid.

6. Pelvic inflammatory disease: Ultrasound differentiation between pelvic inflammatory disease and endometriosis is difficult. Evaluation of laboratory results plus clinical history leads to correct diagnosis. Other entities may have similar ultrasonic presentations and include (1) appendicitis with rupture into the pelvis; (2) chronic ectopic pregnancy; (3) post-trauma with hemorrhage into the pelvis, and (4) pelvic abscesses from various causes such as Crohn's disease or diverticulitis.

7. Bladder distortion: Any distortion of the bladder raises the possibility of an adjacent mass. Tumor, infection, and hemorrhage are the major causes of increased thickness to the urinary bladder wall. Masses such as calculi and catheters may be seen within the bladder lumen. Urinary bladder calculi are highly echogenic. A urinary bladder diverticulum appears as a cystic mass adjacent to the urinary bladder. It may be mistaken for a cystic mass arising from some other pelvic structure, so attempts are made to demonstrate its communication to the bladder.

8. Ultrasound studies can help to determine whether a pelvic mass is mobile.

9. Solid pelvic masses such as fibroids and malignant tumors may be differentiated from cystic masses, which will show sound patterns similar to the bladder.

10. Lesions may be shown to have metastasized.

11. Studies may aid in the planning of tumor radiation therapy.

12. Position of an intrauterine contraceptive device may be determined.

Patient Preparation

1. Explain the purpose and procedure of the test. Fasting is not required.

2. Have the patient drink four glasses of water or liquid 1 hour before the examination. Advise the patient not to void until the test is over.
3. Reassure the patient that there is no pain or discomfort involved.

> **Clinical Alert**
>
> If the patient is NPO or in certain emergency situations, the patient may be catheterized and the bladder filled via the catheter.

Kidney Sonogram

Normal Values
Normal pattern image indicating normal size and position of kidney

Explanation of Test
This noninvasive test, often done to differentiate renal masses, has become an accepted clinical procedure following intravenous pyelography (IVP). It is of value in monitoring the status of the transplanted kidney. Using IVP, the exact location of a renal mass can be located before ultrasonic examinations are performed. However, in the case of impaired renal function and iodine allergies that preclude the use of IVP, renal echograms are fairly reliable and easy to do. They can be used alone or with a nuclear scan to establish a diagnosis. The size of the kidneys can be determined without the need for contrast agents. The location of the kidneys can also be determined. This is particularly useful information in planning radiation therapy for a renal tumor.

Procedure
1. The patient lies quietly in a prone or lateral position on an examining table. However, the right kidney may also be examined with the patient supine, employing the liver as an acoustic window.
2. Warm oil or gel is applied to the back.
3. For visualization of the upper poles of the kidney, the patient must inspire as deeply as possible.
4. The total study time varies from 30 to 45 minutes.

Clinical Implications
1. Abnormal pattern readings reveal
   (a) Cysts
   (b) Solid masses
   (c) Hydronephrosis
   (d) Obstruction of ureters
   (e) Nonopaque calculi
2. Studies can provide information on the size, site, and internal structure of a nonfunctioning kidney.

3. Studies can differentiate between bilateral hydronephrosis, poly-cystic kidneys, and the small, end-stage kidneys of glomerulo-nephritis or pyelonephritis.
4. Ultrasound may be used to follow the kidney development in chil-dren with congenital hydronephrosis. This approach is safer than repeated IVP studies.
5. Perirenal hematomas or abscesses may be discovered.
6. Solid lesions may be differentiated from cystic lesions.

Interfering Factors
Retained barium from x-rays will cause poor results.

Patient Preparation
1. Explain the purpose and procedure of the test.
2. Assure the patient that there is no pain involved; the only discom-fort is that caused by lying quietly for a long period of time.
3. Explain that fasting is usually necessary. Check with your ultra-sound department for guidelines.

Clinical Alert

1. Scans cannot be done over open wounds or dressings.
2. This examination must be performed before barium x-ray. If such scheduling is not possible, at least 24 hours must elapse between barium procedure and renal echogram.
3. Biopsies are often done using ultrasound as a guideline. If a biopsy is done, a surgical permit must be signed by the pa-tient.

Pancreas Sonogram

Normal Values
Normal pattern image on gray scale; B-scan imaging indicating nor-mal size and position of pancreas. The normal gland is an echo-produc-ing structure and will be more echogenic than the normal liver.

Background
The pancreas is an extremely inaccessible abdominal organ; various diagnostic procedures have been attempted to ascertain pathologic conditions of this organ. Ultrasound studies are probably the safest and most accurate procedures available. With gray scale ultrasound equip-ment, the normal pancreas can be visualized 75% to 95% of the time. A sonogram of the pancreas in combination with a pancreas nuclear scan will increase the percentage greatly.

Explanation of Test

Ultrasound studies are done to establish a diagnosis of chronic pancreatitis, pseudocysts, and carcinoma. This is the method of choice in screening suspected pancreatic disease and in monitoring the response of pancreatic tumors to therapy. The results of these studies are used as a guide for percutaneous aspiration and biopsy. Liver and pancreatic ultrasound studies may be done at the same time. The pancreas may be visualized more easily and precisely by echogram than by any other method.

Although sonography is helpful in evaluation of patients who develop complications of acute pancreatitis, it is of little help in evaluation of patients who present with acute pancreatitis. This is primarily due to the associated ileus and gas-filled bowel that prohibits adequate visualization of the pancreas in patients presenting in an acute phase of pancreatitis.

Procedure

1. The patient lies on his back on the examining table.
2. The skin is covered with a layer of mineral oil or scan gel.
3. The patient must inspire deeply before the scans are taken.
4. Total time of the examination is 1 to 1½ hours.

Patient Preparation

1. Explain the purpose and procedure of the test.
2. Check with the individual laboratory to determine whether or not fasting is required.

Clinical Implications

1. Abnormal image patterns can identify the following conditions:
   - (a) Acute and chronic pancreatitis
   - (b) Possible sequelae of pancreatitis
   - (c) Pseudocysts
   - (d) Carcinoma of pancreas
2. In the patient with pancreatitis, the borders of the pancreas are more distinct, and the fibrous tissue septae inside the gland become more apparent.

Clinical Alert

If the patient with pancreatitis has an unusual amount of bowel gas, the scan will need to be repeated or a CT scan done.

3. In ultrasound studies, pseudocysts appear as well-defined masses and usually have echo-free interiors. Pancreatic pseudocysts may not always be echo free. Debris secondary to necrosis and enzy-

matic action on surrounding tissue presents as echogenic regions within a pseudocyst. (A pseudocyst occurs when a portion of the pancreas is deprived of its normal route of drainage through the pancreatic duct. Enzymes continue to be secreted from walled-off cysts with no mucosal lining.)

4. Pancreatic carcinoma may be identified as an irregular mass with scattered internal echoes and poorly defined borders. This condition may easily be confused with lymph node enlargement secondary to lymphoma.

Interfering Factors

1. Air, gas, or bone near the pancreas could interfere with visualization of the organ.
2. If the stomach, costal cartilage, or fat overlies the pancreas, visualization is impeded.
3. The obese patient presents an impediment to visualization because of the difficulty of ultrasound waves passing through layers of fat.
4. Movement of the organ can cause difficulties, but this is less of a problem if real-time imaging techniques are used.
5. Barium from recent radiographic studies will cause problems in visualization.

Gallbladder and Biliary System Sonogram

Normal Values
Normal pattern image reported by B-mode technique; gray scale indicating normal size and position of gallbladder and bile ducts
Normal gallbladder: 3 cm. wide; 7.5–10 cm. long

Explanation of Test
This test is used to differentiate hepatic disease from biliary obstruction. The gallbladder and sometimes the common bile and cystic duct can be identified using echography. This method is the procedure of choice when a patient with poor liver function has an elevated serum bilirubin and contrast x-rays cannot be performed. The test is very helpful in evaluation of a patient with suspected gallstones whose gallbladder fails to opacify during oral or intravenous gallbladder x-rays.

Sonography is an excellent examination in the determination of stones or chronic cholecystitis. A normal study will very likely rule out these conditions. It is a worthwhile initial study in persons with chronic right upper quadrant pain because the common duct, head of pancreas, intrahepatic ducts, liver parenchyma, and porta hepatis can also be seen during gallbladder study.

Procedure
1. The patient lies on his back on the examining table.
2. Generally, scans are performed in supine, decubitus (lateral), or upright positions.

Clinical Implications
1. Abnormal pattern images indicate
   (a) Enlarged gallbladder
   (b) Obstruction of common bile duct
   (c) Thickened gallbladder wall, sometimes a sign of chronic cholecystitis
   (d) Dilatation of biliary tree
   (e) Stones (calculi) in gallbladder and common bile duct

   Note: Gallstones smaller than 2 to 3 mm. in diameter often can be visualized with the new high resolution equipment. These stones are often the most dangerous because they can obstruct the flow of bile by entering the bile ducts. Stones usually cause dense echoes in the gallbladder area.

2. Inflammation of the gallbladder (cholecystitis) will be indicated by a slightly enlarged sonolucent structure with thickened walls.
3. Carcinoma of gallbladder.
4. Polyps within gallbladder.

Patient Preparation
1. Explain the purpose, procedure, and benefits of the test. No ionizing radiation is involved.
2. Instruct the patient not to eat solid food for 12 hours before the examination to allow the greatest dilatation of the gallbladder.
3. Water is permitted.
4. In some instances, enemas will be ordered before testing.

Clinical Alert

When it is difficult to differentiate between an abnormal gallbladder and a normal gallbladder with good contractility, the patient will be given a fatty substance such as Lipomul and another scan will be done to check contractility.

Lymph Node and Retroperitoneal Sonogram

Normal Values
Normal lymph nodes, which are smaller than a fingertip (about 1.5 cm), are not visible with ultrasound. Only when the lymph nodes enlarge, as with tumor, infection, or in a nodal group, are they visible.

Explanation of Test
Ultrasound has made the investigation of the retroperitoneum much easier. Generally, the retroperitoneum is a somewhat inaccessible area for conventional x-ray examination. This test is ordered for patients with aortic or iliac lymph node enlargement when lymphoma is suspected. Lymph node enlargement can be evaluated using ultrasound without the use of contrast agents. Also, retroperitoneal tumor response to therapy can be monitored without lymphangiography. Localization of lymph node masses by this method before radiotherapy is very useful in planning treatment and may be used as a follow-up study to assess shrinkage of the mass. These studies are easy to do and fairly reliable with a 28% chance of error. Ultrasound studies of the lymph nodes are often done in conjunction with lymphangiography.

Procedure
1. The patient lies on his back during the test.
2. Scans in two planes—longitudinal and transverse—must be taken.
3. If scans are taken below the umbilicus, the patient should have a full bladder to push the bowel out of the pelvis.

Clinical Implications
1. Abnormal pattern readings indicate
   (a) Retroperitoneal aden-   (b) Retroperitoneal tumors
       opathy
2. Lymph nodes that have enlarged will be more homogeneous than surrounding structures. However, echoes from enlarged nodes are not always a reliable indicator of their cause.

Patient Preparation
1. Explain the purpose and procedure of the test.
2. A 12-hour fast from solid food before the test is usually required.
3. Water is permitted.

Interfering Factors
With scans taken below the umbilicus, a gas- or feces-filled bowel may cause difficulty in differentiating lymph nodes.

Liver Sonogram

Normal Values
Normal pattern image indicating normal size, shape, and position of liver and normal relationship to adjacent anatomic structures.

Explanation of Test
This noninvasive diagnostic technique is used to determine the cystic, solid, or complex nature of a liver defect. Pleural effusion can be seen

and the intrahepatic ducts and veins can also be visualized. This examination is an excellent guide in evaluating ascites and is used before biopsy. Liver echograms are also used with good results mainly to differentiate cysts and abscesses from tumors. Liver sonograms are extremely useful in conjunction with hepatic radioisotope studies. Unfortunately, liver echograms are not reliable in detecting metastasis, especially in persons whose liver is high and largely under the rib cage.

Procedure
1. The patient lies on his back on the examining table.
2. It is important to have the patient take a deep breath and hold it. Deep inspiration places the liver as caudal as possible and costal margins and ribs are avoided.
3. Scans in several different planes are taken: supine longitudinal, supine transverse, and supine oblique.

Clinical Implications
1. Abnormal pattern readings reveal
   (a) Biliary duct obstruction   (e) Metastasis to liver
   (b) Cirrhosis   (f) Cause of jaundice
   (c) Necrotic tumors
   (d) Liver masses (intrahepatic,
       extrahepatic, subhepatic)
2. Cystic masses, solid masses, and abscesses may be distinguished from one another (cystic lesions have an echo-free nature, while abscesses may contain internal echoes). Solid masses will have internal echoes and will alternate the sound beam more than cystic lesions or abscesses.
3. A cirrhotic liver is more echogenic (contains more echoes) than the normal liver.
4. Serial scans can be used to determine the volume of the liver.
5. Adenocarcinoma and other primary liver tumors will have a dense central echo pattern surrounded by a less echo-producing halo. The image pattern is thus called the *bull's-eye*.

Patient Preparation
1. Explain the purpose and procedure of the test.
2. Check with the laboratory for fasting requirements.

Interfering Factors
Images of the right lobe may be somewhat obscured by rib artifacts.

Spleen Sonogram

Normal Values
Normal pattern image; diffuse, homogeneous, low-level echo pattern

Explanation of Test
This test is useful when the spleen is enlarged, because it is then easily detectable. Ultrasound is often used when a splenectomy is contemplated, such as with thrombocytopenic purpura. This study can be used to estimate spleen size and volume and may spare the patient discomfort from other kinds of diagnostic procedures. It can help to demonstrate the presence of hemostasis or fluid collections in or around the spleen in persons who have had a left upper quadrant injury. Following splenectomy, this test is used to search for a subphrenic abscess. Ultrasound is often used in conjunction with a radioisotope scan, except with pregnant women.

Procedure
1. The patient lies on his back or abdomen on the examining table during the test.
2. The examining time is about 30 minutes.

Clinical Implications
1. Abnormal pattern readings will reveal filling defects associated with an enlarged spleen, splenic metastasis, and cysts.
2. Although splenic metastases are rare, they will produce stronger than normal echoes.
3. Cysts within the spleen are identified because they give off no echoes.
4. In pregnant women who have experienced trauma to the spleen, a splenic hematoma may develop, causing distortion of the border of the spleen; hemorrhagic areas may be separated by a band of echoes.
5. The spleen is often large and echo free in early sickle cell disease, but it shrinks in size and is echo producing in later stages of the disease.

Patient Preparation
1. Explain the purpose and procedure of the test.
2. Fasting from food for 12 hours before the examination is usually necessary.
3. Water is permitted.

Thyroid Sonogram

Normal Values
Normal pattern image of thyroid; echoes are uniformly reflected throughout the gland; boundaries are unevenly displayed. (The normal thyroid is moderately echogenic; on a transverse scan the trachea is posterior to the thyroid gland.)

Explanation of Test

This ultrasound study is used to determine the size of the thyroid, to differentiate cysts from tumors, and to reveal the depth and dimension of thyroid goiters and nodules. The response of a mass in the thyroid to suppressive therapy can be monitored by successive examinations. Theoretically, this technique offers the possibility of a good estimation of thyroid weight—information that is important in radioiodine therapy for Graves' disease.

The examination is easy to do, is done before surgery, and gives 85% accuracy. Often, these studies are done in conjunction with radioactive iodine uptake tests. With pregnant patients, ultrasound studies are the method of choice; radioactive iodine is harmful to the developing fetus.

Procedure

1. The patient lies on his back on the examining table, with his neck hyperextended.
2. Oil is applied to the patient's neck.
3. A pillow is placed under the shoulder for comfort and to bring the transducer into better contact with the thyroid.
4. An alternate procedure involves separation of the neck surface from the transducer by a plastic bag filled with water. The water-filled bag is clipped on a stand and hung over the patient's neck. This water bath device allows for proper transmission of the ultrasound waves through the thyroid.
5. Examining time is about 30 minutes.

Clinical Implications

1. An abnormal pattern reading will present a cystic, complex, or solid echo pattern.
2. Solitary "cold" nodules 1 to 3 cm. in size identified on radioisotope scans can be described as cystic or solid nodules by means of the ultrasound studies. Approximately 20% of these cold nodules prove to be cysts, the great majority of which are benign. Sixty percent are solid benign tumors, and the remaining 20% are solid malignant tumors.
3. Cysts, which are generally benign, are usually echo free with many echoes occurring distal to the posterior wall.
4. Solid tumors generally represent benign adenomas.
5. Thyroid adenoma will be demonstrated by a core of high-amplitude echoes with a halo of low-amplitude echoes.
6. Thyroid carcinomas appear to be lesions that are echo poor with an irregular display or peripheral echoes.

Interfering Factors

1. Nodules less than 1 cm. in diameter may escape detection.
2. Cysts not originating in the thyroid may show the same ultrasound characteristics as thyroid cysts.

3. Lesions of more than 4 cm. in diameter frequently contain areas of cystic or hemorrhagic degeneration and give a mixed echogram that is difficult to correlate with specific disease.

Patient Preparation
Explain the purpose and procedure of the test.

Abdominal and Aorta Sonogram

Normal Values
Normal pattern image of contour and diameter of aorta usually reported in B-mode, gray scale, or real-time. The walls strongly reflect echoes, while the blood-filled lumen is echo free. Normal pattern image of upper abdominal organs indicating no discernible pathology.

Explanation of Test
Abdominal ultrasound includes all the upper abdominal organs from the xiphoid to the umbilicus and includes the gallbladder, liver, pancreas, kidneys, aorta, and spleen, while sonograms may be organ specific, such as pancreas sonogram. They are commonly ordered by region, such as upper abdomen. Aortic echogram's greatest value is in the assessment of abdominal aortic aneurysms. Ultrasound is the least invasive diagnostic procedure available. The aorta is one of the easiest abdominal structures to visualize ultrasonically because of the marked change in acoustic impedance produced by the elasticity of its walls and its blood-filled internal structure. Echograms can evaluate the body tissues from below the xyphoid process to the aortic bifurcation. Ultrasound is an ideal method for serial examinations before and after surgery and in patients with small aneurysms. Clots within the aorta are evaluated by using ultrasound and Doppler in combination. For the pregnant patient, ultrasound studies are the only abdominal diagnostic method used.

Procedure
1. The patient lies on his back or side on the examining table and may also be asked to sit up during the test.
2. The skin surface in the testing area is lubricated with a gel to permit maximum contact between transducer and body surface.
3. The length of examination time is 30 minutes.

Clinical Implications
The typical abnormal pattern readings reveal aortic aneurysms with or without thrombus. See individual organ tests for abnormal results.

Interfering Factors
Retained barium from x-ray procedures will give poor results.

Patient Preparation

1. Explain the purpose and procedure of the test.
2. Explain that there is no pain or discomfort involved.
3. Instruct the patient not to eat solid food for 12 hours before testing.
4. Water is permitted.

Clinical Alert

This examination must be scheduled before barium x-ray procedures. If this cannot be arranged, at least 24 hours must elapse between barium tests and aortic and abdominal echogram.

Heart Sonogram (Echocardiogram)

Normal Values

Normal position, size, movement of heart valves and chamber walls recorded in M-mode and 2-D time. The following values may vary from physician to physician:

Diagnostic Movements and Dimensions	Expected Values
Left ventricular dimensions {diastolic / systolic	3.7–5.6 cm.
Ejection fraction {thickness / motion	0.6–1.1 cm.
Interventricular septum	⅔ LVPW motion
LV posterior wall thickness	0.6–1.1 cm.
Ratio: $\dfrac{\text{IVS}}{\text{LVPW}}$	<1.3
LV outflow tract width (early systolic)	2–3.5 cm.
Right ventricular dimensions	0.7–2.3 cm.
Change	0–0.6 cm.
Aortic root dimension	2–3.7 cm.
Left atrial size	1.9–4 cm.
Mitral valves: amplitude	1.5–2.5 cm.
Diastolic closing velocity (EF slope)	50–150 mm./sec.
Aortic cusp separation	1.6–2.6 cm.
Pre-ejection period	Q wave to aortic opening
Ejection time	Period of aortic opening
Mean V_{cf} (left ventricular velocity of fiber shortening)	1.22–1.73 circm./sec.
Peak V_{cf}	1.15–2.10 circm./sec.

Explanation of Test

This noninvasive technique for examining the heart can provide information about the position, size, and movements of the valves and chambers by means of reflected ultrasound. Echoes from pulsed high-frequency sound waves are used to locate and study the movements and dimensions of cardiac structures such as the valves and chamber walls. Because the heart is a blood-filled organ, sound can be transmitted through it readily to the opposite wall and to the heart–lung interface. This test is commonly used to determine or rule out valvular disease, pericardial effusion, to furnish direction for further diagnostic study, and to follow cardiac patients over an extended period. One of the advantages of this diagnostic technique is that it is a noninvasive procedure that can be performed at the patient's bedside using mobile equipment, or it can be done in the laboratory.

Note: 2-D mode is like the M-mode imaging display, in which the echo lines are displayed in a pie slice shape and recorded on video tape with regard to time.

Procedure
1. A specific diagnosis should accompany the request for the test (*e.g.*, "R/O pericardial effusion" or "determine severity of mitral stenosis").
2. The patient lies on his back, and he may be asked to turn on his left side and sit up, leaning slightly forward. The skin surface is lubricated with a gel. The transducer is held over the fourth left intercostal space apex, and subcostal for scanning.
3. There is no pain or discomfort involved. Electrocardiogram (ECG) leads are attached for a simultaneous ECG and ultrasonic record (see Chapter 15).
4. Examination time is 30 to 45 minutes.

Clinical Implications
Abnormal values help to diagnose

1. Mitral stenosis
2. Mitral valve prolapse
3. Pericardial effusion
4. Subaortic stenosis
5. Tricuspid valve disease
6. Other valvular diseases
7. Congenital heart disease
8. Chamber size variations
9. LV dysfunction
10. Cardiac thrombi

Patient Preparation
Explain the purpose and procedure of the test.

Eye and Orbit Sonograms

Normal Values
Pattern image indicating normal soft tissue of eye and retrobulbar orbital areas, retina, choroid, orbital fat

Explanation of Test

Ultrasound can be used to describe both normal and abnormal tissues of the eye when no alternative visualization is possible because of opacities. This information is of invaluable assistance in the management of eyes with large corneal leukomas or conjunctival flaps and in the evaluation of eyes for keratoprosthesis. Orbital lesions can be detected and distinguished from inflammatory and congestive causes of exophthalmus with a high degree of reliability. An extensive preoperative evaluation before vitrectomy surgery or for vitreous hemorrhages is also done. In this case, the vitreous cavity is examined to rule out retinal and choroidal detachments and to detect and localize vitroretinal adhesions and intraocular foreign bodies. Also, persons who are to have intraocular lens implants after removal of cataracts must be measured for exact length of the eye. These exact measurements must be to the nearest tenth of a millimeter.

Procedure

Two techniques are used: immersion and contact. The immersion technique gives a more sophisticated evaluation because the transducer is placed away from the eye in a water bath.

1. The eye area is anesthetized by instilling eye drops.
2. If the immersion technique is used, the probe is immersed within the fluid, and sound waves are directed along the visual axis.
3. In the contact method, the probe gently touches the corneal surface.
4. If a lesion in the eye is detected, as much as 30 minutes may be required to accurately differentiate pathology.
5. Orbital examination can be done in 8 to 10 minutes.

Clinical Implications

1. Abnormal patterns are seen in
   - (a) Alkali burns with corneal flattening and loss of anterior chamber
   - (b) Detached retina
   - (c) Keratoprosthesis
   - (d) Extraocular thickening in thyroid eye disease
   - (e) Pupillary membranes
   - (f) Cyclitic membranes
   - (g) Vitreous opacities
   - (h) Orbital mass lesions
   - (i) Inflammatory conditions
   - (j) Vascular malformations
   - (k) Foreign bodies
2. Abnormal patterns are also seen in tumors of various types based on specific ultrasonic patterns.
   - (a) Solid, such as meningioma, glioma, neurofibroma
   - (b) Cystic, such as mucocele, dermoid, and cavernous hemangioma
   - (c) Angiomatous, such as diffuse hemangioma
   - (d) Lymphangioma
   - (e) Infiltrative, such as metastatic lymphoma and pseudotumor

Interfering Factors
If at some time the vitreous humor in a particular patient has been replaced by a gas, no result can be obtained.

Patient Preparation
1. Explain the purpose and procedure of the test.
2. Topical anesthetic drops are instilled into the eyes before examination. This is usually done in the examining department.

Patient Aftercare
1. Instruct the patient to refrain from rubbing the eyes until the effects of anesthetic have disappeared. This type of friction could cause corneal abrasions.
2. Advise the patient that minor discomfort and blurred vision may be experienced for a short time.

Urinary Bladder Sonogram

Normal Values
Normal pattern image of the exact dimensions and contour of the bladder and little residual volume

Explanation of Test
This examination is done in the investigation of possible bladder tumor and provides a simple method of estimating postvoid residual urine volume. This test reduces the need for urinary catheterization and risk of subsequent urinary tract infection.

Procedure
1. The patient is placed in a supine position.
2. A gel is applied to the lower abdomen.
3. Total examining time is 20 to 30 minutes.

Clinical Implications
Abnormal results reveal

1. Tumors of bladder
2. Ovarian carcinoma extension to bladder
3. Thickening of bladder wall
4. Masses posterior to bladder
5. Obstruction of lower urinary tract showing residual urine

Interfering Factors
1. Poor technique
2. Overlying gas or fat tissue

Patient Preparation
1. Explain the purpose and procedure of the test.
2. The bladder should be full to start, then emptied to complete the examination.

Patient Aftercare
Return to normal routine of nursing unit.

Intrauterine Contraceptive Device (IUCD; IUD) Localization

Normal Values
An IUD can be visualized ultrasonically if it has not perforated the uterus.

Explanation of Test
Ultrasonography has been found useful for confirming the presence and exact location of an IUD and for identifying the type of contraceptive device within the endometrial cavity. X-ray studies will only indicate that the device is in the pelvis. Most of these devices are sufficiently different in acoustic impedance from the normal uterus, so they are easily detected. The precise appearance depends on the type of device used, the position of the device within the uterus, and the position of the device relative to the transducer.

Procedure
1. The patient lies on her back on the examining table. A full bladder is necessary.
2. A coupling gel is applied to the entire abdomen.
3. The transducer is moved across the area being studied.
4. Total examining time is about 30 minutes.

Clinical Implications
1. A typical pattern will identify the presence of an IUD.
2. If the device has perforated the uterus, it is seldom possible to visualize it ultrasonically because it blends with the surrounding bowel echoes.

Interfering Factors
Overlying gas or obesity interferes with obtaining a satisfactory result.

Patient Preparation
1. Explain the purpose and procedure of the test.
2. Fasting is not required.
3. Instruct the patient to drink three to four glasses of liquid, prefera-

bly water, 1 hour before examination. Advise the patient not to void until the test is completed.
4. The only discomfort involved is the feeling of a full bladder.

Breast Sonogram

Normal Values
Symmetrical echo pattern in both breasts, including subcutaneous, mammary, and retromammary layers

Explanation of Test
Ultrasound mammography is useful for differentiating cystic, solid, and complex lesions, in diagnosing disease in women with very dense breasts, and in the follow-up of women with fibrocystic disease. It is recommended as the initial method of examination in young women with palpable masses and pregnant women with a newly palpable mass. The pregnant patient presents a dilemma because malignancies in pregnancy grow rapidly, and the increased glandular tissue causes difficulties in mammography. Ultrasound may now be used to evaluate women who have silicone-prosthesis (as opposed to silicone-injected) augmented breasts. The prosthesis is readily penetrated by the ultrasound beam. Such prostheses are know to obscure masses on physical examination, and x-ray beams are absorbed by the prosthesis, thus obscuring portions of the breast parenchyma.

When ultrasound is used in combination with x-ray mammography, diagnostic accuracy is improved. In addition, ultrasound mammography is an alternative for women who absolutely refuse to have an x-ray mammogram or those who should not be exposed to diagnostic radiation.

Procedure
1. The patient is asked to lie down on the examining table, which contains a machine with a tank that holds chlorinated, chemically treated, heated water. Visible at the bottom of the tank is a transducer that produces the ultrasound waves and detects their echoes. The patient will hear the sounds of the machine in operation as it records the echoes. (Water is a very good conductor of the ultrasound waves.) One breast at a time is immersed in the water.
2. Total examining time is 15 minutes.

Clinical Implications
Unusual and distinctive echo patterns will indicate the presence of

1. Cysts
2. Benign solids

3. Malignant tumors
4. Tumor metastasis to muscles and lymph nodes

Interfering Factors
1. Women with back problems or those with limited flexibility may have difficulty maintaining the positions necessary for the procedure.
2. Although the tank is built to accommodate breasts of most sizes, 1% of breasts are too large to examine by this method.

Patient Preparation
1. Explain the purpose and procedure of the examination. Tell the patient that nothing will touch her body but the water. There is no discomfort involved. Many diagnostic departments will show the patient a videotape that explains the test.
2. On the day of examination the patient should wear a two-piece outfit because the garments on the torso will be removed prior to examination.
3. No powders, lotions, or other cosmetics should be applied to the upper body on the day of examination.

Patient Aftercare
The breasts are dried and the patient is advised to contact her referring physician for outcomes.

Scrotal Sonogram

Normal Values
Normal scrotal structure

Explanation of Test
This study is useful in diagnosing scrotal abscess, "missed torsion," hydrocele, and spermatocele. Sonography is ideal for evaluating chronic scrotal swelling when the possibility of a testicular tumor exists and is valuable in clarifying ambiguous nuclear studies. It is also the best means of evaluating the clinically normal scrotum when screening for occult disease. Because sonography cannot assess perfusion, it is not the initial examination in an "acute scrotum."

Procedure
1. The patient lies on his back and the penis is gently taped back to the lower abdominal wall.
2. After an acoustical gel is applied to the skin, the transducer is repeatedly passed over the scrotum. Sonographic images are generated.
3. Total examining time is 30 to 60 minutes.

Clinical Implications

Abnormal results are associated with

1. Abscess (cystic and solid pattern)
2. Infarcted testes of missed torsion (solid pattern)
3. Tumor
4. Hydrocele
5. Spermatocele
6. Adherent scrotal hernia
7. Missed torsion
8. Chronic epididymitis

BIBLIOGRAPHY

Athey PA, Hadlock FP: Ultrasound in Obstetrics and Gynecology, 2nd ed. St. Louis, CV Mosby, 1985

Babcock DS, Han BK: Cranial Ultrasound of Infants. Baltimore, Williams & Wilkins, 1981

Barton TB: The thyroid gland: A review for sonographers. Med Ultrasound 4:133, 1980

Callen PW: Ultrasonography in Obstetrics and Gynecology. Philadelphia, WB Saunders, 1983

Fleischer AC, James AE: Real Time Sonography. East Norwalk, CT, Appleton and Lange, 1983

Goldberg BB (ed): Ultrasound in Cancer. New York, Churchill Livingstone, 1980

Hagen–Ansert SL: Textbook of Diagnostic Ultrasonography, 2nd ed. St. Louis, CV Mosby, 1983

Jellens J, Kobayash S (eds): Ultrasonic Examination of the Breast. New York, John Wiley & Sons, 1984

Kremkau FW: Diagnostic Ultrasound—Physical Principles and Exercises, 2nd ed. New York, Grune & Stratton, 1984

McDicken WN: Diagnostic Ultrasonics: Principles and Use of Instruments. New York, John Wiley & Sons, 1981

Sarti DA, Sample WF (eds): Diagnostic Ultrasound Text and Cases. Boston, G. K. Hall Medical Publishers, 1980.

Taylor K: Atlas of Ultrasonography. New York, Churchill Livingstone, 1985

Thijsson JM, Verbeek AM (eds): Ultrasonography in Ophthalmology. The Hague, Dr. W. Junk Publishing, 1982

Thompson HE, Bernstine RL: Diagnostic Ultrasound in Clinical Obstetrics and Gynecology. New York, John Wiley & Sons, 1978

Weill FS, LeMovel A: Exercises in Diagnostic Ultrasonography of the Abdomen. New York, Springer–Verlag, 1983

Weill FS et al: Renal Sonography. New York, Springer–Verlag, 1981

PULMONARY FUNCTION STUDIES; BLOOD GAS ANALYSES

14

Introduction

Pulmonary Physiology
There are three aspects of pulmonary function: perfusion, diffusion, and ventilation. *Perfusion* consists of the passage of blood through pulmonary vessels; *diffusion* consists of exchanging oxygen for carbon dioxide across alveolar capillary membranes; *ventilation* consists of exchanging air between alveolar spaces and the atmosphere.

During breathing, the lung–thorax system acts as a bellows that provides fresh air to the alveoli for adequate gas exchange. Like springs, the lung tissue possesses the property of elasticity. When the inspiratory muscles contract, the thorax and lungs expand, and when the muscles relax and the force is removed, the thorax and lungs recoil to their resting position. In addition, when the thorax and lungs expand, the alveolar pressure is lowered below atmospheric pressure and air flows into the trachea, bronchi, bronchioles, and finally the alveoli. Expiration is mainly passive and is brought about by the recoil of the thorax and lungs to their resting position; alveolar pressure is increased above atmospheric pressure, and air flows out. The primary purpose of the pulmonary blood flow is to conduct mixed venous blood through the capillaries of the alveoli so that oxygen (O_2) can be added and carbon dioxide (CO_2) removed.

Use of Tests
Pulmonary function tests are designed to determine the presence, nature, and extent of pulmonary dysfunction caused by obstruction or restriction, or a combination of both.

When ventilation is disturbed by an increase in airway resistance, the ventilatory defect is called an *obstructive* defect. When ventilation is disturbed by a limitation in chest expansion, the defect is called a *restrictive* defect. When ventilation is disturbed by both increased airway resistance and limitation of chest expansion, the defect is called a *mixed* defect. See Table 14-1 for conditions that affect ventilation.

The results of pulmonary function studies may reveal abnormalities in the airways, alveoli, and pulmonary vascular bed early in the course of disease when physical examinations and x-ray tests are still normal. In addition, the location of an airway abnormality can be determined—for example, upper airway, large airway, or small airway.

Indications for Tests
1. Early detection of pulmonary or cardiac pulmonary disease
2. Differential diagnosis of all patients with dyspnea
3. Assessment of patient's ability to tolerate anesthetics during surgery, particularly if the removal of lung tissue is contemplated

4. Determination of the risk of using certain diagnostic procedures
5. Detection of early respiratory failure
6. To follow course of disease in patients known to have bronchopulmonary disease
7. Periodic examination of workers in industries in which a lung hazard exists
8. Epidemiologic study of populations to provide clues to the causes of pulmonary diseases

Classification of Pulmonary Diseases

1. Restrictive diseases
   Characterized by interference with elastic behavior of lungs, caus-

Table 14-1
Conditions That Affect Ventilation

Diagnosis	Basic Disturbance in Ventilation	Underlying Pathology
Obstructive Defects		
Asthma	Increased airway resistance	Bronchial edema, bronchospasm, and obstructive mucus
Bronchitis	Increased airway resistance	Same as above
Emphysema	Increased airway resistance	Loss in radial traction or respiratory airway due to destruction of alveolar septa
Restrictive Defects		
Kyphoscoliosis	Limitation on chest cavity expansion	Increase in elastic resistance of chest wall due to abnormal curvature of spine
Obesity	Same as above	Increase in elastic resistance of chest wall due to increase in adipose tissue, especially of abdomen
Muscular dystrophy	Same as above	Weakness of inspiratory muscles
Pneumoconiosis	Same as above	Increase in elastic resistance of lung due to fibroses of pulmonary tissue
Mixed Defect		
Pulmonary congestion	Increases in both airway resistance and limitation in expansion of chest cavity	Obstructive due to bronchial edema and compression of respiratory airway due to increased interstitial and intravenous fluid pressure. Restrictive due to increase in elastic resistance of lung due to increased interstitial and intravenous fluid pressure

ing them to be stiff; actual reduction in the volume of air that can be inspired

Examples of Restrictive Diseases	Caused by
Chest wall disease	Injury, kyphoscoliosis, spondylitis, muscular dystrophy, and other neuromuscular diseases
Extrathoracic conditions	Obesity, peritonitis, ascites, and pregnancy
Interstitial lung disease	Interstitial pneumonitis, fibrosis, pneumoniosis, granulomatosis, and edema
Pleural disease	Pneumothorax, hemothorax, pleural expansion, and fibrothorax
Space-occupying lesions	Tumors and cysts

2. Obstructive diseases
   Characterized by need for unusual effort to produce air-flow; respiratory muscles must work with difficulty to overcome resistive forces during breathing. Patient experiences prolongation and impairment of airflow during expiration.

Examples of Obstructive Diseases	Caused by
Peripheral airway disease	Bronchitis, bronchiecstasis, bronchiolites, bronchial asthma
Pulmonary parenchymal disease	Emphysema
Upper airway disease	Pharyngeal and laryngeal tumors, edema, infections, foreign bodies, tracheal tumors, collapse or stenosis of airway.

3. Combined or mixed (a component of both) obstruction and restriction caused by pulmonary congestion.

Classification of Tests

Most pulmonary function tests evaluate the status of the airways, vascular system, and alveoli in an indirect, overlapping way. The patient's age, height, weight, and sex are recorded before testing because they are the basis for the determination of predicted values.

Pulmonary function tests are generally divided into three categories:

1. *Conventional pulmonary function tests*—Usually include spirometry (timed vital capacity) or flow-volume loops, static lung volumes,

diffusing capacity determinations, and arterial blood gas studies at rest

2. *Specialized pulmonary function tests*—Include such procedures as closing volume, isoflow volume, body plethysmography, CO_2 response, maximum voluntary ventilation, bronchial provocation, respiratory stress testing, and exercise arterial blood gas studies

3. *Preoperative pulmonary screening*—Generally includes only the spirometry (before and after bronchodilator administration if indicated)

Pulmonary Function Testing and Spirometry

Lung capacities, volumes, and flow rates are clinically measured by a spirometer. The spirometer has a breathing system that allows gas to be breathed in and out and allows for the addition or removal of accurate amounts of gas. The electrical recording of the amounts of gas breathed in and out forms a spirogram. The values obtained and the predicted values for age, sex, height, and weight are compared by a computer. Spirometers can be grouped into two major categories: the mechanical types such as water-filled, sliding wedge, bellows, and the electronic types such as Fleisch pneumotach and hot-wire anemometer.

The water-seal spirometer has been the basic tool for many years. This spirometer consists of a bell suspended in a container of water (see Figure 14-1). The bell rises and falls in response to the breathing of the patient, who inhales and exhales into a tube connected to the spirometer. The proportional movements of the bell are recorded, either on a kymograph (a rotating drum on which a tracing is made with a stylus) or on an electrical potentiometer. Measured or actual values are then compared with the predicted values by means of regression equations using age, height, weight, and sex and are expressed as a percentage of predicted values.

Spirometry is designed to determine the effectiveness of the various forces involved in the movement of the lungs and chest wall. The values obtained will provide quantitative information about the degree of obstruction to airflow and the restriction of the amount of air that can be inspired.

Screening Spirometry

Screening spirometry is a clinical procedure (see page 748) that takes 15 to 20 minutes to perform and reveals the following values:

1. Forced vital capacity (FVC)

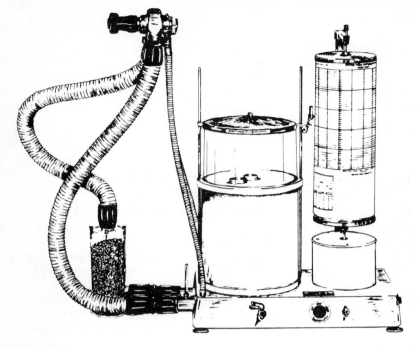

Figure 14-1
The Collins Stead-Wells spirometer. (Courtesy of Warren E. Collins, Inc., Braintree, MA)

2. Forced expiratory volumes FEV_1, FEV_3 (*i.e.*, the volumes exhaled during the first and third seconds of forced vital capacity)
3. Air flow rates (*e.g.*, forced expiratory flow [FEF] 200–1200; FEF 25–75)

Note: Spirometry plus lung volumes will take 40 minutes to complete and includes measurement of spirometry plus functional residual capacity, residual volume, expiratory reserve volume, and total lung capacity.

Procedure for Spirometry
1. The patient is fitted with a mouthpiece that is connected to the spirometer.
2. A nose clip is used so that only mouth breathing is possible.
3. The patient is either sitting down or standing up.
4. The patient is asked to inhale maximally, breath-hold momentarily, and then exhale forcibly and completely.
5. The patient is allowed to rest for a few minutes, and the above step is repeated twice.

6. The procedure takes 15 to 20 minutes to perform.
7. The best tracing from the spirometer is used to provide spirometric measurements of FVC, FEV_1, $FEF_{200-1200}$, and FEF_{25-75}.

Pulmonary Function Testing

Lung Volumes

Lung volumes can be considered as basic subdivisions of the lung (not anatomical subdivisions) and may be subdivided as follows:

1. Total lung capacity (TLC)
2. Tidal volume (VT)
3. Inspiratory capacity (IC)
4. Functional residual capacity (FRC)
5. Expiratory reserve volume (ERV)
6. Vital capacity (VC)
7. Residual volume (RV)

Combinations of two or more volumes are termed *capacities*. There are two basic methods for the determination of lung volumes.

1. The multiple-breath nitrogen washout technique (open circuit)
2. The helium dilution technique (closed circuit)

Both methods employ the use of a gas (oxygen or helium, respectively) to either wash out or dilute the air left in the lung at end tidal expiration.

These volumes and capacities are shown graphically in Figure 14-2. Also shown are values found in normal adult men. Measurement of these values with devices such as the spirometer can provide information about the severity of airway obstruction and can serve as an index of dynamic function.

Flow Rates

Flow rates provide information about the severity of airway obstruction in terms of air trapping and serve as an index of dynamic function. The lung volume at which the flow rates are measured is a most important value.

Diffusion

The measurement of lung diffusion gives information about the amount of functioning capillaries in contact with functioning alveoli. This is the rate of gas transfer across the alveolar capillary membrane and is expressed as *ml./min./mmHg. CO transferred*. These measurements are of value in the diagnosis of pulmonary vascular disease.

Arterial Blood Gases

The measurement of arterial blood gases integrates the whole of respiratory function and allows evaluation of an important factor not ob-

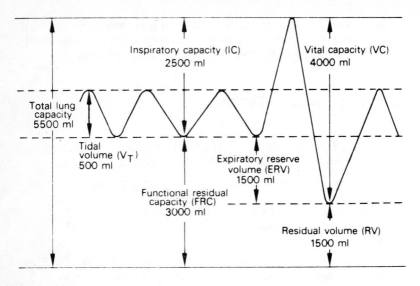

Figure 14-2
Subdivisions of lung volume in the normal adult. (Geschickter CF: The Lung in
Health and Disease. Philadelphia, JB Lippincott, 1973)

tained from routine pulmonary function tests: the degree of ventilation
matched to perfusion. The measurement of the alveolar to arterial oxygen gradient (A-aDO$_2$) gives information about the cause of hypoxemia.

Exercise or Respiratory Stress Tests and Blood Gas Studies
The analysis of bronchogenic and cardiovascular disorders includes
procedures that measure respiratory outcomes and blood gas studies

Table 14-2
Normal Changes in Blood Gas Studies During Moderate Exercise

Value	Change
O$_2$ consumption	Increases
Respiratory quotient	Increases
Ventilation	Increases
Physiologic dead space	Increases
Cardiac output	Increases
Blood lactate	Increases
Arteriovenous O$_2$ content	Increases
V$_D$/V$_T$ ratio	Decreases
Venous-admixturelike perfusion	Decreases
A-aDO$_2$	No change
Arterial blood gas tensions	No change

Table 14-3
Abnormal Changes in Blood Gas Studies During Moderate Exercise

Value	Change	Disorders That Cause Increases or Decreases
Respiratory quotient	Increases	Acidemia develops if person is physically unfit or if cardiovascular system cannot cope with increased demands of the tissues during exercise
Lactate	Increases	
PaO_2	Decreases	Ventilatory impairment
$PaCO_2$	Increases	
P_AO_2	Decreases	Diffusion defect occurs when the area of alveolar surface available for diffusion is reduced. Conditions that cause such a structural change include pulmonary fibrosis, late stages of emphysema, and surgical removal of lung tissue

during exercise. The results of many pulmonary function tests and blood gas studies are normally altered during exercise in healthy persons (see Table 14-2). However, certain specific alterations will be noted when there is cardiovascular or respiratory impairment (see Table 14-3). In virtually all diseases affecting the lungs and circulation, exercise tests are of value in assessing severity and impairment due to an already diagnosed condition. Exercise testing may also allow the recognition of unsuspected abnormalities that are contributing to disability. The diagnosis of psychogenic dyspnea is considered if no expected abnormal response occurs indicative of disease. A new, powerful tool for assessing health uses trace-gases in expired air as an aid in the diagnosis of diseases such as lung cancer and toxic exposure.

Breathalyzer, Breath Analysis

Breathalyzer machines are used to measure how much alcohol is in a person's system. It has additional new uses such as analyzing breath to help in the diagnoses of specific illnesses (liver disorders and cancer) as well as identifying persons who have been exposed to toxic compounds. Expired breath is believed to be at least as good a source of information about a person's metabolic function as urine or blood, but has been largely ignored by modern medicine. In most diseases, a number of compounds may be associated with illness. These abnormal breath compounds occur in extremely low concentrations and scientists are just beginning to be able to identify them. Studies have demonstrated differences in the breath of persons with lung cancer from that of others who do not have this disease. Breath markers have already been identified in liver disease and colon cancer.

A large bag of expired breath is collected after the person has breathed quality compressed air for a sufficient time period. The exhaled gas is pumped through a tightly packed chemical powder that separates out trace gases. The common major components of breath, such as nitrogen, oxygen, water vapor, and carbon dioxide, are allowed to escape. Hot, clean helium carries the trace-gas mixture to a mass spectrometer that separates the gases into distinct components identified by a gas chromatograph.

Procedure Using Breathalyzer To Detect Disease

1. Purified air is breathed for about 10 minutes before an exhaled breath sample is collected.
2. . A nose clamp is applied and the patient is asked to exhale until a sample bag of exhalant is collected.
3. The procedure takes about 20 minutes to complete.

List of Symbols and Abbreviations*

Pulmonary function studies and blood gas analyses measure quantities of gas mixtures and their components, blood and its constituents, and various factors affecting these quantities. The symbolic expression of these quantities was standardized at a conference held in 1950 by American physiologists. The list of symbols and abbreviations given here is based on those standards.

Once you have mastered the meaning of the major and secondary symbols, you should be able to interpret any combination of these symbols. This list will introduce you to general principles and will then apply them to measurements included in the chapter.

General Principles
Gas Volumes
Large capital letters denote primary symbols for gases.

V = Gas volume
$\dot{V}$ = Gas volume per unit time (the dot over the symbol indicates the factor per unit time)
P = Gas pressure or partial pressure of a gas in a gas mixture or in blood
F = Fractional concentration in gas

---

* Adapted from Pace WR, Jr: Pulmonary Physiology in Clinical Practice, 2nd ed. Philadelphia, FA Davis, 1970

Small capital letters indicate the type of gas measured.

A = Alveolar gas
D = Dead space gas
E = Expired gas
I = Inspired gas
T = Tidal gas

Chemical symbols for gases may be placed after the small capital letters listed above.

O_2 = Oxygen
CO = Carbon monoxide
CO_2 = Carbon dioxide
N_2 = Nitrogen

Combinations of Symbols
The following are some of the ways these symbols may be combined in the measurement of gases.

V_T = Tidal volume
V_E = Volume of expired gas
P_ACO_2 = Partial pressure of carbon dioxide in alveolar gas

Blood Gas Symbols
Large capital letters are used in primary symbols for blood.

C = Concentration of a gas in blood
S = Percent saturation of H_gb with CO or O_2
Q = Volume of blood
$\dot{Q}$ = volume of blood per unit time (blood flow)

To indicate whether blood is capillary, venous, or arterial, *lower case letters* are used as subscripts.

v = Venous blood
a = Arterial blood
c = Capillary blood
s = Shunted blood

Combinations of Symbols
Blood gas symbols may be combined in the following ways:

PO_2 = Oxygen tension or partial pressure of oxygen
PvO_2 = Venous oxygen tension or partial pressure of oxygen in venous blood
PaO_2 = Arterial oxygen tension or partial pressure of oxygen in arterial blood
P_AO_2 = Alveolar oxygen tension or partial pressure of oxygen in the alveoli
PCO_2 = Partial pressure of carbon dioxide

$PaCO_2$ = Partial pressure of carbon dioxide in arterial blood
$PvCO_2$ = Partial pressure of carbon dioxide in venous blood
SO_2 = Oxygen saturation
SaO_2 = Percent saturation of oxygen in arterial blood
SvO_2 = Percent saturation of oxygen in venous blood
TCO_2 = Total carbon dioxide content

Lung Volume Symbols
The following list indicates symbols used in measuring lung volumes as well as the units used in expressing these measurements:

FVC = *Forced Vital Capacity*—maximal amount of air that can be exhaled forcibly and completely following a maximal inspiration (units : liters)

FEV_1 = *Forced Expiratory Volume* in 1 second—volume of air expired during the first second of the FVC maneuver (units : liters)

FEV_3 = *Forced Expiratory Volume* in 3 seconds—volume of air expired during the first three seconds of the FVC maneuver (units : liters)

$FEF_{200-1200}$ = *Forced Expiratory Flow* between 200 ml. and 1200 ml.—flow of expired air measured after the first 200 ml. and during the next 1000 ml. of the FVC maneuver (units : liters/sec.)

FEF^{25-75} = *Forced Expiratory Flow* between 25% and 75%—flow of expired air measured between 25% and 75% of the FVC maneuver (units : liters/sec.)

PEFR = *Peak Expiratory Flow Rate*—maximum flow of expired air attained during an FVC maneuver (units : liters/sec. or liters/min.)

PIFR = *Peak Inspiratory Flow Rate*—maximum flow of inspired air achieved during a forced maximal inspiration (units : liters/sec. or liters/min.)

FEF_{25} = Instantaneous flow rate at 25% of lung volume achieved during an FVC maneuver (units : liters/sec. or liters/min.)

FEF_{50} = Instantaneous flow rate at 50% of lung volume achieved during an FVC maneuver (units : liters/sec. or liters/min.)

FEF_{75} = Instantaneous flow rate of 75% of lung volume achieved during an FVC maneuver (units : liters/sec. or liters/min.)

FIVC = *Forced inspiratory vital capacity*—maximal amount of air that can be inhaled forcibly and completely following a maximal expiration (units : liters)

FRC = *Functional Residual Capacity*—volume of gas contained in the lung at the end of a normal expiration (units : liters)

IC = *Inspiratory Capacity*—maximal amount of air that can be inspired from end tidal expiration (unit : liters)

ERV = *E*xpiratory *R*eserve *V*olume—maximal amount of air that can be expired from end tidal expiration (units: liters)

RV = *R*esidual *V*olume—volume of gas left in the lung following a maximal expiration (units: liters)

VC = *V*ital *C*apacity—maximal volume of air that can be expired following a maximal inspiration (units: liters)

TLC = *T*otal *L*ung *C*apacity—volume of gas contained in the lungs following a maximal inspiration (units: liters)

DιCO = Carbon monoxide diffusing capacity of the lung—rate of diffusion of carbon monoxide across the alveolar/capillary membrane (*i.e.*, rate of gas transfer across the alveolar/capillary membrane (units: ml./min./torr)

CV = *C*losing *V*olume—volume at which the lower lung zones cease to ventilate, presumably as a result of airway closure (units: percent of VC)

MVV = *M*aximal *V*oluntary *V*entilation—maximal number of liters of air a patient can breathe per minute by a voluntary effort (units: liters/min.)

$V_{ISO}\dot{V}$ = Volume of isoflow—volume in which flow was the same with air and with helium during an FVC maneuver

Miscellaneous Symbols

The following is an assortment of symbols you may encounter throughout the chapter:

A = Age in years

W = Weight in pounds

H = Height in inches

torr = A unit of pressure equal to 1/760 of normal atmospheric pressure or to the pressure necessary to support a column of mercury one mm. high at 0°C and standard gravity

f = Frequency of breathing

C = Compliance

He = Helium

Hg = Mercury

D = Diffusing capacity

CO = Carbon monoxide

DιO$_2$ = Oxygen diffusing capacity of the lung (ml./min./torr)

A-aDO$_2$ = Alveolar-to-arterial oxygen gradient

BSA = Body surface area (unit: m^2)

H$_2$CO$_3$ = Carbonic acid

HCO$_3$ = Bicarbonate

TGV = *T*horacic *G*as *V*olume (also expressed as V_{TG})

R$_{aw}$ = Airway resistance

F-V = Flow volume

pH = Negative logarithm of the hydrogen ion concentration, used as a positive number to indicate acidity or alkalinity.

V-T = Volume time

BE = Base excess/deficit

TESTS

Functional Residual Capacity (FRC)

Normal Values

Approximately 2400–3000 ml.

Predicted values are based on age, height, weight, and sex.

The observed value should be 75% to 125% of the predicted value.

Explanation of Test

This test is used to evaluate both restrictive and obstructive defects of the lung. Changes in the elastic properties of the lungs are reflected in the FRC. This test measures the volume of gas contained in the lungs at the end of a normal quiet expiration and is expressed mathematically as equal to the sum of the expiratory reserve volume and the residual volume (FRC = ERV + RV).

Procedure

1. The patient is fitted with nose clips and asked to breathe through the mouthpiece on the lung volume apparatus.
2. Depending on the instrument, the patient either
   (a) Breathes 100% oxygen (O_2) until the alveolar nitrogen (A_{N_2}) reaches 1% or 7 minutes elapses (whichever comes first). Calculation of the functional residual capacity (FRC) is based on the fact that 81% of the air in the lung is N_2. The N_2 is "washed" out of the lungs by having the patient breathe 100% O_2 and then measuring the volume of N_2 collected

   or

   (b) Rebreathes a 10% to 12% helium (He) and room-air concentration until equilibrium is reached
3. Results are recorded by either an X–Y recorder on semilog paper or by a respirometer on a kymograph drum (Figure 14-3).
4. At the end of the test, the following values are computed. The choice of the formula depends on the method being used.

$$FRC = \frac{\% \ N_2 \ final \times V_E}{\% \ A_{N_2}}$$

(Nitrogen washout or open circuit technique)

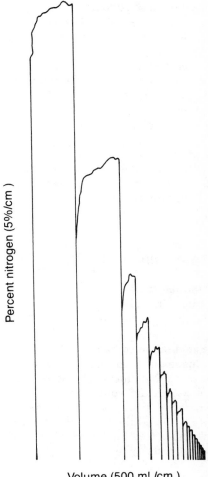

Figure 14-3
Typical tracing of a multiple breath nitrogen washout curve for determining FRC. The patient breathes 100% oxygen until alveolar nitrogen reaches 1%.

Volume (500 ml /cm)

$$FRC = \frac{\% \text{ He initial} - \% \text{ He final}}{\% \text{ He final}} \times \text{initial volume}$$

(Helium dilution or closed circuit technique)

5. The test should be repeated a second time and results between the FRCs should not vary by more than 5% to 10%.

Clinical Implications
1. A value less than 75% is indicative of restrictive disease.
2. Restrictive defects are characterized by normal or decreased FRC.
3. A value of greater than 125% demonstrates air trapping, which is consistent with obstructive airway disease. An increase in the FRC represents hyperinflation, which may result from emphysematous changes, asthmatic or fibrotic obstruction of the bronchioles, compensation for surgical removal of lung tissue, or a thoracic cage deformity.

Patient Preparation
1. Explain the purpose and procedure of the test.
2. Obtain the patient's age, sex, weight, and height and record this information before doing the test.

Total Lung Capacity (TLC)

Normal Values
Approximately 5500 ml.
Predicted values are based on age, height, and sex.

Explanation of Test
This test is used mainly to evaluate obstructive defects of the lungs as well as to delineate restrictive from obstructive pulmonary disease. It measures the volume of gas contained in the lungs at the end of a maximal inspiration. Mathematically, it is the sum of the vital capacity (VC) and the residual volume (RV) or the sum of the primary lung volumes (see Figure 14-2). This value is determined indirectly from other tests.

Procedure
1. There is no procedure to perform.
2. It is a mathematical formula: TLC = VC + RV

Clinical Implications
1. An obstructive defect is characterized by an *elevated* TLC. However, a normal or *increased* TLC does not mean that ventilation or the surface area for diffusion is normal.
2. The TLC may be normal or *increased* in bronchiolar obstruction with hyperinflation and in emphysema.
3. The TLC is *decreased* in edema, atelectasis, neoplasms, pulmonary congestion, pneumothorax, or thoracic restriction.

Vital Capacity (VC)

Normal Values
About 4000–4800 ml.
Predicted values are based on age, sex, and height.

Explanation of Test
This measurement is used to identify defects that can be due to lung or chest wall restriction. It measures the largest volume of gas that can be expelled from the lungs after the lungs are first filled to the maximum extent and then emptied to the maximum extent. The VC is the mathematical sum of the inspiratory capacity (IC) and the expiratory reserve volume (ERV; see Figure 14-2).

Procedure
1. Have the patient inhale as deeply as possible and then exhale completely, with no forced or rapid effort.
2. The inhalation and exhalation are done into a spirometer and the results are recorded on a spirogram.
3. No time limit is set.
4. The procedure should be repeated at least twice, and the VCs should compare within 5% of each other.

Clinical Implications
1. A *reduced* VC is considered to be less than 80% of the predicted value.
2. VC can be lower than expected in either a restrictive or an obstructive disorder.
3. Decreases of VCs can be related to depression of the respiratory center in the brain, neuromuscular diseases, pleural effusion, pneumothorax, pregnancy, ascites, limitations of thoracic movement due to pain, scleroderma, or kyphoscoliosis, and limitation of movement by tumors, ascites, or pregnancy.

Interfering Factors
1. VC increases with physical fitness and height.
2. VC decreases with age after about age 30.
3. VC is generally less in women than in men of the same age and height.
4. VC is decreased by approximately 15% in blacks and 20 to 25% in the oriental populations when compared to whites of the same age, height, and sex.
5. Inadequate patient effort is a cause of lower than expected VC.

Patient Preparation
Explain the purpose and procedure of the test.

Residual Volume (RV)

Normal Values
Approximately 1200–1500 ml.
Predicted values are based on age, sex, and height.

Explanation of Test
This test can be helpful in differentiating between either a restrictive or obstructive ventilatory defect. It is a measurement of the volume of gas remaining in the lungs after a maximal exhalation. Because the lungs cannot be completely emptied and since all the gas cannot be expelled by maximal expiratory effort, it is the only volume that cannot be measured directly from the spirometer. This value is calculated mathematically: Residual volume equals the functional residual capacity minus the expiratory reserve volume (RV = FRC − ERV) (see Figure 13-2).

Procedure
The RV is determined indirectly from other tests. There is no procedure.

Clinical Implications
1. An increase in the RV indicates that in spite of a maximal expiratory effort, the lungs still contain an abnormally large amount of gas. This type of change occurs in young asthmatics and is usually reversible. An increase in RV of predicted value (*i.e.*, >25%) is typically referred to as air trapping.
2. Increases of the RV are also characteristic of emphysema, chronic air trapping, and chronic bronchial obstruction.
3. The RV and the FRC usually increase together, although this is not always true.
4. The RV sometimes decreases in diseases that occlude many alveoli.
5. A RV of less than 75% of predicted value is consistent with restriction.

Interfering Factors
RV normally increases with age.

Patient Preparation
Explain the purpose and procedure of the test.

Expiratory Reserve Volume (ERV)

Normal Values
Approximately 1200–1500 ml.
Predicted values are based on age and height.

Explanation of Test
This test measures the largest volume of gas that can be exhaled following normal resting expiration. This measurement is used to identify lung or chest wall restriction. The ERV can be estimated mathematically by subtracting the inspiratory capacity (IC) from the vital capacity (VC). The ERV comprises approximately 25% of the VC and can vary greatly in subjects of comparable age and height.

Procedure
1. Record the patient's age and height.
2. Have the patient breathe normally for several breaths and then exhale maximally into a spirometer from the end tidal expiratory level.
3. Results are recorded on a spirogram.

Clinical Implications
1. A decreased ERV implies a chest wall restriction due to non-pulmonary causes.
2. Decreased values are associated with elevated diaphragms as seen in massive obesity, ascites, or pregnancy. These decreased values also occur in conjunction with massive enlargement of the heart, pleural effusion, kyphoscoliosis, and thoracoplasty.

Patient Preparation
Explain the purpose and procedure of the test.

Forced Vital Capacity (FVC); Forced Expiratory Volume (FEV); Timed (FEV$_t$)

Normal Values
FVC is approximately 3000–5000 ml. The total FVC should be exhaled in approximately 6 seconds. The FEV$_t$ is expressed in liters.

81%–83% exhaled in 1 second = FEV$_1$
90%–94% exhaled in 2 seconds = FEV$_2$
95%–97% exhaled in 3 seconds = FEV$_3$

Predicted values for a patient of a specific age and height may be determined by use of a nomogram (see Figure 14-4).

Explanation of Test
FEV$_t$ is valuable in quantifying the amount and severity of airway obstruction. The maximum amount of air that can be exhaled rapidly after a maximum deep inspiration is recorded. Three separate exhalations are measured and the highest volume is recorded as the forced vital capacity. The recording is given in liters or as the FVC; VC ratio.

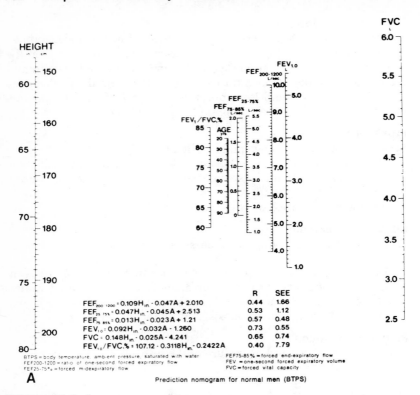

A   Prediction nomogram for normal men (BTPS)

Figure 14-4

Nomogram for determining various expiratory flow rates in normal males (*A*) and normal females (*B*). The values are determined by laying a ruler across the height scale and age scale (corresponding to patient's height and age) and then reading the values where the ruler crosses the other scales. (Burton GG, Gee GN, Hodgkin JE: Respiratory Care: A Guide to Clinical Practice. Philadelphia, JB Lippincott, 1977)

The volumes exhaled within 1 and 3 seconds are referred to as FEV_1 and FEV_3 or timed VCs. These measurements are useful in the evaluation of a patient's response to bronchodilators. If the FEV_1 and/or FEF_{25-75} are below 80% of the predicted, a bronchodilator such as metaproterenol or isoetharine is administered with a mininebulizer and the spirometry is repeated. An increase in the FEV_1 and/or FEF_{25-75} of 20% or more above the prebronchodilator level receives a significant response to the bronchodilator consistent with reversible obstructive airways disease as in asthma. The person with emphysema typically

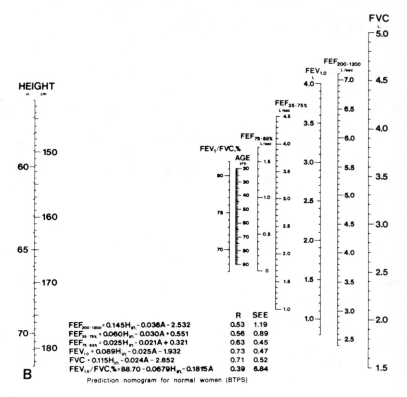

Figure 14-4 (*Continued*)

does not demonstrate a response to bronchodilators because of the nature of the disease state.

Procedure
The patient is asked to breathe normally, inspire maximally, and then exhale as forcefully and as rapidly as possible into the spirometer.

Clinical Implications
1. Obstructive lung disease is a cause of reduced volume and flow rates.
2. Decreased values occur in chronic lung diseases that cause trapping of air, such as emphysema, pulmonary fibrosis, and asthma.
3. In restrictive lung disease, the FVC is reduced; however, the flow rates can be normal or elevated.

Patient Preparation
Explain the purpose and procedure of the test.

Flow-Volume Loops (F-V Loops)

Normal Values
Normal curves or loops are characteristic of absence of lung disease

Explanation of Test
This test is designed to provide both a graphic analysis and a quantitative measurement of flow rates at any lung volume. It is used to evaluate the dynamics of both large and medium size (control) airways and is quite helpful in ruling out peripheral or small airway obstruction. Values obtained in this determination include the FVC, FEV, FEF_{25-75}, PEFR, PIFR, FEF_{25}, FEF_{50}, and FEF_{75}. See Figure 14-5 for an example of a flow-volume loop.

Procedure
The procedure is the same as for spirometry except for the addition of a maximal forced inspiration at the end of the forced expiratory maneuver.

Clinical Implications
Abnormal flow volume loops are indicative of

1. Obstructive lung disease
   (a) Small airway obstructive disease, as in emphysema and asthma
   (b) Large airway obstructive disease, such as tumors of trachea and bronchioles
2. Restrictive diseases when the disease is far advanced.

Patient Preparation
Explain the purpose and procedure of the test.

Peak Inspiratory Flow Rate (PIFR)

Normal Value
An average value of at least 300 liters/min.
Predicted values based on age, sex, and height.

Explanation of Test
This measurement of flow rate is used to identify reduced breathing on inspiration and is totally dependent on the effort the patient makes in inspiration. PIFR is the maximum flow of air achieved during a forced maximal inspiration.

Procedure
1. The PIFR is obtained from the flow-volume loop procedure using the spirometer with an X–Y recorder.

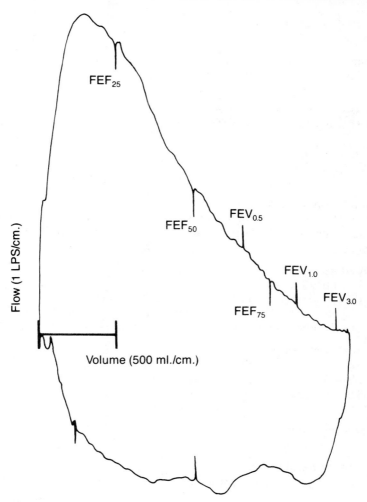

Figure Figure 14-5
Flow-volume loop. $FEV_{0.5, 1.0}$, and $_{3.0}$ = forced expiratory volumes at 0.5 second, 1 second, and 3 seconds, respectively. $FEF_{25, 50}$, and $_{75}$ = forced expiratory flow at 25%, 50%, and 75% of lung volume, respectively.

2. The patient is asked to inspire maximally, exhale forcibly and completely, and then inspire forcibly and completely (see Figure 14-5).

Clinical Implications
1. The value is reduced in neuromuscular disorders, weakness, poor effort, and extrathoracic airway obstruction (*i.e.*, substernal thyroid, tracheal stenosis, and laryngeal paralysis).
2. The PIFR will be altered by upper airway obstruction.

Interfering Factors
Poor patient effort

Patient Preparation
Explain the purpose and procedure of the test.

Peak Expiratory Flow Rate (PEFR)

Normal Values
An average of at least 450 liters/min.
Predicted values are based on age, sex, and height.

Explanation of Test
This measurement of lung volume flow rate is used as an index of large airway function. It is the maximum flow of expired air attained during a forced vital capacity (FVC) maneuver.

Procedure
1. The PEFR is obtained from the flow-volume loop procedure using the spirometer with an X–Y recorder (see Figure 14-5).
2. The patient is asked to inspire maximally, exhale forcibly and completely, and then inspire forcibly and completely.

Clinical Implications
1. The value is normally decreased in obstructive disease such as emphysema when air is trapped.
2. The value is usually normal in restrictive lung disease, except in severe restriction, when it is reduced.

Interfering Factors
Poor patient effort

Patient Preparation
Explain the purpose and procedure of the test.

Carbon Monoxide Diffusing Capacity of the Lung (DLCO)

Normal Values
Approximately 25 ml./min./torr
75% of predicted value based on patient's height, age, weight, and sex
DLCO (in men) = 15.5 (BSA) − 0.238 (A) + 6.8
DLCO (in women) = 15.5 (BSA) − 0.117 (A) + 0.5
(A = age in years; BSA = body surface area in meters squared; factor 15.5 takes into account a normal hemoglobin)

Background

Carbon monoxide (CO) combines with hemoglobin about 210 times more readily than does oxygen (O_2). If there is a normal amount of hemoglobin in the blood, the only other significant limiting factor to CO uptake is the state of the alveolar capillary membranes. Normally there is no CO in the blood to affect the test.

There are two categories of factors that determine the rate of gas (CO) transfer across the lung—physical and chemical. Physical determinants are CO driving pressure, surface area, thickness of capillary walls, and diffusion coefficient for CO. Chemical determinants are red cell volume + reaction rate with hemoglobin.

Explanation of Test

This test is used to diagnose pulmonary vascular disease, emphysema and pulmonary fibrosis, and to evaluate the amount of functioning pulmonary capillary bed in contact with functioning alveoli. During the measurement of this value, alveolar volume (VA) is also determined. D_L measures the diffusing capacity of the lungs for CO. The $D_L O_2$ is obtained by multiplying D_LCO by 1.23 ($D_L O_2 = D_L CO \times 1.23$).

Procedure

1. Record the patient's age, height, weight, and sex.
2. Two techniques are used by laboratories.
   (a) *Single-breath or breathing-holding technique.* With this method, the patient is asked to take a deep breath from a bag containing a mixture of neon (or helium), CO, and air. The helium concentration is approximately .10% and the CO concentration about 0.3%. The patient holds his breath for 10 seconds and exhales (Figure 14-6).
   (b) *Steady-state technique.* The patient is asked to breathe from a bag containing 0.1% to 0.6% CO for several minutes. This method requires an arterial blood sample.
3. During the last 2 minutes, the exhaled air is collected in a neoprine bag and analyzed for O_2, CO_2, and CO concentrations. An arterial blood gas is also drawn during the last 2 minutes.

4. $D_L CO = \dfrac{V_A \times 60}{(BP\text{-}47)x_t} \ln \dfrac{F_A CO_o}{F_A CO_t}$

   $F_A CO_0$ = initial alveolar CO concentrations
   $F_A CO_t$ = alveolar CO concentration at breath-holding time
   V_A = alveolar volume
   60 = conversion factor for seconds to one minute
   t = breath-holding time in seconds

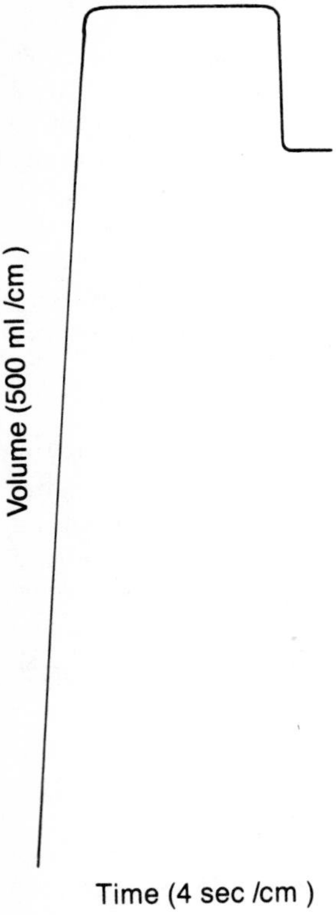

Figure 14-6
Typical tracing for the single-breath carbon monoxide diffusing capacity maneuver. Patient inspires the diffusing gas test mixture maximally, holds breath for 10 to 12 seconds, and then exhales.

Clinical Implications
1. *Decreased values* are associated with
   (a) Multiple pulmonary emboli
   (b) Emphysema
   (c) Lung restriction
   (d) Pulmonary fibroses
       (1) Sarcoidosis   (4) Asbestosis
       (2) Scleroderma   (5) Anemia
       (3) Systemic lupus erythe-   (6) Pulmonary resection
           matosus   (7) Pneumonia
2. *Increased values* are observed in polycythemia, left-to-right shunts, and exercise.
3. The value is relatively normal in chronic bronchitis.

Interfering Factors
Exercise (with an increased cardiac output), polycythemia, and anemia will increase the value. Elevated levels of COHb (as seen in smokers) will decrease the value and decrease the lung volume.

Patient Preparation
Explain the purpose and procedure of the test.

Inspiratory Capacity (IC)

Normal Values
Approximately 2500–3600 ml.
Predicted values are based on age and height.

Explanation of Test
This test measures the largest volume of air that can be inhaled in one deep breath after a normal expiration or that can be inhaled from the end tidal expiratory level. This measurement is used to identify lung or chest wall restriction. This measurement mathematically equals the tidal volume plus the inspiratory reserve volume (V_T + IRV). This value is not commonly measured because many diseases do not affect inspiratory capacity.

Procedure
1. Record the age, sex, and height of the patient.
2. The patient is asked to breathe normally into a spirometer for several breaths and then to inhale deeply or maximally, expanding the lungs as much as possible from end tidal expiration. Normal breathing is then resumed.
3. Step two is usually repeated two or more times and the largest inspired volume is selected.

Clinical Implications
Changes in the IC usually parallel increases or decreases in the vital capacity (VC).

Patient Preparation
Instruct the patient about the purpose and procedure of the test.

Maximum Voluntary Ventilation (MVV)

Normal Values
Approximately 170 liters/min.
Based on age, height, and sex; a healthy person may vary by as much as 25% to 35% of mean group values
MVV (in men) = 3.39 (H) − 1.26 (A) − 21.4
MVV (in women) = 138 − 0.77 (A)
(H = height in inches; A = age in years)

Explanation of Test
This test measures several physiological phenomena occurring at the same time (*e.g.*, thoracic cage compliance, lung compliance, airway resistance, and muscle force available). It is a determination of the liters of air that a person can breathe per minute by a maximum voluntary effort.

Procedure
1. The patient breathes into a spirometer as deeply and rapidly as possible for 10 to 15 seconds. Generally, the frequency is 40 to 70 breaths per minute and tidal volume is 50% of VC (Figure 14-7).
2. Actual value is then extrapolated from the 10- to 15-second time interval to a 1-minute time period.

Interfering Factors
Poor patient effort can be ruled out by using the following formula to predict the MVV of the patient:

$$\text{predicted MVV} = 35 \times FEV_1$$

This is a useful check to determine whether the recorded MVV is indicative of adequate patient effort.

Clinical Implications
1. Obstructive defects, chronic obstructive pulmonary disease (COPD), abnormal neuromuscular control, and poor patient effort are causes of reduced values.
2. In restrictive disease, the value will usually be normal.

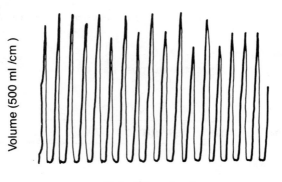

Time (2 sec /cm)

Figure 14-7
Maximum voluntary ventilation. Patient breathes into a spirometer as deeply and rapidly as possible for 10 to 15 seconds.

Patient Preparation
1. Explain the purpose and procedure of the test.
2. Obtain and record the patient's age, height, and sex.

Closing Volume (CV)

Normal Values
Average is about 10% to 20% of vital capacity
Values derived from mathematical regression equations and based on
  age and sex
CV (in men) = 0.562 + 0.357 (A) + 4.15
CV (in women) = 2.812 + 0.293 (A) + 4.90
(A) = age in years

Explanation of Test
In the healthy person, the concentration of N_2 diluted with 100% O_2
rapidly increases near the end of expiration. This rise is due to closure
of the small airways in the lower alveoli. The point at which this closure occurs is termed *closing volume*.

This measurement is used as an index of pathological changes occurring within the small airways (those airways less than 2 mm. in
diameter). The conventional pulmonary function tests are not sensitive
enough to make this determination. The principle of the determination
relies on the fact that the upper lung zones contain a proportionately
larger residual volume of gas than the lower lung zones and that there
is a gradient of intrapleural pressure from the top of the lung to the
bottom of the lung. Additionally, the uniformity of gas distribution
within the lungs can be measured.

Procedure
1. The patient is asked to exhale completely, inhale 100% oxygen, hold
   the breath for a few seconds, and then exhale completely at the rate
   of approximately ½ liter per second.
2. During the exhalation, both volume and percent of alveolar nitrogen are monitored simultaneously on an X–Y recorder. A sudden
   increase in nitrogen represents the closing volume (Figure 14-8).

Clinical Implications
1. The value is increased in diseases in which the airway is narrowed,
   such as bronchitis, and in chronic smokers and the elderly.
2. A change in the slope of the nitrogen curve by more than 2% is
   indicative of maldistribution of inspired air (*i.e.*, uneven alveolar
   ventilation).

Interfering Factors
Value increases with age.

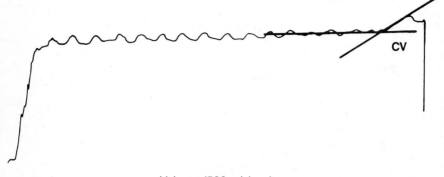

Figure 14-8
Typical single-breath nitrogen washout curve for determination of closing volume (CV). The patient inspires 100% oxygen to total lung capacity and then exhales slowly (0.5 LPS) until the lung is empty.

Patient Preparation
Explain the purpose and procedure of the test.

Volume of Isoflow ($V_{ISO}\dot{V}$)

Normal Values
Values cover a wide range based on age (A).

$$V_{ISO}\dot{V} = 0.450 \, (A) + 4.69$$

Explanation of Test
This test is designed to detect pathological changes occurring in the small airways and may be more sensitive than conventional pulmonary function tests. Helium (He) has the unique property of lowering gas density. Therefore, after breathing a helium-oxygen gas mixture, the effects of convective acceleration and turbulence are negated. Any abnormality observed in the flow-volume loop is due then to an increase in resistance to laminar flow, which is indicative of small airway abnormalities or disease.

Procedure
1. The patient is fitted with nose clips and allowed to breathe into a mouthpiece connected to a spirometer that is interfaced with an X–Y recorder.
2. The patient is instructed to perform a flow-volume loop maneuver.

3. Next, the patient is asked to breathe an 80% He and 20% O_2 gas mix for several breaths and then perform another flow-volume loop maneuver.
4. From the tracings obtained in steps 2 and 3, the flow-volume loops are superimposed and the volume of isoflow is measured at the point in which the two loops intersect.

Clinical Implications

1. An *increased* volume of isoflow is consistent with the diagnosis of mild airway obstruction (*i.e.,* small airways disease).
2. A *decreased* volume of isoflow is normal.

Patient Preparation

Explain the purpose and procedure of the test.

Body Plethysmography

Normal Values

Based on height in inches (H) and weight in pounds (W)
TGV = approximately 2400 ml.
TGV (in men) = 0.081 (H) − 2.94 (W)
TGV (in women) = 0.135 (H) − 0.008 (W) − 4.74
C = 0.2 liters/cm. H_2O
RAW = 0.6 cm.–2.4 cm. H_2O/liter/sec.

Explanation of Test

This test is designed to measure thoracic gas volume (TGV), compliance (C), and airway resistance (RAW). TGV equals all the air contained within the thorax, whether or not it is in ventilatory communication with the rest of the lung. Compliance is an indication of the elasticity of the lung, and airway resistance is a measurement of resistance to airflow in the tracheobronchial tree.

The measurement of TGV via body plethysmography is an application of Boyle's Law, that is, $PXV = PXV^1$ as long as T is constant.

P = pressure
V = volume
T = temperature

$$\text{Compliance} = \frac{\text{change in volume}}{\text{change in pressure}}$$

$$C = \frac{V}{P}$$

Normal C = 0.2L/cmH_2O

$$\text{Airway Resistance} = \frac{\text{change in pressure}}{\text{change in flow}}$$

$$RAW = \frac{P}{F}$$

$$RAW = 0.2 - 2.5 \text{ cmH}_2\text{O/liter/second}$$

Airway resistance increases with decreasing lung volume and decreases at higher lung volumes. Therefore, to provide a volume-standardized Raw measurement, airway conductance (GAW) and specific airway conductance (SGAW) are typically calculated.

$$GAW = \frac{1}{RAW} = 0.4 - 5.0 \text{ liters/second/cmH}_2\text{O}$$

$$SGAW = \frac{GAW}{TGV} = 0.112 - 0.400 \text{ liters/sec/cmH}_2\text{O/liter}$$

Procedure
1. The patient is seated in the body box, fitted with nose clips, and asked to breathe through a mouthpiece connected to a transducer.
2. The box door is secured and the test is not begun for a few minutes, while the box pressure is allowed to stabilize.
3. The patient is instructed to perform a panting maneuver while holding his cheeks rigid and glottis open. The technician makes a recording of box pressure and mouth pressure on the oscilloscope. This recording provides the necessary data for mathematical derivation of TGV.
4. Next, the patient is instructed to breathe rapidly and shallowly. The technician makes a recording of box pressure changes versus flow on the oscilloscope, and this provides the necessary data for mathematical derivation of RAW.
5. For the C determination, a balloon catheter must be passed into the patient's esophagus through the nose. The balloon is then inflated with a few cc. of air, and the patient is instructed to breathe normally. The technician makes a recording of intraesophageal pressure changes during normal respiration (which mimics changes in intrapleural pressure), and this provides the necessary data for the mathematical derivation of C.

Clinical Implications
1. An *increased* TGV demonstrates air trapping, which is consistent with obstructive pulmonary disease.
2. An *increased* RAW demonstrates an increased resistance to airflow through the tracheobronchial tree, which is seen in asthma, emphysema, bronchitis, and other forms of obstruction. RAW is useful in distinguishing between a restrictive ventilatory defect versus an obstructive ventilatory defect, as the former does not increase the resistance to airflow.

3. An *increase* in C (*i.e.*, lung is more distensible) is seen in obstructive diseases.
4. A *decrease* in C (*i.e.*, lung is more stiff) is seen in fibrotic diseases, restrictive diseases, pneumonia, congestion, atelectasis.

Patient Preparation
1. The height, weight, and sex are recorded.
2. Explain the purpose and procedure of the test.

Patient Aftercare
Allow the patient to rest quietly after the test is completed.

Bronchial Provocation

Normal Values
Minimal to no change in airway dynamics (*i.e.*, FEV_1 and/or FEF_{25-75})
Positive response to inhaled antigen is equal to:

>20% decrease in FEV_1
and/or
>30% decrease in FEF_{25-75}

Explanation of Test
Occasionally, the diagnosis of asthma cannot be made with certainty from the history, physical examination, and conventional pulmonary function tests. This is a specific test for bronchial asthma. The asthmatic patient is more sensitive to the bronchoconstrictive effects of cholinergic agents (*e.g.*, methacholine chloride or histamine) than the normal person. Studies indicate that airway resistance tests are sensitive in monitoring the response to bronchoconstrictive agents.

Clinical Implications
A positive response to methacholine or histamine is consistent with a diagnosis of asthma.

Procedure
1. The patient is instructed to perform a forced vital capacity (FVC) maneuver, and the FEV_1 and FEF_{25-75} are measured.
2. The patient is now asked to take an inhalation of 1.25 mg. of methacholine chloride/ml. by means of a nebulizer, to wait 5 minutes, and then repeat the FVC maneuver. A 20% reduction in the FEV_1 or a 30% decrease in FEF_{25-75} is a positive response.
3. If there is no response, the dilution of methacholine chloride is progressively increased (2.50 mg./ml., 5.0 mg./ml., 10.0 mg./ml., and 25 mg./ml.), and the patient repeats step 2. However, once a 20% reduction in the FEV_1 and/or a 30% decrease in FEF_{25-75} is

observed at any dilution ratio, this represents a positive response, and the test is terminated. A bronchodilator is administered.
4. If a patient goes through all five dilution ratios without a 20% reduction in the FEV, and/or 30% reduction in the FEF_{25-75}, this is a negative test.
5. If the methacholine causes no change, the patient can be tested with histamine at a later time. (Usually, the patient is tested first with methacholine, then with histamine.)

Patient Preparation
Explain the purpose and procedure of the test.

Carbon Dioxide (CO_2) Response

Normal Values
Breathing increasing concentrations of CO_2 should result in an increase in minute volume when compared to minute volume when breathing room air (0.03% CO_2).

Explanation of Test
This test is designed to evaluate the respiratory response to increasing levels of inspired CO_2 concentration. As levels of CO_2 increase in alveolar air, so does arterial CO_2. The central chemoreceptors respond by initiating impulses to the respiratory control centers, and this in turn causes an increase in the rate and depth of breathing in the healthy person.

Procedure
1. The patient's minute volume is determined while breathing room air. This is done by allowing the patient to breathe for several minutes into an instrument that records frequency (f) of breathing and tidal volume (V_T). The minute volume is then calculated for 1 minute by computing the value of $F \times V_T$.
2. Next, the patient is instructed to breathe a gas mixture of 2% CO_2 and balanced room air for 5 minutes. During the last 2 minutes, breathing (f) and V_T are recorded.
3. Next, the patient breathes a gas mixture of 4% CO_2 and balanced room air, and the above procedure is repeated. This is also done with 6% CO_2 and sometimes even 8% CO_2 and room air.
4. Finally, a graph is constructed that plots changes in minute volume against increasing inspired CO_2 concentrations.

Clinical Implications
Unresponsiveness to increasing inspired CO_2 concentrations suggests a disturbance in the normal physiological pathway of ventilatory changes to hypercapnia.

BLOOD GASES, ARTERIAL BLOOD GASES, (ABGs)

Introduction

Reasons for obtaining arterial blood gases (ABGs)

1. Assessment of adequacy of oxygenation
2. Assessment of adequacy of ventilation
3. Assessment of the acid–base status by measuring the respiratory and nonrespiratory components

ABGs are used to monitor critically ill patients, to establish base line values, in the preoperational period, to follow up postoperative patients, in the detection and treatment of electrolyte imbalances, and in conjunction with pulmonary function testing.

Reasons for using *arterial* blood rather than *venous* blood to measure blood gases:

1. Arterial blood is a good way to sample a mixture of blood that has come from various parts of the body.
   (a) Venous blood in an extremity gives information mostly about that extremity. The metabolism in the extremity can differ from the metabolism in the body as a whole. This difference is accentuated:
      (1) In shock, when the extremity is cold or under-perfused
      (2) With local exercise of extremity, as opening and closing the fist
      (3) In local infection of the extremity
   (b) Blood from a central venous catheter usually is an incomplete mix of venous blood from various parts of the body. For a sample of completely mixed blood, a sample would have to be obtained from the right ventricle or pulmonary artery, and even then information is not obtained about how well the lungs are oxygenating the blood.
2. Arterial blood gives the added information of how well the lungs are oxygenating the blood.
   (a) If it is known that arterial O_2 concentration is normal (indicating that the lungs are functioning normally), but that the mixed venous O_2 concentration is low, it can be inferred that the heart and circulation are failing.
   (b) Oxygen measurements of central venous catheter blood can tell if the tissues are getting oxygenated, but they do not separate the contribution of the heart from the lungs. If central venous catheter blood has a low O_2 concentration, it means either that
      (1) The lungs have not oxygenated the arterial blood well so that venous blood has a low concentration.

(2) The heart is not circulating the blood well. In this case, the tissues of the body must take more than the usual amount of O_2 from each cardiac cycle because the blood is flowing slowly. This produces a low venous O_2 concentration.

Note: The site of arterial puncture must satisfy three requirements.
1. Available collateral blood flow
2. Superficial or easily accessible
3. Periarterial tissues (should be nonsensitive)

The radial artery satisfies the criteria listed above, although the brachial and femoral are also arteries of choice.

Procedure for Obtaining Arterial Blood Sample
1. Place the patient in either a sitting or a supine position.
2. Perform the Allen's test to assess collateral circulation prior to performing the arterial puncture. If collateral circulation is inadequate, do not puncture the radial artery.
3. Elevate the wrist with a small pillow and ask the patient to extend the fingers downward (this will flex the wrist and move the radial artery closer to the surface).
4. Palpate the artery and rotate the patient's hand back and forth until a good strong pulse is felt.
5. Swab the area liberally with an antiseptic agent such as Betadine.
6. Optional: Anesthetize the area with a small amount of 1% Xylocaine (approximately ¼ ml. or less). This allows a second attempt without undue pain if the first attempt is a failure.
7. Using a 20- or 21-gauge needle, make the puncture and then attach the preheparinized 12-ml self-filling syringe once the artery has been entered, and collect a 3- to 5-ml. sample.
8. Withdraw the needle and place a 4″ × 4″ absorbent bandage over the puncture site and maintain pressure with two fingers for a minimum of 2 minutes.
9. Meanwhile, any air bubbles in the blood sample should be expelled as quickly as possible; the syringe should then be capped and gently rotated to mix heparin with blood.
10. Place the sample on ice and remove to the laboratory. This will prevent alterations in gas tensions because metabolic processes continue after blood is drawn.

Clinical Alert
1. Arterial gases will not indicate to what degree the patient is suffering from an abnormality. For this reason, the vital signs

and mental function of the patient must be used as guides to determine adequacy of tissue oxygenation.

2. The arterial puncture site must have pressure applied and be watched carefully for bleeding.

3. Blood for electrolytes and gases must be drawn without trauma and must be protected from room air at all times. Be aware that air bubbles in the syringe will also change gas values.

4. Include this information in laboratory slip: patient's name, room number, identification number, diagnoses, body temperature, oxygen therapy, and if on ventilation, the fraction of inspired oxygen (FIO_2). Note the time the sample is obtained. Do not use blood for ABGs after 3 hours.

Exercise Pulmonary Function Test

Normal Values
Normal exercise response:
No change in the ECG complex
No systemic hypertension and normal arterial blood pressure
Normal air flow pattern during inspiration and expiration
Normal arterial blood gases and chemistry (CO_2, O_2, pH, HCO_2, lactate), based on an indwelling catheter
Normal pulmonary artery pressure

Background
Respiratory disease reduces the ability to perform exercise. Dynamic exercise employing large muscle groups is accompanied by increases in metabolic oxygen (O_2) consumption and carbon dioxide (CO_2) production. The increase in metabolic demand leads to stresses on all the mechanisms taking part in O_2 and CO_2 transport. Exercise testing allows the measurement of the functional reserve in these mechanisms through the application of the engineering principles of testing under load.

Explanation of Test
Exercise testing of pulmonary function is done to evaluate fitness, to identify work tolerance or intolerance in persons with obstructive and restrictive diseases. Efficiency of the cardiopulmonary system may be quite different during periods of exercise than at rest. For this reason exercise testing is designed to assess ventilation, gas exchange, and cardiovascular function during increased demands. With such tests,

dyspnea due to cardiovascular causes can be differentiated from that due to respiratory causes. Precise information about the mechanisms that influence O_2 and CO_2 transport during exercise can be obtained using a staged approach. This information is important because the ability to exercise or perform work represents an essential part of any definition of health. (Symptoms of limited exercise tolerance include onset of fatigue and shortness of breath.) Patients who require more than the normal amount of O_2 to perform work or exercise can be identified when they are exercised on a cycle ergometer or treadmill.

There are many conditions that an exercise test can detect or exclude, even though the response may be nonspecific. For example, in a person complaining of severe shortness of breath in the presence of a normal exercise response, the likely cause is psychogenic. However, there are a few conditions in which a particular exercise response is strictly diagnostic: exercise-induced asthma and myocardial ischema. Exercise tests are also of value in assessing the severity of impairment due to virtually all diagnosed conditions affecting the lungs and circulation. In addition, exercise testing may uncover unsuspected abnormalities contributing to the person's disability.

The majority of clinical problems can be assessed during the simple procedures included in Stage 1, below. These procedures should always be done before more complex tests are undertaken. An abnormal result is an indication that more precise information is required, using either Stage 2 protocols, which are more complex but bloodless, or Stage 3 protocols, in which arterial blood is sampled. In 75% of cases, only Stage 1 need be performed. One hundred percent O_2 is often used during incremental exercise and is helpful in estimating the magnitude of a hypovolemic stimulus during air breathing exercises to quantify the degree of any right-to-left shunt in known arterial hypoxemia and to determine the degree of O_2 supplementation needed to improve a person's exercise tolerance.

Clinical Alert

Absolute contraindications to exercise testing include

Acute febrile illness	Uncontrolled hypertension
Pulmonary edema	systolic >250 mmMg.
Uncontrolled asthma	diastolic >120 mmMg.
Unstable angina	

Relative contraindications to exercise testing include

Recent MI (less than 4 weeks)	Epilepsy
Resting tachycardia	Respiratory failure
>120 bpm	Resting ECG abnormalities

Procedure
1. Stage 1
   (a) Blood pressure, electrocardiogram (ECG) analysis, and spirometry measurements of expiratory air flow, tidal volume, and frequency of breathing assessments are made using cycle ergometry and incremental exercise.
   (b) Measurements are made at the end of each minute; the test continues to a symptom-limited maximum. O_2 intake and CO_2 output are measured if facilities are available.
   (c) Total examining time is 30 minutes, with two observers.
2. Stage 2
   (a) More complex analytical methods are required.
   (b) Exercise is continued long enough to reach a steady state, usually 3 to 5 minutes.
   (c) Stage 1 measurements plus mixed venous CO_2 tension using a rebreathing technique are done.
   (d) Total examining time is 1 hour, with two observers.
3. Stage 3
   (a) Blood gas sampling and analysis are required.
   (b) An indwelling catheter is inserted in the brachial artery. In some instances, capillary blood is substituted.
   (c) In addition to Stage 2 tests, measurements are obtained for cardiac output, alveolar ventilation, ratio of dead space to tidal volume, alveolar–arterial O_2 tension difference, venous admixture ratio, and lactate.
   (d) Total examining time is 90 to 120 minutes, with three observers.

Clinical Implications
Altered values will reveal

1. Cardiac arrhythmia
2. Cardiac ischemia as related to work rate
3. Degree of impairment in pulmonary restrictive diseases
4. Hypoventilation
5. Work rate at which metabolic acidosis appears
6. Cardiac output if pulmonary artery is catheterized during procedure
7. Decreased work tolerance in chronic obstructive pulmonary disease (COPD)

Interfering Factors
1. The exercise tolerance of any person is affected by the degree of impairment of
   (a) Mechanical factors
   (b) Ventilatory efficiency
   (c) Gas exchange factors
   (d) Cardiac status

    (e) Physical condition
    (f) Sensitivity of the respiratory control mechanisms
2. Obese persons will have a higher than normal V_{O_2} at any given work rate, even though the muscular and work efficiency values are normal.

Alveolar to Arterial Oxygen Gradient (A–aDO$_2$)

Normal Values
9 torr or less in a patient breathing room air

Explanation of Test
This test gives an approximation of the oxygen (O_2) in the alveoli and arteries. It is used to identify the cause of hypoxemia and intrapulmonary shunting: (1) ventilated alveolus but no perfusion; (2) unventilated alveolus with perfusion; or (3) collapse of both alveolus and capillaries.

Procedure
An arterial blood sample is obtained, and the following mathematical formula is solved:

$$A-aDO_2 = P_AO_2 - PaO_2$$
$$P_AO_2 = (BP-47)F_IO_2 - PaCO_2 \times 1.25$$

    BP = barometric pressure
    47 = water vapor pressure
    F_IO_2 = fractional concentration of inspired oxygen (*e.g.,* .21 for room air)
    $PaCO_2$ = partial pressure of arterial carbon dioxide
    1.25 = conversion factor for respiratory quotient
    PaO_2 = Arterial oxygen tension
    P_AO_2 = Alveolar oxygen tension
    D = difference

Clinical Implications
1. *Increased* values may be due to
    (a) Mucus plugs
    (b) Bronchospasm
    (c) Airway collapse as seen in
        (1) Asthma
        (2) Bronchitis
        (3) Emphysema
2. Hypoxemia, due to an increased A-aO$_2$ differences is also caused by
    (a) Atrial septal defects
    (b) Pneumothorax

(c) Atelectasis
(d) Emboli
(e) Edema

Interfering Factors
Value increases with age and increasing O_2 concentration.

Arterial to Alveolar Oxygen Rate (a/A Ratio)

Normal values
75% (regardless of age or F_IO_2)

$$\text{a/A ratio} = \frac{PaO_2}{(BP\text{-}47)F_IO_2 - (PaCO_2 \times 1.25)}$$

Partial Pressure of Carbon Dioxide (PCO₂)

Normal Values
$PaCO_2$ (arterial blood) 35–45 torr
$PvCO_2$ (venous blood) 41–51 torr
Carried in blood in two ways: 10% carried in plasma
                              90% carried in RBCs

Explanation of Test
This test is a measurement of the pressure or tension exerted by dissolved carbon dioxide (CO_2) in the blood and is proportional to the partial pressure of CO_2 in the alveolar air. The test is commonly used to detect a respiratory abnormality and to determine the alkalinity or acidity of the blood. In order to maintain CO_2 within normal limits, the rate and depth of respiration vary automatically with changes in metabolism. The text is an index of the effectiveness of alveolar ventilation and is the most physiologically reflective blood gas measurement. When taken as an arterial sample, it directly reflects how well air is exchanging with blood in the lungs.

CO₂ tension in the blood and in cerebrospinal fluid (CSF) is the major chemical factor regulating alveolar ventilation. When the CO_2 of arterial blood rises from 40 torr to 45 torr, it causes a threefold increase in alveolar ventilation. A CO_2 of 63 torr in arterial blood increases alveolar ventilation tenfold. When the CO_2 concentration of breathed air exceeds 5%, the lungs can no longer be ventilated fast enough to prevent a dangerous rise of CO_2 concentration in tissue fluids. Any further increase in CO_2 begins to depress the respiratory center, causing a progressive decline in respiratory activity rather than an increase.

Procedure
1. Obtain an arterial blood sample.
2. Do not expose the sample to air.
3. A small amount of blood is then introduced into a blood gas analyzing machine (*e.g.*, Radiometer, Corning, IL) and the CO_2 tension is measured with a silver–silver chloride electrode (Severinghaus electrode).

Clinical Implications
1. A *rise* in PCO_2 is usually associated with hypoventilation; a *decrease*, with hyperventilation. Reduction in PCO_2 through its effect on plasma bicarbonate concentration decreases renal bicarbonate reabsorption. For each mEq./liter fall in HCO_3, the PCO_2 falls by 1 to 1.3 mm. of Hg. Because HCO_3 and PCO_2 bear this close mathematical relationship, and this ratio in turn defends the hydrogen ion concentration, the outcome is that the steady state PCO_2 in simple metabolic acidosis is equal to the last two digits of the *p*H. Also, addition of 15 to the bicarbonate level also equals the last two digits of the *p*H. Failure of the PCO_2 to achieve predicted levels defines the presence of superimposed respiratory acidosis on alkalosis.
2. The causes of *decreased* PCO_2 include
   (a) Hypoxia
   (b) Nervousness
   (c) Anxiety
   (d) Pulmonary emboli
   (e) Pregnancy
   (f) Other cause of hyperventilation
3. The causes of *increased* PCO_2 include
   (a) Obstructive lung disease
      (1) Chronic bronchitis
      (2) Emphysema
   (b) Reduced function of respiratory center
      (1) Overreaction
      (2) Head trauma
      (3) Anesthesia
   (c) Other more rare causes of hypoventilation, such as pickwickian syndrome

Clinical Alert

Increased PCO_2 may occur even with normal lungs if the respiratory center is depressed. Always check laboratory reports for abnormal values. In interpreting laboratory reports remember that PCO_2 is a gas and is regulated by the lungs, not the kidneys.

Oxygen Saturation (SO$_2$)

Normal Values
Arterial blood saturation (SaO$_2$) = 95% or higher
Mixed venous blood saturation (SvO$_2$) = 75%

Explanation of Test
This measurement is a ratio of the actual oxygen (O$_2$) content of the hemoglobin compared to the potential maximum O$_2$ carrying capacity of the hemoglobin. The percentage of SO$_2$ is a measure of the relationship between O$_2$ and hemoglobin. The percentage of saturation does not indicate the O$_2$ content of arterial blood. The maximum amount of O$_2$ that can be combined with hemoglobin is called the O$_2$ capacity. The combined measurements of O$_2$ saturation, partial pressure of O$_2$, and of hemoglobin will indicate the amount of O$_2$ available to the tissue (tissue oxygenation).

Procedure
Obtain an arterial blood sample. Two methods for determining oxygen saturation are used.

1. The blood sample is introduced into the oximeter, which is a spectrophotometric device for determining the oxygen saturation of the blood. The value is measured directly with an oximeter.
2. Oxygen saturation is calculated from the oxygen content and oxygen capacity determinations.

$$\text{Percentage saturation} = \frac{100 \times O_2 \text{ content volume \%}}{O_2 \text{ capacity volume \%}}$$

That is

$$\text{Percentage saturation} = 100 \times \frac{\text{vol. of } O_2 \text{ actually combined with hemoglobin}}{\text{vol. of } O_2 \text{ with which hemoglobin is capable of combination}}$$

The O$_2$ content of the blood sample is measured before and after exposure to the atmosphere.

Oxygen (O$_2$) Content

Normal Values
Arterial blood: 15%–22 vol. %
Venous blood: 11%–16 vol. %
(Vol % = volume percentage = ml./100 ml. of blood)

Explanation of Test

The actual amount of oxygen (O_2) in the blood is termed the *oxygen content*. Blood can contain less O_2 than it is capable of carrying. About 98% of all O_2 delivered to the tissues is transported in chemical combination with hemoglobin. One gram of hemoglobin can carry or is capable of combining with 1.34 ml. of O_2, whereas 100 ml. of blood plasma can carry only up to 0.3 ml. of O_2. This measurement is determined mathematically by multiplying the number of grams of hemoglobin in 100 ml. of blood by 1.34 times the saturation, plus the PaO_2 times .003.

Clinical Implications

Decreased arterial blood O_2 associated with increased arterial blood CO_2 can be due to

1. Chronic obstructive lung disease
2. Patients with respiratory complications postoperatively
3. Flail chest
4. Kyphoscoliosis
5. Neuromuscular impairment
6. Obesity hypoventilation

Procedure

1. An arterial or venous blood sample is obtained.
2. Mathematical formula

$$O_2 \text{ content} = SaO_2 \times Hgb \times 1.34 + PaO_2 \times 0.003$$

Partial Pressure of Oxygen (PO$_2$)

Normal Values

PaO_2 80 torr or greater: arterial sample
PvO_2 30–40 torr: venous or peripheral blood sample

Background

Oxygen (O_2) is carried in the blood in two forms: dissolved and in combination with hemoglobin. Most of the O_2 in the blood is carried by hemoglobin. It is the partial pressure of a gas that determines the force it exerts in attempting to diffuse through the pulmonary membrane. The partial pressure reflects the amount of O_2 passing from the pulmonary alveoli into the blood and is directly influenced by the amount of O_2 being inhaled.

Explanation of Test

This is a measure of the pressure exerted by the amount of O_2 dissolved in the plasma. It is a test that measures the effectiveness of the lungs to oxygenate the blood, and is used to assess the effectiveness of oxygen therapy. The severity of impairment of the ability of the lungs to diffuse O_2 across the alveolar membrane into the circulating blood is indicated by the level of partial pressure of oxygen (PO_2).

Procedure
1. An arterial blood sample is obtained.
2. A small amount of blood is then introduced into a blood gas analyzing machine and the O_2 tension is measured with a polarographic electrode (Clark electrode).

Clinical Implications
1. *Increased levels* are associated with
   (a) Polycythemia
   (b) Hyperventilation during arterial blood sampling
   (c) Increased F_1O_2
2. *Decreased levels* are associated with
   (a) Anemias
   (b) Cardiac decompensation
   (c) Insufficient atmospheric O_2
   (d) Intracardiac shunts
   (e) Chronic obstructive disease
   (f) Restrictive pulmonary disease
   (g) Hypoventilation due to neuromuscular disease
3. *Decreased* arterial PO_2 with normal or decreased arterial blood PCO_2 tension is associated with
   (a) Diffuse interstitial pulmonary infiltration
   (b) Pulmonary edema
   (c) Pulmonary embolism
   (d) Postoperative extracorporeal circulation

Carbon Dioxide (CO_2) Content or Total Carbon Dioxide (TCO_2)

Normal Values
23–30 mmol/liter

Background
In normal blood plasma, more than 95% of the total CO_2 content is contributed by bicarbonate (HCO_3^-), *which is regulated by the kidneys.* The other 5% of CO_2 is contributed by the dissolved CO_2 gas and carbonic acid (H_2CO_3). Dissolved CO_2 gas, which is regulated by the lungs, therefore contributes little to the total CO_2 content. Total CO_2 content gives little information about the lungs.

HCO_3^- in the extracellular spaces exists first as CO_2, then as H_2CO_3, and thereafter, much of it is changed to sodium bicarbonate ($NaHCO_3$) by the buffers of the plasma and red cells.

Explanation of Test
This test is a general measure of the alkalinity or acidity of the venous, arterial, or capillary blood. This test measures CO_2 from

1. Dissolved CO_2
2. Total H_2CO_3
3. HCO_3^-
4. Carbamino carbon dioxide

$$\text{Total carbon dioxide} = HCO_3^- + 0.03 \times PCO_2$$

Procedure
1. A venous or arterial blood sample of 6 ml. is collected in a heparinized syringe.
2. If the collected blood sample cannot be studied immediately, the syringe should be placed in an iced container.

Clinical Implications
(See also Table 14-4)

1. *Elevated* CO_2 content levels occur in
   (a) Severe vomiting
   (b) Emphysema
   (c) Aldosteronism
   (d) Use of mercurial diuretics
2. *Decreased* CO_2 content levels occur in
   (a) Severe diarrhea
   (b) Starvation
   (c) Acute renal failure
   (d) Salicylate toxicity
   (e) Diabetic acidosis
   (f) Use of chlorothiazide diuretics

   Note: In diabetic acidosis the supply of ketoacids exceeds the demands of the cell. Blood plasma acids rise. Blood plasma HCO_3 decreases because it is used in neutralizing these acids.

Clinical Alert

1. A double use of the term CO_2 is one of the main reasons why understanding acid–base problems may be difficult. Use the terms *CO_2 content* and *CO_2 gas* to avoid confusion. Remember the following:
   (a) *CO_2 content* is mainly bicarbonate and a base. It is a solution and is regulated by the kidneys.
   (b) *CO_2 gas* is mainly acid. It is regulated by the lungs.
2. Panic value is 6.0 or less and is usually associated with severe metabolic acidosis, with the *p*H often less than 7%. This is a medical emergency.

Interfering Factors
There are a number of drugs that may cause increased or decreased levels.

Blood *p*H

Normal Values
Arterial blood: 7.35–7.45
Venous blood: 7.31–7.41

Background
The *p*H is the negative logarithm of the hydrogen ion concentration in the blood. The sources of hydrogen ions are: (1) volatile acids, that can vary between a liquid and a gaseous state, and (2) nonvolatile acids that cannot be volatilized and are fixed (*e.g.*, dietary acids, lactic acids, and ketoacids).

Explanation of Test
This is a measurement of the chemical balance in the body and is a ratio of acids to bases. A determination of the blood *p*H is one of the best ways to tell if the body is too acid or too alkaline. Low *p*H numbers (<7.35) indicate an acid state, and higher *p*H numbers (>7.45) indicate an alkaline state. This balance is extremely intricate and must be kept within the very slight margin of 7.35 to 7.45 *p*H (alkaline) in the extracellular fluid. (Recall that 1–7 represents acidity; 7 is neutrality; and 7–14 represents alkalinity.) *p*H limits compatible with life are 6.9 to 7.8.

Procedure
1. An arterial blood sample is obtained.
2. Two methods of determining the *p*H are used: the direct method and the indirect method.
   (a) *Direct method:* A small amount of blood is introduced into a blood gas machine and the *p*H is measured.
   (b) *Indirect method:* The Henderson–Hasselbalch equation is solved.

$$pH = p\kappa' + \log \frac{(H_2CO_3^-) \text{ major blood base}}{(H_2CO_3) \text{ major blood acid}}$$

Clinical Implications
1. Generally speaking, the *p*H is *decreased* in acidemia because of increased formation of acids. *p*H is *increased* in alkalemia because of a loss of acids.
2. When attempting to interpret an acid–base abnormality, one must
   (a) Check the *p*H to see if there is an alkalemia or an acidemia
   (b) Check PCO_2 to see if there is a respiratory abnormality

(c) Check HCO_3^- or base excess to see if there is a metabolic abnormality.

3. See Table 14-4 for a more complete explanation of the changes occurring in respiratory and metabolic acidemia and respiratory and metabolic alkalemia (alkalosis).
4. Metabolic acidemia (acidosis)
   (a) Renal failure
   (b) Ketoacidosis in diabetes and starvation
   (c) Lactic acidosis
   (d) Strenuous exercise
5. Metabolic alkalemia (alkalosis)
   (a) Deficient potassium
   (b) Hypochoremia
   (c) Gastric suction or vomiting
   (d) Massive administration of steroids
   (e) Sodium bicarbonate administration
   (f) Aspirin intoxication
6. Respiratory alkalemia (alkalosis)
   (a) Acute pulmonary disease
   (b) Myocardial infarction
   (c) Chronic and acute heart failure
   (d) Adult cystic fibrosis
   (e) Third trimester pregnancy
   (f) Anxiety, neuroses, psychoses
   (g) Pain
   (h) CNS diseases
   (i) Anemia
   (j) Carbon monoxide poisoning
   (k) Acute pulmonary embolus
   (l) Shock
7. Respiratory acidemia (acidosis)
   (a) Acute respiratory distress syndrome
   (b) Ventilatory failure

Clinical Alert

1. Ventilation failure is a medical emergency. Aggressive and supportive measures must be taken immediately.
2. Observing the rate and depth of respiration may give a clue to blood pH.
   (a) Acidosis usually *increases* respirations.
   (b) Alkalosis usually *decreases* respirations.

Interfering Factors

There are a number of drugs that may cause increased or decreased levels.

Base Excess/Deficit

Normal Values (± 3 mEq./liter)
Positive value indicates a base excess (*i.e.*, nonvolatile acid deficit)
Negative value indicates a base deficit (*i.e.*, nonvolatile acid excess)

Explanation of Test
This determination is an attempt to quantify the patient's total base excess or deficit so that clinical treatment of acid–base disturbances (specifically those that are nonrespiratory in nature) can be initiated. It is also referred to as the whole blood buffer base and is the sum of the concentration of buffer anions (in mEq./liter) contained in whole blood. These buffer anions are the bicarbonate (HCO_3^-) ion in plasma and red blood cells, and the hemoglobin, plasma proteins, and phosphates in plasma and red blood cells.

Total quantity of buffer anions is 45 to 50 mEq. per liter or about twice that of HCO_3^-, which is 24 to 28 mEq. per liter. Thus, the quantity of HCO_3^- ions accounts for only about half of the total buffering capacity of the blood. Therefore, the base excess/deficit measurement provides a more complete picture of the buffering taking place and is a critical index of nonrespiratory changes in acid–base balance versus respiratory changes.

Procedure
Calculation is made from the measurement of pH, $PaCO_2$, and hematocrit. These values are plated on a nomogram and the base excess/deficit is read.

Clinical Implications
1. Negative value (below 3 mEq./liter) reflects a nonrespiratory or metabolic disturbance. It indicates a true base deficit or a nonvolatile acid accumulation due to
   (a) Dietary intake of organic and inorganic acids
   (b) Lactic acid
   (c) Ketoacidosis
2. Positive value (above 3 mEq./liter) reflects a nonvolatile acid deficit or true base excess.

Anion Gap or R Factor

Normal Values
$< \pm 12$ mEq./liter
< 16 mEq./liter if potassium concentration is used to calculate the anion gap

Table 14-4
Summary of Changes in Four Basic Forms of Acid–Base Imbalances

Form	pH	Bicarbonate (HCO$_3^-$)	pCO$_2$	Occurrence	Compensatory Mechanism
1. Respiratory acidosis due to decreased alveolar ventilation and retention of CO$_2$	→	←	←	1. *Depression of respiratory centers* (a) Drug overdose (b) Barbiturate toxicity (c) Use of anesthetics *Interference with mechanical function of thoracic cage* (a) Deformity of thoracic cage (b) Kyphoscoliosis *Airway Obstruction* (a) Extrathoracic tumors (b) Asthma (c) Bronchitis (d) Emphysema *Circulatory Disorders* (a) Congestive heart failure (b) Shock	Renal reabsorption of the bicarbonate ion.
2. Respiratory alkalosis due to increased alveolar ventilation and excessive blowing off of CO$_2$ and water	←	→	→	2. *Hyperventilation* *Hysteria* *Lack of oxygen* *Toxic stimulation of the respiratory centers* (a) High fever (b) Cerebral hemorrhage (c) Excessive artificial respiration (d) Salicylates	Glomerular filtration of the bicarbonate ion.

3. Metabolic acidosis due to accumulation of fixed body acids or loss of HCO_3^- (bicarbonate) from the extracellular fluid

3. *Acid addition*
   (a) Renal failure
   (b) Diabetic ketoacidosis
   (c) Lactic acidosis
   (d) Anaerobic metabolism
   Hypoxia
   Base subtraction
   (a) Diarrhea
   (b) Renal tubular acidosis

Hyperventilation through stimulation of central chemoreceptors.

4. Metabolic alkalosis due to loss of fixed body acids or gain in bicarbonate (HCO_3^-) in the extracellular fluid

4. *Acid subtraction*
   (a) Loss of gastric juice
   (b) Vomiting
   Potassium or chloride depletion
   Base addition
   (a) Excessive bicarbonate or lactate administration

Hypoventilation

Heavier arrows indicate the primary abnormality

NOTE: 1. Although these four basic imbalances occur individually, a combination of two or more is observed more frequently. These disturbances may have an antagonistic or a synergistic effect upon each other.

2. Compensation is most efficient in respiratory and nonrespiratory acidemia.

3. The degree of hypoventilation is precisely related to the degree of hypobicarbonatemia. For each mEq./liter fall in bicarbonate, PCO_2 falls by 1–1.3 torr. A close mathematical relationship prevails between bicarbonate and PCO_2. Their ratio (HCO_3 and PCO_2) defines the prevailing hydrogen ion concentration. For this reason, the steady state PCO_2 in simple metabolic acidosis is equal to the last two digits of the pH. Failure of the PCO_2 to rech predicted levels defines the presence of superimposed respiratory acidosis or alkalosis.

Explanation of Test

This test is a measurement of the difference between sodium (Na^+) and potassium (K^+) ion concentrations (the measured cations) and the sum of chloride (Cl^-) and bicarbonate (HCO_3^-) (the measured anions). This difference reflects the concentration of anions that are present in the extracellular fluid. These components include phosphates, sulfates, ketone bodies, lactic acid, and proteins. Increased amounts of these unmeasured anions are produced in the acidotic state.

Primary hypocarbonatemia is brought about by any combination of these three mechanisms: (1) overproduction of acids, which causes replacement of $NaHCO_3$ by the Na salt of the offending acid (e.g., Na lactate replaces HCO_3 in lactic acidosis); (2) loss of $NaHCO_3$ through diarrhea along with renal retension of dietary NaCl, which causes hyperchloremic metabolic acidosis; (3) generalized renal failure or specific forms of renal tubular acidosis, which causes retention of acids that are normally produced by intermediary metabolism or by urinary excretion of alkali (see Table 14-5).

Hyperbicarbonatemia with sustained increases of HCO_3^- levels is brought about by a source of *new* alkali and the presence of factors that stimulate renal retension of excess HCO_3^- (see Table 14-6). These mechanisms include contraction alkalosis, excessive gastrointestinal loss of acid, exogenous alkali in persons whose kidneys avidly retain $NaHCO_3$, and renal synthesis of HCO_3^- in excess of daily consumption. Other pathophysiological factors that affect renal reabsorption of more than 25 mEq. of HCO_3^- and contribute to sustained hyperbicarbonatemia include extracellular fluid volume contraction, hypercapnia, hypokalemia, hyperaldosteronemia, and hypoparathyroidism.

Procedure

This measurement is obtained by determining the difference between the sum of the serum cations and the sum of the serum anions.

Table 14-5
Subclassification of Anion Gap Metabolic Acidosis
(Hypobicarbonatemia) Into High- and Low-Potassium Forms*

Hyperkalemic Form	Hypokalemic Form
Acidifying agents	Diarrhea
Mineralocorticoid deficiency	Ureteral sigmoidostomy and
Renal diseases such as SLE interstitial nephritis, amyloidosis, hydronephrosis, sickle cell nephropathy	malfunctioning
	Ileostomy
Early nonspecific renal failure	Renal tubular acidosis, both proximal and distal

* All metabolic acidoses can be classified on the basis of how they affect the anion gap. (After Narins RG et al: Diagnostic strategies in disorders of fluid, electrolyte, and acid–base homeostasis Am J Med 72[3]:510, 1982)

Table 14-6

Classification of Anion Gap Metabolic Alkalosis (Hyperbicarbonatemia) on the Basis of Urinary Chloride Excretion

Saline-Responsive Urinary Chloride Excretion of Less Than 10 mEq./Day	Saline-Unresponsive Urinary Chloride Excretion of Less than 10 mEq./Day

1. Excess body bicarbonate content
  (a) Renal alkalosis
    Diuretic therapy
    Poorly reabsorbable anion therapy, such as carbenicillin, penicillin, sulfate, phosphate
    Posthypercapnia
  (b) Gastrointestinal alkalosis
    Gastric alkalosis
    Intestinal alkalosis such as chloride diarrhea
  (c) Exogenous alkali
    Baking soda
    Sodium citrate, lactate, gluconate, acetate
    Transfusions
    Antacids
2. Normal body bicarbonate content
  Contraction alkalosis—This means that the urinary loss of sodium chloride and water without bicarbonate loss will cause extracellular fluid contraction around an unchanged body content of alkali, resulting in hyperbicarbonatemia. This is especially important in persons with edema and persons who have excess body stores of water, sodium, bicarbonate, and chloride.
	1. Excess body bicarbonate content
	  (a) Renal alkalosis—normotensive conditions
	    Bartter's syndrome
	    Severe potassium depletion
	    Refeeding alkalosis
	    Hypercalcemia and hypoparathyroidism
	  (b) Hypertensive conditions—Endogenous mineralocorticoids
	    Primary aldosteronism
	    Hyperreninism
	    Adrenal enzyme deficiency: 11- and 17-hydroxylase
	    Liddle syndrome
	  (c) Exogenous mineralocorticoids
	    Licorice
	    Carbenoxolone
	    Chewing tobacco

(After Narins, RG et al: Diagnostic strategies in disorders of fluid, electrolyte, and acid–base homeostasis. Am J Med 72[3]:511, 1982)

Clinical Implications

1. An anion gap occurs in acidosis due to excess metabolic acids and excess serum chloride levels. If there is no change in sodium content, anions such as phosphates, sulfates, and organic acids will increase the anion gap because these components replace bicarbonate.

2. *Increased* anion gap is associated with an increase in metabolic acid when there is an excessive production of metabolic acids as in

(a) Alcoholic ketoacidosis
(b) Diabetic ketoacidosis
(c) Fasting and starvation
(d) Ketogenic diets

(e) Lactic acidosis
(f) Salicylate, ethylene glycol (anti-freeze), and methanol poisoning

3. *Increased* anion gap is also associated with decreased loss of metabolic acids as in renal failure
4. *Increased* bicarbonate loss with resulting normal anion gap is associated with
   (a) *Decreased* renal losses as in
      (1) Renal tubular acidosis
      (2) Use of acetazolamide
   (b) *Increased* chloride levels as in
      (1) Altered chloride reabsorption by the kidney
      (2) Parenteral hyperalimentation
      (3) Administration of sodium chloride and ammonium chloride
   (c) Loss of intestinal secretions as in
      (1) Diarrhea
      (2) Intestinal suction or fistula
      (3) Biliary fistula

Lactic Acid

Normal Values
0.5–2.2 mEq./liter venous blood
0.5–1.6 mEq./liter arterial blood

Background
Lactate is a product of carbohydrate metabolism. Lactic acid is produced during periods of anaerobic metabolism when cells do not receive adequate oxygen to allow conversion of fuel sources to carbon dioxide and water. Lactic acid will accumulate because of excess production of lactate and decreased removal of lactic acid from blood by liver.

Explanation of Test
This measurement contributes to the knowledge of acid–base volume in the body and is used to detect lactic acidosis in persons with underlying risk factors that predispose them to this imbalance, such as cardiovascular and renal disease. Lactate will be elevated in a variety of conditions in which hypoxia is present and in liver disease. Lactic acidosis can occur both in diabetics and nondiabetics, and it is an often fatal form of metabolic acidosis.

Procedure
A venous or arterial blood sample of at least 4 ml. is obtained. The specimen must be brought to the laboratory immediately.

Clinical Implications
1. Values will be *increased* in
   (a) Lactic acidosis   (e) Diabetes
   (b) Cardiac failure   (f) Shock
   (c) Pulmonary failure   (g) Liver disease
   (d) Hemorrhage
2. Lactic acidosis can be distinguished from ketoacidosis by the absence of severe ketosis and hyperglycemia.

Interfering Factors
Lactic acid levels normally rise during strenuous exercise when blood flow and oxygen cannot keep pace with increased needs of exercising muscle.

Clinical Alert

The presence of an unexplained fall in *p*H associated with a hypoxia-producing condition is reason to suspect lactic acidosis.

BIBLIOGRAPHY

Altose MD: The physiological basis of pulmonary function testing. Clin Symp 31(2):1–39, 1979

American Thoracic Society: Guidelines for bronchial inhalation challenges with pharmacologic and antigenic agents. ATS News, Spring:11–19, 1980

Bass H: The flow-volume loop: Normal standards and abnormalities in chronic obstructive pulmonary disease. Chest 63:171–176, 1973

Boren H, Kory R, Snyder J: The Veterans Administration–Army cooperative study of pulmonary function: II—Lung volume and its subdivisions in normal men. Am J Med 41(1):96–114, 1966

Borrows B, Kasik JE, Niden AH et al.: Clinical usefulness of the single-breath pulmonary diffusing capacity test. Am Rev Resp Dis 84:789–806, 1961

Brust SA, Ross BB: Predicted values for closing volumes using a modified single-breath nitrogen test. Am Rev Resp Dis 107:744, 1973

Cherniack RM: Pulmonary Function Testing. Philadelphia, WB Saunders, 1977

Chusid EL: Diagnostic procedures in bronchopulmonary diseases. Hosp Pract 16(7):99–108, 1981

Clausen JL: Pulmonary Function Testing, Guidelines and Controversies. New York, Academic Press, 1982

Cohen S: Pulmonary function tests in patient care. Am J Nurs 80:1135–1161, 1980

Cropp G: The exercise bronchoprovocation test: Standardization of procedures and evaluation of response. J Allergy Clin Immunol 64:627–633, 1979

Eggleston P: Exercise challenge: Indications, techniques, and data analysis. J Allergy Clin Immunol 64:604–608, 1979

Fishman AP: Assessment of Pulmonary Function. New York, McGraw-Hill, 1980

Fraser RG, Pare JA: Organ Physiology: Structure and Function of the Lung, 2nd ed. Philadelphia, WB Saunders, 1977

Geschickter CF: The Lung in Health and Disease. Philadelphia, JB Lippincott, 1973

Gilb AF, Molony PA, Klein E et al: Sensitivity of volume of isoflow in the detection of mild airway obstruction. Am Rev Resp Dis 112:401–405, 1975

Goldman HO, Becklake MR: Respiratory function tests. Normal values at median altitudes and the prediction of normal results. Am Rev Tuberculosis Pulm Dis 79:457, 1979

Guenter C, Welch MH (eds): Pulmonary Medicine, 2nd ed. Philadelphia, JB Lippincott, 1982

Halsted CH, Halsted JA (eds): The Laboratory in Clinical Medicine, 2nd ed. Philadelphia, WB Saunders, 1982

Isselbacher KJ et al (eds): Harrison's Principles of Internal Medicine, 11th ed. New York, McGraw–Hill, 1987

Jones NL: Exercise testing in pulmonary evaluation: Rationale, methods, and the normal respiratory response to exercise. N Engl J Med 293(11):541–544, 1975

Jones NL: Exercise testing in pulmonary evaluation clinical application. N Engl J Med 293(13): 647–652, 1975

Kenasewitz GT: Pulmonary Function Testing Principles and Practice. New York, Churchill Livingstone, 1984

Keogh BA et al: Clinical significance of pulmonary function tests. Chest 78(6): 856–865, 1980

Narins RG: Diagnostic strategies in disorders of fluid, electrolyte, and acid–base homeostasis. Am J Med 72:496–520, 1982

Ruppel G: Manual of Pulmonary Function Testing, 3rd ed. St. Louis, CV Mosby, 1982

Schoenberg JB, Beck GJ, Bouhuys A: Growth and decay of pulmonary function in healthy blacks and whites. Respir Physiol 33:367–393, 1978

Slonim NB, Hamilton LH: Respiratory Physiology, 4th ed. St. Louis, CV Mosby, 1981

Victor LD, Chmielinski MA: Pulmonary function and exercise stress testing. Hosp Pract 17(7):125–132, 1982

Williams MH: Essentials of Pulmonary Medicine. Philadelphia, WB Saunders, 1982

Wilson AF: Pulmonary Function Testing: Indications and Interpretations. Orlando, Grune & Stratton, 1985

Woolf CR: The Clinical Core of Respiratory Medicine. Philadelphia, JB Lippincott, 1981

West JB: Respiratory Physiology, 3rd ed. Baltimore, Williams & Wilkins, 1985

SPECIAL SYSTEM AND ORGAN FUNCTION STUDIES

Introduction

These special tests of the eye, body fat estimates, and of the cardiovascular, peripheral vascular, cerebrovascular, and nervous and muscle systems have been selected for discussion in this chapter because of their great importance in diagnosing alterations in the functions of these vital systems and organs.

Electroencephalography (EEG)

Normal Values
Normal symmetrical pattern of alpha activity

Explanation of Test
This test measures and records electrical impulses from the cortex of the brain. Electrodes are placed outside the cranial vault to record the electrical manifestations of brain activity. This test is used to help diagnose epilepsy and as an aid in identifying brain tumors, abscesses, and subdural hematomas; to help diagnose cerebrovascular diseases, such as cerebral infarcts and intracranial hemorrhages; and to help diagnose cerebral diseases such as narcolepsy and Alzheimer's disease.

It is common practice to use the EEG pattern to define cerebral death. A record that is flat is usually the result of cerebral hypoxia or ischemia, and the brain is largely necrotic. When this EEG pattern is recorded, there is no chance of neurologic recovery and the patient may be considered dead, despite the preservation of cardiovascular functions supported by mechanical respiration.

Procedure
1. An EEG is usually scheduled early in the day.
2. The technician places electrodes in the form of small discs on the scalp, fastening them with skin glue or paste. Nineteen to 25 electrodes are attached according to an internationally accepted design called the *10–20 System*. This system correlates both standardization of electrode placement and anatomical structure of the brain. Conduction gel is placed in the electrode itself.
3. The patient sits in an easy chair or lies on a bed or couch.
4. The patient is instructed to keep the eyes closed and to relax.
5. Near the beginning of the examination, the patient may be asked to breathe deeply through the mouth 20 times a minute for 3 minutes. This hyperventilation may cause dizziness or numbness in hands or feet, but it is nothing to be alarmed about. Rapid, shallow breathing contributes to alkalosis causing vasoconstriction, which may activate a seizure pattern.

6. A flashing light may be used over the face at frequencies of 1 to 30 times per second with the eyes opened or closed. This technique, called *photic stimulation,* may cause an abnormal discharge not otherwise recorded in the EEG.
7. Some patients may be sleep-deprived before the test to promote rest and sleep. Sleep is especially helpful in bringing out abnormalities, especially different forms of epilepsy.
8. The technician removes the discs after the test and removes the ointment or paste from the scalp.
9. Total examining time is 1 hour 15 minutes.

Clinical Implications
1. Abnormal pattern readings will reveal generalized seizures (*e.g.,* grand mal and petit mal epilepsy), provided the EEG is recorded during the seizure. If a patient suspected of having epilepsy shows a normal EEG, the test may have to be repeated with sleep deprivation and special electives.
   (a) The EEG is also abnormal during other types of seizure activity (*e.g.,* focal [psychomotor], infantile myoclonic, and Jacksonian seizures).
   (b) Between seizures, 20% of patients with petit mal epilepsy and 40% with grand mal epilepsy show a normal pattern.
   (c) The diagnosis of epilepsy can be made only by correlating the clinical history with the EEG abnormality, if one exists.
2. An EEG may often be normal in the presence of cerebral pathology.
   (a) However, most brain abscesses and glioblastomas cause EEG abnormalities.
   (b) EEG changes due to cerebrovascular accidents (CVAs) depend on the size and location of the infarcts or hemorrhage.
   (c) Following a head injury, a series of EEGs may be helpful in identifying the prospect of epilepsy as a result of the trauma if a previous EEG is on record.
   (d) In dementia, the EEG may be either normal or abnormal.
   (e) In later stages of metabolic disease, the EEG will be abnormal; in the early stages, it will be normal.
3. The EEG is abnormal in most disease in which there is an impairment of consciousness. The more profound the change in consciousness, the more abnormal the EEG pattern.

Interfering Factors
1. Sedative drugs and mild hypoglycemia may affect the normal EEG.
2. Oily hair or hair spray interferes with the placement of leads and a true tracing.
3. Artifacts may appear even in technically well done EEGs. Eye movements and body movements cause changes in the wave pat-

tern and must be noted so that they will not be mistaken for brain waves.

Patient Preparation

1. Explain the purpose and procedure of the test. Some persons are very fearful of this test, even though it involves no pain or discomfort. Emphasize that it is not a test of thinking or intelligence, that no electrical impulses pass from the machine to the patient, and that the test has no relation to any type of shock treatment.
2. Food may be taken if the patient is sleep deprived, but no coffee, tea, or cola is permitted within 8 hours of the test. Emphasize that food should be eaten to prevent hypoglycemia.
3. Smoking is usually allowed before the test.
4. Hair should be shampooed the evening before the test so that leads will remain firmly in place.
5. If a sleep study is ordered, an adult patient should sleep as little as possible the night before (up past midnight) so he will be tired enough to fall asleep during the test.
6. If a sleep-deprivation study is ordered for a child, call the diagnostic department for special instructions.

Patient Aftercare

1. The hair should be shampooed after the test to remove the substance used to fasten the discs. Oil can be of some help before the shampoo.
2. If the patient received a sedative during the test, allow him to rest with bedside rails in raised position.

Evoked Responses or Potentials

Brainstem auditory evoked potentials (BAEP): Absolute latency measured in milliseconds (msec.) of the first five wave forms at a stimulation rate of 11 clicks/second sound

Wave	Mean	SD (Standard Deviation)
I	1.7	0.15
II	2.8	0.17
III	3.9	0.19
IV	5.1	0.24
V	5.7	0.25

Visual-evoked response (VER): Absolute latency measured in milliseconds of the first major positive peak (P_{100})

Wave	Mean	Range	SD
P_{100}	102.3	89–114	5.1

Somatosensory-evoked response (SER): Absolute latency of major wave forms measured in milliseconds at a stimulation rate of 5 impulses/second

Wave	Mean	SD
E.P.	9.7	0.7
A	11.8	0.7
B	13.7	0.8
II	11.3	0.8
III	13.9	0.9
N_2	19.1	0.8
P_2	22	1.2

Normal Values
Depend on waveform latency and are established by each individual laboratory due to varying factors such as instrument type and laboratory environment. Values vary between persons and in the same person over time.

Explanation of Test
Potentials evoked by stimulation of a sensory path are used to test conduction through that sensory pathway. The most important abnormal clinical finding is an increase of the latency of response components, which indicates a delay in conduction and implies damage to nerve fibers of the sensory system under study. Evoked potentials can be divided by sensory modality into visual, auditory, and somatosensory responses.

Somatosensory-Evoked Response (SER)

This test is used in the assessment of patients with spinal cord lesions, stroke, and complaints of numbness and weakness of the extremities. It is done to study the conduction of impulses through the somatosensory pathway. Electrical stimuli are applied to the median or peroneal nerve at an intensity near that which produces thumb or foot twitches. With this procedure, it is possible to measure in milliseconds the time it takes for the current to travel along the nerve to the cortex of the brain.

Visual-Evoked Response (VER)

This test of visual pathway function is valuable in the diagnosis of lesions involving the optic nerves and optic tracts, multiple sclerosis, and other disorders. It is known that visual stimulation excites retinal pathways and initiates impulses that are conducted through the central visual path to the primary visual cortex. Fibers from this area project to the secondary visual cortical areas on the occipital convexity. Through this path, a visual stimulus to the eyes causes an electrical response in the occipital regions, which can be recorded with electrodes placed along the vertex and occipital lobes.

Auditory Brain Stem Response (ABR)

This test uses conventional EEG recording techniques along with computer data processing to evaluate the electrophysiologic integrity of the central auditory pathway of the brain stem, including the peripheral nerve. Special recording and stimulating methods have been developed that permit recording of signals generated by subcortical structures in the auditory pathway. Stimulation of either ear evokes potentials that can reveal lesions in the brain stem involving the auditory pathway without affecting hearing. Evoked potentials of this type are also used to evaluate hearing in infants, children, and adults, which is called *electrical response audiometry*.

This study is also helpful in the evaluation of suspected peripheral hearing loss, cerebellopontine angle lesions, brain stem tumors, infarcts, and multiple sclerosis. It is also useful in evaluating the mechanisms of coma as well as in monitoring the cause of disorders associated with coma.

Procedure
1. Electrodes that pick up a visually evoked response are placed on the scalp along the vertex and occipital lobes. The patient is asked to watch a checkerboard pattern flash for several minutes, first with one eye, then with the other.
2. Somatosensory-evoked responses are obtained from recordings of several pairs of pick-up electrodes. Electrical stimuli are applied to the median nerve at the wrist or the peroneal nerve at the knee with electrodes placed over the sensory cortex of the opposite hemisphere in the scalp. This procedure measures in milliseconds the time it takes for the current to travel along the nerve to the cortex of the brain.
3. Auditory brain stem responses are obtained from scalp electrodes placed on the vertex and each earlobe. Stimuli consisting of clicking noises or tone bursts are delivered to one ear through earphones. Because sound waves delivered to one ear can be heard by the opposite ear, a continuous masking noise is simultaneously delivered to the opposite ear.

Clinical Implications
1. Abnormal visual-evoked responses are associated with
   (a) Demyelinating disorders such as multiple sclerosis
   (b) Lesions of the optic nerves and eye (prechiasmal defects)
   (c) Lesions of the optic tract and visual cortex (postchiasmal defects)

(d) Abnormal visual-evoked potentials may also be found in persons without a history of retrobulbar neuritis, optic atrophy, or visual field defects. However, many patients with proven damage to the postchiasmal visual path and known visual field defects may have normal evoked potentials.

2. Abnormal somatosensory-evoked responses are associated with
   (a) Spinal cord lesions
   (b) Cerebrovascular accident (CVA)
   (c) Multiple sclerosis
   (d) Cervical myelopathy
3. Abnormal auditory brain stem-evoked responses are associated with
   (a) Acoustic neuroma
   (b) CVA
   (c) Multiple sclerosis
   (d) Lesions affecting any part of the auditory nerve or brain stem area

   Note: Some difficulty of interpreting brain stem-evoked potentials may arise in persons with peripheral hearing defects that alter the evoked potential results.

Patient Preparation
1. Explain the purpose and procedure of the test.
2. Hair should be shampooed before testing.

Patient Aftercare
Assist the patient in washing the hair (if so desired) to remove gels applied to the scalp. Also, be sure that gel is carefully washed from any other area of the body to be tested.

Cognitive Tests (Event-Related Potentials [ERPs])

Normal Values
No shift of P_3 components to longer latencies
ERP: absolute latency of P_3 waveform

Wave	Mean	SD
P_3	294	21

Explanation of Test
ERPs are being used more frequently as objective measures of mental function in neurological diseases that produce cognitive defects. These measurements use the method of auditory-evoked response testing (see page 804) in which sound stimuli are presented through earphones. A rare tone is associated with a prominent endogenous P_3 component

that reflects the differential cognitive processing of that tone. Although a systematic neurological increase in P_3 component latency occurs as a function of increasing age in normal persons, in many instances of neurologic diseases producing dementia, the latency of the P_3 component has been reported to exceed substantially the normal age-matched value.

This test is useful in evaluating persons with dementia or decreased mental functioning. It is also helpful in differentiating persons with real organic defects in cognitive function from those who are unable to interact with the examiner because of motor or language defects and those who are unwilling to cooperate because of problems like depression or schizophrenia.

Procedure

1. The procedure is the same as that used in obtaining auditory brain stem responses (see page 804).
2. Patients are asked to count the occurrences of rare tones.

Interfering Factors

Latency of P_3 component normally increases with age.

Clinical Implications

An increased or abnormal P_3 latency is associated with neurological diseases producing dementia such as

1. Alzheimer's disease
2. Metabolic encephalopathy such as hypothyroidism and alcoholism with severe electrolyte disturbances
3. Brain tumor
4. Hydrocephalus

Patient Preparation

Explain the purpose and procedure of the test.

Electrocardiography (ECG or EKG) (With Brief Description of Vector Cardiogram)

Normal Values

Normal positive and negative deflections in an electrocardiographic record. One cardiac cycle is represented by the P wave, QRS complex, and T wave. This cycle is repeated continuously. P = Atrial systole Contraction/Depolarization; QRS = Ventricular Contraction Systole; T = Ventricular Repolarization/Resting Stage between beats (Table 15-1).

Waves

Capital letters refer to relatively large waves (over 5 mm) and small letters refer to relatively small waves (5 mm).

1. The P wave is upright and represents *atrial* depolarization and the electrical activity associated with the original impulse from the sinoatrial (SA) node and its subsequent spread through the atria.

    If P waves are present and of normal size, shape, and deflection, it can be assumed that the stimulus began in the SA node.
2. T_a wave is a deflection produced by atrial depolarization and is usually not seen in the 12-lead ECG. There is a pause after the QRS complex, then a T wave appears. The T wave is a period of no cardiac activity, before the ventricles are again stimulated. It represents the recovery phase after contraction.
3. The Q(q) wave is an initial downward negative deflection resulting from ventricular depolarization.
4. The R(r) wave is a true upright/positive deflection resulting from ventricular depolarization.
5. The S(s) wave is the first downward/negative deflection that follows the first positive deflection.
6. QS wave. A negative deflection that does not rise above the baseline.
7. $R^1(r')$ wave. The 2nd upward/positive deflection or the first positive/upward deflection during ventricular depolarization that follows the S wave. The negative deflection following the r' is termed the s'.
8. T wave is a deflection produced by ventricular polarization.
9. U wave is a deflection (usually positive, following the T wave, but preceding the next P wave; it is thought to be caused by repolarization of Purkinje's (intraventricular) conduction system.

Intervals

1. RR interval is the distance between two successive R waves. In regular ventricular rhythm, the interval in seconds (or fractions of seconds) between .2 successive R waves, then divided into 60 seconds, will give the heart rate per minute.
2. PP interval will be the same as the RR interval in regular sinus rhythm.
3. PR interval measures conduction tone and includes time for atrial depolarization, normal conduction delay in the AV node, and the passage of impulse through the bundle of His and the bundle branches to the onset of ventricular depolarization. The impulse has traversed the atria and the AV node. It is the period from the start of the P wave to the beginning of the QRS complex. This interval represents the time taken for the original impulse to reach the ventricles and initiate ventricular contraction (depolarization).

Table 15-1
Normal Measurements and Ranges of Components of
P–Q–R–S–T–U Cycle*

	P Wave		PR Interval	Q Wave Q% of R	
	Amplitude	Width			
	Maximum	Maximum	0.12 sec.–0.20 sec.	Width	Depth
	2.5 mm.	0.10 sec.		Less than 0.04 sec.	QR ratio
L₁					15% of R wave
L₂				↓	20% of R wave
L₃				Up to 0.08 sec.	25% of R wave
ᴀVR				Up to 0.08 sec.	
ᴀVL				Less than 0.04 sec.	25% of R wave
ᴀVF				↓	
V₁				Up to 0.08 sec.	
V₂				↓	
V₃				Less than 0.04 sec.	
V₄					
V₅					
V₆	↓	↓	↓	↓	↓

* For practical purposes, these are the upper and lower limits of the normal ECG. However, there are "gray zones," and variation from these limits may not necessarily imply abnormality.

Table 15-1
Normal Measurements and Ranges of Components of
P–Q–R–S–T–U Cycle* (Continued)

QRS Interval	R-Wave Amplitude	ST Segment	T Wave	U-Wave Amplitude	Width
0.10 sec.	Maximum to minimum	1 mm.	1mm.–5 mm.	1.5 mm.	0.24 sec.
	5 mm.–16 mm.	Above or below			
		1 mm. elevation			
	Less than +4 mm.		Except in this lead (T is neg.)		
	5 mm.–13 mm. Transverse heart				
	5 mm.–21 mm. Vertical heart				
	5 mm.–27 mm.		13 mm.		
0.11 sec.					
0.11 sec.					

ST Segment vertical annotations: 1 mm. elevation · 1 mm.–2 mm. depression · 2 mm.–4 mm. elevation

(Ritota MC: Diagnostic Electrocardiography, 2nd ed. Philadelphia, JB Lippincott, 1977)

The normal range is related to heart rate; the higher the heart rate, the shorter the PR interval; the slower the heart rate, the longer the PR interval.

4. QRS interval is ventricular depolarization/contraction time and represents the electrical impulse as it travels from the AV node to the Purkinje's fibers and into the myocardial cells. Normal waves consist of an initial downward deflection (Q wave), a large upward deflection (R wave), and a second downward wave (S wave). It is measured from the onset of the Q wave (or R if no Q is visible) to the termination of the S wave and is evidence that the ventricles have been stimulated in a normal manner.

Segments and Junctions
1. PR segment is normally isoelectric and is that portion of the ECG tracing from the end of the P wave to the onset of the QRS complex.
2. RST (J) junction is the point at which the QRS complex ends and the ST segment begins.
3. ST segment or RST segment is that part of the ECG from the J point to the onset of the T wave. It is elevated or depressed in comparison with that portion of the baseline between the end of the T wave and the beginning of the P wave or when related to the PR segment.
   This segment represents the period between the completion of depolarization and repolarization (recovery) of the ventricular muscles.
4. TP segment is that portion of the ECG record between the end of the T wave and the beginning of the next P wave. It is usually isoelectric at normal heart rate.

Voltage Measurements
1. Upright deflection voltage is measured from the upper part of the baseline to the peak of the wave.
2. Negative deflection voltage is measured from the lower portion of the baseline to the nadir of the wave.

Explanation of Test
An electrocardiogram (ECG) is a recording of the electrical impulses that stimulate the heart to contract and is an important indicator of how well the heart is functioning. The ECG is helpful in diagnosing the following: origins of and monitoring of pathological rhythms; myocardial ischemia and infarction; atrial and ventricular hypertrophy; conduction delay of atrial and ventricular electrical impulses, and pericarditis. It is also helpful in diagnosing systemic diseases that affect the heart; determination of effect of cardiac drugs, especially digitalis and antiarrhythmic agents; disturbances in electrolyte balance, especially potassium and calcium, and evaluation of cardiac pacemaker function.
   The heart is unique among the muscles of the body in that it pos-

sesses the properties of automatic impulse formation and rhythmic contraction. Formation and conduction of these electrical impulses produces weak electrical current that spreads through the body. Each normal heart beat begins with an electrical impulse that originates in a specialized area of the right atrium called the sinoatrial (SA) node. This island of tissue serves as a battery for the heart and normally discharges an electrical force 60 to 100 times a minute in rhythmic fashion. Because the SA node controls the rate of the heart beat, it is designated as the pacemaker. (All areas of the myocardium have the potential ability to serve in this capacity, but they assume this role only under abnormal circumstances.) The original impulse is transmitted through the heart in an orderly path. When it reaches the ventricular muscles, contraction occurs. After contracting, the muscles rest and recover while the ventricles fill with blood. The next impulse normally arrives when filling is complete and ventricular contraction again occurs. The combined periods of contraction (depolarization) and recovery (repolarization) constitute the cardiac cycle.

Recording provides a continuous picture of the electrical activity during a cycle. Heart cells are charged or polarized in the resting state but when electrically stimulated, they depolarize and contract. The body fluid is an excellent conductor of electrical current. When the depolarization (stimulation) process sweeps in a wave across the cells of the myocardium, the electrical current generated is conducted to the body's surface where it is detected by special electrodes placed on the patient's limb and chest. An ECG tracing also shows the voltage of the waves and the time duration of both waves and intervals. By studying the amplitude and time duration of the waves and intervals, disorders of impulse formation and conduction can be diagnosed.

Recording the Electrical Impulses
1. Because the electrical forces extend in several directions at the same time, a comprehensive view can be obtained only if the flow of current in different planes is recorded.
2. Twelve leads are used simultaneously.
    (a) Limb leads—I, II, III, AVF, AVR—record events in the frontal plane of the heart.
    (b) Chest leads—V, V_2, V_3, V_4, V_5, and V_6—record a horizontal view of the heart's electrical activity.

ECG vs. Vectorcardiogram
The vectorcardiogram, like the ECG, records the electrical forces of the heart. The major difference between these methods is the way in which these forces are displayed. A vectorcardiogram records a *three-dimensional* display of the heart's electrical activity, whereas the ECG shows activity in a *single plane*.

The three planes of the vectorcardiogram are as follows:

1. Frontal plane (combines the Y and X axes)
2. Sagittal plane (combines the Y and Z axes)
3. Horizontal plane (combines the X and Z axes)

Briefly, the two records of the heart's electrical activity may be compared as follows:

ECG	*Vectorcardiogram*
Records electrical forces as deflections on a scale	Depicts electrical forces as vector loops, thereby showing the *direction* of electrical activity
Recorded in the frontal and horizontal planes of the body	Recorded on the frontal, horizontal, and sagittal planes of the body
	The term *vector* is used to indicate the direction of electrical activity.

Clinical Implications of ECG

1. The ECG *does not* depict the actual mechanical state of the heart or function of the valves.
2. An ECG may be quite normal in the presence of heart disease unless the pathologic process disturbs the electrical forces.
3. Final conclusions from an ECG should be done only with a full knowledge of the clinical status of the patient.
4. Abnormalities of an ECG are categorized into five general areas:
   (a) heart rate
   (b) heart rhythm
   (c) axis or position of the heart
   (d) hypertrophy
   (e) infarction

   Certain specific abnormalities in these areas are typical of
   (1) Pathological rhythms
   (2) Conduction system diseases
   (3) Myocardial ischemia
   (4) Myocardial infarction
   (5) Hypertrophy of the heart
   (6) Pulmonary infarction
   (7) Aortic stenosis
   (8) Electrolyte changes in potassium, calcium, and magnesium
   (9) Pericarditis
   (10) Effects of drugs (*e.g.*, digitalis and quinidine)

Clinical Implications of Vectorcardiogram

1. The vectorcardiogram is more sensitive than the ECG in the diagnosis of myocardial infarction, but it is probably not more specific.
2. Vectorcardiography is more specific than the ECG in the assess-

ment of hypertrophy or dilatation of the ventricles of the heart in children.
3. Intraventricular conduction abnormalities can possibly be differentiated from a variety of causes.

Clinical Considerations
1. If chest pain is experienced on a lead run, it should be noted on the involved ECG strip.
2. The presence of a pacemaker and whether or not a magnet was used in testing should be indicated.
3. Reproducibility of precardial lead placement should be ensured by proper positioning and by marking the position on the chest wall in ink when indicated.

Procedure
The following steps apply to both the ECG and the vectorcardiogram.
1. The patient is placed in a supine position on a table, bed, or couch. The recording can also be done during exercise or the patient can be ambulatory, in which case a Holter device is used for a continuous 24–48 hour recording.
2. The skin is prepared (including shaving if there is excess hair) by the application of contact paste or prejelled discs.
3. Electrodes are placed anywhere on the four extremities and on the chest. The right leg is the ground.
4. The operator then records the ECG through machine setting.
5. The test may take only a few minutes or as long as 24–48 hours if a Holter recording has been ordered.

Interfering Factors
1. Race: ST elevation with T wave inversion is more common in blacks, but disappears with maximal effort exercise.
2. Food intake: high carbohydrate content, especially, is associated with an intracellular shift of K in association with intracellular glucose metabolism; nondiagnostic ST depression and T wave inversion may occur.
3. Anxiety: episodic anxiety and hyperventilation are associated with PR prolongation, sinus tachycardia, and ST depression with or without T wave inversion. May be due to an imbalance of autonomic nervous system input.
4. Deep respiration: position of the heart in the chest becomes more vertical with deep inspiration and horizontal with deep expiration.
5. Exercise/Movement: strenuous exercise before the test can produce a misleading record. Muscle twitching by the patient can alter the record.
6. Position of heart within thoracic cage: there may be anatomic cardiac rotation in both horizontal and frontal planes.

7. Position of precardial leads: inaccuracy of placement of the bipolar chest leads will affect test results and the interchange of right and left arm and left leg electrodes. In normal persons, this will produce the typical ECG findings of dextrocardia in frontal plane leads and can mimic an MI pattern.

8. Weight: in conjunction with excess body weight, there is a leftward shift in the QRS axis.

9. Age: at birth and infancy there is hypertrophy of the right ventricle because, in the fetus, the right ventricle performs more work than the left ventricle. T wave inversion in leads V_{1-3} persists into the second decade of life and into the third decade in blacks.

10. Sex: slight ST segment depression in women.

11. Chest configuration and dextrocardia: in this congenital anomaly the procedure leads must be recorded over the right side of the chest.

12. There are many medications that affect ECG results: severe drug overdose, especially when barbiturates are involved.

13. The serious effects of electrolyte balance on the ECG record can be seen in clinical considerations of individual electrolytes: K_1, page 253, Ca, page 244, and magnesium, page 251. (Blood chemistry)

14. Mechanical: poor contact between the skin and the electrode can result in a less than optimum record. Incorrect standardization of the electrocardiographic machine will produce inaccurate voltage of the complexes that can lead to false interpretations.

15. Arbitrary limits of normal are in the 95th to 98th percentile based on 100th percentile range for each measurement. Two to five percent will fall outside the normal and be considered abnormal ECGs.

Patient Preparation

1. Explain the purpose and procedure of the test and the factors that interfere with an accurate test result, emphasizing that it is painless and that there is no current flow to the body. It must be kept in mind that a resting ECG (without stressing the heart) is no more than a one-minute record of the electrical activity of the heart.

2. The patient must be completely relaxed in order to ensure a satisfactory tracing.

3. Ideally, the person should be at rest for 15 minutes prior to ECG recording, with no recent meal, and no smoking for 30 minutes before testing.

Patient Aftercare

In patients with heart symptoms, it is important that the limitations of an ECG are recognized. A normal ECG does not rule out coronary artery disease or areas of ischemia in the heart. On the other hand, an abnormal ECG in and of itself does not signify heart disease.

It is most important that the patient does not become a cardiac "cripple" solely on the basis of an ECG. On the other hand, a person may receive unwarranted assurance of the absence of heart disease solely on the basis of the normal ECG. Patients need to know that the resting ECG is usually normal for patients with only angina and no other heart problems. It can, however, provide evidence of prior heart attack of which the person may not have been aware.

Clinical Alert

1. When an ECG shows changes indicating ischemia, injury, or infarction, these changes must be reported and acted upon immediately to increase myocardial blood supply and reduce oxygen demand.
   (a) When ECG changes representing stages of ischemia, injury, or necrosis are seen and symptoms of possible MI appear, the first concern is to correct the imbalance between myocardial oxygen supply and demand.
       (1) Give ordered nitroglycerine to dilate blood vessels
       (2) Sedate with narcotics to limit size of infarction
       (3) Administer calcium channel blocks to relieve coronary spasm
       (4) Start oxygen to increase supply of oxygen
       (5) Beta-blocking drugs to slow rapid heart rate
       (6) Antiarrhythmics to correct abnormal rhythms
       (7) Constant reassurance to reverse panic
   (b) Special Alerts: In patients with inferior MI, observe for AV block, increased likelihood of vasovagal episodes, and poor right ventricular compliance. Use vasodilators such as nitroglycerine and morphine sulfate with caution because they encourage venous pooling and reduced venous return.
2. Serious diagnostic error can be made if the ECG is not interpreted in the light of history and signs and symptoms.
3. When looking at the ECG interpretation of heart position, keep in mind that this refers to a pattern resulting from electrical spread of excitation. The electrical axis is not synonymous with the anatomic position of the heart.

Holter Continuous ECG Monitoring

Normal Values
Normal sinus rhythm

Explanation

Holter monitoring is a method of continuously recording the electrocardiograph (ECG) on magnetic tape for prolonged periods of time. Twenty-four and forty-eight hours are the common recording durations. The tape recorder is a battery powered device with very slow (3¾ in/min) tape speeds and is small enough to be carried on a strap over the shoulder or around the waist. Two ECG channels recorded simultaneously are graphic records of the electrical impulses that are generated by contraction and recovery of the myocardium.

The Holter recorder is equipped with a digital clock, which is synchronized to the tape recorder and this allows for accurate time marking. The patient carries a diary with him in which he enters any symptoms experienced during the monitoring period, his activity status, and the time at which the symptoms occurred. When a symptom occurs, the patient pushes an event-marker button on the recorder. This marks one of the channels for easy recognition during playback.

A 24-hour recording contains over 100,000 cardiac cycles. Playback and tape analysis are done at 60, 120, or 180 times real time. The tape may be rapidly analyzed by computers that can provide summaries of heart rates, frequency of premature atrial or ventricular extrasystoles, coupling intervals and other variations in pattern. Another method of scanning the tapes superimposes each QRS complex on the preceding complex. This makes any variations in the QRS contour become apparent and arrhythmias are found in this way. In either method of scanning, segments of the tape recording can be reproduced on electrocardiographic paper. The diary the patient kept is also used to see if there is a correlation between symptoms and ECG findings. A report is then produced which provides ECG strips and a summary of arrhythmias that were found during the recording.

Indications for Holter Monitoring

Holter monitors are placed on patients for a variety of reasons.

1. They are used for documentation of a suspected rhythm disturbance. The recording, along with the diary the patient keeps, can be used to correlate rhythm disturbances with patient symptoms of syncope, palpitations, chest pain, lightheadedness, and unexplained dyspnea. If these symptoms have no obvious cause, a Holter recording can be used to detect the presence of unsuspected arrhythmias in patients, such as supraventricular and ventricular tachycardias, bradycardia-tachycardia in patients with sick sinus syndrome, and other ventricular and supraventricular arrhythmias.
2. The recording of the onset and termination of a rhythmic disturbance may provide insight into the electrophysiologic mechanisms responsible for the arrhythmia.
3. Pacemaker functioning can be checked.

4. The efficiency of antiarrhythmic therapy and lack of toxicity can be documented in a Holter report.

Procedure

1. The patient is placed in a supine position on a table.
2. The skin is prepared. This involves shaving the chest, if necessary, cleansing the skin with alcohol, and reddening the skin by rubbing it with gauze or similar rough material. These preparations are important for good electrode contact.
3. Electrodes are placed: two for each channel, and one ground. Electrodes are positioned over bony prominences. The two negative electrodes are placed on the manubrium, while their corresponding positive electrodes (for the two channels) are placed in the V_1 and V_5 positions.
4. Loose wires are taped down and everything is secured. The recorder is started and calibrated. The patient is then free to pursue all activities except bathing.
5. After the required (24-to-48 hours) amount of time, the recorder is stopped and the electrodes are removed from the patient's chest.
6. The tape is scanned by a technician.

Interfering Factors

1. Incomplete diary and/or event: marker not pushed during symptoms
2. Interference caused either mechanically or by patient scratching electrode area

Clinical Implications

Abnormal results include:

1. Rhythm disturbances such as
   (a) Supraventricular tachycardia
   (b) Ventricular tachycardia
   (c) Bradycardia-tachycardia in patients with sick sinus syndrome
   (d) Other ventricular and supraventricular abnormal rhythms

---

Phonocardiography

Normal Values

Normal heart sounds

Explanation of Test

This test graphically records the occurrence, timing, and length of sounds of the heart cycle. Heart murmurs can be both visualized and accurately timed. Sounds that originate in the heart and large vessels are recorded from the body's surface and correspond to what is heard through a stethoscope. This diagnostic technique involves the electronic detection, amplification, and recording of cardiac sounds. A specially designed microphone is placed on the patient's chest for recording purposes. This device picks up the low-frequency cardiac vibrations for amplification and recording. The phonocardiograph is recorded simultaneously with carotid pulse, ECG, and respiration.

Phonocardiography provides information about underlying hemodynamics that is not obtainable through physical examination. It also provides a permanent objective record of events with which subsequent comparison may be made. It is useful in detecting abnormalities in valvular function and can be used in conjunction with other cardiovascular monitoring techniques to assess specific portions of the cardiac cycle such as systolic ejection time and pre-ejection time. It is a valuable teaching aid.

Procedure
1. The test should be done in a quiet room.
2. The patient is placed on a table in a supine position with pillows under his head.
3. Electrocardiographic leads are placed on all four extremities and standard lead two (2) is recorded throughout the procedure. A neck cuff for the indirect carotid pulse is secured in place and inflated to 15 to 20 mm. Hg. Microphones (small, round, bell-like devices) for sound recording are placed over the pulmonary area and apex.
4. The patient is instructed to inhale deeply and to allow most of the air to escape from the lungs. At this point in expiration, he is instructed to suspend breathing for a few seconds without tensing the muscles. Then the patient is asked to breathe quietly through the mouth, and a recording is made.
5. The pulmonary area microphone is then removed and placed over the aortic area and a recording made during held expiration.
6. Next, the neck cuff is removed and the patient's upper body is lowered to one pillow. The upper microphone is placed over the left sternal border in the fourth intercostal space, and a jugular pulse recording is made during held expiration.
7. The patient is turned on his left side and another recording is made.
8. Total examining time is about 30 minutes.

Clinical Implications
Phonocardiography can be used to augment, but not replace, auscultation.

Cardiac Catheterization and Angiography
(Angiocardiography; Coronary Arteriography)

Normal Values
Normal heart and coronary arteries
Normal pressure and cardiac output
Normal percentage of oxygen saturation

Explanation of Test
This is a method of studying and diagnosing defects in the chambers of the heart, its valves, and its vessels by inserting arterial and venous catheters carrying contrast material into the right and left sides of the heart. As the catheters are advanced, fluoroscopy and rapidly taken x-ray pictures projected on TV monitors show the action of the heart under study. The injected dye or contrast medium provides definition of the cardiac structures. Each coronary artery is filmed as well. An oscilloscope near the TV monitor shows the patient's heart rate, rhythm, and pressures.

Coronary arteriograms are highly useful in diagnosing heart disease, determining the extent of damage, diagnosing congenital abnormalities, identifying cardiac structure and function before surgery, and measuring pressures within heart chambers and great vessels. They are also useful in determining cardiac output (using dye dilatation, thermodilution, and Fick method), and obtaining blood samples directly from the heart to measure oxygen content of blood and oxygen saturation.

Cardiac catheterization with angiography is indicated in patients with angina, incapacitating chest pain, syncope, valvular and ischemic disease; in patients with cholesteremia and familial heart disease who are experiencing chest pain; in patients with abnormal resting ECGs; in patients who have had cardiac revascularization with recurring symptoms; in young patients with a history of coronary insufficiency and ventricular aneurysm, and in patients with coronary neurosis who can be assured that their arteries are normal. This test can be done in the acute stage of myocardial infarction and, if necessary, the patient can be sent to surgery immediately.

Although it is an examination with some risks, it is highly accurate as a diagnostic technique.

Procedure
1. The test is usually done in a darkened room.
2. To decrease fear of the procedure, the patient is continuously told what is being done.
3. The patient lies on an x-ray table; ECG leads are attached to the chest. During the procedure, the patient will be turned from side to

side and may be asked to exercise (optional) to evaluate heart changes of any kind during activity. Atrial pacing can also be done as part of a cardiac catheterization in persons who cannot walk (paraplegics) or cannot use a treadmill. In these instances there is a sequence of events in which the heart is stressed, a rest period follows, measurements are taken, the heart is paced again, and another rest period follows.

4. The catheterization procedure is done under sterile conditions. The skin is prepared with an antiseptic solution. A local anesthetic is injected before making small incisions for the insertion of the catheter into an artery and vein. (Incisions are not always made.) Catheters are gently pushed into the heart and great vessels.
5. The patient may be able to watch all procedures on a screen of brightened heart image with "instant replay"; usually the screens are placed so that the examiner can see them.
6. After x-ray films have been taken at all angles, catheters are removed and skin incisions (if any) are closed with a few stitches. A sterile pressure bandage is applied. The procedure takes about 1 hour, or a little longer if the patient must exercise.

Clinical Implications

1. Abnormal results
    (a) Advancing catheters will reveal altered intracardiac pressures
    (b) Injecting contrast will reveal altered ventricular contractibility and blocked coronary arteries
    (c) Analyzing blood oxygen will confirm cardiac or arterial irregularities
2. Abnormal pressures are indicative of
    (a) Valve stenosis or insufficiency
    (b) Left and/or right ventricular failure
    (c) Idiopathic hypertrophic subaortic stenosis (IHHS)
    (d) Rheumatic fever
3. Abnormal blood oxygen samples are indicative of
    (a) Congenital or acquired shunting of blood
    (b) Septal defects
    (c) Leakage or abnormal sequential circulation of blood through the heart
4. When contrast is injected into the ventricles, abnormal size, bulging, ejection fractions, aneurysms of the heart, leaks, stenosis, and altered contractibility of the heart can be detected.
5. When contrast is injected into coronary arteries, abnormal circulation through coronary circulation can be detected.

Patient Preparation

1. Explain the purpose, procedure, benefits, and risks of the test. A legal permit must be signed before the examination.

2. Usually, a bland meal is eaten the evening before the examination, but nothing can be consumed for at least 3 hours before testing.
3. Analgesics, sedatives, or tranquilizers are administered before the examination.
4. Have the patient void before going to the catheterization laboratory.
5. Allow the patient to wear dentures.
6. The patient should be aware that he will be asked to breathe deeply and cough during the test, and that he will experience certain sensations that are common to the procedure.
   (a) A slight shock (like hitting the "funny bone") might be felt if the nerve lying next to the artery is touched, and a tiny bump in the neck is experienced as the catheter is inserted and pushed through the artery into the chest. Neither of these sensations is very painful.
   (b) When contrast is injected, a pumping sensation (with palpitations and warm flashes) lasts 30 to 60 seconds. The injection causes skin vessels to vasodilate, and warm systemic blood rises to the skin surface, returning again as the heat fades.
   (c) Nausea, vomiting, headaches, and cough are side-effects that some patients may experience.

Patient Aftercare
1. Bed rest is maintained for 2 to 12 hours after the test. Time limits are based on the exact procedure used, the physician's desires, and patient status.
2. Check vital signs and dressing for swelling or bleeding. Some discomfort at the puncture site can be expected.
3. Antibiotics may be administered before or after the examination to prevent infection.
4. Encourage fluids after testing.
5. Keep the affected extremity extended (not elevated) and immobilized with a sandbag to decrease discomfort and bleeding, and apply ice to the site, if ordered. Analgesics, if ordered, can be administered for pain at insertion sites.
6. Sutures, if used, are removed in 7 days.

Clinical Alert

1. This procedure is contraindicated in patients with gross cardiomegaly.
2. Complications that can occur include
   (a) Arrhythmias

(b) Allergic dye reactions (evidenced by urticaria, pruritus, and conjunctivitis)
(c) Thrombophlebitis of cutdown vein
(d) Infection at cutdown site
(e) Pneumothorax
(f) Hemopericardium
(g) Embolism
(h) Tears in liver, especially in infants and children (results from poor technique)
3. Notify attending physician if there is any increased bleeding or a drastic fall or increase in blood pressure.
4. When angiography is performed, the following equipment should always be available for complications:
(a) Resuscitation equip-   (e) Cardiac drugs (epineph-
    ment   rine, norepinephrine,
(b) DC fibrillator   isoproterenol)
(c) External pacemaker
(d) Electrocardiographic
    monitor
5. Diabetics who need insulin will usually get half the early dose (because an IV is running) prior to cardiac catheterization and electrophysiology studies.

Electrophysiology Procedure
(EP; His Bundle Procedure)

Normal Values
Normal conduction intervals
Normal refractory periods
Normal recovery times
No arrhythmias induced

Explanation of Test
An electrophysiology procedure (EP) is an invasive test used in the diagnosis and treatment of ventricular arrhythmias; it is very similar to cardiac catheterization. The difference lies in the fact that an EP study measures the electrical conduction system of the heart through solid electrode catheters instead of the open-lumen catheters used to measure pressures. The electrode catheters are almost always inserted into veins because of the greater risk in the arterial system. Using fluoroscopy as a guide, the catheters are advanced into the right atrium and the right ventricle. Besides an x-ray monitor that shows the loca-

tion of the catheter, there is also a physiological monitor that shows the patient's surface ECG leads as well as intracardiac electrograms from the catheters.

An EP study is highly useful in diagnosing diseases of the heart's conduction system and to point the direction toward optimal treatment. Besides measuring control resting values for the patient, the electrode catheters are also used to pace the heart in an attempt to induce any arrhythmia that may be giving the patient problems. If the patient is on medication such as quinidine, procainamide, lidocaine or phenytoin to control arrhythmia, the EP study can determine how well the medication is working by how easily the arrhythmia can be induced. This is in contrast to the trial and error method in which there is no way to know that a particular drug is ineffective until that drug has failed.

An EP procedure is indicated for patients with disorders of impulse formation (supraventricular versus ventricular rhythms). EP studies are also used to provide diagnostic insight into the etiology and mechanism of conduction disorders (AV block, bypass tracts). EP studies are often used as a work-up for syncope or sick sinus syndrome. Finally, EP studies are indicated in testing the effectiveness of an antiarrhythmic drug.

Procedure

1. The test is usually done in a darkened room.
2. To decrease fear of the procedure, the patient is continuously told what is being done.
3. The patient lies on an x-ray table; ECG leads are attached to the chest.
4. The procedure is done under sterile conditions. The skin is prepared with an antiseptic solution. Usually one or two sites are chosen (right and/or left antecubital area, right and/or left groin). The sites chosen depend on where in the heart the catheters will have to be placed and also upon the patency and size of the patient's veins. A local anesthetic is injected into the skin before a needle is inserted into the vein. (An incision is usually not needed.) The catheters are gently pushed into the heart.
5. Baseline values are recorded. Some baseline values require pacing. (For example: sinus node recovery times require pacing the atrium until the sinus is fatigued and then measuring the time it takes to recover.)
6. After baseline values have been determined, pacing is used to induce arrhythmias that may have been giving the patient problems. If a sustained arrhythmia is induced, an attempt will usually be made to capture the heart by pacing to terminate the arrhythmia. If the patient's cardiovascular system cannot compensate for the ar-

rhythmia so that the patient starts to lose consciousness, an external defibrillator will be used to terminate the arrhythmia.
7. A quiet conversation is continuously held with the patient in order to assess his level of consciousness.
8. After the procedure, the catheters are removed and a sterile pressure bandage is applied (no stitches).
9. The procedure takes a minimum of one hour for a repeat study of drug effectiveness to a maximum of four hours to evaluate a complex arrhythmia such as the pre-excitation syndromes. Each drug has certain effects that must be anticipated during the loading phase—for example, hypotension with quinidine and procainamide and abdominal cramping with quinidine, and pain in vein used for phenytoin as well as a state of "happy drunkeness." IV saline is used to support blood pressure.

Clinical Implications
Abnormal results of an EP procedure will reveal
1. Conduction intervals that are longer or shorter than normal.
2. Refractory periods that are longer than normal.
3. Recovery times that are prolonged.
4. The induction of an arrhythmia that would not have been induced in a normal subject with an identical protocol.

Abnormal results are indicative of:

1. Long AH intervals indicate disease in the AV node if sympathetic and vagal influences have been eliminated.
2. Long HV intervals indicate disease in the His–Purkinje's system.
3. Prolonged sinus node recovery times indicate sinus node dysfunction, such as sick sinus syndrome.
4. Prolonged sinoatrial conduction times can indicate sinus exit block.
5. A wide or split His bundle deflection indicates that a His bundle lesion is present.
6. The induction of sustained ventricular tachycardia by using one or two premature stimuli confirms the diagnosis of recurrent ventricular tachycardia.

Patient Preparation
1. Explain the purpose and procedure of the test. A description of possible sensations that may be experienced, even more than procedural steps, will help to reduce anxiety. The patient should be aware that he might experience certain sensations that are common to the procedure.
   (a) A peculiar sensation in the arm and neck as the catheter is advanced. The sensation feels like a "bug crawling."
   (b) Palpitations or heart racing may be felt when the heart is paced.
   (c) Lightheadedness or dizziness may be experienced. This is not a

common sensation to be ignored. The patient must tell the nurse or doctor any time he feels lightheaded or dizzy.
2. Obtain a legal, signed permit before the procedure. The patient needs to know the reason for the study: that there is a high degree of suspicion that he may be susceptible to a dangerous tachycardia. Patients who are not in full agreement that this method is the best approach to the patient's problem should not be tested. Be certain that the patient has been informed of the major risks and benefits of the study.
3. Blood samples for potassium level (and drug levels if the effectiveness of a drug is to be determined) are drawn.
4. A standard 12-lead EKG should be taken before the test.
5. Usually, a bland meal is eaten the evening before the procedure, but nothing can be consumed for at least three hours before testing.
6. Analgesics, sedatives, or tranquilizers are not usually given before the procedure, but *nothing* can be consumed for at least three hours before testing.
7. Have the patient void before going to the EP laboratory.
8. Allow the patient to wear dentures.

Patient Aftercare
1. Bedrest with no leg bending is maintained for 6 to 8 hours after the procedure.
2. Check vital signs and the insertion site for swelling or bleeding, q. 15 min × 4, 30 min × 2 and q. 1 h × 2.
3. Keep the affected extremity extended (not elevated) to decrease discomfort and bleeding. Analgesics, if ordered, can be administered for pain at the insertion site.
4. Keep the head of bed elevated less than 45 degrees for 6 hours.
5. Encourage side-to-side turning.
6. Infection control. If an electrode catheter is left in place for sequential studies, it is sutured in place and covered with a sterile dressing. Scrub the site and length of the catheter with a povidone-iodine solution, dry with sterile sponges, and recover with a sterile dressing.

Clinical Alert

1. Contraindications: although the unstable clinical setting of acute myocardial infarction may limit detailed and prolonged EP procedures, brief but clinical useful procedures can be safely performed.
2. Observe the patient for complications that can occur, which include

(a) Hemorrhage, particularly from the femoral site when the femoral artery has been punctured.
(b) Thromboembolism. Thrombosis at the puncture site or thromboembolism from the catheter.
(c) Phlebitis
(d) Hemopericardium
(e) Atrial fibrillation, usually transient
(f) Ventricular fibrillation
3. Notify the attending physician if there is any bleeding, fall in blood pressure, or life-threatening arrhythmia. Be aware of drug studies carried out and monitor for effects of that pharmaceutical.
4. If the series of tests is successful, reinforce to the patient that, with compliance to prolonged drug therapy, there should be no recurrence of tachycardia.
5. When an adverse reaction to a drug is found, ECG monitoring is the major requirement for the elimination time of the drug.

Stress/Exercise Testing (Graded Exercise Tolerance Test)

Normal Values
Negative when patient has no significant symptoms, arrhythmias, or other ECG abnormalities and when patient reaches 85% of maximum heart rate predicted for age and sex.

Explanation of Test
This test measures the efficiency of the heart during a dynamic exercise stress period on a motor driven treadmill or ergometer. It is valuable in diagnosing ischemic heart disease and in investigating physiologic mechanisms underlying cardiac symptoms such as angina, arrhythmias, inordinate blood pressure rise, and functional valve incompetence. Exercise testing is also done to measure functional capacity for work, sport, or participation in a rehabilitation program, and to estimate response to medical or surgical treatment.

The systolic blood pressure normally increases with exercise, and the diastolic normally remains essentially unchanged. Stress exercise testing takes place in a controlled environment that requires a low temperature (68°) and low humidity.

Procedure
There are many different types of stress tests in use today. Most of them include the following steps:

1. Recording electrodes are placed on patient's chest (see description of ECG) and attached to a monitor. A blood pressure recording device is also used.
2. While the patient walks on a motor-driven treadmill, a computerized ECG and heart monitoring device records the performance. The patient walks at progressive speeds and elevations in an effort to increase heart rate and workload.
3. ECG, heart rate, and blood pressure are recorded at rest. The patient is asked to report any symptoms such as chest pain or shortness of breath that are experienced during the test. Normal persons are symptom free at submaximal efforts. At peak or maximal efforts, symptoms expected in normal persons are exhaustion, fatigue, and sometimes nausea or dizziness.
4. The patient is stressed in stages. Each stage consists of a predetermined level of the treadmill (in miles per hour) and an elevation of the treadmill (in percent grade).
5. ECG, heart rate, and blood pressure are constantly monitored for any signs of abnormality and any unusual symptoms such as intolerable dyspnea, chest pain, and severe cramping (claudication) in the legs.
6. Usually, a 3-minute and 10-minute recovery stage are recorded while the patient is seated. The test is terminated if there are ECG abnormalities, fatigue, weakness, abnormal blood pressure changes, or intolerable symptoms.
7. Commonly used criteria for stopping a test include attainment of
   (a) Maximum possible performance
   (b) End point based on emergence of signs or symptoms indicative of a disease process
   (c) Predetermined end point such as 85% of age-related maximal heart rate, arbitrary work load (one that raises heart rate to 150), or diagnostic ECG change
8. Total examination time is about 30 minutes; however, the patient should plan to be in the laboratory for 1 to 1½ hours.

Clinical Implications
Abnormal responses to exercise testing include

1. Alterations in blood pressure such as
   (a) Failure of systolic pressure to rise
   (b) Progressive fall in systolic pressure
2. Alterations in heart rate such as
   (a) Excessive tachycardia
   (b) Bradycardia
3. Changes in ECG such as
   (a) Ischemic deviation of ST segments; can be depression or elevation

(b) Dysrhythmia, ventricular tachycardia, multifocal ventricular premature contractions, atrial tachycardia, atrioventricular block greater than first degree

4. Ectopic rhythms, either ventricular or supraventricular, must be considered abnormal responses but not necessarily ischemic responses.

5. Ischemic ST segment displacement >0.1 mm. of 80 msec. duration or longer is the most common abnormality found. Men aged 40 to 59 who develop ST depression during exercise that is not present at rest have five times the risk of developing overt coronary heart disease as do men who do not develop ST depression.

6. Unusual symptoms such as
   (a) Anginal pain
   (b) Inappropriate breathlessness
   (c) Faintness, dizziness, light-headedness, confusion
   (d) Claudication, leg pain

7. Unusual signs such as
   (a) Cyanosis, pallor, mottling of skin
   (b) Cold sweat, piloerection
   (c) Ataxia, glassy stare
   (d) Gallop heart sounds
   (e) Valvular regurgitative murmur
   (f) Abnormal cardiac impulse

Interfering Factors

Common causes of false-positive exercise ECG responses include

1. Syndrome X in women
2. Left ventricular hypertrophy
3. Digitalis
4. ST segment abnormality at rest
5. Hypertension
6. Valvular heart disease
7. Left bundle branch block
8. Anemia
9. Hypoxia
10. Vasoregulatory asthenia
11. Lown–Ganong–Levine syndrome
12. Pletus excavatum

Patient Preparation

1. Explain the purpose and procedure of the test. No food, coffee, or cigarettes are allowed prior to testing. Water is allowed.

2. A legal consent form must be signed.

3. Have the patient wear flat walking shoes or tennis shoes; bedroom slippers are not suitable. Men should wear gym shorts or loose-fitting light trousers. Women should wear a bra, a short-sleeved blouse that buttons in front, and slacks, shorts, or pajama pants (no one-piece undergarments or panty hose).

4. Some medications should be discontinued before testing. Beta-adrenergic blocking agents such as propranolol should be reduced or tapered gradually before stopping. Check with the laboratory for specific protocols for digoxin, isordil, and other drugs.

Patient Aftercare
The patient should not leave the premises until the physician is satisfied what pretest baseline levels of heart rate, blood pressure, and ECG wave form have been met.

Clinical Alert

Stress/exercise testing can be risky for patients with chest pain of recent onset or attacks of angina several times a day. The test is usually not given to these patients at this time, but it may be rescheduled in 4 to 6 weeks.

Noninvasive Tests of the Peripheral and Cerebral Vascular Systems

Noninvasive diagnostic techniques provide objective physiologic information about blood flow for the detection and localization of peripheral arterial, venous, and extracranial cerebrovascular diseases. A combination of examinations is used to localize obstruction, assess collateral circulation, and determine a need for angiography. The results of these tests provide complementary and additional data that are used to confirm diagnoses, to predict therapeutic results, to monitor therapy, and to follow the progression of peripheral vascular disease. These tests are usually done before invasive diagnostic procedures in the determination of hemodynamically significant vascular disease. It is important to keep in mind that reports and values of noninvasive vascular studies must be correlated with history and physical examination. Tests are not meant to replace these assessments. Because there are many modalities available for testing with laboratories across the country having different machines and methods, it is necessary that the caregiver become familiar with the user-testing laboratory policies and its reports. Tests are performed by highly trained vascular technologists.

Indications for testing for evaluation and medicolegal documentation can be divided into use in arterial, venous, and cerebrovascular disease.

Blood flow studies can be grouped into three main categories: tests for arterial disease, tests for venous disease, and tests for cerebrovascular disease. See Tables 15-2, 15-3, and 15-4. The major testing methods incorporate Doppler and plethysmographic instruments, duplex scanner, and spectral analyzer (see Table 15-5).

Table 15-2
Noninvasive Tests To Detect Peripheral Artery Disease

Test	Normal or Expected Values
Arterial Doppler examination of lower extremities; ankle site	Multiphasic signal with prominent systolic component and one or more diastolic sounds
Pressures with Doppler blood flow detection = ankle–arm index or ankle–brachial (AB) index, and Segmental limb pressures	Ankle pressure equal to or greater than arm pressure. Proximal thigh pressure of 20–60 mmHg or more above arm pressure. Less than 20–30 mmHg pressure gradient between adjacent levels of measurement in leg. Arm segmentals-forearm pressures equal to or higher than that of brachial pressure/20 mmHg.
Duplex scannings and spectral analysis	No stenosis based on spectral analysis of wave and no plaque
Plethysmography	Pulse wave form shows a steep upslope, narrow peak, dicrotic wave on downslope concave toward baseline
Pulse volume recordings (PVR)	Normal sympathetic vasoconstrictive reflex with attenuation of pulse amplitude in response to deep breath indicative of intact sympathetic vasomotor innervation

1. *Arterial Disease*
   (a) Arteriosclerosis
   (b) Symptoms of arterial insufficiency and digital ischemia
   (c) Diabetic foot ischemia differentiated from neuropathy
   (d) Reynaud's phenomenon and disease
   (e) Documentation of arterial reconstruction results
   (f) Healing potential for skin lesions and amputation sites
   (g) Acute embolic phenomena
   (h) Thoracic outlet syndrome
   (i) Trauma to vascular system
   (j) Vasculogenic impotences
   (k) Evaluation of iatrogenic arterial injury
   (l) Symptoms due to spinal, arthritic, or muscular disorders, that may mimic arterial disease

2. *Venous Disease*
   (a) Acute deep vein thrombosis

Table 15-3

Noninvasive Tests To Detect Peripheral Venous Disease

Test	Normal or Expected Values
Venous Doppler examination is used primarily to rule out presence of deep venous thrombosis. Doppler flow is evaluated at posterior tibial, popliteal, superficial femoral, and common femoral veins to detect presence of lower extremity deep venous thrombosis, or at the radial, brachial, axillary and subclavian veins, to rule out upper extremity deep venous thrombosis.	Doppler flow should be spontaneous and phasic with respiration in the presence of patient veins. Augmentation of flow velocity with limb compression maneuvers Competent valves Signals that fluctuate with respiration, not heartbeats
Plethysmographic studies: Venous outflow plethysmography; Determination of venous outflow using SPG, IPG, or air (PVR).	Maximal venous capacitance to maximal venous outflow is plotted on a graph.
Phleborrheography (PRG): Determination of venous responses in thigh, calf, and foot to respiration, foot compression, and calf compression. An air-filled cuff transducer is applied to chest to record respiration.	Limb volume fluctuates in phase with respiration No significant increase in limb volume in response to foot or calf compression Decrease in foot volume in response to calf compression
Toe and finger pressures	Normal toe pressure of at least 80% of ankle pressure or greater; finger pressure usually 80% of wrist pressure or greater
Treadmill exercise to assess collateral circulation and functional impairment with or without ECG monitor. Measure ankle pressure with a Doppler before and after treadmill exercise.	No drop in ankle pressure, exercise test normal
Reactive hyperemia test: ankle pressure before and after 3-minute application of proximal thigh tourniquet	Ankle pressure after cuff release falls no more than 35% below preischemia value and returns to baseline within 1 minute.
Venous reflux plethysmography: To identify incompetent valves in either deep or superficial venous systems and to determine refilling time of calf veins after exercise or manual compressions. An SPG is placed around each calf on a seated patient. Test may also be repeated with rubber tourniquets below knees to prevent reflux in incompetent superficial veins. A photoplethysmography transducer (PPG) may also be used to record skin blood content response to leg exercise.	Normal reflux. No valvular incompetence. Calf volume decreases by at least 1% during exercise and returns to baseline in 10–30 seconds. Recovery time not significantly affected by tourniquets

Table 15-4
Noninvasive Carotid Tests of Extracranial Cerebrovascular Disease

Test	Normal or Expected Values
Carotid periorbital indirect Doppler exam: determination of flow at branches of internal carotid artery; frontal or supraorbital artery evaluated by applying compression at branches of the external carotid	Normal antegrade flow out of periorbital artery branches of ophthalmic artery; unaffected by compression
Supraorbital photoplethysmography: determination of supraorbital pulse from terminal branches of ophthalmic artery, branches of external carotid artery, and common carotid arteries.	Normal supraorbital pulse amplitude not significantly affected by compression of external carotid branches; affected only by compression of ipsilateral common carotid artery.
Oculoplethysmography: ocular pulse delay methods	Eye-to-eye pulse delay of less than 10 msec
Oculopneumoplethysmography	Ocular systolic pressures: Special criteria applies for normal/abnormal reports
Carotid phonoangiography (CPA): identification of carotid bruits differentiates bruits from subclavian arteries, common carotid, and carotid bifurcation.	No bruits recorded
Carotid direct neck exam with Doppler: determination of blood flow from each common, external, and internal carotid artery using a directional Doppler probe	External carotid artery signal multiphasic and similar to other peripheral arteries
	Internal carotid acting signal has high-pitched flow velocity in both systole and diastole. Common carotid artery signal has intermediate characteristics between the internal and external carotid signals.
	A normal image similar to oblique view on contrast arteriogram of carotid artery bifurcation with no occlusion or calcification
Duplex of scan of carotid arteries shows plaque or absence of plaque. Spectral analysis shows stenosis of artery.	Normal arteries pulsate, nonturbulent arterial blood flow. Absence of plaque and no stenosis
Optional carotic evaluation is a combination of a direct and indirect exam.	

Table 15-5
Basic Noninvasive Testing Methods and
Application in Vascular Disease

Instrument Used	Applications
1. *Doppler:* ultrasound blood flow detector sensitive to frequency shift reflected from moving blood cells	In *peripheral arterial diseases:* to obtain waveforms and segmental pressures. To monitor pressures before and after treadmill. In *Extracranial cerebrovascular disease* (carotid): to obtain periorbital flow direction. In *Venous disease:* to obtain venous flow signals to detect patency and competence of deep system and superficial veins
2. *Plethysmography:* record of volume dimensional changes of a finger, toe, arm, leg, eye, or other part of the body. Various transducers are used such as impedence, air, water, and photoelectric (PPG)	In *Peripheral artery disease:* using digital plethysmography and pulse volume recorder (PVR), to obtain digital blood pressure and limb blood flow. In *Extracranial cerebrovascular disease:* using oculopneumoplethysmographic (air-filled OPG), oculoplethysmography (fluid filled OPG). In *Venous disease with tests:* to obtain venous outflow with strain gauge (SPG) or impedence (IPG), venous volume changes using a PRG, and venous reflux using SPG or photoelectric.
3. *Duplex scanning:* used with Doppler to give anatomic and physiologic data with image and spectral analyzer processes. Doppler arterial blood flow electrical signals into frequency of components and power spectrum for study. In addition to the spectral analyzer, Fast Fourier Transform analysis (FFT) is a frequency spectrum of Doppler signal displayed on a screen for real-time study.	Used for study of any system: artery, vein or carotids, to detect vessel wave abnormalities associated with ulcerative plaque, to evaluate patency of grafts, and determine outcome of other reconstructive surgery. It is valuable in the follow-up management of peripheral vascular disease.

(b) Postphlebotic syndrome
(c) Superficial thrombophlebitis
(d) Primary differentiated from secondary varicose veins
(e) Incompetent perforator
(f) Screening for source of emboli in pulmonary embolism

3. *Cerebrovascular Disease*
   (a) Extracranial occlusive disease with asymptomatic carotid bruits
   (b) Amaurosis fugax (total blackout of vision in one eye)
   (c) Transient ischemic attacks (TIA)
   (d) Upper extremity pulse deficits
   (e) CVA
   (f) Carotid screening in high risk stroke-prone patients, diabetics, hypertensives, and those with cardiac disease
   (g) Reversible neurologic ischemia defint (RIND); lasts longer than TIA
   (h) Vertebral basilar insufficiency

Clinical Responsibilities for Peripheral Arterial Blood Flow Studies

Patient Preparation

1. Explain the purpose, method of testing, and benefits of the tests and that there are no known risks. Emphasize that the examinations are painless.
2. Help the patient to relax. A relaxed patient is required for these tests. A tense and nervous patient will provide inaccurate readings.
3. If the patient is in pain, the pain should be controlled before the patient is sent for the test.
4. Explain that studies must be performed at rest for baselines.
5. Because nicotine constricts vessels, no smoking is permitted two hours prior to testing. Emphasize that all patients with arterial disease should discontinue smoking.

Clinical Alert

1. No tests can be performed on a cold, cyanotic, or waxen extremity because there may not be an available blood flow.
2. Notify the technologist if the patient is in isolation. If the patient is too ill to stay in the laboratory, notify the examining department. These tests can be done at bedside if necessary.
3. Diabetics develop a medial artery disease that reduces elasticity of vessels and eventually prohibits compression of these vessels.
4. Clinical implications of ankle brachial AB index.
   (a) The highest ankle pressure is divided by the highest arm pressure to obtain the index.

(b) In persons with an ischemia or AB index of .30 or less, caregivers must be careful to protect the foot because breakdown can occur very rapidly. This patient must have pain medication administered promptly and is usually in too much pain to do self-care. Most of these patients cannot tolerate any leg elevation, and most can hardly bear to stay in bed at night.

Normal ankle pressures are the same or higher than the arm pressure. As peripheral resistance (arterial obstruction) increases, ankle pressures decrease with peripheral vascular disease. Different levels of ischemia cause different symptoms and the symptoms vary even from patient to patient. Diabetes complicates the peripheral vascular problem; in such persons, the ankle pressures are not always indicative of the severity of the problem.

0.96 and above—normal	No significant peripheral vascular occlusion in the legs at rest. If there is leg pain, other causes must be found.
0.85–0.95	Mild ischemia, usually mild or no symptoms. Claudication after walking distances.
0.51–0.84	Moderate ischemia. Persons usually contact health-care system because of symptoms of leg cramping on walking (claudication). Trophic skin changes become clinically evident.
0.26–0.50	Severe ischemia. Increased claudication, decreased walk distance. May experience rest pain with dependent rubor, as the values numbers decrease into the .30 category.
0.25 and below	Gangrene or ischemic ulcers often present. Limb salvage. Patient will need bypass or amputation depending on other test results.

Clinical Responsibilities for Peripheral Venous Blood Flow Studies

Patient Preparation
1. Explain the purpose, method, benefits, and risks (no known) of the test.

2. Stress that no pain is involved in testing and no needles or catheters are inserted.
3. Use measures to promote relaxation. Tenseness will result in inaccurate outcome.
4. Pain should be controlled before the patient goes to the testing department.

Clinical Alert

1. Notify the testing laboratory if the patient is in isolation.
2. Test can be done at bedside if assessment reveals the patient is too ill to transport.
3. Cold extremity and vasoconstriction inhibits examination.

Clinical Responsibilities for Carotid Extracranial Cerebrovascular Blood Flow Studies

Patient Preparation

1. Explain the purpose of the test and that assessment of cerebral blood flow is based on an indirect evaluation of carotid artery blood flow. There are no known risks, except that in oculoplethysmography (OPG) there is a 3% risk of conjunctival hemorrhagic irritation. Inform the patient that tests are painless.
2. Assess the range of motion. The patient must be able to be on his back.
3. Help the patient to relax. A nervous patient may provide inaccurate results.
4. A complete eye examination is done before the OPG examination. No OPG examination is done for lens implants, systolic BP over 200, allergies to local anesthetic, detached retina and eye surgery, or infection.

Clinical Alert

1. Some persons are not candidates for direct neck carotid study due to abnormal neck size (too large) and abnormal anatomy.
2. Notify the testing laboratory if the patient is isolated.
3. Clinical implications of abnormal, spectral value, and duplex score:

(a) 1%–15% reduction in diameter may or may not be
     16%–49% reduction in diameter hemodynamically
                                     significant
(b) 50%–75% reduction in diameter: moderate stenosis
(c) >75% reduction in diameter: high grade stenosis
(d) Significance of abnormal values depends on whether the
    patient shows symptoms. For example, if a person has no
    symptoms, but with evidence of stenosis, it is not clini-
    cally significant. However, evidence of plaque in a person
    who has symptoms can be very serious.

Tests of Eye Function

Fluorescein Angiography (FA)

Normal Values

Normal retinal vessels, normal retina, normal choroidal circulation as
seen in color photographs.

Explanation of Test

The purpose of this test is to detect vascular disorders of the retina that
may be the cause of poor vision. Fluorescein, a contrast substance, is
injected intravenously over a 3-minute time period. Films of the eye
taken by a special camera are studied to detect the presence of retinal
disorders.

Procedure

1. A series of three drops is given at 5-minute intervals to dilate the
   pupil of the eye.
   (a) Complete dilatation occurs within 30 minutes of giving the last
       drop.
   (b) When dilatation is complete, a series of color photographs of
       both eyes is taken.
2. The patient sits with the head immobilized in a special frame in
   front of a fundus camera and indirect ophthalmoscope.
3. Fluorescein dye is slowly injected intravenously; the brachial vein
   is the site usually chosen.
4. Another series of photographs is taken as the dye flows through the
   retinal blood vessels (a period of approximately 3 minutes).
5. A final series of photographs is taken 15 to 60 minutes after the
   injection.

Clinical Implications

Abnormal results reveal

1. Diabetic retinopathy
2. Aneurysm
3. Hemorrhagic macular degeneration
4. Diabetic neovascularization

Patient Preparation

1. Determine whether the patient has any known allergies to medications or contrast substance.
2. Instruct the patient about the purpose, procedure, and side-effects of the test. A legal consent form must be signed.
3. Some persons experience nausea for a short period after the injection.
4. Inform the patient that eye drops may sting or cause a burning sensation as they are instilled.
5. Advise the patient that pre-examination films are often taken to familiarize him with bright lights, necessity of fixation, and other aspects of the procedure.

Patient Aftercare

1. Educate the patient about color changes in the skin (yellow) and urine (bright yellow or green) that may be apparent for 36 to 48 hours after the test.
2. Advise the patient to wear dark glasses and not to drive while his pupils remain dilated (4–8 hours). During this time, persons are unable to focus on nearby objects and react abnormally to changes in light intensity.

Electro-oculography (EOG)

Normal Values

2

1.80–2 is probably normal; values vary with laboratory methods used; bright light will cause the ratio to be larger.

Explanation of Test

This test of retinal function is used in the study of suspected hereditary and acquired degeneration of the retina. As a measurement of retinal function, the test serves primarily to complement electroretinography (ERG) by determining the functional state of retinal pigment epithelium, as in retinitis pigmentosa. This test determines the electrical potential of the eye at rest in both darkness and light. Normally, the potential between the front and back of the eye should grow as light is increased.

Clinical Implications
1. A value of 1.60 to 1.79 is probably abnormal; 1.20 to 1.59 is definitely abnormal; less than 1.20 is flat, based on normal values reported above. The outcome is usually reported as normal or abnormal.
2. The EOG ratio decreases in most retinal degeneration such as retinitis pigmentosa; this sometimes parallels the decrease on the electroretinography (ERG) examination.
3. In Best's disease (congenital macular degeneration), the EOG is abnormal, but the ERG is normal.
4. In retinopathy due to toxins such as antimalarial drugs, the EOG may show abnormalities earlier than the ERG.
5. Supernormal EOGs have been noted in albinism and aniridia in which the common factor seems to be chronic excessive light exposure with resultant retinal damage.

Procedure
1. The patient sits in the examining chair.
2. Skin electrodes are placed in the inner and outer canthi of the eye, and an instrument similar to a bowl is used for adaptation. The results are recorded on a polygraph unit.
3. Two procedures are carried out. First, the patient is tested for 15 minutes in total darkness, and eye movement through a known angle is measured. Second, with the integrating sphere lighted, the patient is asked to move the eyes through the same angle, and the electrical potential is recorded.
4. Total examining time is 30 minutes.

Patient Preparation
1. Explain the purpose and procedure of the test.
2. No discomfort will be experienced.

Patient Aftercare
No special aftercare is needed.

Clinical Alert

If FA and EOG are both ordered, the EOG must be done first because the eye must be dilated for the FA but not for the EOG. However, when an ERG and an FA are performed on the same day, the FA should be done first to avoid corneal edema caused by the corneal electrode used in ERGs. The waiting time between FA and ERG should be at least 2 hours.

Electroretinography (ERG)

Normal Values
Normal A and B waves

Explanation of Test
This test is used in the study of hereditary and acquired disorders of the retina including partial and total color blindness (achromatopia), night blindness, retinal degeneration, and detachment of the retina in cases where the ophthalmoscopic view of the retina is prohibited by some opacity, such as vitreous hemorrhage, cataracts, or corneal opacity. When these disorders exclusively involve either the rod systems or the cone systems to a significant degree, the ERG shows corresponding abnormalities.

In this test, an electrode is placed on the eye to obtain the electrical response to light. When the eye is stimulated with a flash of light, the electrode will record electric change that can be displayed and recorded on an oscilloscope. This test is indicated when surgery is considered in cases of questionable retinal viability.

Clinical Implications
1. Changes in ERG are associated with
   (a) Diminished response in ischemic vascular disease
      (1) Arteriosclerosis
      (2) Giant cell arteritis
   (b) Siderosis (poisoning of the retina when copper is imbedded intraocularly). This is not associated with stainless steel foreign bodies.
   (c) Drugs such as chloroquine or quinine that produce retinal damage (decreased ERG response).
   (d) Retinal detachment
   (e) Opacities of ocular media
   (f) Decreased response
      (1) Vitamin A deficiency
      (2) Mucopolysaccharidosis
2. Diseases of the macula do not affect the standard ERG. Macular disorder can be detected using a focal ERG.

Procedure
1. Eyes are propped open during the procedure.
2. The patient may be sitting up or lying down.
3. Topical anesthetic eye drops are instilled.
4. Bipolar cotton wick electrodes saturated with saline rest on the cornea.
5. Two states of light adaptation are used to detect rod and cone disorders along with different wavelengths of light to separate rod

and cone function. Normally, the more intense the light, the greater the electrical response.

   (a) Room light

   (b) Room darkened for 20 minutes, then a white light is flashed

   (c) Bright flash (in cases of trauma when there is vitreous hemorrhage, a much more intense flash of light must be used)

6. In infants and small children who are being tested for a congenital abnormality, chloral hydrate or a general anesthetic may be used.

7. Total examining time is 1 hour.

Patient Preparation

1. Explain the purpose and procedure of the test.

2. No discomfort is experienced; the electrode may feel like an eyelash in the eye.

Patient Aftercare

1. Caution the patient not to rub his eyes for 1 hour after testing to prevent accidental corneal abrasion.

2. Usually, anesthetic effects disappear in about 20 minutes.

Electromyography, Electromyoneurogram (EMG)

Normal Values

1. Normal nerve conduction

2. Normal muscle action potential

   (a) On insertion

   (b) At rest

   (c) During minimum voluntary muscle contraction

   (d) During maximum voluntary muscle contraction

Explanation of Test

Electromyoneurography is the combined use of electromyography and electroneurography. These studies, done to detect neuromuscular abnormalities, measure nerve conduction and electrical properties of skeletal muscles. These tests, along with evaluation of range of motion, motor power, sensory defects, and reflexes, can differentiate between neuropathy and myopathy. The electromyogram is useful in defining the site and cause of muscle disorders such as myasthenia, muscular dystrophy, and myotonia as well as lesions involving the motor neurons in the anterior horn of the spinal cord. Electromyogram is helpful in localizing the site of peripheral nerve disorders such as radiculopathy and axonopathy. Skin and needle electrodes are used to measure and record electrical activity. Sound equivalents of electrical activity are heard over a loudspeaker and recorded. The tape can be played later and restudied as often as necessary.

Procedure
1. The test is done in a copper-lined room to screen out interference.
2. The patient lies and/or sits during the test.
3. A surface disk is applied to ground the patient. The muscles and nerves the examiner checks are dependent on the patient's signs and symptoms, history, and physical condition (certain nerves innervate specific muscles).
4. Instructions are given to relax (the examiner may massage certain muscles to get the patient to relax) and to contract certain muscles (*e.g.*, to point toes, when directed).
5. The test consists of two parts. The first test is done to determine *nerve conduction*.
   (a) The metal surface electrodes are coated with electrode paste and firmly fixed over the body part that is being tested. Electrodes may be taped to the involved areas. The metal electrode is placed over a specific nerve area and electrical current is passed through the patient. This will cause sensations directly proportional to the time involved.
   (b) The amplitude wave is read on an oscilloscope.
   (c) Electrical current leaves no mark but can cause an unusual and surprising sensation, not usually considered unpleasant. Measurement can be made of how fast and how well a nerve transmits messages. Nerves in the face, arms, or legs may be tested in this way.
6. The second test is done to determine *muscle potential*.
   (a) A monopolar electrode (½-in.–3 in. very fine needle) is inserted and a pricking sensation may be felt as the needle pierces the skin. The needle is advanced into the muscle by increments. The examiner may move the needle around without removing it to see if readings change, or he may reinsert the needle in another muscle area.
   (b) The electrode causes no pain unless the end of the needle is near a terminal nerve; then it can cause considerable pain. Ten or more insertions may be made. No shocks are given because the needle detects the electricity normally present in muscle.
   (c) The examiner watches the oscilloscope for a normal wave and listens to a loudspeaker for a normal quiet sound at rest. A "machine-gun" popping sound or rattling sound like hail on a tin roof is normally heard when the patient is asked to contract the muscles.
   (d) If the patient complains of pain, the examiner removes the needle because pain yields false results.
   (e) Total examining time is 45 to 60 minutes if testing is confined to a single extremity, and up to three hours for more than one

extremity. There is no completely "routine" EMG. The length of the test depends on the clinical problem.

Clinical Implications

Abnormal results are indicative of muscle or nerve disorders. Any spontaneous, involuntary electrical activity that occurs while the muscle is in a resting state, together with abnormal waveforms, is indicative of neuromuscular abnormality. Abnormal conduction velocity rates and terminal latency or slowing are associated with nerve disorders.

1. Diseases or disturbance of striated muscle fibers or cell membrane.
   (a) Muscle fiber disorder such as muscular dystrophy
   (b) Cell membrane hyperirritability such as myotonia and myotic disorders such as polymyositis, hypocalcemia, thyrotaxicosis, tetanus, and rabies
   (c) Myasthenia
      (1) Myasthenia gravis
      (2) Cancer due to nonpituitary ACTH secretion by tumor
         (a.) Bronchial cancer   (b.) Sarcoid
      (3) Deficiencies
         (a.) Familial hypokalemia   (b.) McArdle's phosphorylase
      (4) Hyperadrenocorticism
      (5) Acetylcholene blockers
         (a.) Curare   (c.) Kanamycin
         (b.) Botulism   (d.) Snake venom
2. Disorders or diseases of lower motor neuron.
   (a) Lesion involving motor neuron on anterior horn of spinal cord (myelopathy)
      (1) Tumor   (6) Anterior poliomyelitis
      (2) Trauma   (7) Amyotrophic lateral
      (3) Syringomyelia   sclerosis
      (4) Juvenile muscular dys-   (8) Peroneal muscular atro-
          trophy   phy
      (5) Congenital amyotonia
   (b) Lesion involving nerve root (radiculopathy)
      (1) Guillain-Barré
      (2) Entrapment
         (a.) Tumor   (d.) Hypertrophic spurs
         (b.) Trauma   (e.) Spinal stenosis
         (c.) Herniated disk
   (c) Damage or disease to peripheral or axial nerve
      (1) Entrapment
         (a.) Carpal and tarsal tunnel

(b.) Facial, ulnar, radial, and peroneal palsy
(c.) Meralgia paresthetica
(2) Endocrine
(a.) Hypothyroidism   (b.) Diabetes
(3) Toxic
(a.) Heavy metals   (d.) Chemotherapy
(b.) Solvents   (e.) Antibiotics
(c.) Antiamebicides
(d) Early peripheral nerve degeneration and regeneration

Interfering Factors

1. Conduction can vary with age; conduction is normally decreased in the elderly.
2. Pain can yield false results.
3. Electrical activity from extraneous persons and objects can yield false results.
4. The test is ineffective in the presence of edema, hemorrhage, or thick subcutaneous fat.

Patient Preparation

1. Explain the purpose and procedure of the test. There is a risk of hematoma if the patient is on anticoagulant therapy.
2. Sedation or analgesia may be ordered.

Patient Aftercare

1. If the patient has experienced pain or is in pain, provide relief.
2. Provide restful, relaxing activities. The patient may be exhausted if the examination time is lengthy.

Clinical Alert

1. When ordering the test, provide the examiner with all available pertinent information. The more data given, the more precise will be the interpretation of findings.
2. Enzyme levels that reflect muscle activity (AST, LDH, CPK) must be determined before testing because EMG will cause misleading elevation of these enzymes for up to 10 days.
3. Although it is rare, hematomas may form at needle insertion sites. Notify the physician if this occurs.

Electronystagmogram (ENG)

Normal Values
Normal vestibular-ocular reflex
Nystagmus accompanying head turning is expected

Explanation of Test
This study aids in the differential diagnoses of lesions in the brainstem and cerebellum, unilateral hearing loss of unknown origin, and helps identify the cause of vertigo or ringing in the ears. Evaluation of the vestibular system and muscles controlling eye movement is based on measurements of the nystagmus cycle. In health, the vestibular system maintains visual fixation during head movements through *nystagmus*, the involuntary back and forth eye movement caused by the initiation of the vestibular-ocular reflex.

Procedure
1. The test is usually done in a darkened room, with the patient sitting or lying on an examination table.
2. If there is wax in the ears, it should be removed prior to testing.
3. Five electrodes are taped to the face in locations around the eye.
4. During the study, the patient is asked to look at different objects, open and close the eyes, and to change position.
5. Near the end of the test, air is gently blown into the external ear canal, first on the affected side. Water may also be used to irrigate the ears during the test.
6. Total examining time is one hour.

Clinical Implications
Prolonged nystagmus following a head turn is abnormal and can be caused by lesions of the vestibular or ocular system.
1. Cerebellum disease
2. Brain stem lesion
3. Peripheral lesion occurring in the elderly, head trauma, and middle ear disorders
4. Congenital disorders

Interfering Factors
1. Test results are altered by an inability of the patient to cooperate, by poor eyesight, blinking of the eyes, and poorly applied electrodes.
2. Anxiety of the patient and some medications such as CNS depressants and stimulants and antivertigo agents can be the cause of false-positive test results.

Patient Preparation

1. Explain the purpose and procedure of the test. There is no discomfort or shock associated with the recording. There are no known risks.
2. No face makeup should be applied prior to testing.
3. Advise that no heavy meal should be eaten before the test and all caffeine and alcoholic beverages should be avoided for at least 48 hours before the test.
4. In most cases, medications such as tranquilizers, stimulants, or antidizziness medications are withheld for 5 days. However, a withholding check should be discussed with the attending physician.

Clinical Alert

1. The test is contraindicated in persons with pacemakers.
2. Water irrigation should not be done in persons who have perforated eardrums. However, a fingercot may be inserted into the ear canal to protect the middle ear.

Patient Aftercare

1. Allow the patient to rest comfortably for an hour before returning to his home or hospital room.
2. Nausea, vertigo, and weakness may be present for some time after the test is completed.

Body Fat Distribution

Normal Values

Normal waist-to-hip fat distribution ratio (WHR)
Approximate ratios indicate that waist size is a percentage of hip girth.
   The ratio will be higher in men.

Explanation of Test

This study, used in estimating the distribution of a person's body fat and/or adipose tissue, is helpful in the management and understanding of obesity. It is a good marker for determining if further diabetes testing should be done in women and a predictor of ischemic heart disease in both women and men. Excess body fat accumulation is one of the most important medical and public health problems of our time.

There are a number of methods used to estimate body fat: skin impedance and skin folds measure the amount of body fat; CT scan measures the amount of body fat and can also evaluate its distribution;

and waist–hip ratio (WHR) gives information about body fat distribution but not directly about the amount of fat.

Procedure
The patient stands while measurements are taken to determine minimum waist circumference and maximum hip circumference. The waist is divided by the hip for the mathematical ratio.

Clinical Implications
1. Increasing WHR is associated with a greater prevalence of diabetes, gout, and atherosclerosis.
2. A high ratio of waist- to hip-circumference is associated with a high proportion of intra-abdominal fat and with elevated triglycerides, glucose, insulin concentrations, and insulin resistance.
3. Women with upper-body fat concentration have large abdominal fat cells and have a significantly greater chance of undiagnosed diabetes than women whose excess fat is located below the waist. Lower-body obese women have increased numbers of normal size thigh cells and are at low risk of having diabetes. It is believed that upper-body obese women may have a relatively high male-to-female hormone ratio.
4. Although upper-body obese men have a greater risk of health disorders, it is generally believed that they are more likely to have an easier time losing weight. It seems that lower-body obese women have a harder time losing weight.

Patient Preparation
Explain the purpose and procedure of the test. There are no risks.

BIBLIOGRAPHY

Basmajiar JV: Muscles Alive, Their Functions Revealed by Electromyography, 4th ed. Baltimore, Williams & Wilkins, 1978

Bernstein EF (ed): Noninvasive Diagnostic Techniques in Vascular Disease. St. Louis, CV Mosby, 1985

Bjorntorp P: Morphological classifications of obesity. Int J Obes 8:525–533, 1984

Dubin D: Rapid Interpretation of EKGs. Tampa, FL, C.O.V.E.R. Co., 1974

ECG. Rapid ECG Interpretation Patient Care Flow Charts. Danen, CT, Roche, Miller & Fink Corp, 1974

Ellestad MH: Stress Testing Principles and Practice, 2nd ed. Philadelphia, FA Davis, 1980

Gallen IR (ed): Symposium on noninvasive cardiac diagnosis. I. Med-Clin North Am 64:1–146, 1980

Garrow JS: Indices of adiposity. Rev Clin Nutr 53(8):697–706. John Wiley & Sons, 1980

Grossman W (ed): Cardiac Catheterization and Angiography, 2nd ed. Philadelphia, Lea & Febiger, 1980

Hatle L, Angelson B: Doppler Ultrasound in Cardiology: Physical Principles and Applications. Philadelphia, Lea & Febiger, 1982

Johnson EW (ed): Practical Electromyography, 4th ed. Baltimore, Williams & Wilkins, 1980

Jones NL, Campbell EJ: Clinical Exercise Testing, 2nd ed. Philadelphia, WB Saunders, 1982

Niedermeyer E, Lopes da Silva F (eds): Electroencephalography: Basic Principles, Clinical Applications and Related Fields. Baltimore, Urban and Schwarzenberg, 1982

Race GJ (section ed): Laboratory Methods/Diagnostic Procedures. Vol. 2 of Spittell JA, Jr (ed): Practice of Medicine. Hagerstown, Harper & Row, 1978

Raines J, Traad E: Noninvasive evaluation of peripheral vascular disease. Med Clin North Am 64(2):283–304, 1980

Shahrokhi F, Chiappi K, Young R: Pattern shift visual evoked responses. Arch Neurol 35(2):65–71, 1978

Spiegel MB: Electromyoneurography. AFP 119–130, 18 November 1978

Squires N, Donchin E, Squires K, et al: Biosensory stimulation: Inferring decision-related processes from the P300 component. J Exp Psychol (Hum Percept) (3):299–315, 1977

Stoner EK: Electromyography and nerve conduction studies. In Spittell, JA, Jr (ed): Practice of Medicine, Vol. 2. Hagerstown, Harper & Row, 1978

Teasley D: Don't let cardiac catheterization strike fear in your patient's heart. Nursing 12(3):52–56, 1982

Weisberg J: Doppler today. Appl Radiol Nuclear Med 9(1):100–109, 1980

PRENATAL DIAGNOSIS AND TESTS OF FETAL WELL-BEING

Introduction

Tests in this chapter are used to monitor changes in the status of the maternal-fetal unit, to identify the fetus at risk for intrauterine asphyxia and, in the early diagnosis of infection, to identify genetic and biochemical disorders, together with all major anomalies.

The fetal biophysical profile is often referred to in the literature. This profile is a collection of information about fetal tone, movements, measurements, and amniotic fluid volume, based on real-time ultrasound (see Chapter 13) and the nonstress test. Tests done to predict normal fetal outcome and to identify the fetus at risk for asphyxia during labor are outlined in Table 16-1.

Hormonal Testing

Normally, all steroid hormones increase in amount as pregnancy progresses. Serial testing is done to monitor a particular hormone over a period of time for a continuing rise in level. The significance of decreasing values indicates that the maternal-placental-fetal unit is not functioning well. The mother is not adversely affected by a decrease in steroids because the hormone level already exceeds her nonpregnant level. For the infant it is different. The infant is maintained in a closed environment, and can be quite susceptible to maternal system adjustments. Biochemical analyses of several hormones are used to monitor changes in the status of the maternal-fetal unit. (See Chapters 3 and 6.)

1. In early pregnancy, human chorionic gonadotropin (HCG) provides evidence of a viable pregnancy.
2. HCG, along with prolactin and the luteinizing hormone (LH), prolongs the life of the corpus luteum once the ovum is fertilized. HCG stimulates the ovary for 6 to 8 weeks of pregnancy, prior to the placental synthesis of progesterone. Its function later in pregnancy is unknown.
3. Late in pregnancy, estriol and human placental lactogen (HPL) reflect fetal homeostasis.

HPL is a protein hormone produced by the placenta. HPL testing only evaluates placental functioning. Blood testing of the mother usually begins after the 30th week and may be done weekly thereafter. A level of 1 mcg./ml. may be detected by 6 to 8 weeks of gestation. HPL slowly increases throughout pregnancy, reaching a level of 7 mcg./ml. at term, and dropping abruptly to zero after delivery. A value of 4 mcg./ml. after 30 weeks of gestation is an indication of probable fetal distress. However, falsely high values are common. Low HPL values indicate the

Table 16-1
Tests Done To Predict Normal Fetal Outcome and Identify Fetus at Risk for Intrauterine Asphyxia

Name of Test & Normal Values	Reason for Performing Test
Breast Stimulation Test (BST) Normal Values: Reactive; negative Implies that placental support is adequate and that the fetus is probably able to tolerate the stress of labor should it begin within a week. There should be a low risk of intrauterine death due to hypoxia.	After 26 weeks' gestation, the nipples are stimulated to release oxytocin that causes uterine contractions similar to labor contractions.
Oxytoxic Challenge Test (OCT) Normal Values: Reactive; negative Implies placental reserve is sufficient should labor begin within one week	Intravenous oxytocin is administered to produce three (3) good quality contractions of at least 45 seconds each in 10 minutes, and the FHR is monitored for reaction to this stress. It is performed when a nonstress test is nonreactive or a BST is either positive or unsatisfactory.
Acoustic Stimulation Normal Values: Reactive	Using an electronic fetal monitor and sound source on the maternal abdomen, an evaluation of fetal movement in response to stimulation is done.
Nonstress Test Normal Values: Reactive; at least two (2) episodes of fetal movement associated with a rise in FHR Provides a baseline status and implies an intact CNS and autonomic N-S that are not being affected by intrauterine hypoxia	It determines fetus' ability to respond to environment by an increase in FHR associated with movement where not under the stress of labor.

need for further assessment with nonstress testing, and amniocentesis to corroborate results.

Fetoscopy

Explanation

Fetoscopy is a technique for observing the fetus directly and obtaining a sample of fetal blood or skin. Fetoscopy permits direct visualization of the fetus in 2 to 4 cm. segments so that developmental defects can be identified. A fetal blood sample permits the diagnosis of disorders such as hemophilia A and B that are not presentable by other means.

Procedure
1. Real-time ultrasound locates the area through which to insert a cannula and trocar transabdominally into the uterus.
2. Following insertion, an endoscope (fetoscope), consisting of a fiberoptic light source and self-focusing lens, is inserted into the desired part of the fetus for viewing and sampling.
3. Skin biopsies and blood samples may be obtained.

Clinical Alert
1. There is an increased risk of spontaneous abortions (5% to 10%) and of preterm delivery (10%).
2. It is offered only to those women who have a significant risk of producing a child with a birth defect that can be diagnosed only by fetoscopy.

Chorionic Villus Sampling (CVS)

Chorionic villus sampling (CVS) is a procedure done between 8 and 12 weeks of pregnancy for early fetal diagnosis of genetic and biochemical disorders.

A sample of villi is obtained by suction via a catheter placed through a speculum in the vagina, using ultrasound as a guide. The catheter is inserted into the cervix and uterine cavity, into the area within the villi of the chorion frondosum. A sample of tissue is obtained from several chorionic villi by suction aspiration. Fetal in origin, chorionic villi are a source of fetal genetic information because these cells reflect the chromosome analysis, enzyme determination, and DNA analysis of the fetus. It is not as safe, reliable, and accurate as amniocentesis.

AMNIOTIC FLUID STUDIES

Introduction

The origin of amniotic fluid is not completely understood, but it is believed to be primarily a product of fetal pulmonary secretions, urine, and metabolic products from the intestinal tract.

Initially, amniotic fluid is produced from the cells of the amniotic membrane, but later, most of it is derived from the maternal blood. The volume increases from about 30 ml. at 2 weeks' gestation to 350 ml. at 20 weeks' gestation. After 20 weeks, the volume ranges from 500 ml. to 1000 ml. There is constant change in the amniotic fluid as a result of fluid movement in both directions through the placental membrane. Later in pregnancy, the fetus contributes to the volume of amniotic fluid by excretion of urine, and, by swallowing amniotic fluid, the fetus absorbs up to 400 ml. every 24 hours through its gastrointestinal tract and bloodstream and by the umbilical arteries exchanged across the placenta. Some fluid probably is also absorbed in direct contact with the fetal surface of the placenta. Amniotic fluid contains cast-off cells from the fetus and resembles extracellular fluid in which undissolved material is suspended. Amniotic fluid is slightly alkaline and contains albumin, urea, uric acid, creatinine, lecithin, sphingomyelin, bilirubin, fat, fructose, epithelial cells, leukocytic enzymes, and lanugo hair.

Amniotic Fluid Analysis
When amniocentesis is advised early in pregnancy (15 to 18 weeks), it is for the purpose of studying the genetic makeup of the fetus, and determining developmental abnormalities. Fetal cells are separated from the amniotic fluid by centrifugation and placed in tissue culture medium so that they can be grown and harvested for subsequent karyotyping to identify chromosome disorders. Testing in the third trimester is for the purpose of determining fetal age and well-being, studying blood groups, or detecting amnionitis.

Amniocentesis

Explanation of Test
Amniotic fluid for analysis is aspirated using a needle inserted through the abdominal and uterine walls into the amniotic sac. This method of prenatal diagnosis is preferably performed after the 15th week. By this time, the amniotic fluid level has expanded to 150 ml. to supply an adequate specimen of 10 ml. It also appears to be the best time, based on uterine size and number of viable cells. If a determination of fetal maturity is to be made, it should be done after the 35th week of gestation.

Amniocentesis gives high-risk couples the opportunity to have healthy children, provided the parents are willing to terminate pregnancy in the event an abnormal fetus is detected. The test is used in the evaluation of hematologic disorders, fetal infections, inborn errors of metabolism, and in the determination of fetal sex for the purpose of diagnosing sex-linked disorders. It is *not* used to determine sex simply out of curiosity.

Identification of chromosomal abnormalities and neural tube defects such as anencephaly, encephalocele, spina bifida, and myelomeningocele can be done as well as the estimation of fetal age, well-being, and pulmonary maturity.

High-Risk Parents Who Should Be Offered Prenatal Diagnosis

1. Women of advanced maternal age (35 or over). 90% fall in this category; at risk for children with chromosome abnormality, especially trisomy 21 (at age 35 to 40, the risk for Down's is 1% to 3%; at age 40 to 45, there is a 4% to 12% risk; and over age 45, the risk is 12% or greater.
2. Women who have previously borne a trisomic child, or clients who previously had a child with any kind of chromosome abnormality.
3. Parents of previous child with spina bifida or anencephaly or family history of neural tube disorders.
4. Couples in which either parent is a known carrier of a balanced translocation chromosome for Down syndrome.
5. Couples, of which both partners are carriers for a diagnosable metabolic or structural autosomal recessive disorder. Presently, over 70 inherited metabolic disorders can be diagnosed by amniotic fluid analysis.
6. Couples, of which either partner or a previous child is affected with a diagnosable metabolic or structural dominant disorder.
7. Women who are presumed carriers of a serious x-linked disorder.
8. Couples and families whose medical history reveals mental retardation, ambiguous genitalia, parental exposure to environmental agents (drugs, irradiation, infections).
9. Couples and families whose medical history reveals multiple miscarriage or stillbirths, infertility.
10. Anxiety about potential offspring.

Clinical Implications

1. Elevated level of alpha-fetoprotein is an indicator of possible neural tube defects.
2. Creatinine levels are reduced in prematurity.
3. Increased and decreased total volume of amniotic fluid is associated with certain developmental arrests.
4. Increased bilirubin levels are associated with impending fetal death.
5. Color changes of fluid are associated with fetal distress and other disorders.
6. Sickle cell anemia and thalassemia can be detected by examination of fibroblast DNA obtained by amniocentesis.

7. X-linked disorders are not routinely diagnosable *in utero*. However, because they affect only males, the sex of the fetus may be determined in a woman who is a carrier of a deleterious x-linked gene, as in hemophilia or Duchenne's muscular dystrophy. In these cases, if desired, a male fetus may be aborted.

8. Cystic fibrosis.

9. The presence of some of the over 100 detectable metabolic disorders. Examples of these are Tay–Sachs disease, Lesch–Nyhan syndrome, Hunter syndrome, Hurler syndrome, and various hemoglobinopathies. Hereditary metabolic disorders are caused by the absence of an enzyme due to a gene deletion, the alteration of an enzyme structure due to a gene mutation, or a mutation of the gene that regulates the synthesis of the enzyme. If the enzyme in question is expressed in amniotic fluid cells, it can be used potentially for prenatal diagnosis. An unaffected fetus would have normal levels of the enzyme, a clinically normal "carrier" of the mutant gene defect would have approximately half the enzyme level, and an *affected* fetus would have very small amounts or no enzyme levels.

10. For disorders in which an abnormal protein is not expressed in amniotic fluid cells, other test procedures are necessary, such as *DNA restriction endonuclease analysis.*

Interfering Factors

1. Fetal blood contamination can cause false-positive levels of alphafetoprotein.

2. False-negative and false-positive errors in karyotyping occur.

3. Polyhydramnios may falsely lower bilirubin values by dilution.

4. Hemolysis of specimen can alter test results.

5. Oligohydramnios may increase falsely some values in amniotic fluid analysis, especially bilirubin, which can lead to error in predicting the clinical state of the fetus.

Procedure (In Combination with Ultrasound)

1. The patient is asked to lie on her back with arms behind her head to prevent touching the abdomen and the sterile field during the procedure.

2. The position of the fetus is determined by palpation and should always be combined with real time ultrasound to locate the placenta, various fetal parts, and to establish that there is only one fetus present.

3. The skin is thoroughly cleansed with antiseptic solution such as Betadine. Sterile drapes are placed around the puncture site. A local anesthetic is injected slowly under the skin and then into the subcutaneous tissues.

4. A 3½-inch spinal needle (20–22 gauge) with stylet is inserted through the abdominal wall into the amniotic sac. The fetus and

placenta are avoided. If the fetus moves, the needle may have to be withdrawn and reinserted.

5. After the stylet is removed, a syringe is attached to the needle so that a 20 ml. to 30 ml. specimen can be obtained.

6. An adhesive bandage is placed over the puncture site when aspiration is completed.

7. The specimen is placed in a sterile brown or foil-covered silicone container that protects fluid from light and prevents breakdown of bilirubin. The container is labeled with the patient's name, date, and expected date of delivery or estimated weeks of gestation.

8. Amniotic fluid should be delivered to the laboratory immediately.

9. The actual procedure time is about 20 minutes. However, the laboratory work for genetic diagnoses takes at least 2 weeks and perhaps as long as 4 weeks to complete. Specimens done for fetal age, such as creatinine, take 1 to 2 hours; L/S and phosphotidyl glycerol take 3 to 4 hours; Gram stain to rule out infection takes ½ hour, and cultures take 24 to 48 hours.

10. The procedure may have to be repeated if no amniotic fluid is obtained or if there is failure of cell growth or negative culture.

11. Record the type of procedure done, date, time, name of physician performing the test, mother-fetal response, and disposition of specimen.

Patient Preparation

1. Genetic counseling that is elective, not mandatory, should include a discussion of the risk of having a genetically defective infant, risk of a positive test result, and problems (depression and guilt) resulting from a selective abortion. The father should be present for the counseling and be a partner in the decision-making process. In genetic counseling, persons must not be coerced into undergoing abortion or sterilization; this should be an individual choice.

2. Explain the purpose, procedure, and risks of the test.

3. A legal consent form must be signed by the patient and her husband.

4. Instruct the patient to void just before the test so that the bladder will be empty.

5. Obtain baseline data on maternal blood pressure, pulse, respiration and fetal heart rate. Monitor natal signs for 15 minutes.

6. The patient should be made aware of short-lived feelings of nausea, vertigo, and mild cramps that may occur during the procedure.

7. Help the patient to relax.

Patient Aftercare

1. Check blood pressure, pulse, respiration, and fetal heart tone every 15 minutes for the first half hour after completion of the test. Palpate the fundus to assess fetal and uterine activity.

2. Have the patient rest on her left side to counteract supine hypotension and to increase venous return and cardiac output.
3. Instruct the patient to notify her physician if she experiences amniotic fluid loss, signs of onset of labor, abdominal pain, bleeding, elevated temperature, chills, unusual fetal activity, or lack of movement.

Clinical Alert

1. Fetal loss is less than 0.5%. Repeat amniocentesis is necessary in 0.1 of all amnios.
2. Fetal complications include
   (a) Spontaneous abortion as a possible consequence of test
   (b) Injury to fetus (fetal puncture)
   (c) Hemorrhage
   (d) Infection
   (e) Rh sensitization if fetal blood enters mother's circulation
3. Maternal complications include
   (a) Hemorrhage
   (b) Hematomas
4. This test is contraindicated in women with a history of premature labor or incompetent cervix and in the presence of *placenta previa* and *abruptio placentae*. If the amniotic fluid is bloody (blood is usually of maternal source), and if a significant number of fetal cells (Kleibauer Betke smear) are present in an Rh-negative mother, the use of human anti-D globulin (RhoGAM) should be considered. Some doctors prefer to administer RhoGAM to all Rh-negative mothers following amniocentesis, provided they are not already sensitized at that time.
5. Families should be counseled that prenatal diagnoses based on amniotic fluid assay are not infallible, and that sometimes results may not reflect the true fetal status. Amniocentesis cannot guarantee a normal child. It can only determine the presence or absence of specific disorders and within the limits of laboratory error. Some conditions cannot be determined by this method; for example, nonspecific mental retardation, cleft lip and palate, and PKU.
6. Excellent results from amniocentesis are possible only if these safety factors are established.
   (a) Gestation of 15 weeks or greater
   (b) Ultrasound monitoring to locate suitable pools of amniotic fluid, to outline the placenta, to exclude the presence

of multiple pregnancy, and to estimate maturity accurately. This is necessary for the correct interpretation of alpha₁-fetoprotein (AFP) levels in amniotic fluid and in maternal blood.

   (c) Excellent amniocentesis technique
   (d) Needle gauge of 20 or 21
   (e) Not more than 2 needle insertions for one tap
   (f) Anti-D immunoglobulin for Rh-negative women
7. The level of accuracy is 99.8% for cytogenetic analysis.
8. The technique has been developed to allow for successful amniocentesis in triplet pregnancy.

Alpha₁-Fetoprotein (AFP)

Normal Values
Vary considerably depending on age of fetus and laboratory method. A peak is reached at 13 to 15 gestational weeks at 30 to 43 μg./ml.; at 40 weeks, the value is 0.8 μg./ml.

Background
Alpha₁-fetoprotein (AFP) is synthesized by the embryonic liver and is the major protein (glycoprotein) in fetal serum. It resembles albumin in molecular weight, amino acid sequence, and immunologic characteristics. It is not detectable in normal persons after birth. Normally, a fetoprotein is a substance found in high levels in a developing fetus and in low levels in maternal serum and amniotic fluid.

Explanation of Test
This prenatal measurement of AFP in the amniotic fluid is used to diagnose neural tube defects (malformation of the central nervous system). In pregnancies in which the fetus has a neural-tube defect, fetoprotein leaks into the amniotic fluid, causing elevated levels. Causes of neural tube defect are not known, but a genetic component is assumed because there is an increased risk of recurrence. Neural-tube defects are usually polygenic (multifactional) traits. In cases of anencephaly and open spina bifida, both maternal blood and amniotic fluid AFP levels are abnormal by the 18th week of gestation. In addition, measurement of AFP has been used as an indicator of fetal distress when it can be increased in both amniotic fluid and maternal serum. However, confirmation must come from further studies.

Total Volume **859**

Clinical Implications
Increased levels are associated with

1. Neural-tube defects such as anencephaly (100% reliable), encephalocele, spina bifida, and myelomeningocele (90% reliable).
2. Congenital Finnish nephrosis
3. Omphalocele
4. Turner syndrome with cystic hydromas
5. Obstructions of the gastrointestinal tract
6. Missed abortion
7. Fetal distress
8. Imminent or actual fetal death
9. Severe Rh immunization
10. Esophageal and duodenal atresia

Interfering Factors
1. Fetal blood contamination will cause increased levels.
2. Increased levels are associated with multiple pregnancies.
3. Some false positives (0.1 to 0.2%) are associated with fetal death, twins, or anomalies. Sometimes no explanation is available.

Clinical Alert
1. Any couple delivered of a child with a neural-tube defect should be offered antenatal detection in future pregnancies. If one parent has spina bifida, the pregnancy should be monitored.
2. Cases of elevated AFP must be confirmed with high-resolution ultrasound.

Total Volume

Normal Values
Corrected level of amniotic fluid equals measured level of specific substance times actual volume divided by average volume.

Average volumes are approximately 350 ml. at 15 weeks, 450 ml. at 20 weeks, 750 ml. at 25 weeks, 1500 ml. at 30 and 35 weeks; volume then decreases to 1250 ml. at term.

Explanation of Test
Measurement of the total volume of amniotic fluid is helpful in estimating the changes in total amounts of certain imported substances that circulate in the amniotic fluid such as bilirubin pigment, creatinine, and surface-active agents. Knowledge of total volume is important because marked changes in amniotic fluid can decrease the predictive

value of serial concentration measurements of specific substances. This measurement is most important ,when the results of testing do not agree with the clinical picture.

Procedure
In the laboratory, a sample of amniotic fluid is studied using a solution of para-aminohippuric acid (PAH) for absorbency and dilution to calculate probable amniotic fluid volume in milliliters.

Clinical Implications
1. Increased amniotic fluid, over 2000 ml. (polyhydramnios), is suggested by a total intrauterine volume greater than standard deviations above the mean for a given gestational age. It is estimated that 18% to 20% of fetuses with polyhydramnios will have congenital anomalies. Esophageal atresia and anencephaly are the two most common anomalies. The remainder of fetuses will have involvement secondary to Rh disease, diabetes, and unknown causes. Polyhydramnios is also associated with multiple births (*e.g.*, twins).
2. Oligohydramnios (reduction in the amount of amniotic fluid to under 300 ml.) is suggested by a total intrauterine volume value of two standard deviations below the mean that is seen before the 25th week of gestation. A disturbance of kidney function due to renal agenesis or kidney atresia may cause oligohydramnios. After this time, premature rupture of membranes, intrauterine growth retardation, and post-term pregnancies are suspected causes of decreased amniotic fluid levels.

Clinical Alert

If either polyhydramnios or oligohydramnios is suspected, the fetus should be screened with ultrasound to detect the presence of structural anomalies.

Creatinine

Normal Values
1.5–2 mg./dl. or greater indicates fetal maturity. Laboratory dependent.

Background
Creatinine, a byproduct of muscle metabolism in amniotic fluid, is a reflection of increased fetal muscle mass and the ability of the mature

(glomerular filtrating system) kidney to excrete creatinine into the amniotic fluid. Amniotic creatinine increases progressively as pregnancy advances. The mother's blood creatinine should be known before the amniotic fluid creatinine value is interpreted.

Explanation of Test
Measurement of this substance is used as an indicator of fetal physical maturity and correlates reasonably well with pulmonary maturity. As pregnancy progresses, creatinine levels increase. A value of 2 mg./dl. is accepted as an indication that pregnancy is 37 weeks or more. However, the use of this value alone to assess maturity is not advisable for several reasons. A high creatinine value may be a reflection of muscle mass in a fetus and does not necessarily indicate kidney maturity. For example, a macrosomatic fetus of a diabetic mother may have high creatinine levels due to increased muscle mass. In addition, a small, growth-retarded infant of a hypertensive mother may have low creatinine levels due to decreased muscle mass. Creatinine levels can be misleading if used without other data. As long as maternal blood creatinine is not elevated, measurement of amniotic creatinine has a certain degree of reliability when used in conjunction with other maturity studies.

Procedure
1. A 0.5 ml. specimen of amniotic fluid is needed for this measurement.
2. Protect the specimen from direct light.

Clinical Implications
1. Decreased values are associated with prematurity and small, growth-retarded infants of hypertensive mothers, due to decreased muscle mass.
2. Creatinine levels lower than expected may be due to the following:
    (a) gestation less advanced   (c) fetal kidney abnormalities
    (b) fetus smaller than normal

Interfering Factors
There is a 5% false-positive rate

Lecithin/Sphingomyelin Ratio
(L/S) (Surfactant Components)

Normal Values
Ratio of 2 : 1 or greater indicates pulmonary maturity, and 1 : 2 dilution on shake test indicates lung maturity.

Background

Lecithin and sphingomyelin have detergent gravity. These substances, produced by lung tissue, stabilize the neonatal alveoli and prevent their collapse on expiration and consequential atelectasis. Lecithin in amniotic fluid will be less than sphingomyelin until 26 weeks; at 30 to 32 weeks, the two lipids are about equal. At about 35 weeks, the amount of lecithin rises abruptly, but the sphingomyelin stays constant or decreases slightly.

Explanation of Test

The relationship of the phospholipids and surface-active agents, lecithin and sphingomyelin, is used as an index of fetal lung maturity. If early delivery is indicated due to conditions such as diabetes, premature rupture of membranes, maternal hypertension, placental insufficiency, or erythroblastosis, a measurement of the L/S ratio can be used to determine a mature fetal lung that might be expected to function properly at birth. Unfortunately, early delivery may be necessary for fetal welfare, but the result may be prematurity, pulmonary immaturity, and perinatal mortality. A measurement of the L/S ratio should also be performed on all repeat cesarean sections before the time of delivery to determine when fetal lungs are mature.

Clinical Implications

1. Decreased levels are often associated with pulmonary immaturity and respiratory distress syndrome (RDS).
2. An L/S ratio greater than 2 : 1 signifies fetal lung maturity, and the occurrence of RDS is extremely unlikely.
3. An L/S ratio of 1.5 to 1.9 : 1 indicates possible mild or moderate RDS.
4. An L/S ratio of 1 to 1.49 : 1 indicates immaturity of the fetal lungs with moderate to severe RDS.
5. An L/S ratio of less than 1 indicates severe RDS.

Clinical Alert

1. If the L/S ratio is less than 1.2 : 1, it is preferable to delay induced delivery until the lung has become more mature.
2. The maturation of the fetal lung appears to be regulated by a number of hormonal factors, some stimulatory and some possibly inhibitory. For this reason, hormones such as celestone will be given in 12 mg. dosages for two doses and administered 12 to 18 hours apart in combination with other therapy in instances of premature labor.
3. Under certain conditions of acute and chronic stress, premature maturation of fetal lungs may be seen. Conditions in

which one may see accelerated maturation of the lungs include

(a) Premature rupture of the membranes. (Prolonged rupture of the membranes after 72 hours has an acute effect on lung maturation.)

(b) Acute placental infarction

(c) Placental insufficiency

(d) Chronic *abruptio placentae*

(e) Renal hypertensive disease due to degenerative forms of diabetes.

(f) Cardiovascular hypertensive disease in clients with history of drug abuse

(g) Severe pregnancy-induced hypertension

This accelerated maturation of the fetal lungs is thought to be a protective mechanism for preterm fetus if delivery actually does occur.

4. Delayed maturation of fetal lungs may be seen in

(a) Infants born to mothers with class A, B, and C diabetes

(b) Infants born to mothers with nonhypertensive glomerulonephritis.

(c) Hydrops fetalis

In these instances, no higher L/S ratio (3 : 1) may be necessary to ensure adequate lung maturity.

5. A lung profile of amniotic fluid to evaluate lung maturity looks for not only lecithin but also for two other phospholipids—PG or phosphatidylglycerol or PI or phosphatidylinositol. PI increases in the amniotic fluid after 26 to 30 weeks, peaks at 35 to 36 weeks, and then decreases gradually. PG appears after 35 weeks, and continues to increase until term. Results are classified as positive PG or negative PG. The lung profile is a useful adjunct to evaluating L/S ratio. It appears that lung maturity can be confirmed in most pregnancies, if the PG is present in conjunction with an L/S ratio of 2 : 1. The PG may provide stability that makes the infant less susceptable to respiratory distress syndrome when experiencing hypoglycemia, hypoxia, or hypothermia. More research is being done on using PI in the same manner as the PG. The PG measurement is especially useful in borderline cases and in class A, B, and C diabetes where pulmonary maturation is delayed.

Interfering Factors

1. High false-negative rates
2. Unpredictability or borderline values

3. Unpredictability of contaminated blood specimens
4. Occasional false-positive values associated with conditions such as Rh diseases, diabetes, and severe birth asphyxia

Shake Test

The shake test is a qualitative measurement of the amount of pulmonary surfactant contained in the amniotic fluid. It is quick and inexpensive. It is a bedside test of lung maturity and, in an obstetrical emergency, an immediate decision can be made about delivery. The advantage of this functional test over the L/S ratio is that it can be performed easily by a physician, technician, or nurse, and results are highly reliable. The test is based on the ability of the surfactant in the amniotic fluid to form a complete ring of bubbles on the surface of the fluid in the presence of 95% ethanol. Exact amounts of 95% ethanol, isotonic saline, and amniotic fluid are shaken together for 15 seconds. The L/S ratio is normally not done when the shake test is positive because the shake test also indicates fetal maturity. A dilutionable table is available from which determinations can be made of various stages of lung maturity. There is a high false-negative, but a low false-positive rate.

Foam Stability Index (FSI)

The foam stability is similar to the shake test. In this test, 0.5 ml. of amniotic fluid is added to various amounts of 95% ethanol. The sample is shaken and observed for foam, which indicates maturity. This test seems as reliable as the L/S ratio in normal pregnancy, and seems to have a lower false-positive rate than the shake test.

Fern Test

Normal Values
Positive test for amniotic fluid

Background
Fern production is the result of activity of electrolytes in the cervical glands under the control of estrogen. Close to term, amniotic fluid will show a typical fern pattern in the laboratory that is similar to that seen in cervical mucus, indicating a predominantly estrogen effect; urine will not produce any kind of fern pattern.

Explanation of Test
This study differentiates urine from amniotic fluid. It is done to determine whether the fluid passed by a woman is urine, or to test for prematurely ruptured membranes.

Procedure
1. A vaginal examination using a sterile speculum is done.
2. Only a few drops of fluid on a slide are necessary.

Clinical Implications
1. A positive test shows a fern pattern that is indicative of amniotic fluid.
2. A negative test shows no ferning or crystallization, indicating little or no estrogen effect.
3. If the specimen is urine, no fern pattern is seen.

Interfering Factors
Blood in the specimen inhibits fern formation.

Clinical Alert

Urine can also be differentiated from amniotic fluid when it is tested for the presence of urea and potassium. However, urine samples are usually detected by lack of alpha-fetoprotein (AFP) and by odor and appearance.

Color of Amniotic Fluid

Normal Values
Colorless or pale straw color

Explanation
Amniotic fluid specimens may vary in color from no color to a pale straw color. White particles of vernix caseosa from the skin of the fetus may be present, as well as lanugo hair. The color of the amniotic fluid changes in the presence of certain disorders such as missed abortion, chromosomally abnormal fetus, and fetus with anencephaly.

Procedure
Every specimen should be inspected for color change from normal.

Clinical Implications
1. Yellow is indicative of blood incompatibility and the presence of bile pigment released from red blood cell hemolysis.
2. Dark yellow aspirate indicates probable fetal involvement.

3. Red color indicates contamination with blood. In this instance, a determination must be made in the laboratory whether the source of the blood is from the mother or fetus. If the origin is from the fetus, a danger exists.
4. Green opaque fluid indicates contamination with meconium. Meconium is passed as a result of hyperperistalsis in response to a stressor that can be of a transient, one-time nature or of a more serious nature, such as hypoxia. A very good correlation is that the more meconium present, the more severe and immediate the stress. Additional assessments, such as amnioscopy and amniography, must be made to determine if the fetus is suffering ongoing episodes of hypoxia. Green color can also be suggestive of erythroblastosis but is not indicative of it.
5. Yellow-brown opaque fluid may indicate intrauterine death, although not necessarily from erythroblastosis.

Clinical Alert

1. Before the amniotic membranes have ruptured, color change and staining can be observed by amnioscopy. During this procedure, an amnioscope is placed in the vagina and against the fetal presenting port. The amniotic fluid is visualized through the amniotic membranes. Problems with amnioscopy include inadvertent rupturing of membranes, insufficient dilatation of the cervix and difficulty in inserting the amnioscope, intrauterine infection, and occasional difficulty in interpreting the color of the amniotic fluid. The test may also be difficult to perform if a patient is in active labor.
2. Meconium staining may also be observed when an amniocentesis is done. After the membranes have ruptured, meconium staining may be observed in the drainage from the vagina. Once meconium staining is identified, more assessments (such as fetal heart rate patterns) must be made before delivery is contemplated, to determine if the fetus is suffering ongoing episodes of hypoxia.
3. The presence of meconium in the amniotic fluid is normal in breech presentations.

Bilirubin Optical Density (ΔOD)

Normal Values
ΔOD of 0.02 or less is indicative of maturity
<0.28 mg./dl. or a 1+ is normal or possibly slightly affected

Background
Bilirubin is a pigment that is acquired by the amniotic fluid during its circulation through the gastrointestinal tract. It is not excreted by the mother as is fetal serum bilirubin. Bilirubin may be found in amniotic fluid as early as the 12th week of pregnancy, and it reaches its highest concentration between 16 and 30 weeks of pregnancy. As the pregnancy continues, the amount of bilirubin progressively decreases, finally disappearing near term. Bilirubin is known to be increased in the amniotic fluid of erythroblastotic fetuses and fetuses with anencephaly and intestinal obstruction.

Explanation of Test
This measurement is used to monitor the condition of a fetus in a Rh_o-negative pregnant woman who has a rising anti-Rh_o antibody titer. A rising titer is synonymous with Rh erythroblastosis fetalis or hemolytic disease of the newborn (HDN). This determination is usually not made before 20 to 24 weeks because no therapy is available to the fetus before that time. Close to term, the concentration of bilirubin pigment in the amniotic fluid will normally decrease in the absence of Rh sensitization.

Optical density is a laboratory method of measuring bilirubin and is reported as the deviation (Δ) or difference between the expected and plotted curves at 450 nm. on a spectrophotometer. Optical density levels can be interpreted by realizing that a value of 0.1 ΔOD (deviation of optical density) corrected will correspond to approximately 0.14 mg./dl. of bilirubin. The degree of hemolytic disease falls into three zones in testing.

1. If the optical density falls into zone 1 (low zone) at 28 to 31 weeks, the fetus will not be affected or will have very mild hemolytic disease.
2. If the optical density falls on zone 2 (mid zone), there is moderate involvement of the fetus. The age of the fetus and the trend in optical density indicate the necessity for intrauterine transfusion and premature delivery.
3. If the optical density falls into zone 3 (high zone), the fetus is severely affected and death is a possibility. In this case, a decision concerning delivery or intrauterine transfusion dependent on the age of the fetus should be made. After 32 to 33 weeks of gestation, early delivery and extrauterine treatment are preferred.

Procedure
1. Ten milliliters of amniotic fluid should be collected in a brown tube and then placed in a light-proof container.
2. Fluid should be sent to the laboratory immediately.
3. The specimen may be kept up to 24 hours in the refrigerator. It can be frozen if a longer time will elapse before analysis.

4. Avoid including any blood in the specimen, If initial aspiration produces a bloody fluid, the needle should be repositioned to obtain a specimen free of red cells. A bloody specimen must be examined at once before hemolysis occurs.

Clinical Implications
1. ΔOD greater than 0.04 is indicative of prematurity.
2. A value of 0.28 to 0.46 is 2+, zone 1, and the fetus is affected by hemolytic disease but is not in danger. Amniocentesis should be repeated in two to three weeks.
3. A value of 0.47 is 3+, zone 2, and the fetus is moderately affected and in danger. Amniocentesis is repeated frequently so a trend can be determined.
4. A value of 0.95 is 4+, zone 3, and indicates impending fetal death.

Interfering Factors
Blood in the specimen can be the source of inaccurate results.

Clinical Alert
1. Difficulty in the interpretation of this value occurs if the measurement is between 0.03 and 0.04 or if the bilirubin concentration unexpectedly decreases early in pregnancy.
2. If the bilirubin level fails to decline as expected or the level increases, this is an indication that the fetal condition is deteriorating.

Cytologic Examination of Fetal Cells for Maturity (Lipids)

Normal Values
Interpretive report

Explanation of Test
This determination of fetal maturity is done by staining fetal fat cells from the amniotic fluid with Nile blue sulfate. The fetus sheds cells during its intrauterine life. In the last weeks of pregnancy, the sebaceous glands begin to function, and the cells are sloughed into the amniotic fluid. These sebaceous cells contain lipid globules. The number of these fat cells increases as the fetus matures, and the percentage of these cells in the amniotic fluid gives an indication of gestational age.

Procedure

An amniotic fluid specimen is obtained and examined.

Clinical Implications

1. When the number of sebaceous cells is less than 2%, the prematurity rate is 85%.
2. If more than 20% of cells in the fluid stain orange, the infant should weigh at least 2500 g. and have a gestational age of 35 weeks or greater.
3. If less than 10% of cells in the fluid stain orange, the gestational age is less than 35 weeks.

BIBLIOGRAPHY

Auvenshine MA, Enriquez MG: Maternity Nursing, Dimensions of Change. Belmont, CA, Wadsworth Publishing, 1985

Copel JA et al: Contraction stress testing with nipple stimulation. J Reprod Med 30(6):465–470, June 1985

Graham D, Jacques S, DeGeorges V: The role of ultrasound in the diagnosis and management of the obstetrical patient. J Obstet Gynecol Neon Nurs, September/October, 1983

Griffith-Kenney J: Contemporary Women's Health, A Nursing Approach. Menlo Park, CA, Addison–Wesley, 1986

Hill, WC: Characteristics of uterine activity during the breast stimulation stress test. Obstet Gynecol 64(4):459–492, October 1984

Hogge WA, Schonberg SA, Golbus MS: Prenatal Diagnosis by Chorionic Villus Sampling: Lessons of the First 600 Cases. New York, John Wiley & Sons, 1985

Hogge WA, Schonberg SA, Golbus MS: Chorionic villus sampling. J Obstet Gynecol Neon Nurs January/February, 1986

Ladewig PA, London L, Olds B: Essentials of Maternal-Newborn Nursing. Menlo Park, CA, Addison–Wesley, 1986

MacMillen JB, Hale RW: Contraction stress testing with mammary self-stimulation. J Reprod Med 29(4):219–221, April 1954

Manning FA: Fetal biophysical profile scoring predicts trouble—When it counts. Obstet Gynecol, January 1985

Manning FA, Lange IR, Morrison I, Harman CR: Fetal biophysical profile score and the non-stress test: A comparative trial. Obstet Gynecol 64:326, 1984

Platt LD, Eglinton GS, Sipes L, Broussard P, Paul RH: Further experience with the fetal biophysical profile. Obstet Gynecol 61:480, 1983

San Francisco General Hospital: Standardized Procedures for Nonstress, Oxytocin Challenge Test, and Breast Stimulation Tests in the Prenatal Testing Center. August/September, 1985

Vintzileos AM, Campbell WA, Ingardia CJ, Nochimson DJ: The fetal biophysical profile and its predictive value. Obstet Gynecol 62:271, 1983

APPENDIX ONE:
TABLE OF VITAMINS

Substance Tested Reference Range (RR) and Critical Range (CR)	Clinical Significance of Values	
	Increase	*Decrease*
Vitamin A		
Retinol (serum) *RR:* 30–65 μg./dl. or 1.22–2.62 μ./mol./ liter *CR:* <10 μg./dl. indicates severe deficiency Carotene (serum) *RR:* 48–200 mcg./dl. 50–300 μg./100 ml. 100–300 iu./100 ml.	Excessive dietary intake and toxicity Hyperlipemia Hypercholesterolemia Uncontrolled diabetes mellitus Chronic nephritis Oral contraceptives Pregnancy Idiopathic hypercalcemia in infants	Fat malabsorption syndrome Steatorrhea Celiac disease Liver disease Protein–calorie malnutrition Febrile disease Insufficient dietary intake Hypothyroidism Disseminated TB Carcinoid syndrome Very low protein Sterility
Vitamin B₁		
Thiamine (Urine) *RR:* >100 μg./24 hr. >377 nmol/d.	Leukemia Polycythemia vera Hodgkin's disease	Inadequate dietary intake Thyrotoxicosis Malabsorption syndrome Beriberi Liver disease Maple syrup urine disease Alcoholism Diuretic therapy Increased metabolic demands, *i.e.*, fever, exercise, pregnancy Peripheral neuropathy Wernicke's Encephalopathy CHF Hyperthyroidism Pyruvate carboxylose deficiency

(Continued)

Substance Tested Reference Range (RR) and Critical Range (CR)	Clinical Significance of Values	
	Increase	Decrease

Vitamin B₂
(Urine)
RR: 80–269 μg./g. or
24–81 μmol./mol.

| | | Insufficient dietary intake B₂ Malabsorption syndrome Stress, neuropathy, dermatitis, anemia, pregnancy, hyperthyroidism, alcoholism, infections, malignancy, pellegra |

Vitamin B₆
(Pyridoxine)
(Urine: Pyridoxal, Pyridoxamine)
Measure xanthurenic acid after tryptophan challenge <50 mg./24 hrs.
>100 mg./24 hrs. indicates B₆ deficiency
(Plasma)
RR: 3.6–18.0 ng./ml. or
14.6–72.8 nmol./liter

Malnutrition
Malabsorption
Malignancy
Kwashiorkor
Pregnancy
Oral contraceptives
Uremia
Neuritis
Anemia: hypochromic; microcytic
Chronic alcoholism
Industrial exposure to hydrozene

Vitamin C
Ascorbic Acid
(Plasma)
RR: 0.6–2.0 mg./dl. or
34–114 μmol./liter
Males lower than females; level decreases with age.

Excessive dietary intake or megadoses of vitamin
Oxalic acid calculi

Insufficient dietary intake
Pregnancy, esp. postpartum
Anemia
Infection and fever
Scurvy
Stress
Smokers
Impaired iron absorption
Duodenal ulcers
Decreased WBCs
Postoperative state

Vitamin D (Cholecalciferol)
(Serum)
25-Hydroxy, D₃ and 1-25 Dihydroxy, D₃
Metabolite: 25-(OH)D₃
RR: Winter: 14–42 ng./ml. or
37.4–199.7 nmol./liter

Hypervitaminosis D
Excessive sun exposure

Inadequate dietary intake
Hepatic disorders
Malabsorption diseases
Biliary and portal cirrhosis
Thyrotoxicosis
Dietary and anticonvulsant osteomalacia

(Continued)

Substance Tested Reference Range (RR) and Critial Range (CR)	Clinical Significance of Values	
	Increase	*Decrease*
Summer: 15–80 ng./ ml. or 34.9–104.8 nmol./ liter Most active form: Metab- olite 1,25-$(OH)_2D_3$ *RR:* 24–45 pg./ml. or 60–180 pmol./liter	1.25-$(OH)_2D_3$ Hyperparathyroidism Hypothyroidism Idiopathic hypercalce- mia Acromegaly Tumor calcenosis Pregnancy and lacta- tion	1,25-$(OH)_2D_3$ Chronic renal failure Osteomalacia (tumor induced) Vitamin D—rickets Pseudohypoparathyroidism Hyperthyroidism Some drugs Adolescents needing insulin
Vitamin E Tocopheral (serum) *RR:* 0.5–2.0 mg./dl. or 11.6–46.4 μmol./liter	Increased dietary intake or increased vitamin E supple- ment	Fat malabsorption dis- eases Premature infants Protein–calorie mal- nourishment Acanthocytosis Vitamin E deficiency Hemolytic anemia Diet high in unsaturated fatty acids A-beta Lipoproteinemia
Vitamin K (phylloquinone menaquinone) *RR:* Serum: prothrombin time: normal indirect	Increased dietary intake or adminis- tered vitamin K preparations Premature infant— hyperbilirubinemia following parenteral vitamin K	Coagulation disorders due to faulty forma- tion of Factors II, VII, IX, and X Conditions that limit absorption or synthe- sis of vitamin K (ob- structive jaundice, pancreatic disease, colitis, antibacterial therapy, salicylates), mineral oil Hemorrhagic disease of newborn (HDN) Infants with diarrhea, esp. breast fed

APPENDIX TWO: TABLE OF TRACE MINERALS

Substance Tested *Specimen Needed,* *Reference Range (RR),* *and Critical Range (CR)*	Clinical Significance of Values
Aluminum (Serum) *RR:* 0.4 µg./dl. or 0.15 umol./liter	*Increase:* excessive occupational exposure, lung diseases, Shaver's disease (abrasives from aluminum oxide) *Toxicity not seen* normally, except in renal failure, when aluminum-containing antacids are used; long-term intermittent dialysis
Antimony (Urine [24 hr./100 ml.]) *RR:* <50 mcg./liter *CR:* >1 mg./liter	*Increase:* excessive occupational exposure (ore mining, bronze, ceramic)
Arsenic (Blood [20 ml.]) (Urine [24 hr./50 ml.]) (Hair [0.5 g.]) (Nails) *RR* Blood: <3 mcg./100 ml. *RR* Urine: <100 mcg./liter/d. *CR* Urine: >850 mcg./liter/d. *RR* Hair: <65 mcg./100 g. *CR* Hair: >100 µg./100 g. *RR* Nails: 90–180 µg./100 g.	*Increase:* accidental or intentional poisoning. Excessive occupational exposure (ceramics, agriculture)
Beryllium (Urine [24 hr.]) *RR:* 0.05 µg./d. *CR:* >20 µg./liter or >2.22 µmol./liter	*Increase:* excessive occupational exposure, metal extraction, refinery, rocket base, nuclear plants, extensive coal burning. Acute lung irritation, pneumonitis, berylliosis, secondary polycythemia

(Continued)

Substance Tested *Specimen Needed,* *Reference Range (RR),* *and Critical Range (CR)*	Clinical Significance of Values
Bismuth (Urine [24 hr.]) *RR:* <20 μg./liter or <95.7 nmol./liter *RR* Plasma: <1.0 μg./dl. or <47.9 nmol./liter	*Increase:* excessive occupational exposure to cosmetic disinfectant, pigment, and solder resulting in osteosclerosis
Boran (Blood [4 ml. serum]) *RR:* 1 mg./dl. *CR:* 10 to 20 mg./dl. (Urine [24 hr./5 ml.]) *RR:* 0.3 mg./dl.	*Increase:* excessive occupational exposure (glass, soap, fireproofing). Accidental ingestion of boric acid or boric salts

Cadmium
(Blood [1 ml.])
RR: 0.1–0.5 μg./dl. or
    0.89–4.45 nmol./liter
CR: 10–300 μg./dl. or
    0.89–26.70 μmol./liter
RR: 10 to 580 mcg./l. (after exposure) 20 mcg./l. (without exposure)
	Increase: (tissue) in prostatic and renal cancer; (urine) in hypertension, industrial exposure; (blood) poisoning from foods prepared in cadmium-lined vessel, inhaling of cadmium fumes, and hypertension

Chromium
(Blood [Serum])
RR: 14 ng./ml. or
    2.7 nmol./liter
(Urine)
RR: 0.8 μg./d. or
    15.4 nmol./d.
(Hair)
RR: 0.21 ± 0.14 μg./g. or
    4.0 ± 2.7 nmol./g.
	Increase: industrial overexposure to the metal, such as in tanning, electroplating and steel making. High levels normal at birth—previous (recent) radioactive tests with chromium may affect test results.
	Decrease: impaired ability to metabolize glucose suggested as causal factor in atherosclerosis, pregnancy, diabetic children; hair decreased in diabetics.

Cyanide (Blood [5 ml.]) *RR:* 0.004 mg./liter or 0.15 μmol./liter (nonsmokers) *CR:* >0.1 mg./liter or >3.84 μmol./liter	*Increase:* Industrial exposure (pesticides, metallurgy). Inhalation of hydrocyonic acid and fumes from burning nitrogen-containing products. Ingestion of salts, some fruit seeds and laetrile
Cobalt—Part of Vitamin B₁₂ (Blood [Serum—metal-free container]) *RR:* 0.12–0.20 μg./dl. or 20.4–33.9 nmol./liter	*Decrease:* insufficient dietary intake and hematopoiesis imbalance *Increase:* excessive ingestion of beer containing cobalt as a stabilizer; dermatitis and red blood cell disease from industrial exposure with inhalation of cobalt dust

(Continued)

Substance Tested *Specimen Needed,* *Reference Range (RR),* *and Critical Range (CR)*	Clinical Significance of Values
Copper (Blood [Serum or plasma— metal-free container]) *RR:* male: 70–140 μg./dl. or 10.99–21.98 μmol./liter Female: 85–155 μg./dl. or 12.56–24.34 μmol./liter (Urine [24 hr.]) *RR:* 15–30 μg./24 hr. or 0.24–0.47 μmol./liter	*Increase (Serum):* leukemia, hemochro- matosis, myocardial infarction, rheu- matoid arthritis, biliary cirrhosis of liver, typhoid fever, Hodgkin's, pelle- gra, tuberculosis, anemia (megaloblas- tic and aplastic) thalassemia, brain infarction, ankylosing spondylitis, hypo- and hyperthyroidism, collagen diseases, SIE, complications of renal dialysis and neonatal transfusions, cancer of bone, GI system, lung, breast and cervix *Decrease:* Wilson's disease, nephroses, hypoproteinemia, sprue, Menkes' syndrome, some iron-deficiency dis- eases, burns, chronic ischemic heart disease, ACTH or prednesone Rx of leukemia *Increase (Urine):* Wilson's disease, chronic active hepatitis, biliary cir- rhosis, rheumatoid arthritis, protein- uria *Decrease:* protein malnutrition
Fluoride (Blood [5 ml.]) *RR:* 0.01–0.20 mg./liter or 0.5–10.5 μmol./liter (Urine [10 ml.]) *RR:* 0.2–1.1 mg./liter or 10.5–57.9 μmol./liter *CR:* 4.0–5.0 mg./liter or 2.10.4–263.0 μmol./liter	*Increase:* excessive industrial and insec- ticide exposure (aluminum, yeast, welding, fertilizers); possibly elevated with fluoride treatment for osteoporo- sis
Gold (Blood [<10 μg./dl. or <0.51 μmol./liter]) Therapeutic: 38–500 μg./dl. or 1.93–25.40 μmol./liter	*Increase:* rheumatoid arthritis if gold sodium thiomalate given
Iron (Blood [3 ml.]) *RR:* (diagnostic) Male: 50–160 μ./dl. or 8.95– 28.64 μmol./liter Female: 40–150 μg./dl. or 7.16– 26.85 μmol./liter *CR:* 280–2550 μg./dl. or 50.12–456.5 μmol./liter	*Increase:* pernicious anemia, aplastic and hemolytic anemia, hemochroma- tosis, B_6 deficiency, thalassemia, acute hepatitis, repeated transfusions, ne- phritis, excessive iron therapy *Decrease:* iron-deficiency anemia, acute and chronic infection, cancer, postop- eratively, kwashiorkor, remission of pernicious anemia

(Continued)

Substance Tested *Specimen Needed,* *Reference Range (RR),* *and Critical Range (CR)*	Clinical Significance of Values
Serious Iron Poisoning: >1800 µg./dl. or >322.2 µmol./liter	
Lead (Blood [2 ml.]) *RR:* <30 µg./dl. or 1.45 µmol./liter (children) <40 µg./dl. or 1.93 µmol./liter (unexposed adults) <60 µg./dl. or <2.90 µmol./ liter (accepted industrial exposure) *CR:* >100 mg./dl. or >4.83 (Urine [24 hr.]) *RR:* <80 µg./liter or <0.39 µmol./liter <120 µg./liter or 0.58 µmol./ liter (accepted industrial exposure)	*Increase:* industrial exposure (lead, Pb paints, plumbing, ceramics, insecticides, gasoline)
Manganese (Blood [15 ml.]) *RR:* 0.4–1.14 µg./dl. or 73–255 nmol./liter (Hair) 0.23 ± 0.11 ug. or 4.2 ± 2.0 µmol./kg.	*Increase:* industrial exposure (drugs, welding, glass, ceramics), estrogens, acute hepatitis, myocardial infarction *Decrease:* deficient dietary intake. High calcium and phosphorous dietary intake interferes with manganese absorption; reproduction dysfunction
Mercury (Urine [24 hr.]) *RR:* <20 µg./liter or <0.1 µmol./liter *CR:* >150 µg./liter or >0.75 µmol./liter (Blood [5 ml.]) *RR:* <5 µg./dl. or <0.25 µmol./liter (Hair) Approximately 300× blood level	*Increase:* industrial exposure (agriculture, amalgams and dyes); excessive therapeutic intake
Nickel (Urine [24 hr.]) *RR:* Male: 2.6 ± 1.3 µg./dl. or 44.2 ± 22.1 µmol./dl. Female: 2.2 ± 0.8 µg./dl. or 37.4 ± 13.6 nmol./dl. (Blood [metal-free container]) *RR:* Male: 0.45 ± 0.14 µg./dl. or 76.5 ± 23.8 nmol./liter	*Increase:* industrial and environmental exposure (incl. electroplating, ceramics, magnets, spark plugs, paints, stainless steel, enamels, batteries, glass and alloys); after myocardial infarction *Decrease:* hepatic cirrhosis, chronic anemia

(Continued)

Substance Tested *Specimen Needed,* *Reference Range (RR),* *and Critical Range (CR)*	**Clinical Significance of Values**
Female: 0.53 ± 0.11 µg./dl. or 90.1 ± 18.7 nmol./liter	

Selenium
(Urine [24 hr.—metal-free container])
RR: 10–100 µg./liter or
 0.13–1.27 µmol./liter
CR: >400 µg./liter or
 >5.08 µmol./liter

Increase: industrial exposure (glass, developing films, paints, dyes, electronic equipment, fungicides, rubber and semiconductors)
Decrease: anemia, Keshan disease

Silica
(Lung Tissue [10 g.])
RR: 0.2% of dry weight lung tissue

Increase: industrial exposure (clay, cement and mining)

Silver
(Serum [metal-free container])
RR: 0.21 ± 0.15 µg./dl. or
 19.47 ± 13.90 nmol./liter

Increase: industrial exposure (associated with argyria [bluish-gray skin]). Silver salts are used as bacteriostatics and antiseptics

Thallium
(Blood [metal-free container])
RR: 0.5 µg./dl. or 24.5 nmol./liter
CR: 10–800 µg./dl. or
 0.5–39.1 µmol./liter
(Urine [metal-free container])
RR: <2.0 µg./liter or
 <9.78 nmol./liter
CR: 1.0–2.0 mg./liter or
 4.9–97.8 µmol./liter

Increase: industrial exposure (diamonds, dyes, and optical glass, rodentocides). Used in medications, cosmetics and pesticides

Zinc
(Serum)
RR: 55–150 µg./dl. or
 10.7–22.9 µmol./liter
(Urine [24 hr.])
CR: >800 µg./d. or
 >12.2 µmol./d.
(Hair cut close to scalp in 2–5 cm lengths)
RR: 216 ± 87 µg/g (ISD) or
 3.30 ± 1.33 µmol/g (ISD)

Serum Increase: coronary heart disease, arteriosclerosis, osteosarcoma, inhalation of zinc oxide (industrial exposure)
Serum Decrease: Tuberculosis, metastatic cancer to liver, sprue, thalassemia major, acute M.I., acute infection, alcoholic cirrhosis, hypogonal dwarfism, leukemia, lymphoma, pernicious anemia, Danboldt syndrome, and typhoid fever
Urine Increase: Hyperparathyroidism
Urine Decrease: Hypogonadal dwarfism
Hair Decrease: Diabetes, celiac disease, protein malnutrition

INDEX

The letter *f* after a page number indicates a figure;
t following a page number indicates tabular material.